Histology and Comparative Organology:

a text-atlas

Histology and Comparative Organology:

a text-atlas

WILLIAM J. BANKS, Ph.D.

Associate Professor of Anatomy
Director, University Electron Microscopy Training Center
College of Veterinary Medicine and Biomedical Sciences
Colorado State University
Fort Collins, Colorado, USA

The Williams & Wilkins Company, *Baltimore*

428 E. Preston Street
Baltimore, Md. 21202, U.S.A.

Made in the United States of America

Library of Congress Catalog Card Number 73-8808
SBN 683-00409-3

Composed and printed at the
Waverly Press, Inc.
Mt. Royal and Guilford Aves.
Baltimore, Md. 21202, U.S.A.

Dedicated
to
B.F.B. & G.P.E.

Preface

The effectiveness of teaching microanatomy is predicated upon numerous factors. Of these, the availability to the student of diverse histological preparations is an important contribution to success. Notwithstanding the wealth of specimens available to students of animal histology, one significant teaching aid has been lacking, i.e., a concise compilation of diagrams, micrographs and text that presents an integrated and broad spectrum approach to the subgross architecture of domestic animals and related species, as well as birds. This book is an attempt to fill this void.

Although the inclusions in this text are directed specifically toward veterinary students, the approach is sufficiently broad to be applicable to the training of all students in microanatomy. Specimens from numerous organisms, encompassing veterinary, avian, laboratory and wildlife species, have been included. The text, however, is by no means all-inclusive.

The integrated approach begins with the light and electron microscopic characteristics of cells. Emphasis is placed on those features, common and unique, that account for the functional significance of the cells, as well as the higher degree of organization that typifies the mammalian and avian soma. This naturally leads to the presentation of the four basic tissue types. A concerted attempt has been made to present the detailed morphology of these tissues within the framework of comprehension of function. For the attainment of this end, therefore, the significant modifications and specializations of the tissues are presented as variations of a basic scheme.

Organology, introduced early in the presentation, is expanded upon in the later chapters. The common morphological features of specific organs are presented, and species differences apparent in these organs are included when appropriate. Similarly, organs unique to various species are included in the appropriate sections on systems.

The unified approach has been influenced by the author's experience in teaching histology to veterinary and biology students. Despite the laboratory aids that may be available, comprehension of microscopic organization is predicated upon proceeding from that which is familiar and readily comprehensible to that which is unfamiliar and less comprehensible. For this reason, diagrams and low power micrographs have been utilized to increase understanding.

The accompanying textual material is sufficiently broad to permit the use of this book as the text and atlas for introductory undergraduate histology courses. Over 450 diagrams, light micrographs and electron micrographs are included in the presentation. It also has value as a supplemental atlas for advanced histology courses. Its greatest value as a supplemental study aid is that it presents details of structure that, except for the materials available through individual professors, are not readily available to the students.

Routine staining preparations have been used primarily, but special staining has also been included to illustrate specific characteristics at various levels of microscopic organization. Unless otherwise specified, all light microscopic sections have been stained with hematoxylin and eosin. All electron micrographs have been stained with uranyl acetate and lead citrate. Further, all micrographs in the text have been reproduced at 100%. The stated original magnifications of light micrographs permits the student to associate these magnifications with those used in his practical laboratory work.

The author realizes that no text, this one included, is able to give *in toto* coverage of such a vast and rapidly expanding field. It is, however, a positive step toward satisfying the needs of students in this specialized area of histology. The book is an adaptation of materials that have been used effectively in teaching histology to veterinary and biology students. It should aid the professional student in establishing a firm foundation in normal histology so that histopathology will be more meaningful. Moreover, it should aid in the establishment of a clear understanding of subgross organization for the veterinary and biology student.

I am indebted to numerous people who have contributed directly or indirectly to this book.

The technical staffs of the Histology Preparation Laboratories of the Western College of Veterinary Medicine, University of Saskatchewan, and Department of Anatomy, College of Veterinary Medicine and Biomedical Sciences, Colorado State University, were most helpful. They were always willing to obtain, prepare or retrieve specimens that eventually were used in the book.

The stimulating conversations with Dr. F. Hrudka, Dr. W. K. Latshaw and Dr. A. Horowitz of the Department of Veterinary Anatomy, Western College of Veterinary Medicine, University of Saskatchewan, were significant during the formative stages of the book.

The negatives supplied by Dr. G. P. Epling, Ms. A. M. Sheppard and Mr. W. Todd were appreciated.

The suggestions of my colleagues, Dr. J. Bowman, Dr. H. Nornes, Dr. R. Frandson and Dr. Y. Z. Abdelbaki, were most helpful.

The suggestions and comments by Mr. J. Newbrey, Mr. J. Latham and Mr. D. Goldner were most helpful. Mr. Newbrey's assistance with the references was especially valuable.

The technical assistance of my associate, Ms. A. M. Sheppard, was most appreciated. She spent many long and arduous hours in the darkroom and cutting room. The technical assistance of Ms. L. Mayberry was appreciated also.

The assistance and patience of my wife, Mrs. B. F. Banks, made the accomplishment of the task much easier.

The expert assistance of my secretary, Miss Karla Kohnen, is gratefully acknowledged. Her help with all aspects of the manuscript was extremely valuable. The assistance with the index by my sister, Miss Eileen K. Banks, was most helpful.

To Dr. R. A. Kainer, Associate Professor of Anatomy, and Dr. G. P. Epling, Professor and Chairman of the Department of Anatomy, I owe a special expression of appreciation. Besides offering many helpful suggestions and stimulating interesting conversation about the subject matter, these academicians spent many hours proofreading the manuscript and discussing micrographs with me.

The editorial staff of Williams & Wilkins, especially Miss S. Finnegan, made this task easier by their patience and many helpful suggestions.

To my numerous colleagues and students, from whom I have learned so much, my sincerest appreciation is expressed.

W. J. Banks
Fort Collins, Colorado

Contents

SECTION 1: CYTOLOGY

1 Cytology

General Cellular Characteristics

As the structural and functional unit of living organisms, the cell is responsible for the complex organization that is apparent in all metazoa. This organization is predicated on a division of labor and specialization among the component cells. The specialization is so precise that functional inferences can be made from structure alone. The reverse is also true. Although cells possess many common properties (irritability, growth, reproduction, etc.), generalizations about cells are very difficult.

Cellular Shape. The shape of an animal cell is often described as spheroidal; this is a misleading and poor generalization. Specialization has a profound influence on cell shape. Cellular contact and pressure, as well as the inherent ability to alter shape, are determinants of morphological configuration. Thus, a cell may be round (Fig. 1-1), stellate (Fig. 1-2), spindle-shaped (Fig. 1-3), elongated (Fig. 1-4), columnar (Fig. 1-5), squamous (Fig. 1-6), cuboidal (Fig. 1-7) and myriad other shapes. Some cells may progress through a number of these shapes before a definitive shape is attained. Also, cellular shape is influenced in such a way as to indicate the type and amount of specific functional activity taking place within the cell.

Cellular Polarity. Despite the diversity of cellular shape, the constituent parts of cells (*plasma membrane*, *cytoplasm* and *nucleus*) generally possess a spatial distribution that is reasonably predictable. Round or spheroidal cells usually possess rounded and centrally located nuclei (Fig. 1-8). As a cell becomes elongated, the nucleus becomes more ovoid and oriented parallel to the long axis (Figs. 1-9, 1-10). Also, nuclear shape and position are correlated with the position of other organelles, as well as with the shape of the cell. Thus, some cells are spatially polarized (Fig. 1-11).

Cellular Size. Cells vary not only among the various groups of animals (*interspecific*) but even within the body of a specified organism (*intraspecific*). There is no correlation, however, between the size of the organism and the size of its cells; i.e., the cells of the horse will not be significantly larger than the cells of the dog. Some cells are *macroscopic* (visible with the unaided eye), whereas others exhibit a wide range of *microscopic* sizes (visible only with the aided eye). The *perikaryon* of a microgliocyte may be a few micrometers (1 μm = 10,000 A) in diameter; the red blood corpuscle (RBC) ranges from 4 to 7 μm in diameter depending on the species, while the ovum may be as large as 300 μm in diameter. (Incidentally, since RBC's will appear in most sections examined, they can serve as a "built-in micrometer.") The length of a striated muscle cell may be in inches, while the length of a nerve cell extending from the ventral horn of the spinal cord to the tip of an appendage may be several feet long. Even within the narrow limits of microscopic observation, there may be a wide diversity of size in at least one dimension. Giant cells, such as the megakaryocytes, are appreciably larger than developing red blood corpuscles (Fig. 1-12). Similarly, striated mus-

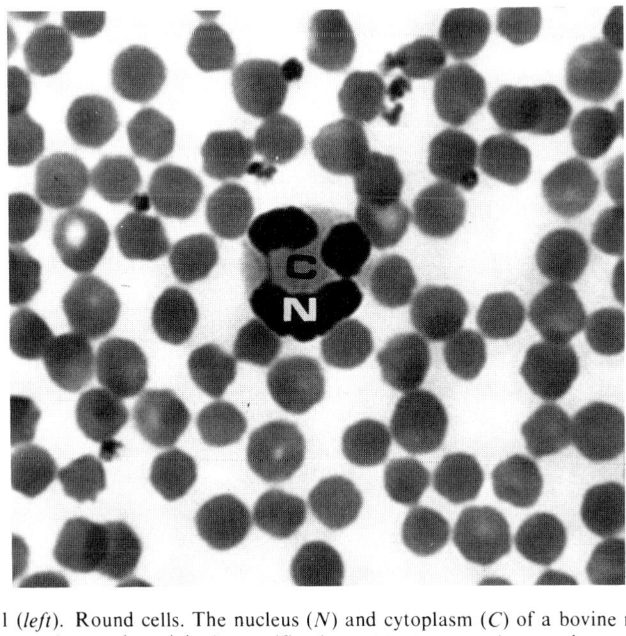

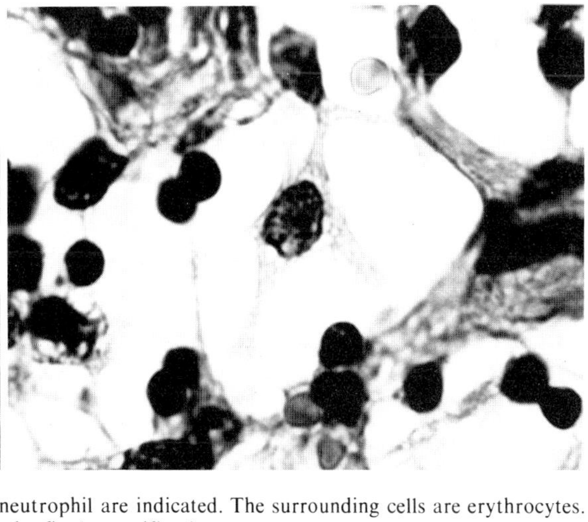

Fig. 1-1 (*left*). Round cells. The nucleus (*N*) and cytoplasm (*C*) of a bovine neutrophil are indicated. The surrounding cells are erythrocytes. ×400. All light micrographs are the original magnifications. All electron micrographs are the final magnifications.

Fig. 1-2 (*right*). Stellate cell. A reticular cell from a lymph node is in the center of the field. ×160.

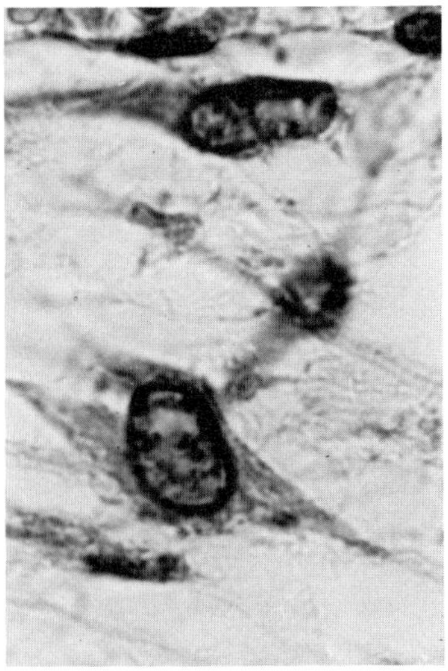

Fig. 1-3. Spindle-shaped cell. These are mesenchymal cells from loose connective tissue. ×400.

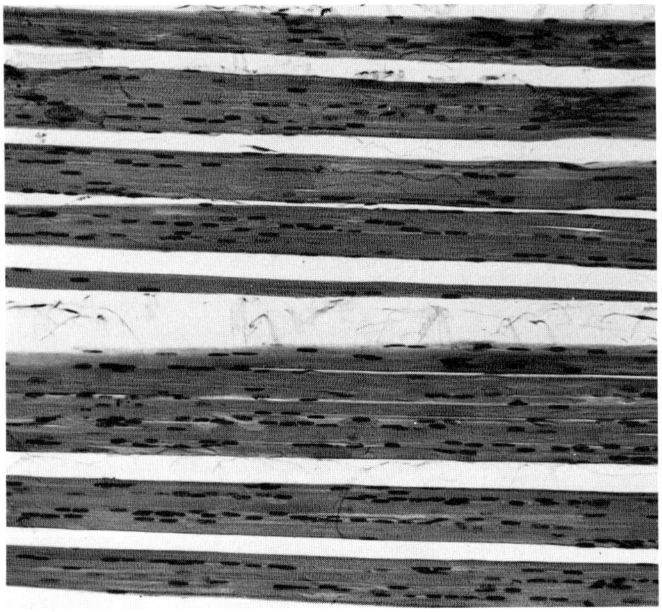

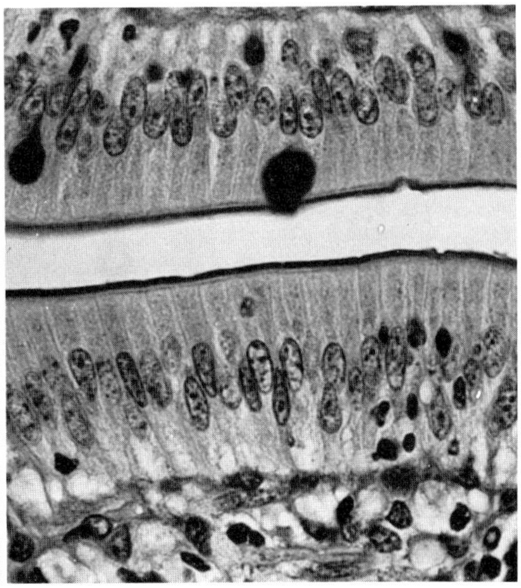

Fig. 1-4 (*left*). Elongated cells. The multinucleated cells are skeletal muscle cells. ×40.
Fig. 1-5 (*right*). Columnar cells. These lining cells are longer than they are wide. ×160.

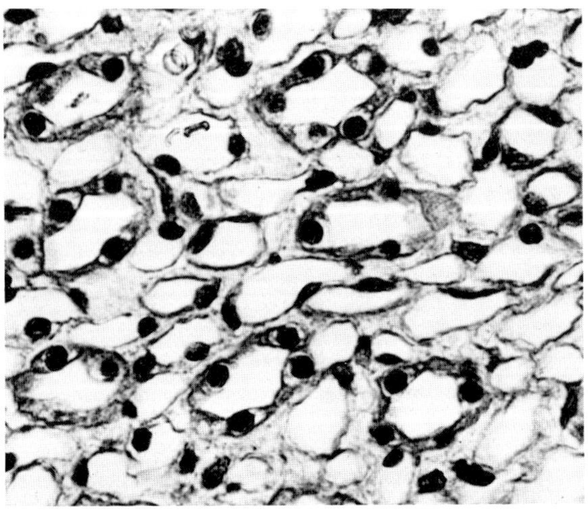

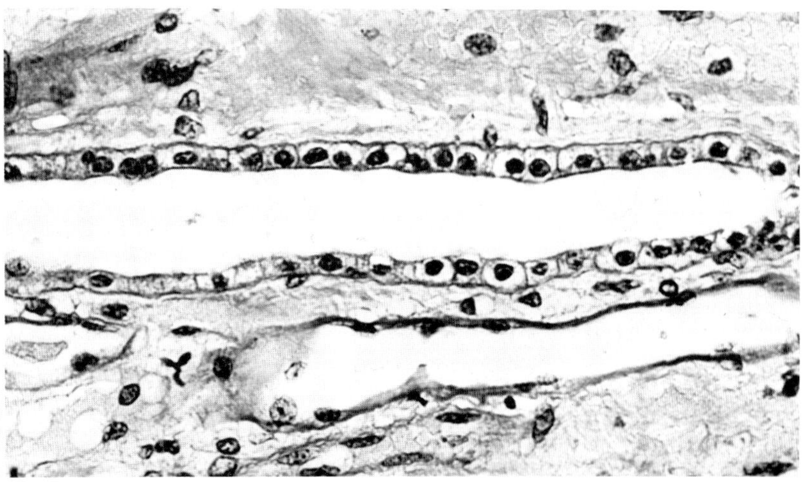

Fig. 1-6 (*left*). Squamous cells. All of the tubules depicted are lined by these flattened cells. ×160.
Fig. 1-7 (*right*). Cuboidal cells. The lining cells of this tubule are square. Their three-dimensional configuration, however, is cuboidal. ×100.

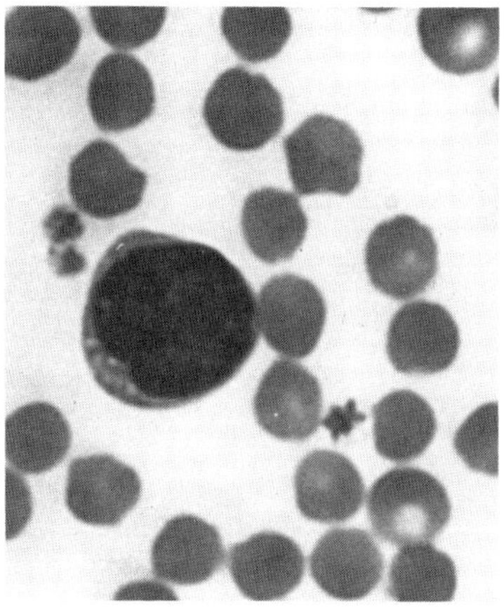

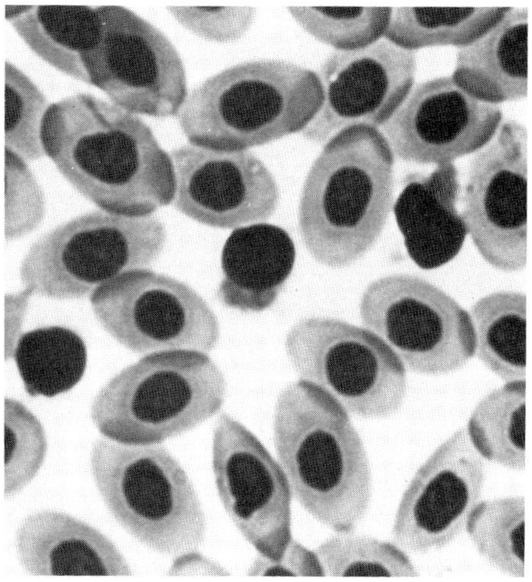

Fig. 1-8 (*left*). A bovine lymphocyte. The round cell contains a round nucleus. ×400. Fig. 1-9 (*right*). Avian RBC's. The slightly elongated cells contain elongated nuclei. ×400.

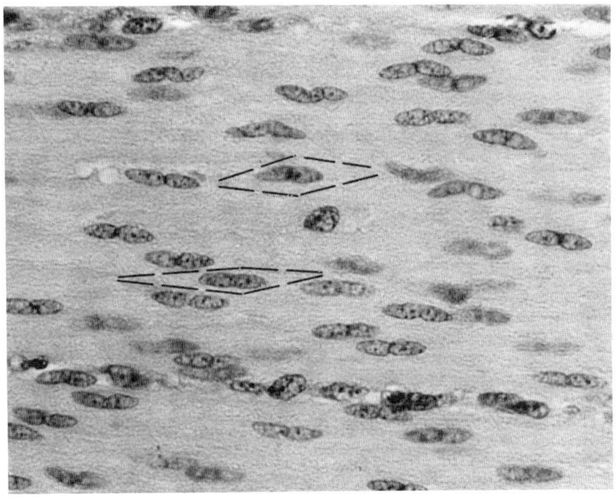

Fig. 1-10. Smooth muscle cells. The margins of the cells are indicated by *dashed lines*. The elongated cells contain elongated nuclei. ×160.

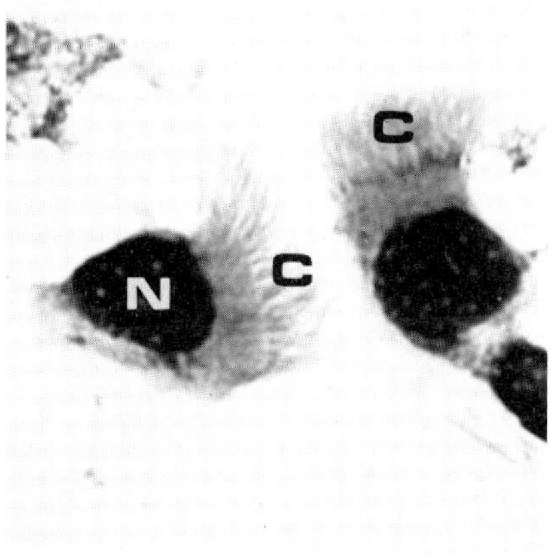

Fig. 1-11. Polarized cells. These are ciliated cells that have been removed individually from an epithelial lining. The nuclei (*N*) are basally displaced. The apical border has cilia (*C*). ×160.

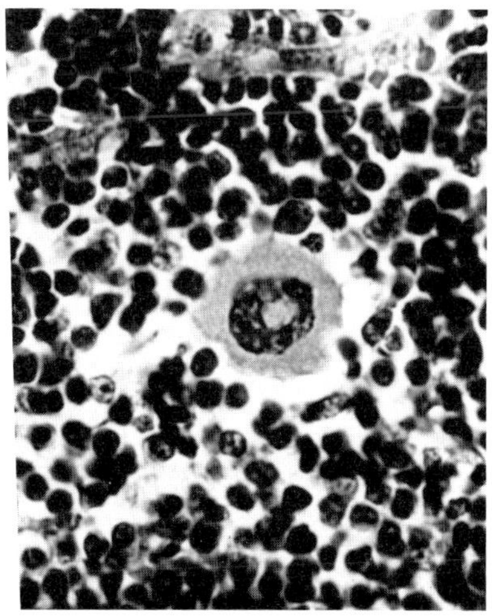

Fig. 1-12. A megakaryocyte and other bone marrow cells. The megakaryocyte is in the center of the field. ×100.

cle cells are much larger than the fibroblasts associated with them. Generally, most mammalian cells will range between 10 and 30 μm.

Nucleus

The nucleus, as a constantly occurring and required component of most cells, is responsible for the control and mediation of numerous cellular activities. These include metabolism, synthesis, reproduction and cellular homeostasis. Some functional correlations with nuclear morphology are possible. The most distinguishable of these are the morphological criteria associated with a dividing (*mitotic*) and nondividing (*intermitotic*, *interphase* or *vegetative*) cell. Since the greatest number of cells encountered in the body will be performing vegetative functions, the interphase nucleus will be discussed first.

In the interphase nucleus, four distinct components may be identified: *nuclear membrane*, *karyolymph*, *chromatin* and *nucleolus* (Fig. 1-13).

Number. Most often a cell will be mononucleated (Figs. 1-1, 1-2, 1-3, 1-5, 1-7, 1-8, 1-9). Some, however, may be *binucleated*, while others may be *multinucleated* (Fig. 1-14). Other extremes may range from enucleation, as in the mammalian erythrocyte (Figs. 1-1, 1-8) and certain cells of the lens, to the case of the spermatozoon, in which the bulk of the cell is composed of a nucleus.

Shape. Nuclear morphology varies with the shape of the cell. Round to oval cells usually possess a similarly shaped nucleus (Figs. 1-2, 1-7, 1-8). Elongated cells usually possess an elongated nucleus (Figs. 1-4, 1-5, 1-9, 1-10). Others, however, may possess nuclei that are crescent-shaped or lobulated (Fig. 1-1).

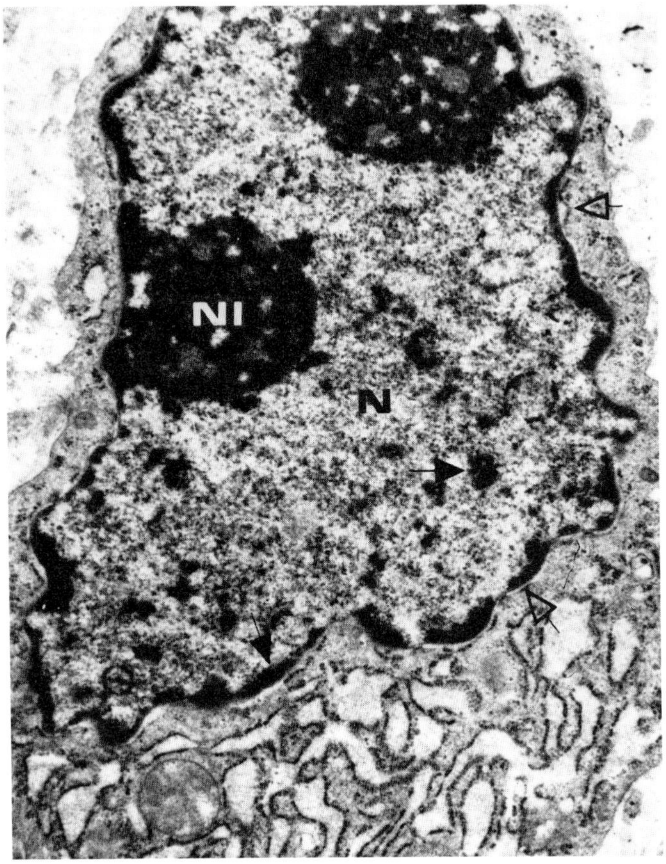

Fig. 1-13. Nuclear components. The nucleus (*N*) contains two nucleoli (*Nl*). Heterochromatin (*solid arrows*) is interspersed with euchromatin. The nuclear envelope (*open arrows*) surrounds the nucleus. ×16,000.

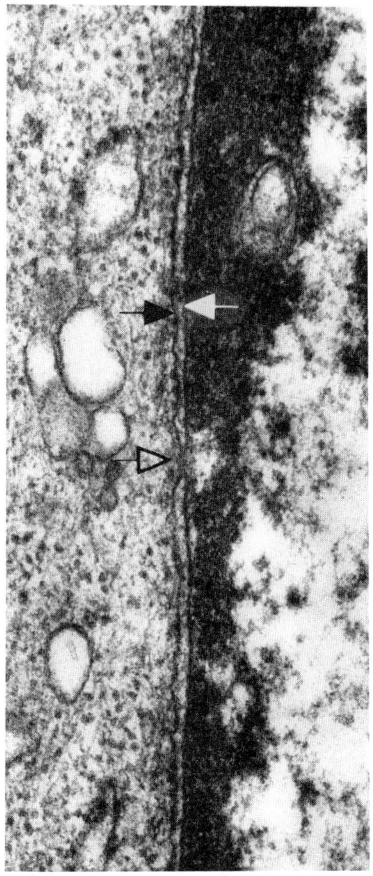

Fig. 1-15. Nuclear membrane. The outer nuclear membrane (*black arrow*) is separated from the inner nuclear membrane (*white arrow*) by the nuclear cistern. A nuclear pore (*open arrow*) is apparent. ×52,000.

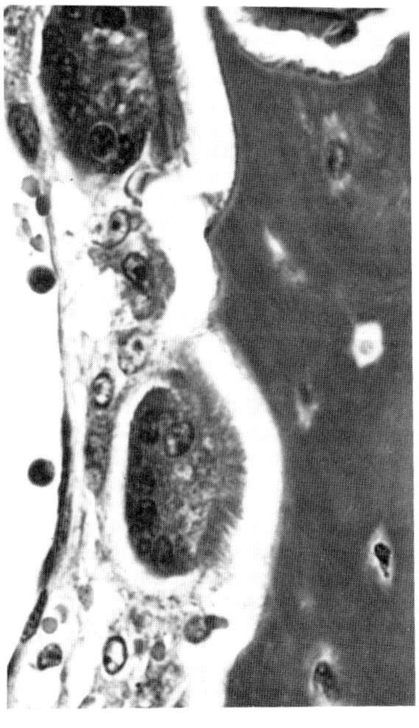

Fig. 1-14. Multinucleated cells. These osteoclasts contain a variable number of nuclei. ×100.

Position. The position of the nucleus will also reflect the degree of polarity in a particular cell type (Fig. 1-11).

Nuclear Envelope. A darkly basophilic (blue-staining with hematoxylin) line of demarcation between the nucleus and surrounding cytoplasm is apparent in light microscopic sections (Figs. 1-1, 1-2, 1-3). This limiting membrane represents a condensation of nuclear and cytoplasmic components, as well as stain, on either side of the *nuclear membrane* or *nuclear envelope*. The electron microscope (Fig. 1-15) reveals two membranes comprising the nuclear envelope, the *inner* and *outer nuclear membranes*. Each of these measures approximately 7.5 nm (1 nm = 10 A), and they are separated from each other by a *perinuclear space* or *cisterna* which varies from 40 to 70 nm wide. The perinuclear space, and thus the outer nuclear membrane, is continuous with profiles of the rough endoplasmic reticulum. *Ribonucleic protein* or *ribosomes* are often attached to the outer nuclear membrane. The inner nuclear membrane is sometimes associated with filaments that form a *fibrous lamina* along its nuclear (inner) margin. The nuclear envelope is not a continuous, uninterrupted, structural entity. Rather, the inner and outer nuclear membranes are continuous and reflected at certain points (Fig. 1-15). Points of discontinuity or fusions between the inner and outer membranes are manifested as openings or *nuclear pores* (Fig. 1-16). These pores are covered by a diaphragm, which probably allows for the selective passage of materials between nucleus and cytoplasm.

Nuclear Matrix. The aforementioned limiting membrane encloses the *matrix of the nucleus*. This ***nuclear sap*** or ***karyolymph*** is the soluble phase of nuclear material. With the information gained from electron micrographs it is apparent that it is more than simply a fluid material. Accordingly, the terms ***nuclear matrix*** and ***nuclear ground*** *substance* have been proposed to describe it more precisely.

Chromatin. *Chromatin* is contained within the confines of the nuclear envelope and is suspended in the nuclear matrix. The term, chromatin, is actually used to describe any area in the nucleus suspected of containing *deoxyribonucleic acid* (DNA) and its bound protein. Different types of chromatic ma-

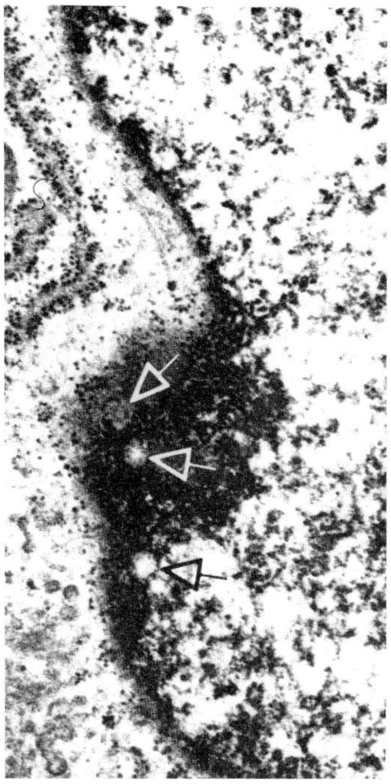

Fig. 1-16. Face view of nuclear pores. *Arrows*, nuclear pores. ×23,000.

terial are recognizable during the interphase. *Heterochromatin* is that chromatin which is deeply stained with basic dyes and is condensed (Fig. 1-17). It is metabolically inert. *Euchromatin* stains lightly, is dispersed and is believed to be the metabolically active form of DNA (Fig. 1-17). Various ratios of heterochromatin/euchromatin will appreciably alter the appearance of a nucleus from *condensed* (much heterochromatin) to *open* or *vesicular* (little heterochromatin). In some instances, the spatial distribution of one to the other is a diagnostic feature of some cell types. Most significantly, the amount of euchromatin is an indicator of the potential protein-synthetic activity of a cell. The more heterochromatin, the less active is the cell; the more euchromatin, the greater will be the potential protein synthesis (Figs. 1-13, 1-17).

Nucleolus. The *nucleolus*, or "little nucleus," is a prominently staining, highly refractive, smooth-surfaced body found in the nucleus (Fig. 1-17). It may occur singly or there may be more than one. It is readily identifiable in those cells involved in protein synthesis. Experimental evidence has implicated it as a center for *ribonucleic acid* (RNA) synthesis. Although the nucleolus is generally basophilic, depletion of RNA through natural or artifactual causes will cause the nucleolus to appear acidophilic, a function of the basic proteins associated with RNA.

At the ultrastructural level, the nucleolus contains a *pars amorpha* and a threadlike *nucleolonema* (Fig. 1-18). Chromatin may be contained within the confines of the nucleolonema or associated with the peripheral portions of the nucleolus.

Cytoplasm

General Characteristics. The cytoplasm, which is composed of numerous biochemical and morphological entities, is present (in varying amounts) in all living cells. The types, kinds and numbers of morphologically and biochemically identifiable components are responsible for the specializations that contribute to histological identification.

The bulk of the cytoplasm, or *ground substance*, is an admixture of water, protein, carbohydrates, organic salts and inorganic salts. The physical characteristics of the cytoplasm are in a constant state of flux. Thus sol-gel properties are apparent. Although this is not generally apparent in somatic cells, some cells (egg cells, amoeboid cells) possess a clear, peripheral *ectoplasm* and an internal, granular *endoplasm*. The former is more viscous (gel-like) and relatively free of organelles compared to the more fluid, granular (sol-like) and organelle-rich endoplasm.

The cytoplasm of mature somatic cells is generally *acidophilic*; however, it may be totally or focally *basophilic*, as well as totally or focally *chromophobic* or *neutrophilic*. Acidophilic components are basic and have an affinity for acid dyes. Basophilic components are acidic and have an affinity for basic dyes. These staining characteristics contribute to the overall light microscopic appearance of a cell, enabling the microscopist to identify numerous cell types. Numerous cytoplasmic components contribute to the general characteristics of a cell. Among these are the organelles, vacuoles, granules, crystals, droplets, amount and distribution of cytoplasm, amount and distribution of organelles and inclusions. The size, shape, location and number of nuclei, as well as the distribution of chromatin contained therein, are additional aids to the cellular morphologist.

Plasma Membrane. The *plasma membrane* (*plasmalemma*, *cell membrane*) encloses the entire cytoplasm and is that portion of the cell exposed to the extracellular environment. It is approximately 8.0 nm thick. Since the limit of resolution of the

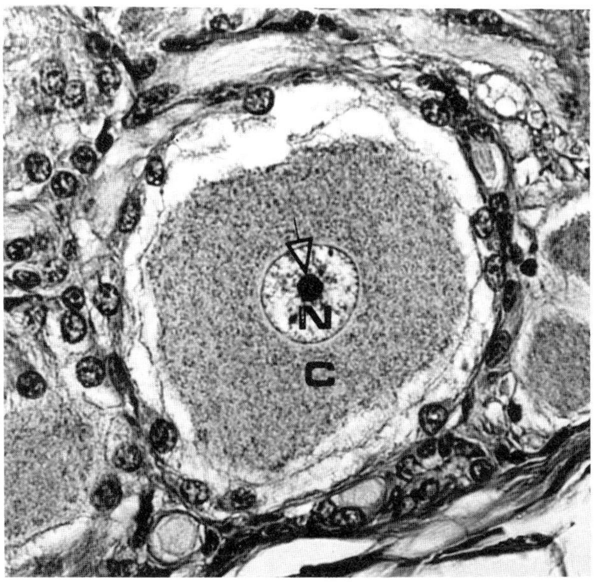

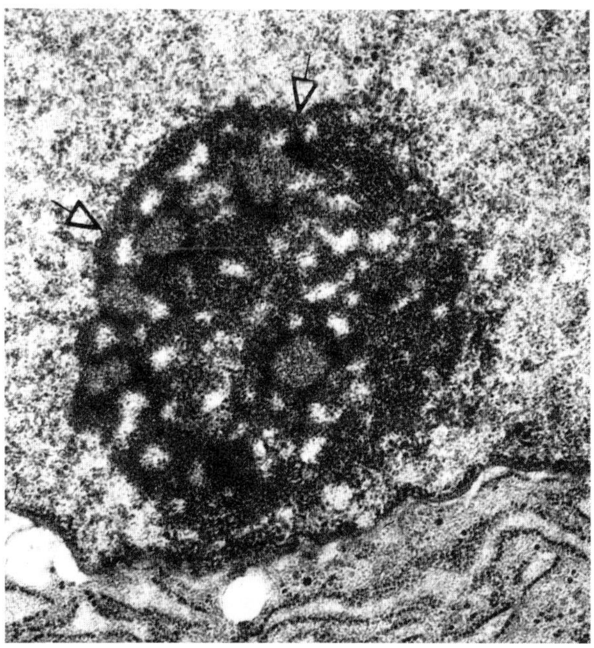

Fig. 1-17 (*left*). A ganglion cell. The cytoplasm (*C*) contains a vesicular nucleus (*N*). The nucleus has a prominent nucleolus (*arrow*). ×100.
Fig. 1–18 (*right*). An electron micrograph of a nucleolus. The nucleolonema (*arrows*) is the prominent feature of this section. ×25,000.

white light microscope is approximately 200 nm, it is impossible for the plasmalemma to be resolved. Despite this, *cellular limits* are discernible within the aforementioned limits of resolution. This is due to a condensation of structural protein, addition of stain and the condensation of contiguous materials at the interfaces, as well as the presence of a *cell coat*. The plasma membrane is not seen with light microscopy, but the cell limit does define the peripheral extent of the cell.

Despite the ability of the electron microscope to resolve the plasmalemma, no concise and definitive structure has been determined for this entity. It appears as a trilaminar structure composed of two *osmiophilic* bands separated by an *osmiophobic* band (Fig. 1-19). Each band is approximately 2.5 nm wide. This is supposed to correspond to a sandwich-like relationship in which two layers of protein are laid upon a layer of lipid (protein-lipid-protein). This structural design comprised the unit membrane concept and was supposed to be applicable to the structural configuration and biochemical composition of all membrane systems. Too many variations, structurally and chemically, have been observed (Fig. 1-20). Recently, a repeating subunit model has been proposed as being the most reasonable representation of membrane systems. In this model, globular proteins are immersed in layers of lipids. Further investigations will be necessary before definitive statements about membrane structure are possible.

The *glycocalyx* (*cell coat*) is peripheral to, attached on and probably intimately integrated with the structural moieties of the plasmalemma (Fig. 1-21). It is a glycoprotein- and carbohydrate-rich substance which is highly periodic acid-Schiff (PAS)-positive (Fig. 1-22). Its structure varies with the free, lateral or basal surfaces of cells. It has been implicated in a variety of functions: cell recognition, absorption, adhesion, antigenicity and contact inhibition.

Ribosomes and Granular Endoplasmic Reticulum. The cytoplasm of many cells possesses either a total or focal basophilia. These areas are referred to as the *ergastoplasm*. These areas of basophilia contain high quantities of RNA. This chemical is complexed with a protein and is manifested as small granules, *ribosomes*, which are approximately 15 nm in diameter. They occur singly in the cytoplasm as *free ribosomes* or as multiple units called *polyribosomes* (Fig. 1-23). The individual units of the polyribosomes are believed to be connected by a thread of messenger RNA. These single and multiple free ribosomes are responsible for

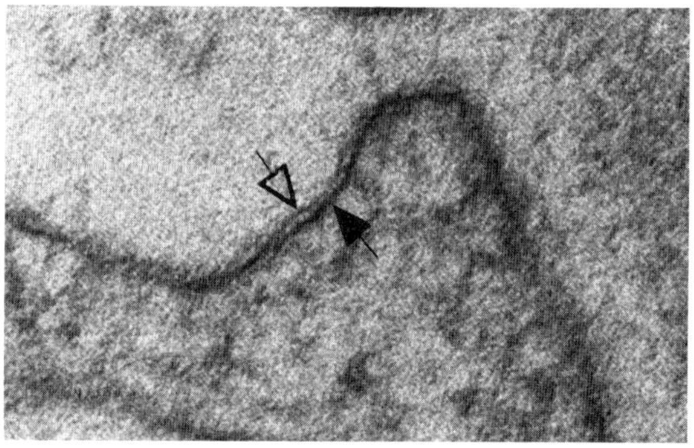

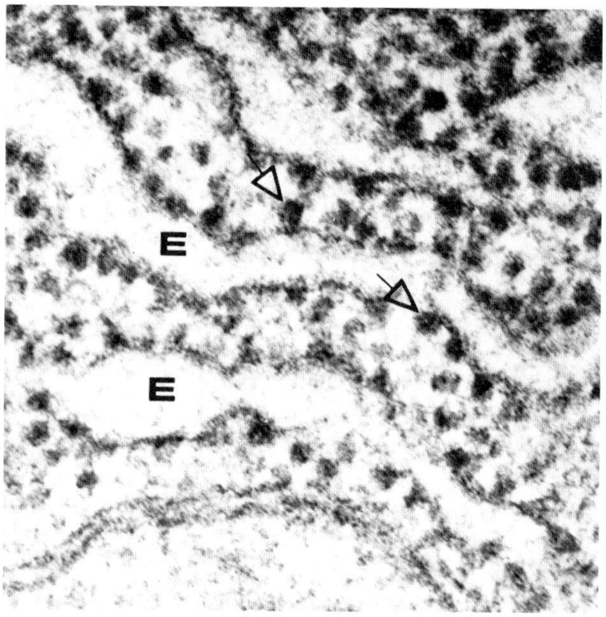

Fig. 1-19 (*left*). Trilaminar cytoplasmic membrane. The outer, thinner lamina (*open arrow*) is separated by a translucent space from the inner thicker lamina (*solid arrow*). ×215,000.

Fig. 1-20 (*right*). Globular cytoplasmic membranes. The cisterns (*E*) of the granular endoplasmic reticulum are membrane-bound and studded with ribosomes (*open arrows*). The membranes are globular. ×156,000.

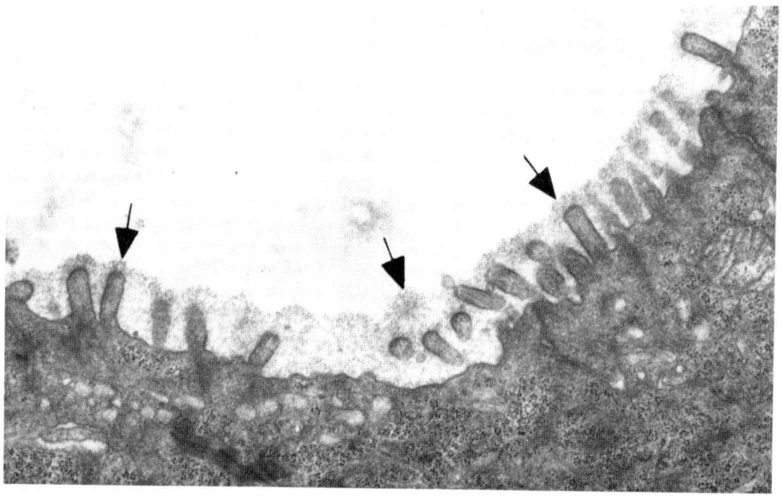

Fig. 1-21. An electron micrograph of the glycocalyx. The glycocalyx (*arrows*) covers the microvilli of mouse intestinal cells. ×14,000. (Courtesy of A. M. Sheppard)

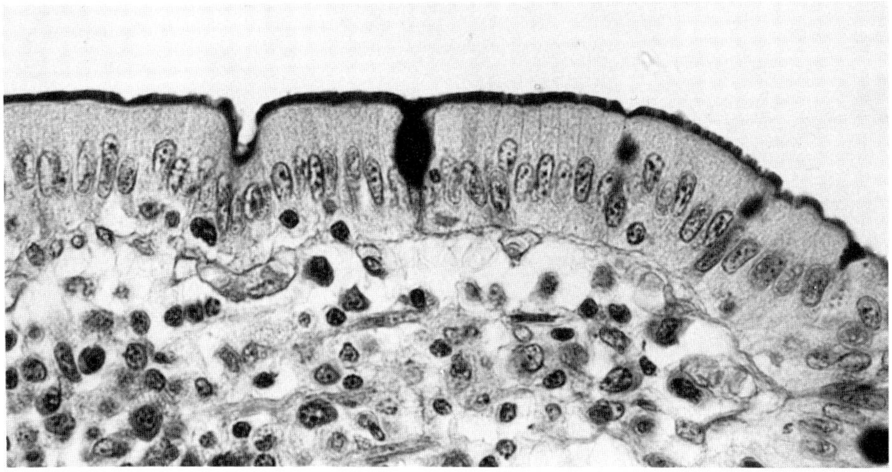

Fig. 1-22. The glycocalyx with special staining. The apical, striated border is covered by a dark-staining glycocalyx. ×160 (PAS).

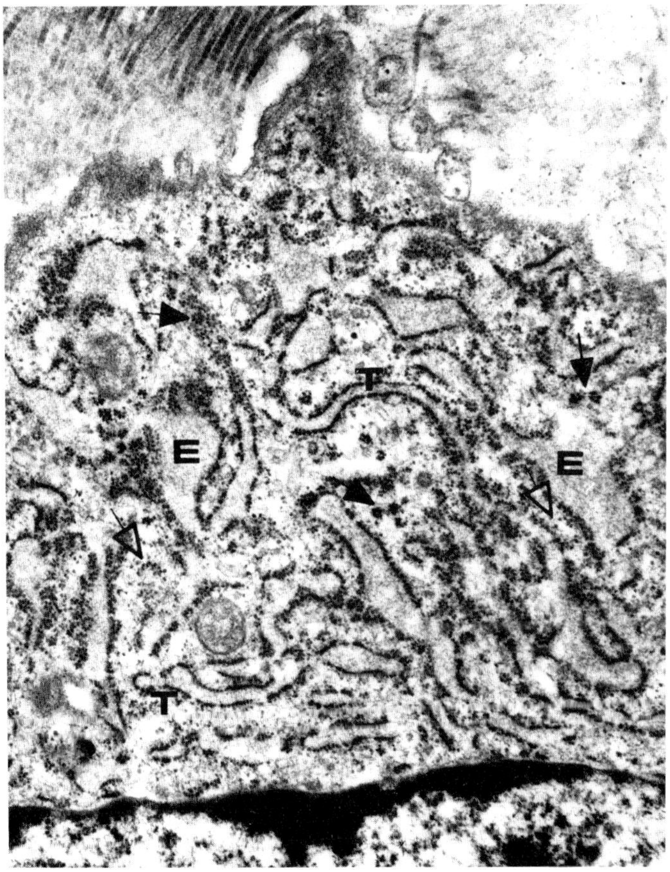

Fig. 1-23. An electron micrograph of a fiber-forming cell. The cytoplasm contains numerous profiles of granular endoplasmic reticulum. Some are tubular (*T*) while some are cisterns (*E*). Ribosomes (*open arrows*) and polyribosomes (*solid arrows*) are abundant. ×20,000.

the production of proteins for use within the cell.

An extensive network of tubules, flattened vesicles and cisternae extends throughout the cytoplasm of many cells. In those instances in which ribosomes or polyribosomes are attached to this ***network*** (***reticulum***), the organelle is referred to as the *rough* (*granular*) *endoplasmic reticulum* (Fig. 1-23). This organelle is also continuous with the outer nuclear membrane. In light microscopy, rough endoplasmic reticulum is also partially responsible for the cytoplasmic basophilia referred to previously. As in the pancreatic acinar cell (Fig. 1-24), it may appear as a basally located basophilia. In the plasma cell it is manifested as total cytoplasmic basophilia. The proteins produced by the ribosomal material associated with the granular endoplasmic reticulum are primarily for extracellular use.

The type, quantity and distribution of ribosomal material give valuable insights into cell function. Cells with high quantities of *free ribosomes* and *free polyribosomes* are involved in synthetic activity for intracellular utilization. Mesenchymal cells (cells that are undifferentiated) have numerous free ribosomes and free polyribosomes and a paucity of granular endoplasmic reticulum. Conversely, cells like plasma cells which are involved in protein synthesis for extracellular use have a preponderance of granular endoplasmic reticulum.

Nuclear and nucleolar morphology can be correlated with cytoplasmic properties to gain insights about protein synthetic potential.

Agranular Endoplasmic Reticulum. The *smooth* (*agranular*) *endoplasmic reticulum* is not as extensive as its granular counterpart, except in certain types of cells. The smooth, anastomosing, tubular profiles do not have ribosomes associated with their membranes (Fig. 1-25). These profiles are similar to and often continuous with, as well as indistinguishable from, the Golgi profiles. Functionally, they are associated with glycogen metabolism and synthesis, lipid metabolism, ion concentration and distribution and detoxification of certain substances. They are found in large quantities in cells in which ion balance is essential in maintaining electrical potential and in liver cells. The latter play an important role in glycogen metabolism and the detoxification of various substances.

Golgi Complex. The *Golgi complex* is demonstrable with osmium, silver and other heavy metal stains. This pleomorphic complex is impregnated with these metals and appears as a dark-staining, juxtanuclear reticulum (Fig. 1-26). With routine staining, however, an extensive Golgi complex appears as a ***chromophobic*** or ***negative*** Golgi area. In those cells in which a polarity is apparent, the position of the Golgi complex will reflect this polarization.

At the electron microscopic level, the Golgi complex consists of an aggregate of membrane-bound components of various types (Fig. 1-27). The most prominent is the parallel array of flattened *saccules* or *cisternae*. The others are small vesicles and large secretory vesicles. A series of these saccules and associated vesicles will often assume a semilunar configuration. The *convex face* (*immature* or *formative*) is generally associated with small vesicles, while the *concave face* (*mature*) is often associated with secretion vesicles in various stages of maturation.

Functionally, the Golgi complex is involved in packaging of secretory units for intracellular and extracellular use, synthesis of polysaccharides and the formation of the cell coat and plasmalemma.

Mitochondria. At the light microscopic level, *mitochondria* appear as threads or granules with various staining techniques. Special staining techniques, however, stain them specifically; e.g., the supravital stain, Janus green B. Their shape is quite varied;

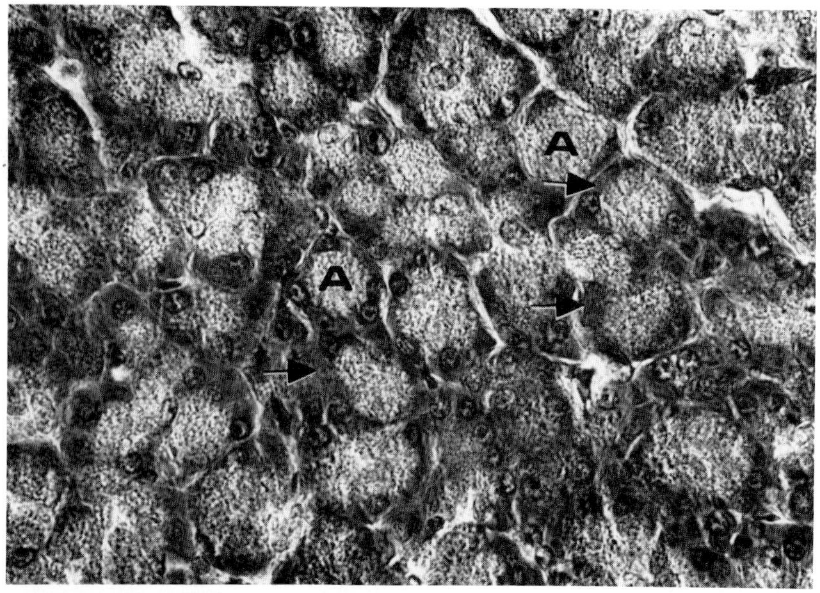

Fig. 1-24. Ergastoplasm of a pancreatic acinar cell. The apical margins of the cell (*A*) are light (acidophilic). The basal portions (*arrows*) are dark (basophilic). ×40.

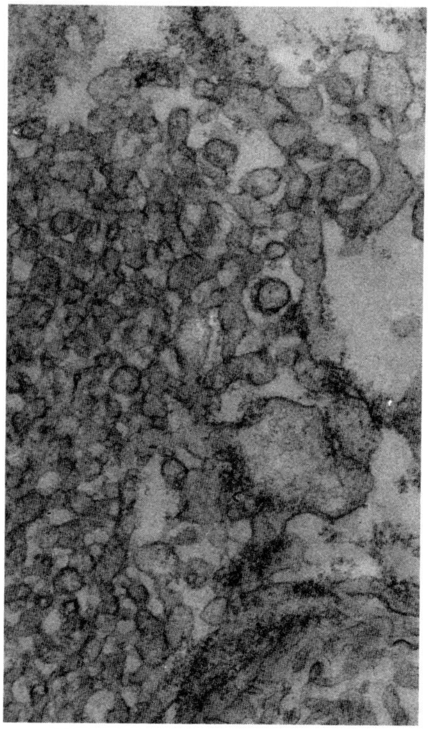

Fig. 1-25. An electron micrograph of smooth endoplasmic reticulum. ×41,000.

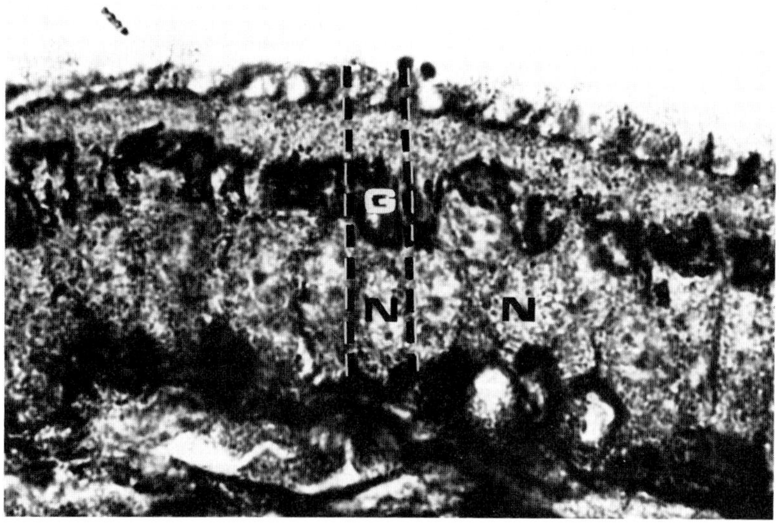

Fig. 1-26. Golgi apparatus of cells of the ductus epididymidis. The approximate lateral limits of one cell are defined by *dashed lines*. The nucleus (*N*) is basally positioned and the silver-impregnated Golgi apparatus (*G*) is supranuclear. ×400 (silver stain).

even within a specific cell type they are extremely pleomorphic, ranging from round to oval or from elongated to filamentous. The number of mitochondria in a cell varies with the energy requirements of the cell. The size of mitochondria is also quite varied. Although most may be 2–3 μm long, they may exceed a length of 10 μm.

At the electron microscopic level, mitochondria are demonstrable as a double-membrane system (Fig. 1-28). The *outer mitochondrial membrane* has a smooth contour, is approximately 7.0 nm thick and defines the peripheral limits of the organelle. The ***inner mitochondrial membrane*** is approximately 8.0 nm thick and is modified into platelike or tubular folds (*cristae mitochondriales*). The cristae are separated by a *mitochondrial matrix* which is homogeneous and finely granular but of varying density. Electron-dense granules, *mitochondrial granules*, occur within the matrix.

In vitro studies have determined that mitochondria are capable of changing shape. A change in shape or conformation has been linked with *coupled* or *uncoupled oxidative phosphorylation*. The *orthodox conformation* is associated with coupled oxidative phosphorylation and is represented morphologically by the "typical" picture of mitochondria (Fig. 1-28). The *condensed conformation* is associated with an uncoupled oxidative phosphorylation and is represented by mitochondria with enlarged cristae and a condensed mitochondrial matrix (Fig. 1-29).

The inner mitochondrial membrane and mitochondrial matrix contain all the enzymes of the citric acid cycle and those in-

Fig. 1-27. (*left*). An electron micrograph of the Golgi apparatus. The Golgi apparatus (*G*) is positioned close to the nucleus (*N*). ×20,000.

Fig. 1-28 (*right*). Typical mitochondria. These mitochondria are in the orthodox conformation. The cristae are prominent, while the mitochondrial matrix is electron-dense. ×27,000.

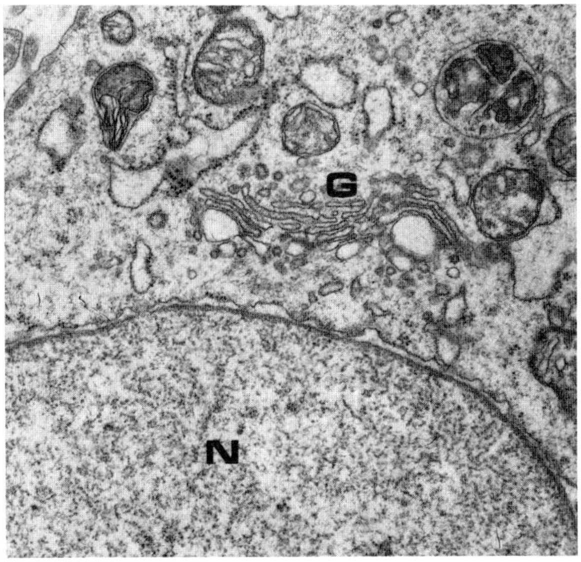

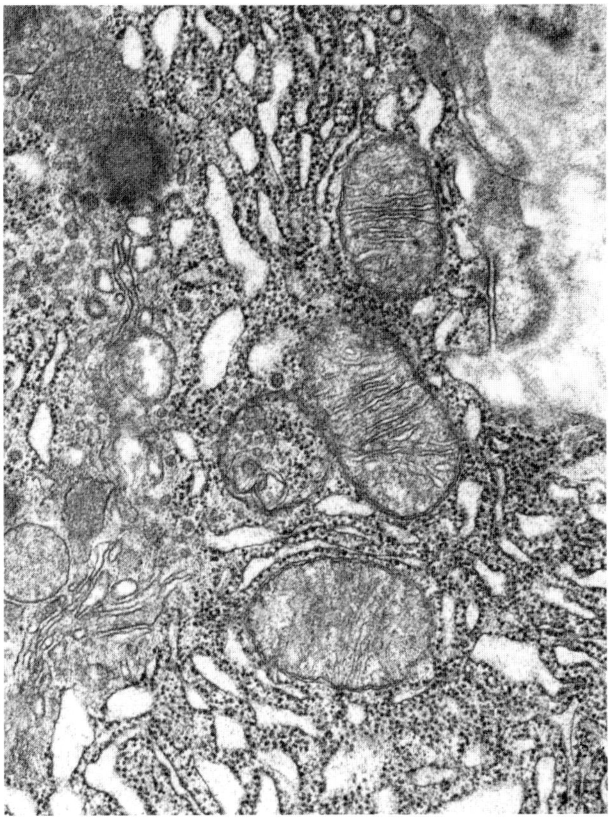

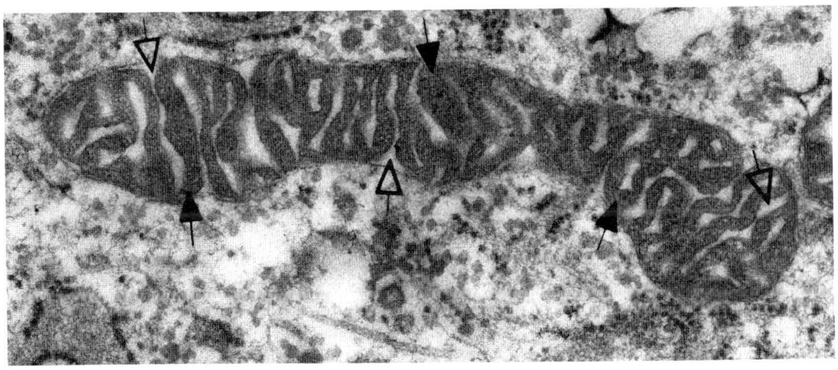

Fig. 1-29. A mitochondrion in the condensed conformation. The cristae (*open arrows*) are separated from each other by a condensed matrix (*solid arrows*). ×48,000.

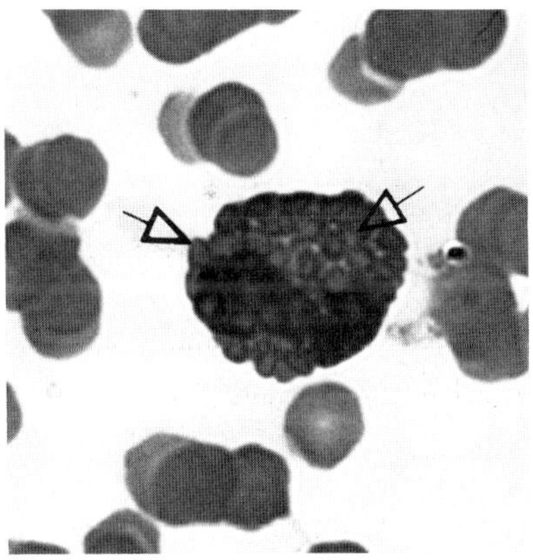

Fig. 1-30. Lysosomes of an equine eosinophil. The lysosomes (*arrows*) are the predominant cytoplasmic organelles. ×400.

volved in oxidative phosphorylation, as well as those involved in fatty acid oxidation. The primary role of mitochondria, therefore, is the production of energy. Mitochondria, however, also contain DNA and RNA. They therefore possess some genetic and protein-synthetic potential.

Lysosomes. *Lysosomes* are membrane-bound particles that are rich in *hydrolytic enzymes*. There is no single description applicable to these particles. They are represented morphologically by numerous shapes and sizes. Except in a few instances, the histochemical demonstration of specific hydrolases (*acid phosphatase, arylsulfatase*) is necessary for the absolute identification of these organelles. At the light microscopic level, the specific granules of basophils, eosinophils (Fig. 1-30) and neutrophils are representative of lysosomes and clearly demonstrate the range of structure and staining properties associated with these particles.

Although the concept of lysosomes was initially derived from biochemical investigations, electron microscopic studies have added appreciably to an understanding of their structure and relationship to cell function. Lysosomes are particles in various stages of formation, maturation and activity. This continuum is represented by particles of varying morphological configuration.

The adjoining scheme represents the relationship of lysosomal particles in various stages of activity (Fig. 1-31). Vacuoles bud from the Golgi complex and are transformed into *dense bodies* (*primary lysosomes, inactive lysosomes*). The fate of these primary lysosomes is dependent upon the subsequent activity with which they are associated. Two distinct types of activity are associated with lysosomes, *endocytosis*

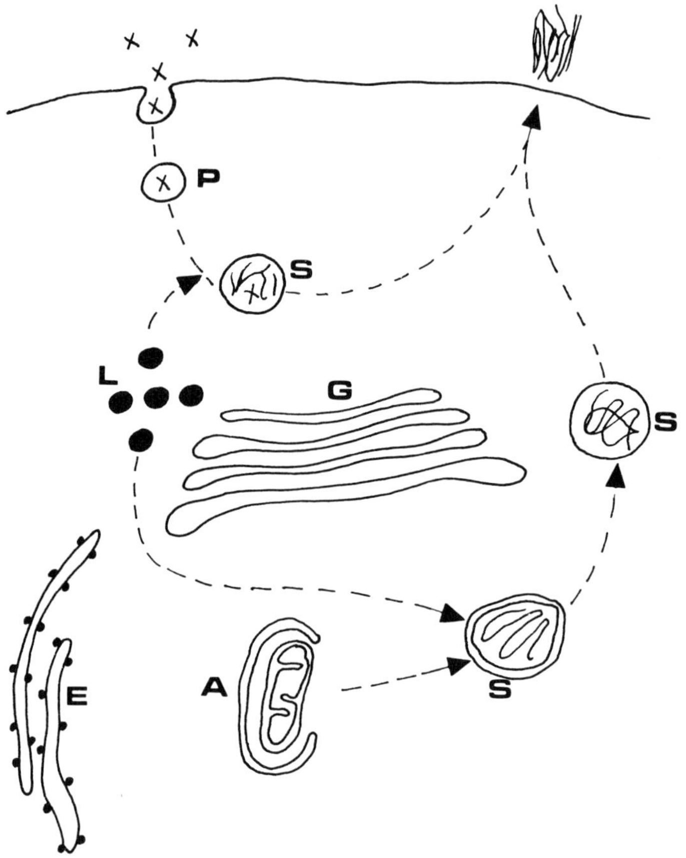

Fig. 1-31. Relationship of lysosomes to hydrolytic activity. Particulate matter (X) is picked up by endocytotic vesicles as phagosomes (P). These fuse with primary lysosomes (L) derived from the Golgi apparatus (G) to form secondary lysosomes (S). Upon completion of the hydrolytic activity, residual bodies are formed. These may be retained or extruded. In autophagocytosis, the initial membrane of the autophagosome (A) may be formed from the granular endoplasmic reticulum (E). The subsequent events are similar to those just described.

and *autophagocytosis*. Endocytotic activity may be further subdivided into *phagocytosis* or *pinocytosis*.

In *phagocytosis*, particulate matter is engulfed by the cell in the form of membrane-bound vesicles (*phagosomes*). The union of a primary lysosome with a phagosome produces a *secondary* or *active lysosome*, often referred to as a *phagolysosome*. Upon completion of the digestive activity of this newly formed structure, or during an arrest in the activity, a resulting *residual body* is formed. The latter, upon completion of the digestive function, is extruded from the cell.

In *pinocytosis*, fluid material is engulfed by the cell in *pinocytotic vesicles*. These vesicles fuse with primary lysosomes, but their integrity is not lost; i.e., they appear within a dense body as vesicles. At this point, the primary lysosome and engulfed pinocytotic vesicles are referred to as a ***multivesicular body***. Following the completion of the digestive process, it is assumed that the multivesicular body is converted to a primary lysosome for future functioning or, as in the case of phagocytosis, a residual body is formed.

In ***autophagocytosis***, a sequence of events occurs that is similar but not identical to that associated with phagocytosis. Various organelles, as well as insoluble portions of cytoplasm, tend to degenerate or become functionless. These are represented as *foci of cytoplasmic degeneration*. These degenerative or functionless cytoplasmic components are engulfed by primary lysosomes and are referred to as *autophagic vacuoles* or *cytolysosomes*. The fate of cytolysosomes is similar to the fate of phagolysosomes.

Numerous other terminologies have been applied to lysosomes. It should be clear that the complexity and diversity of lysosomal function accounts for the heterogeneity of these particles. The significance of lysosomes in cellular function cannot be overstated. They are extremely important organelles. Not only are they responsible for routine digestive properties of cells, but they are also important organelles through which protective functions of cells are mediated. They are responsible for protecting cells, and hence the body, against foreign materials, and also for destroying cells. These organelles account for *autolytic processes*. Under normal conditions, routine cellular death (*necrobiosis*) is mediated through autolysosomal function (*autolysis*). In pathological conditions, lysosomes can account for abnormal cell death (*necrosis*) via autolytic processes as well.

Centrioles and Basal Bodies. The *centrioles* of resting cells are two small bodies contained within an area of gelatinous material referred to as the *centrosphere*. Although these bodies are usually inconspicuous in resting cells, special staining techniques can be utilized to demonstrate them at the light microscopic level.

The two small dots or bodies shown by the light microscope are resolved with the electron microscope as cylindrical units which are 150 nm in diameter and approximately 500 nm long (Fig. 1-32). They are oriented perpendicular to each other. Each cylinder is composed of nine groups of three tubules. Although cylindrical, the nine groups of tubules are oriented eccentrically to each other. Fibrous material connects the terminal tubules of each group to the terminal tubules of adjacent groups. Also, fibrous material connects the peripherally located groups to the center of the centriole. Ideal sections and good resolution are requisite to demonstrate this fibrillar substructure.

Centrioles play a significant role in the mitotic process, at which time they are duplicated and are associated with the microtubules of the spindle apparatus. Recently, a dense cytoplasmic region adjacent to the centrioles within the centrosphere has been associated with microtubule formation. This dense region has been implicated as either a ***microtubular subunit aggregation center*** or a ***subunit synthesizing center***. The functional relationship of this dense region to the centrioles is not clear.

The basal bodies are structurally similar

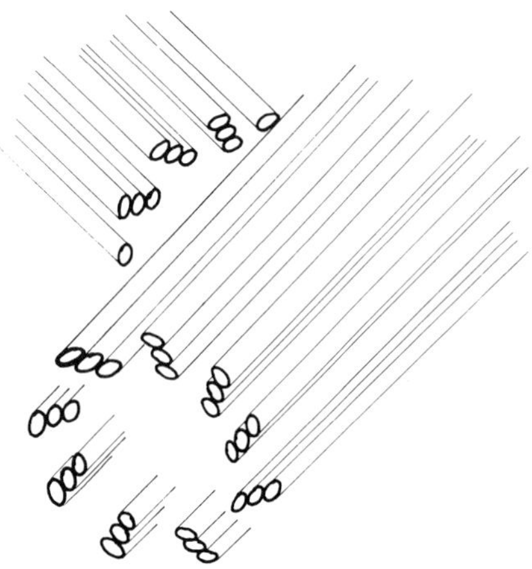

Fig. 1-32. Diagram of centrioles. The centrioles are paired structures oriented perpendicular to each other. They consist of nine groups of three tubules.

to the centrioles. The former are structurally associated with cilia and are responsible for the formation of cilia.

Microbodies. *Microbodies* or *peroxisomes* are spherical or ovoid organelles that are smaller than mitochondria. Special staining techniques are required for their demonstration at the light microscopic level. They can be identified on the basis of the presence of the following enzymes: uricase, catalase and *d*-amino oxidase. Some investigators have proposed that they are developing mitochondria (not widely accepted), while others claim that they are related to lysosomes. It appears as though they are specific organelles, the specific function of which is yet to be elucidated.

At the electron microscopic level of examination, microbodies are bound by a single membrane that encloses a matrix, the granularity and homogeneity of which have been compared to the mitochondrial matrix. A central density, core or crystalloid particle may be present within the matrix. The size, shape and nature of these particles, as well as the presence or absence of same, is species-dependent. These organelles, most commonly with a diameter of 300–600 nm, are closely associated with smooth endoplasmic reticular profiles.

Microbodies have been identified in liver cells and the epithelial lining cells of the proximal convoluted tubules of the kidney. They are, however, of variable occurrence in other cells of various animals.

Microtubules. *Microtubules* occur in a variety of cells and subserve various functions. Except in the case of the mitotic spindle apparatus, microtubules are difficult to identify at the light microscopic level. Even then, they appear as fibers rather than being resolved as tubules.

With the electron microscope, they are resolved as tubules with an outside diameter of 20–26 nm and a wall 5–7.0 nm thick (Fig. 1-33). It is proposed that globular monomeric subunits are arranged in a helical array to form microtubules. They are found scattered throughout the cytoplasm of many cell types, as well as being preferentially distributed throughout the cytoplasm in certain cells. It is believed that they are significant contributors to the maintenance of cell shape; thus, they may be considered a part of the cytoplasmic skeleton. They are found in cilia, in flagella and in the manchette of spermatids. They are significant, therefore, in the development of and motility associated with these structures. Also, they are longitudinally oriented along the axoplasm of neurons, wherein they serve as a transport medium for various secretory products.

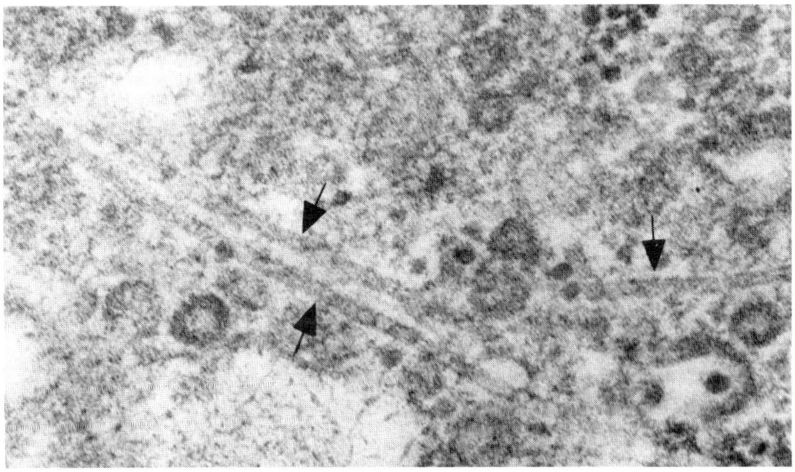

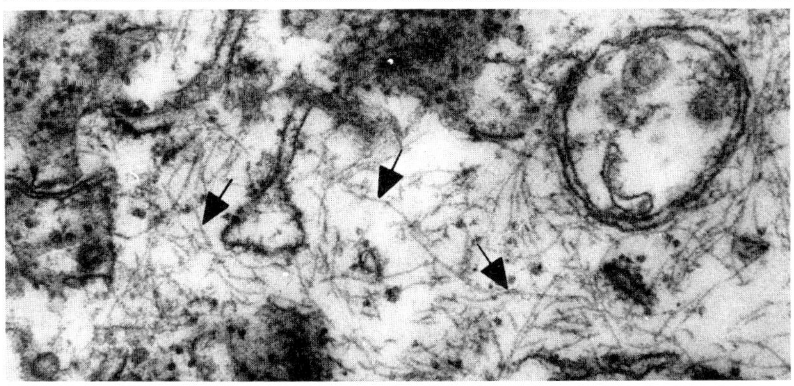

Fig. 1-33 (*top*). A electron micrograph of microtubules. The microtubules (*arrows*) are scattered among other cytoplasmic components. ×94,000.

Fig. 1-34 (*bottom*). An electron micrograph of cytofilaments. The cell was ruptured and has lost much of its normal cytoplasmic matrix components. As a result, the cytofilaments (*arrows*) are easily observed. ×52,000.

Filaments and Fibrils. *Cytofilaments* or *tonofilaments* are scattered throughout the cytoplasm and constitute the *cell web* (Fig. 1-34). These cytoplasmic components are 4–5.0 nm thick and are of variable lengths. They serve as supportive or skeletal components of the cytoplasm. Although individually beyond the limits of resolution with the light microscope, they are resolved when they are grouped together as *tonofibrils*. These tonofibrils constitute the *terminal web* of some cells and are associated with plasmalemmal modifications utilized in cellular attachments.

In those cells modified for contractile functions (smooth muscle, skeletal muscle, cardiac muscle, myoepithelial cells), filaments with contractile properties are either randomly dispersed throughout the cytoplasm or are oriented into highly organized contractile units. These *myofilaments* are divisible into two distinct subgroups. *Myosin myofilaments* are approximately 10 nm in diameter, while *actin myofilaments* are about 6.0 nm in diameter (Chapter 8). Although not resolved as individual units at the light microscopic level, they are observable as larger *myofibrils*.

Secretory Inclusions. The secretory products of cells are varied and include such products as enzymes, acids, proteins and mucus. In some instances, the morphology of a given cell may be altered significantly through its involvement in a specific secretory function or through the accumulation of its secretory products. In other instances, the synthesis and/or elaboration of a secretory product is not accompanied by a change in cellular morphology. Specific examples of the aforementioned conditions follow in subsequent chapters. A few general examples will serve to illustrate cellular secretory activity.

The morphological configurations of the secretory products are as diverse as the products themselves. Lysosomes, as secretory products for intracellular use, have already been described. *Zymogen* granules, membrane-bound packets of enzymes for extracellular use, typify many protein-secreting cells. As in the case of the pancreatic acinar cell, these secretory products appear as granules in a subluminal position. The granules are derived from the mature face of the Golgi complex, mature as they move toward the lumen and are individually secreted at the apical cell surface (Fig. 1-35).

Some cells that secrete ***mucoid sub-***

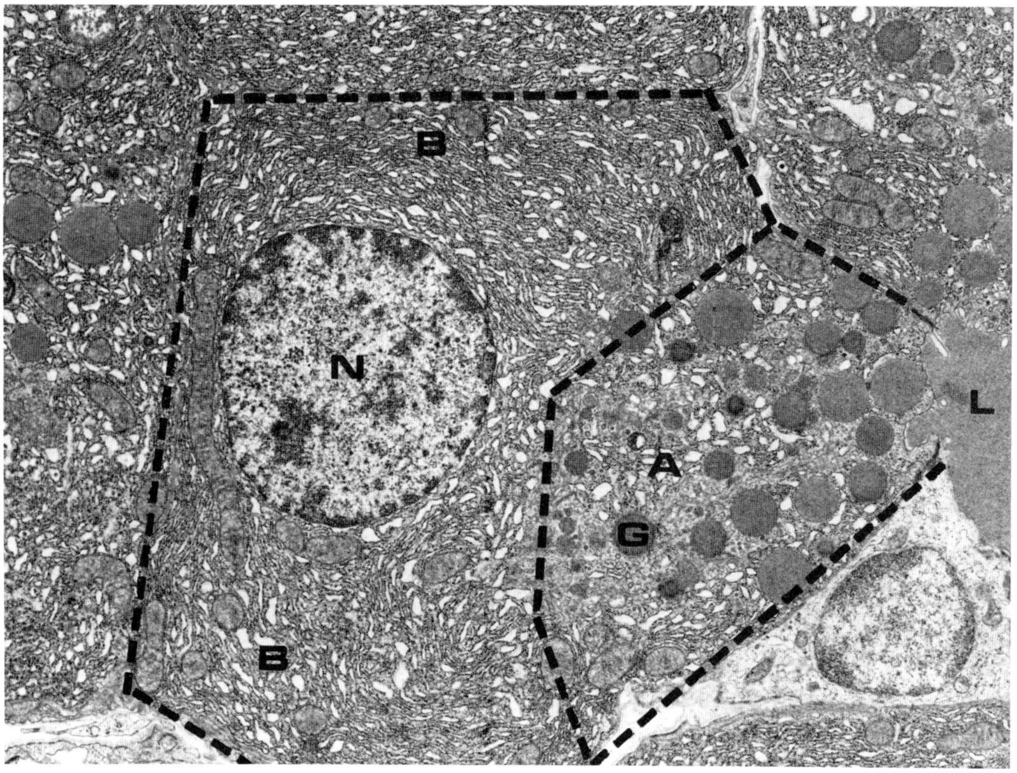

Fig. 1-35. An electron micrograph of a pancreatic acinar cell. The approximate limits of the cell (*outer dashed line*) are indicated. The apex (*A*) of the cell borders the lumen (*L*). The apex (***inner dashed line***) contains numerous zymogen granules (*G*). The basal portion (*B*) contains the nucleus (*N*), granular endoplasmic reticulum and mitochondria. ×7,000.

stances (mucus) are characterized, as in the case of the ***goblet cell*** depicted (Fig. 1-36), by a very foamy cytoplasm. The cytoplasm is basophilic and the nucleus is displaced basally. The foamy appearance is attributed to the packets of mucous precursor material contained within the cytoplasm.

The secretion of lipid material is normally associated with cells that possess a foamy but acidophilic cytoplasm. In these cases, however, the foamy appearance is a result of lipids having been leached from the cytoplasm. Cells from the cortex of the adrenal gland exemplify this type of secretory inclusion product (Fig. 1-37).

As mentioned previously, other cells secrete various products that are not visible at the light microscopic level. Among these are the numerous cells of connective tissues. They secrete mucopolysaccharides and proteins without any definitive, routine light microscopic evidence of this activity.

In some cells, a watery or *serous* secretion is accompanied by attendant alterations at the secretory surface. However, the accumulation of light microscopically visible products is not evident. The serous cells of some glands, characterized as cells with a finely granular and acidophilic cytoplasm and centrally or paracentrally located nuclei, exemplify another variation in cellular secretory activity and resulting products (Fig. 1-38).

Cellular secretory methods and products are discussed in Chapter 2.

Nutritive Inclusions. Most cells possess the ability to store various products that subserve a nutritive function. The most common of these that are readily visible at the light microscopic level are *glycogen* and *lipids*. Glycogen is especially apparent in the liver, skeletal muscle and cells of cartilage. A carmine stain is used specifically to identify glycogen, but the use of PAS and diastase is also an acceptable demonstration method. At the electron microscopic level, glycogen may appear as single particles which range from 15.0 to 30.0 nm in diameter with an irregular outline (the *beta particles*) (Fig. 1-39). Accumulations in the form of *rosettes* (*alpha particles*) are also demonstrable (Fig. 1-40).

Lipid droplets within cells represent the storage of triglycerides. Various cells store these lipids to varying degrees. The ultimate storage of lipids is manifested in fat cells. The large vacuities do not represent lipids, rather the foci from which they were leached from the cytoplasm by the fat solvents used routinely in the preparatory techniques. Special handling and staining techniques are necessary for the demonstration of lipids. At the electron microscopic level, lipid inclusions appear as osmiophilic bodies of varying density (Fig. 1-41). The degree of dark staining (uptake of osmium) is a function of the lipid composition of the droplet. Although they appear to be membrane-bound, they actually occur free in the cytoplasm. The precipitation of osmium at the lipid-cytoplasmic interface may be misinterpreted as a membrane. In specific instances, however, triglycerides in intestinal lining cells are membrane-bound.

Miscellaneous Inclusions. Numerous types of other inclusions occur within a large variety of cells. The most notable of these are the ***pigment granules***.

Melanin is the brown pigment responsible for that coloration in a variety of foci scattered throughout the body. It is produced in *melanoblasts* and is transferred to *melanophores*.

Lipofuscin is a gold-brown pigment, the origin and function of which is debatable. Absent in the cells of young animals, it appears with progressive age. It is often referred to as the "wear and tear" pigment, but some believe, on the basis of the presence of esterase activity, that these granules are active in cell metabolism as part of the lysosomal system.

Hemosiderin is a red-brown pigment resulting from the degradation of hemoglobin. Since the body cannot store iron, this is the mechanism whereby iron is recycled through the body. Although this pigment can be found in numerous intracellular and extracellular foci throughout

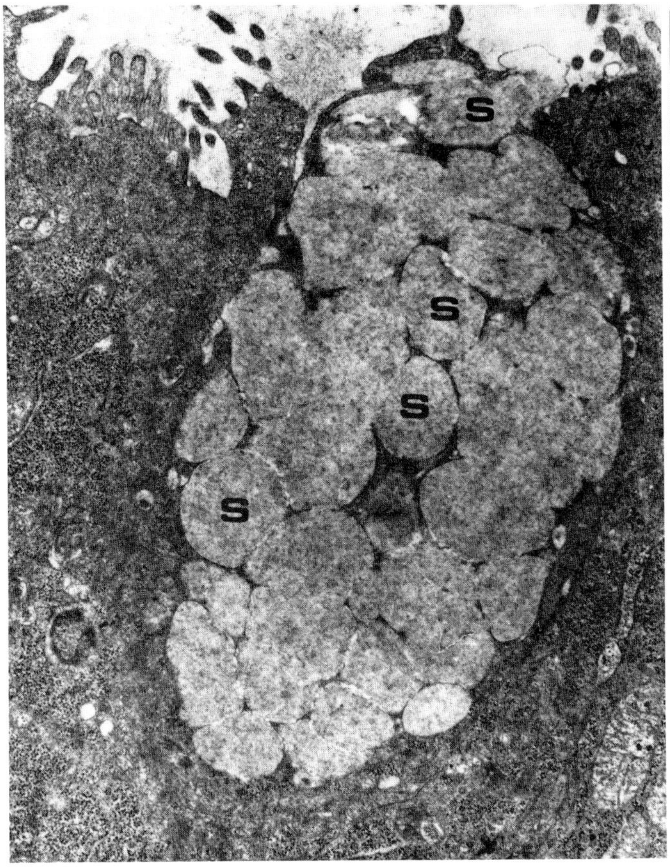

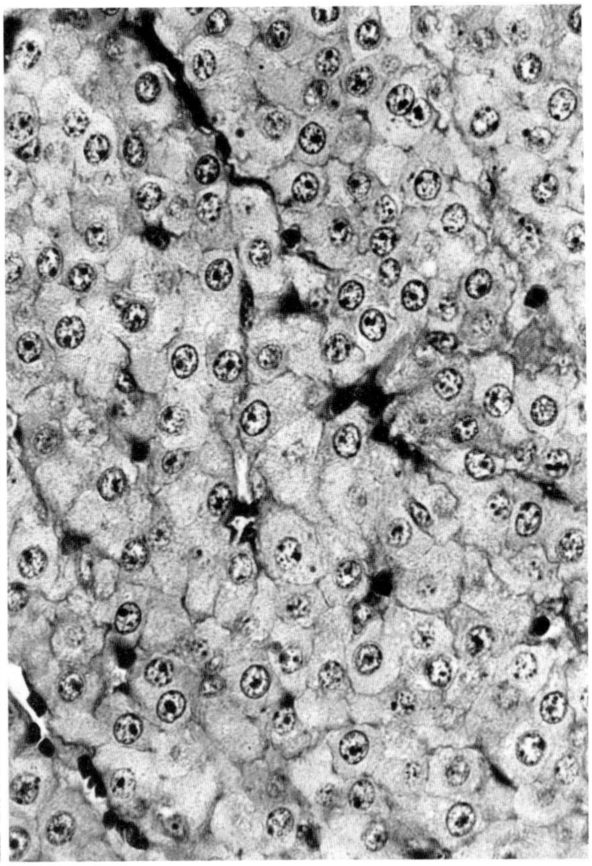

Fig. 1-36 (*left*). An electron micrograph of a goblet cell. The cytoplasm has been displaced peripherally by the numerous secretory droplets (*S*). The nucleus is not in the plane of section. ×14,000. (Courtesy of A. M. Sheppard)

Fig. 1-37 (*right*). Lipid containing cells from the adrenal gland. These pyramidal cells have a foamy appearance due to their content of lipid materials. ×160.

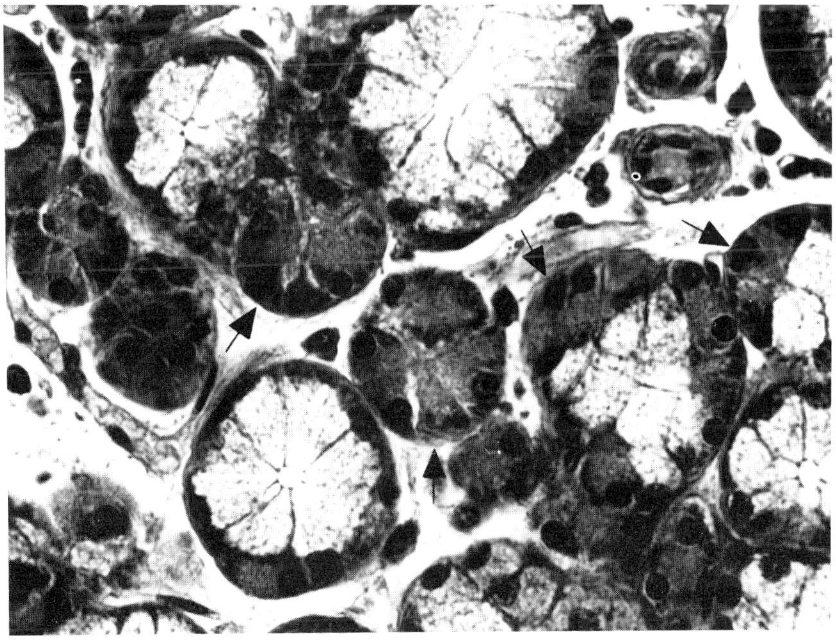

Fig. 1-38. Serous cells from a salivary gland. The dark cells (*arrows*) are the serous cells. The light cells are mucous cells. ×160.

the body, it is especially prominent in the phagocytes of the spleen.

Numerous crystalline inclusions occur in a variety of cell types. These will be discussed with the specific cells involved in subsequent chapters.

Cell Division

Cell Cycle. The necessity of adding new cells to the body during prenatal and postnatal growth phases should be apparent. However, the addition of new cells to the somatic complement does not cease with the termination of growth. Rather, the *replacement* of old or dead cells with new ones is a constant but variable occurrence. Some cells, as those of the skin, are replaced at regular intervals; others, such as the muscle cells of the heart, are not replaced. Generally, however, the body has the means to replace most cells. Besides the ability to replace worn out cells, one other criterion must be satisfied; i.e., *the ability to replace a given cell with an identical cell.* The mechanism responsible for this faithful replication is *mitosis*.

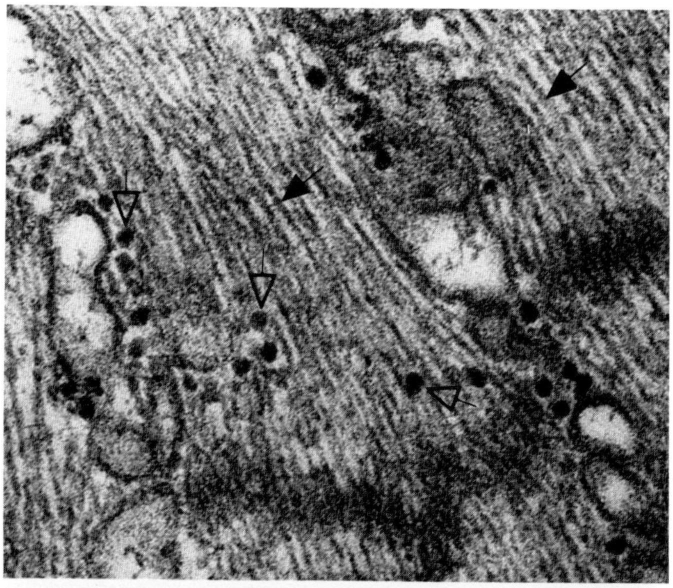

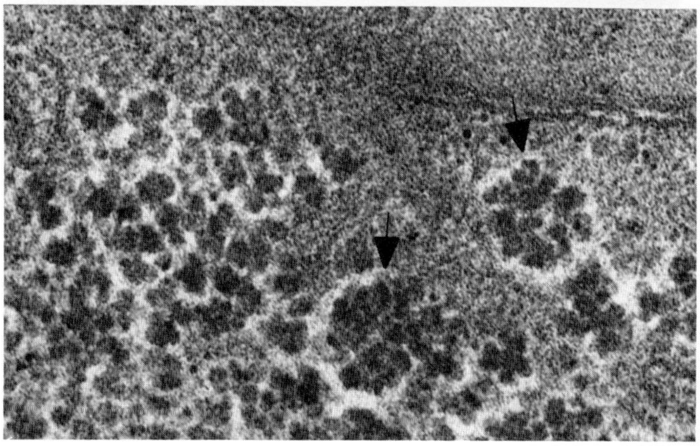

Fig. 1-39 (*top*). An electron micrograph of glycogen particles. The beta particles (*open arrows*) are scattered among myofilaments (*solid arrows*) of a striated muscle cell. ×51,000.

Fig. 1-40 (*bottom*). An electron micrograph of glycogen particles. *Arrows*, alpha particles. ×133,000.

This built-in replacement mechanism implies that cell lives are finite. This, of course, is true, but the longevity of a cell is variable and specific for different cell types. Within the framework of a finite existence for various cell types, a definitive *cell cycle* can be defined. The cell cycle is defined as the passage of a cell through the interphase and mitosis, while the *generation time* is the time period required to complete one cycle.

Although routine histological staining techniques allow only for the recognition of interphase and mitotic cells, autoradiographic techniques add valuable insights relative to interphase activity. Through the use of tritiated thymidine (a DNA precursor), subdivisions of the interphase are apparent. The *preduplication* or *presynthetic phase* (G_1) represents the period prior to the uptake of the labeled thymidine. This phase may be referred to as the *vegetative phase*. It is the stage during which time the cell will conduct its routine functions. Also, if the cell has a potential for mitosis, it is during this stage that the metabolites necessary to support mitosis will be accumulated. Most of the cells or accumulation of cells examined in histology will be in this stage.

The *duplication phase* (S) is the stage during which time DNA replication takes place, as evidenced by the nuclear uptake of the labeled thymidine. Not all the chromatic material is labeled (or duplicated) simultaneously. *Telomeric* (near the chromosome ends) replication occurs prior to *centromeric* (near the middle of chromosomes) replication. The end result, however, is the duplication of the chromosomes and a doubling of the DNA complement.

The *postduplication phase* (*postsynthetic phase*) is the G_2 stage. The naming of this phase refers only to the termination of DNA replication. Much synthetic, and therefore duplicative, activity characterizes this stage. The synthesis of histones, as well as that of RNA, occurs in this stage.

The interphase of the cell cycle is an extremely active phase responsible for a variety of cellular functions and events: increase in the total mass of a cell, increase in nuclear and nucleolar mass, duplication of chromatic material, synthesis of RNA and proteins and the conduction of routine cellular functions. In comparison with the interphase, the mitotic phase of the cell cycle is extremely short.

Differentiation and Mitotic Potential. During early stages of embryonic and fetal growth, most of the cells of the body have a high potential for division as well as the potential to become a variety of cells. As development ensues, the *differentiation* of varied cell populations is apparent. A consequence of this *specialization* (differentiation) is the *reduction or loss of cell potentiality* and a *reduction or loss of reproductive capacity* (*mitotic potential*).

Generally, highly specialized cells possess a low capacity for or an inability to duplicate themselves. Neurons (Fig. 1-17) and cardiac muscle cells are examples of these.

Specialized cell populations usually have specific cells associated with them from which other members of their population arise. These are referred to generally as *stem cells*. The basal layer of cells of the epidermis (stem cell or germinative cell layer) is an example of a residual cell population within a community of specific cells that retains the ability to replace cells lost from the skin. These cells are capable only of forming "epidermal" cells. Other examples will be included in subsequent sections.

The *mesenchymal cell* of the body represents a cell similar to the aforementioned. It is a stem cell. However, this cell possesses a high potentiality and reproductive capacity. It is an undifferentiated cell capable of specializing into a variety of cell types: muscle cells, bone cells, cartilage cells, blood cells, etc. It is scattered throughout the body in association with numerous cell populations wherein it retains this ability for mitosis and multiple expression. It is especially apparent around small blood vessels in the *perivascular space*. It is a stellate or fusiform cell with a scant cytoplasm and a large, vesicular nucleus. Its ultrastructural features conform to the relationships discussed regarding euchromatin, ribosomes, polyribosomes and granular endoplasmic reticulum.

Some cells, despite their high degree of differentiation, still retain a high reproductive capacity under certain conditions. One example of this apparent paradox is the *hepatocyte*. The cells of the liver, following an injury, become highly mitotic.

In order to maintain the reproductive capacity described, the dividing cells will commit one cell to the differentiated state and retain the other in an undifferentiated condition for future division.

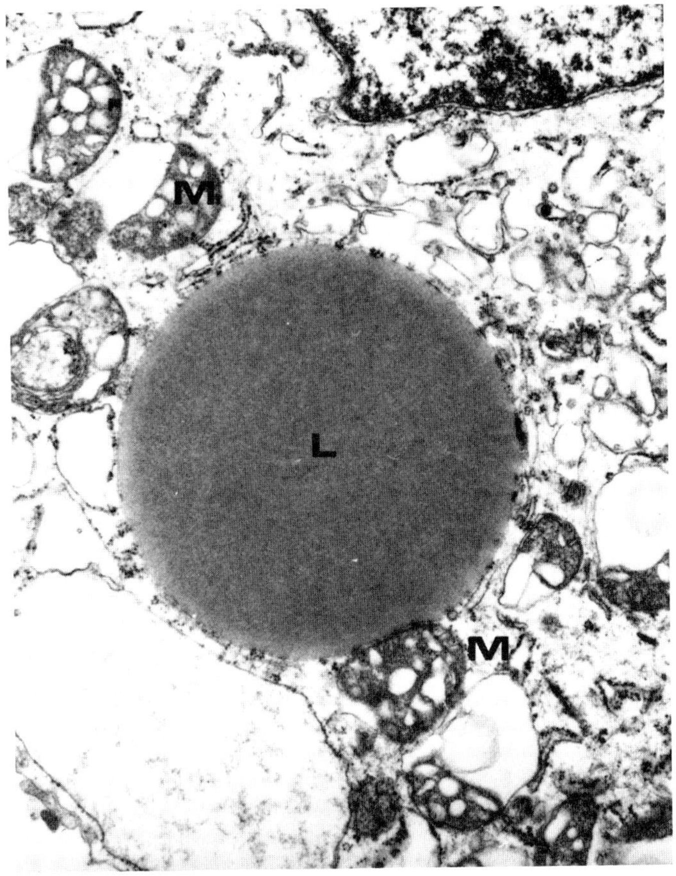

Fig. 1-41. Lipid droplets from a tumor cell (electron micrograph). The lipid droplet (*L*) is not membrane-bound. Condensed mitochondria (*M*) are present also. ×20,000.

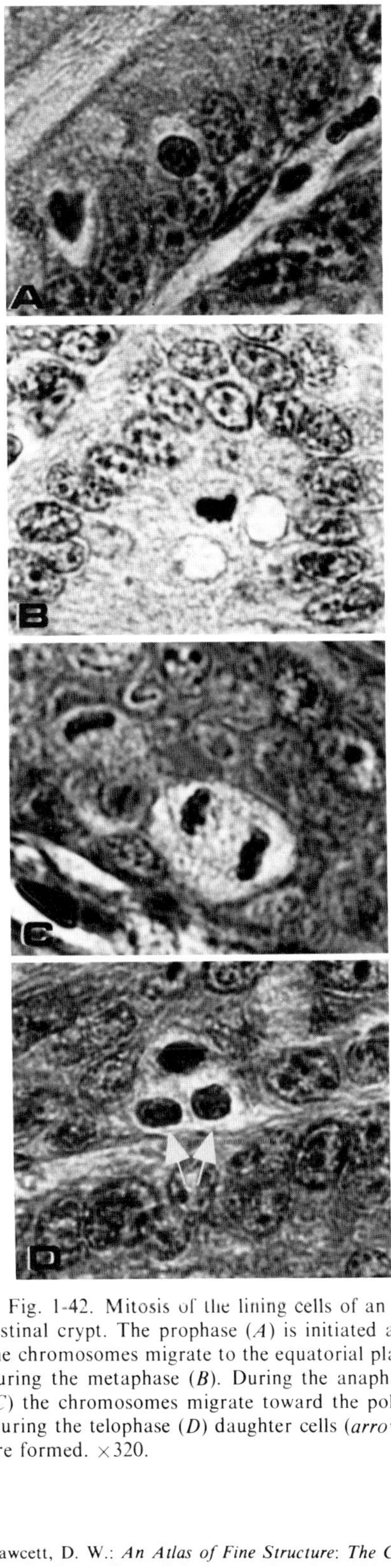

Fig. 1-42. Mitosis of the lining cells of an intestinal crypt. The prophase (*A*) is initiated and the chromosomes migrate to the equatorial plane during the metaphase (*B*). During the anaphase (*C*) the chromosomes migrate toward the poles. During the telophase (*D*) daughter cells (*arrows*) are formed. ×320.

Divisional Sequence. The continuum of the divisional process has been arbitrarily divided into five stages: *interphase*, *prophase*, *metaphase*, *anaphase* and *telophase*. The last four stages actually comprise *mitosis*; however, the significance of the interphase cannot be neglected and has been elaborated upon previously.

During the *prophase* (Fig. 1-42), the chromatic material undergoes a progressive condensation which culminates with the chromosomes becoming distinct entities in late prophase. During the latter part of prophase the nuclear membrane disintegrates. At the same time, the nucleolus disappears. In the cytoplasm, the *centrosphere* divides, each part containing a pair of *centrioles*, and the centrioles move toward opposite poles of the cell. *Spindle fibers*, composed of microtubules, are apparent between the migrating centrospheres.

During the *metaphase* (Fig. 1-42), the chromosomes migrate toward and align themselves along the *equatorial plane* of the cell. Microtubules attach themselves to the *centromere* and each chromosome is composed of two *chromatids* attached at the centromere. The alignment along the equatorial plane is random and *homologous chromosomes* do *not* align themselves one next to the other as pairs. This is an important distinction between *mitosis* and *meiosis*.

With the splitting of the two chromatids at the centromere, daughter chromosomes begin to migrate to the opposite cellular poles. These events mark the initiation of the *anaphase* (Fig. 1-42). Thus, the anaphase is characterized by the initiation of *karyokinesis*.

The reconstitution of the nuclear membrane marks the initiation of the *telophase* (Fig. 1-42). The chromosomes become dispersed while the nucleus enlarges. *Cytokinesis*, initiated peripheral to the equatorial plane, is completed and two identical daughter cells result.

References

General References

Bloom, W. and Fawcett, D. W.: *A Textbook of Histology*. 9th ed. Saunders, Philadelphia, 1968.

Brachet, J. and Mirsky, A. E.: *The Cell: Biochemistry, Physiology and Morphology*. 6 Vols. Academic Press, New York, 1959–1964.

Bresnick, E. and Schwartz, A.: *Functional Dynamics of the Cell*. Academic Press, New York, 1968.

DeRobertis, E. D. P., Nowinski, W. W. and Saez, F. A.: *Cell Biology*. 4th ed. Saunders, Philadelphia, 1965.

DuPraw, E. J.: *Cell and Molecular Biology*. Academic Press, New York, 1968.

Fawcett, D. W.: *An Atlas of Fine Structure: The Cell, Its Organelles and Inclusions*. Saunders, Philadelphia, 1967.

Ham, A. W.: *Histology*. 6th ed. Lippincott, Philadelphia, 1969.

Lentz, T. L.: *Cell Fine Structure: An Atlas of Drawings of Whole-Cell Structure*. Saunders, Philadelphia, 1971.

Matthews, J. L. and Martin, J. H.: *Atlas of Human Histology and Ultrastructure*. Lea and Febiger, Philadelphia, 1971.

Porter, K. R. and Bonneville, M. A.: *Fine Structure of*

Cells and Tissues. 3rd ed. Lea and Febiger, Philadelphia, 1968.

Sandborn, E. B.: *Cells and Tissues by Light and Electron Microscopy*. 2 Vols. Academic Press, New York, 1970.

Nucleus

Bennett, H. S.: Fine structure of cell nucleus, chromosomes, nucleoli and membrane. Rev. Mod. Phys. *31*:297, 1959.

Dalton, A. J. and Haguenau, F.: *Ultrastructure in Biological Systems: The Nucleus*. Vol. 3. Academic Press, New York, 1968.

Monneron, A. and Bernard, W.: Fine structural organization of the interphase nucleus in some mammalian cells. J. Ultrastruct. Res. *27*:266, 1969.

Moses, N. J.: Studies on nuclei using correlated cytochemical, light and electron microscopic techniques. J. Biophys. Biochem. Cytol. *2*:397, 1956.

Nuclear Envelope

Barnes, B. G. and Davis, J. M.: The structure of nuclear pores in mammalian tissues. J. Ultrastruct. Res. *3*:131, 1959.

Franke, W.: Isolated nuclear membranes. J. Cell Biol. *31*:619, 1966.

Franke, W. and Kartenbeck, J.: Structure of nuclear membranes isolated from brain cells. Experientia. *25*:396, 1969.

Kessel, R. G.: Fine structure of the pore-annulus complex in the nuclear envelope and the annulate lamellae of germ cells. Z. Zellforsch. *94*:441, 1969.

Wiener, J., Spiro, D. and Lowenstein, W. R.: Ultrastructure and permeability of nuclear membranes. J. Cell Biol. *27*:107, 1965.

Yoo, B. Y. and Bayley, S. T.: The structure of pores in isolated pea nuclei. J. Ultrastruct. Res. *18*:651, 1967.

Chromatin

Barr, M. L.: The significance of the sex chromatin. Int. Rev. Cytol. *19*:35, 1966.

Bujard, H.: Electron microscopy of single stranded DNA. J. Molec. Biol. *49*:125, 1970.

Dales, S.: A study of the fine structure of mammalian somatic chromosomes. Exp. Cell Res. *19*:577, 1960.

Osgood, E. E., Jenkins, D. P., Brooks, R. and Lawson, R. K.: Electron micrographic studies of the expanded and uncoiled chromosomes from human leukocytes. Ann. N. Y. Acad. Sci. *113*:717, 1963.

Priest, J. H. and Shikes, R. H.: Distribution of labeled chromatin. J. Cell Biol. *47*:99, 1970.

Nucleolus

Bernhard, W. and Granboulan, N.: Electron microscopy of the nucleolus in vertebrate cells. In *Ultrastructure in Biological Systems: The Nucleus*, edited by A. J. Dalton and F. Haguenau. Vol. 3. Academic Press, New York, p. 81, 1968.

Vincent, V. S. and Miller, O. J., Jr. (eds.): The nucleolus, its structure and function. Nat. Cancer Inst. Monogr. *23*: 1965.

Cellular Membranes

Bolis, L. and Pethica, B. A.: *Membrane Models and the Formation of Biological Membranes*. North Holland Publishing, Amsterdam, 1968.

Dalton, A. J. and Haguenau, F. (eds.): *Ultrastructure in Biological Systems: The Membranes*. Vol. 4. Academic Press, New York, 1968.

Davson, H.: Growth of the concept of the paucimolecular membrane. Circulation *26*:1022, 1962.

Finean, J. B.: The molecular organization of cell membranes. Progr. Biophys. *16*:143, 1966.

Korn, E. D.: Structure of biological membranes. Science *153*:1492, 1966.

Robertson, J. D.: The ultrastructure of cell membranes and their derivatives. Biochem. Soc. Sympos. *16*:3, 1959.

Sjostrand, F. S.: A comparison of plasma membranes, cytomembranes and mitochondrial membrane elements with respect to ultrastructural features. J. Ultrastruct. Res. *9*:561, 1963.

Sjostrand, F. S.: A new repeat structural element of mitochondrial and certain cytoplasmic membranes. Nature *199*:1262, 1963.

Vanderkooi, G. and Green, D. E.: New insights into biological membrane structure. Bioscience *21*:409, 1971.

Ribosomes and Granular Endoplasmic Reticulum

Alfrey, V. G.: Nuclear ribosomes, messenger RNA and protein synthesis. Exp. Cell Res. *9*:183, 1963.

Haguenau, F.: The ergastoplasm: Its history, ultrastructure and biochemistry. Int. Rev. Cytol. *7*:425, 1958.

Palade, G. E.: A small particulate component of the cytoplasm. J. Biophys. Biochem. Cytol. *1*:59, 1955.

Porter, K. R.: Observations on a submicroscopic basophilic component of the cytoplasm. J. Exp. Med. *97*: 727, 1953.

Rich, A.: Polyribosomes. Sci. Amer. *209*:44, 1963.

Agranular Endoplasmic Reticulum

Christensen, A. K.: Fine structure of testicular interstitial cells in the guinea pig. J. Cell Biol. *26*:911, 1965.

Christensen, A. K. and Fawcett, D. W.: The fine structure of the interstitial cells of the mouse testis. Amer. J. Anat. *118*:551, 1966.

Ito, S.: The endoplasmic reticulum of gastric parietal cells. J. Biophys. Biochem. Cytol. *11*:333, 1961.

Remmer, H. and Merker, H. J.: Effects of drugs on the formation of smooth endoplasmic reticulum and drug metabolizing enzymes. Ann. N. Y. Acad. Sci. *123*:79, 1965.

Golgi Complex

Beams, H. W. and Kessel, R. G.: The Golgi apparatus: Structure and function. Int. Rev. Cytol. *23*:209, 1968.

Berlin, J. D.: The localization of acid mucopolysaccharides in the Golgi complex of intestinal goblet cells. J. Cell Biol. *32*:760, 1967.

Caro, L. G. and Palade, G. E.: Protein synthesis, storage and discharge in the pancreatic exocrine cell. An autoradiographic study. J. Cell Biol. *20*:473, 1964.

Hodge, A. J., McLeon, S. D. and Mercer, F. V.: A possible mechanism for the morphogenesis of lamellar systems in plant cells. J. Biophys. Biochem. Cytol. *2*:597, 1956.

Jamieson, J. D. and Palade, G. E.: Intracellular transport of secretory proteins in the pancreatic exocrine cell. I. Role of the peripheral elements of the Golgi complex. J. Cell Biol. *34*:597, 1967.

Neutra, M. and Leblond, C. P.: Synthesis of the carbohydrate of mucus in the Golgi complex as shown by electron microscope radioautography of goblet cells from rats injected with glucose-H^3. J. Cell Biol. *30*: 119, 1966.

Mitochondria

Ashwell, M. and Work, T.: The biogenesis of mitochondria. Ann. Rev. Biochem. *39*:251, 1970.

Claude, A. and Fullom, E. F.: Electron microscopic study of isolated mitochondria. J. Exp. Med. *81*: 51, 1945.

Fernandez-Moran, H., Oda, T., Blair, P. V. and Green, D. E.: A macromolecular repeating unit of mitochondrial structure and function. J. Cell Biol. *22*: 63, 1964.

Green, D. E. and Young, J. H.: Energy transduction in membrane systems. Amer. Sci. *59*:92, 1971.

Hackenbrock, C. R.: Ultrastructural basis for metabolically-linked mechanical activity in mitochondria. I. Reversible ultrastructural changes in metabolic steady state in isolated liver mitochondria. J. Cell Biol. *30*:269, 1966.

Hackenbrock, C. R.: Ultrastructural basis for metabolically-linked mechanical activity in mitochondria. II. Electron transport-linked ultrastructural transformations in mitochondria. J. Cell Biol. *37*:345, 1968.

Hall, D. and Palmer, J.: Mitochondrial research today. Nature *221*:717, 1969.

Lehninger, A. L.: *The Mitochondrion*. Benjamin, New York, 1964.

Wagner, P.: Genetics and phenogenetics of mitochondria. Science *163*:1026, 1969.

Weber, N. E. and Blair, P. V.: Ultrastructural studies of beef heart mitochondria. I. Effects of adenosine diphosphate on mitochondrial morphology. Biochem. Biophys. Res. Commun. *36*:987, 1969.

Lysosomes

DeDuve, C.: Lysosomes. Sci. Amer. *208*:5, 1963.

Gahan, P. B.: Histochemistry of lysosomes. Int. Rev. Cytol. *21*:1, 1967.

Gordon, G. B., Miller, L. R. and Bensch, K. G.: Studies on the intracellular digestive process in mammalian tissue culture cells. J. Cell Biol. *25*:41, 1965.

Novikoff, A. B., Essner, E. and Quintana, N.: Golgi apparatus and lysosomes. Fed. Proc. *23*:1010, 1964.

Centrioles and Basal Bodies

Randall, J. and Hopkins, J. M.: Studies on cilia, basal bodies and some related organelles. II. Problems of genesis. Proc. Linnean Soc. London *174*:37, 1963.

Szollosi, D.: Centrioles, centriolar satellites and spindle fibers. Anat. Rec. *148*:343, 1964.

Yamada, E.: Some observations on the fine structure of the centriole in the mitotic cell. Kurume Med. J. *5*:36, 1958.

Microbodies

Hruban, Z. and Rechcigl, M., Jr.: Microbodies and Related Particles: Morphology, Biochemistry, and Physiology. Int. Rev. Cytol. Suppl. 1. Academic Press, New York, 1969.

Microtubules, Filaments and Fibrils

Brody, I.: The ultrastructure of the tonofilaments in the keratinization process. J. Ultrastruct. Res. *4*:265, 1960.

Huxley, H. E.: Electron microscopic studies in the structure of natural and synthetic protein filaments from striated muscle. J. Molec. Biol. *7*:281, 1963.

Ledbetter, M. C. and Porter, K. R.: Morphology of microtubules of plant cells. Science *144*:872, 1964.

Sandborn, E., Koen, P. F., McNabb, J. D. and Moore, G.: Cytoplasmic microtubules in mammalian cells. J. Ultrastruct. Res. *11*:123, 1964.

Slautterback, D. B.: Cytoplasmic microtubules. I. Hydra. J. Cell Biol. *18*:367, 1963.

Inclusions

Billingham, R. E. and Silvers, W. K.: The melanocytes of mammals. Quart. Rev. Biol. *35*:1, 1960.

Bjorkerud, S.: The isolation of lipofuscin granules from bovine cardiac muscle. J. Ultrastruct. Res. *5*:5, 1963.

Napolitano, L.: The differentiation of white adipose cells. An electron microscope study. J. Cell Biol. *18*: 663, 1963.

Revel, J. P.: Electron microscopy of glycogen. J. Histochem. Cytochem. *12*:104, 1964.

Cell Division

Flemming, W.: Contributions to the knowledge of the cell and its vital processes. J. Cell Biol. *25*:3, 1965. (A translation of the 1880 work.)

Mazia, D.: How cells divide. Sci. Amer. *105*:101, 1961.

Mazia, D.: Fibrillar structure in mitotic apparatus. In *Formation of Cell Organelles*, edited by K. B. Warren. Academic Press, New York, 1967.

SECTION 2 HISTOLOGY

2 Epithelia

General Characteristics

Form and Function. Epithelial tissue, one of the four basic tissues of the body, consists of those aggregations of cells that line the surfaces of the body. Epithelia are generally composed of similar cells, or cells closely related one to another, that are in intimate contact with each other. There is, therefore, very little *intercellular* material between them. As a consequence, epithelial tissues have a *high cellular density*. Varying degrees of cellular polarity are usually apparent. The *apical* or *luminal* border is quite distinct from the *basal* border. The former is free and may be in contact with the external (integumentary, respiratory systems) or internal environment (coelom, digestive tube). The basal border is associated with the underlying connective tissue space which contains blood vessels, lymphatics and nerves. Epithelia, however, are separated from the connective tissue space by a *basement membrane*. As a result of this relationship, epithelial tissues are avascular and are dependent upon diffusion to and from the underlying connective tissue compartment for the movement of metabolites and waste products.

The apical, lateral and basal borders of epithelial cells possess numerous modifications: desmosomes, microvilli, basal lamina and cilia. Although not all these modifications are unique to epithelial cells, they occur with sufficient frequency to be described as epithelial characteristics.

Epithelial cells are sufficiently modified, as cells and as populations, to subserve a variety of functions. *Protection* from various insults—mechanical, bacterial, desiccative—is an important function. The external portion of the body, as well as the body orifices, are covered by thick layers of epithelial cells. The *transport* of various materials along the apical borders of epithelial tissues is accomplished by ciliary action. The *secretion* of various materials is an important function of these tissues. Epithelial tissues are modified in numerous ways to accomplish this specific function. Some secretory products are specifically used to serve as *lubricants*. Modifications of the urinary, integumentary and respiratory epithelia are such as to subserve an *excretory* function—urine, sweat and carbon dioxide. The *absorption* of various materials through the lungs, gastrointestinal organs and kidney tubules also represents another morphological and physiological modification of epithelia. High degrees of specialization may be achieved in those epithelial cells modified as *sensory receptors*. Olfactory, gustatory and auditory functions are mediated through such cells. Lastly, specific cells are reserved in the soma for the perpetuation of the species. These special cells of the gonads are reserved for a *reproductive* function.

Classification. The classification and naming of epithelial tissues is based on two criteria: the number of cells layered upon each other and the predominant or surface cell shape. An epithelial lining is either *simple* (one cell layer), *stratified* (more than one cell layer), *pseudstratified* (one cell layer appearing as more than one) or *transitional* (layers subject to change).

Simple epithelia are named according to the predominant cell type accordingly: *squamous*, *cuboidal*, *columnar* or *pseudo stratified*. Stratified epithelia, however, are named on the basis of the shape of the apical or luminal cell type accordingly: *squamous*, *cuboidal* or *columnar*. Although current indications are that transitional epithelium actually represents a pseudostratified condition, it is worthy of special consideration since it is capable of varying the number of layers that are apparent. Some authors, however, may also refer to it as a stratified cuboidal epithelium.

Most epithelial tissues are derived from two embryonic germ layers, *endoderm* and *ectoderm*. The derivatives of these germ layers account for the ubiquitous and variable nature of most epithelia. The lining cells of the cardiovascular system, lymphatic system and kidney, however, are derived from *mesoderm*. These lining cells, which are morphologically simple squamous, are referred to as *endothelium*. Similarly, the mesoderm gives rise to simple squamous cells which line the body cavities (coelomic spaces). These cells are specifically referred to as *mesothelium*. Also, renal tubular epithelium is derived from mesoderm.

Other variations in epithelial or epithelial-like tissues will be discussed with the specific organs that comprise subsequent sections.

Simple Epithelia

Simple Squamous Epithelium. This type of tissue is characterized by extremely thin cells, the cytoplasm of which is barely visible with light microscopy (Fig. 2-1). Often there is a prominent bulge into the free surface at the location of the nucleus. The cytoplasm is expansive, and nuclei are generally quite a distance from each other. In many instances the cytoplasm, although expansive, is thin and gives the appearance of being absent. However, an electron micrograph verifies its presence and nature (Fig. 2-2). In surface view the cells composing this tissue are polygons, but they appear spindle-shaped when cut perpendicular to the free surface or basal border.

Occurrence: Lining of coelomic spaces (mesothelium); lining of cardiovascular and lymphatic systems (endothelium); functional lining of lung; small ducts of numerous glands; specific portions of kidney tubules and Bowman's capsule; membranous labyrinth of the inner ear.

Simple Cuboidal Epithelium. The general shapes of the cells of this type of tissue are described as cubes. In actuality, they appear as squares in sections perpendicular to the apical border (Fig. 2-3). From surface views they appear as hexagons. Nuclei are usually *central* or *paracentral* in position. Lateral cell borders may or may not be distinct. Naming of this tissue is sometimes difficult, since there is a continuum of cellular conformation from squamous to columnar. Some histologists will use modifiers such as "high cuboidal" or "low columnar."

Occurrence: Secretory and duct portions of numerous glands; certain tubules of the kidney; specific portions of the respiratory tree; surfaces of the lens and iris; surface epithelium of the ovary; specific tubules of the testis; pigmented epithelium of the retina.

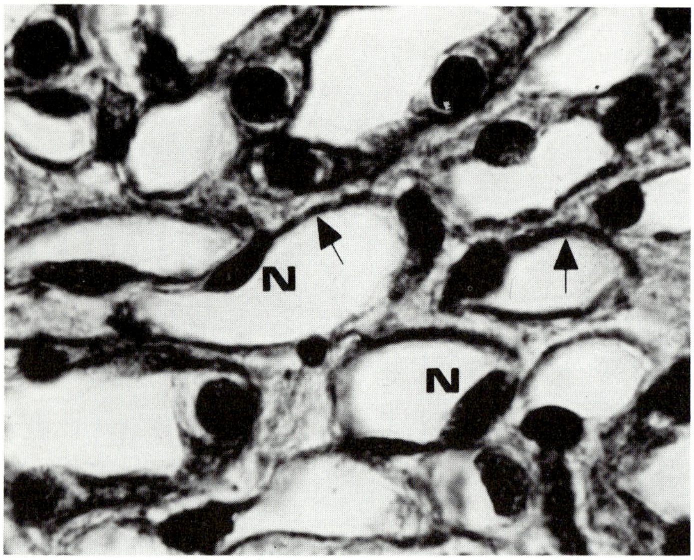

Fig. 2-1. Simple squamous epithelium lining tubules of a canine kidney. The dark nuclei (*N*) are contained within a cytoplasm which is barely visible (*arrows*). ×160. All light micrographs are the original magnifications. All electron micrographs are the final magnifications.

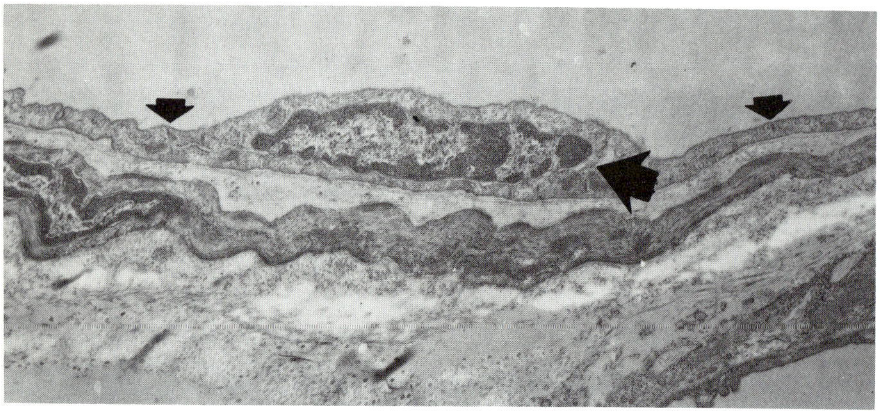

Fig. 2-2. An electron micrograph of an alveolar lining cell. The nucleus (*large arrow*) protrudes into the lumen. The lateral projections (*small arrows*) are attenuated. ×12,000. (Courtesy of G. P. Epling)

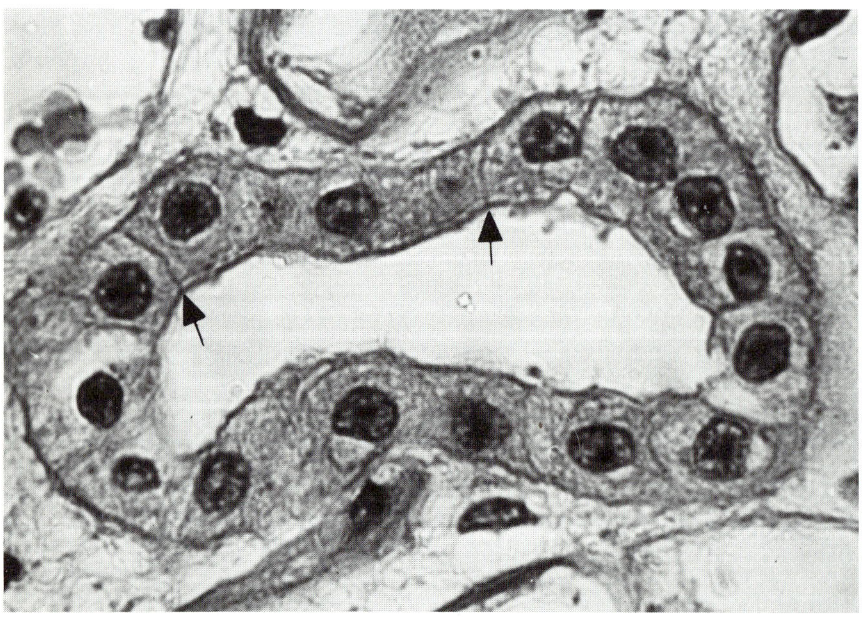

Fig. 2-3. Cuboidal epithelium of a collecting tubule of an equine kidney. The nuclei are contained within a homogeneous cytoplasm. Some cellular limits are apparent (*arrows*). ×320.

Simple Columnar Epithelium. The basic morphological feature of this tissue is that the cells are taller than they are wide (Fig. 2-4). The nuclei, similarly, are elongated and generally displaced toward the basal border. There is, therefore, a distinct cellular polarity. Usually the nuclei will form a distinct row; occasionally they may form two rows due to a crowding of cells.

Occurrence: Lining of glandular stomach, small and large intestine; middle portions of the respiratory tree; lining of the uterus and uterine tubes; lining of the secretory and conducting portions of many glands; lining of the cholecyst.

Pseudostratified Epithelium. All of the cells of this type of epithelium reside on the basement membrane. Not all of them, however, reach the free surface. Only the columnar cell component reaches the luminal surface. In section this epithelial type appears to be overcrowded with cells (Figs. 2-5, 2-34). The basal and middle part of the lining is congested with the nuclei of the three cell types that comprise this epithelium—basal cells, fusiform cells and columnar cells. A fourth type of cell, a *goblet cell*, is present in certain loci. Surface modifications, *cilia*, are often found on the luminal surfaces of the columnar cells. This epithelial type is most precisely referred to as *pseudostratified columnar* or *pseudostratified ciliated columnar epithelium*.

This epithelium is most often confused with simple columnar epithelium which has been cut on a plane oblique to the surface (Fig. 2-6). However, careful examination of the sections will show that, even in an oblique plane, simple columnar epithelium does not possess the degree of nuclear congestion mentioned previously.

Occurrence: Lining of upper respiratory tract; lining of specific regions of urogenital system; ducts of glands at points of transition between simple and stratified epithelium.

Stratified Epithelia

Stratified Squamous Epithelium. Characterized by many cellular layers which are derived from a single basal layer, this type of epithelium is found where protection of the underlying tissues is an important functional consideration (Fig. 2-7). The thickness of this tissue type may vary from quite thin to exceedingly thick.

The basal layer of cells (*stratum basale*) consists of a single layer of cuboidal or columnar cells which are extremely basophilic due to the extensive ergastoplasm (Fig. 2-8). As the name implies, this cell layer resides on the basement membrane and is partially responsible for giving rise to subsequent cellular components.

The cells of the *stratum spinosum* are lighter in staining affinity than those of the basal layer and are progressively more flattened toward the luminal surface.

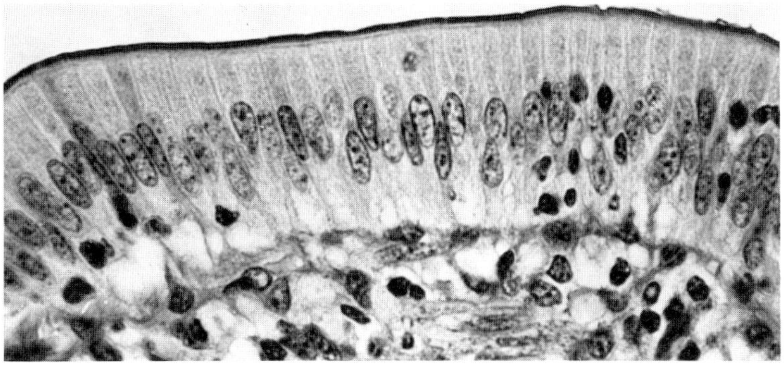

Fig. 2-4. Columnar cells from the duodenum of a bird. ×320.

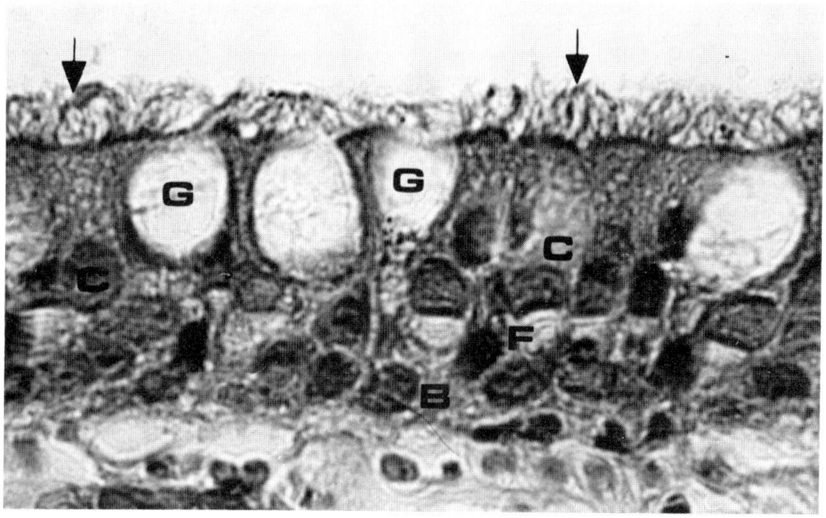

Fig. 2-5. Pseudostratified ciliated columnar epithelium from an ovine trachea. The basal (*B*), fusiform (*F*) and columnar (*C*) cell nuclei are apparent. Goblet cells (*G*) are present. Cilia (*arrows*) line the luminal border. ×320.

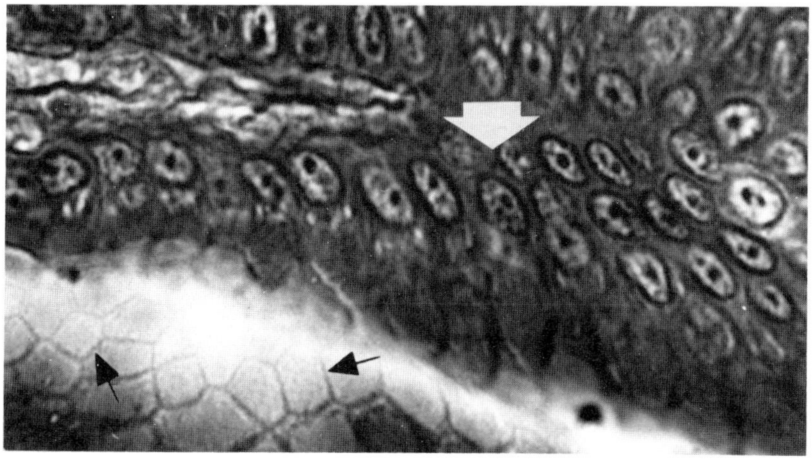

Fig. 2-6. Oblique section of simple columnar epithelium from the duodenum of a bird. The cells to the left of the large white arrow are cut normal to their long axis; to the right, they are cut oblique to the long axis. Note the hexagonal appearance of the cells on surface view (*arrows*). ×320.

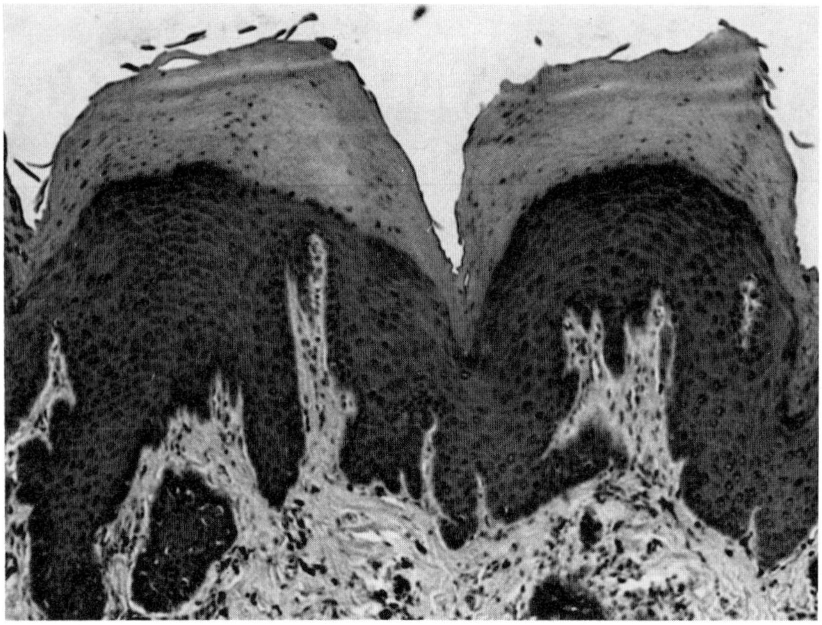

Fig. 2-7. Stratified squamous epithelium of the canine muzzle. ×25.

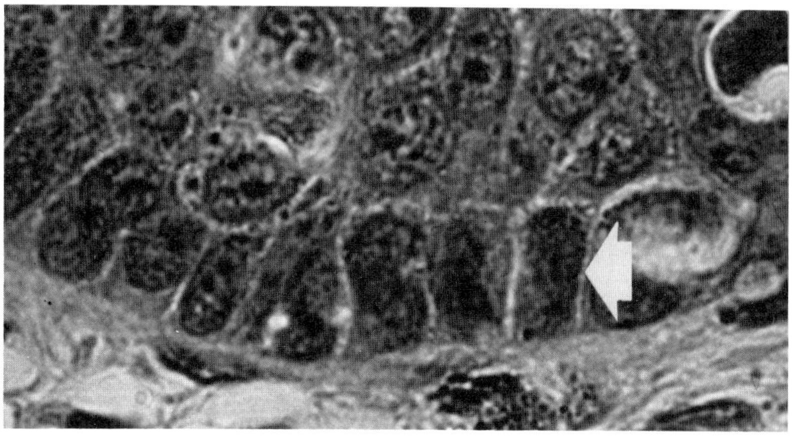

Fig. 2-8. The stratum basale (*arrow*) of stratified squamous epithelium of the canine muzzle. ×400.

Shrinking of cells by processing techniques demonstrates intercellular spaces in which numerous cellular processes from adjacent cells are in contact with one another (Fig. 2-9). These processes (*spines* or *prickles*) are not actually intercellular bridges but represent two cellular processes joined by a *desmosome*. This configuration is responsible for the naming of this layer as *spinous cell layer* or *prickle cell layer*.

Together, the *stratum basale* and the *stratum spinosum* are referred to as the *stratum germinativum* or *Malpighian layer*. Mitoses within the germinal layer are responsible for the replacement of cells lost at the luminal surface.

The *stratum granulosum*, depending upon the specific location of the epithelium, may be several cell layers thick or may be totally absent. The granularity of the spindle cells of this layer is attributable to the basophilic *keratohyalin* granules (Fig. 2-10). These are precursor substances to *keratin*. Degenerative changes in the cells, as evidenced by pyknotic nuclei, are also characteristic of the cells of this layer.

The cells of the *stratum lucidum* are extremely flattened, pale-staining or slightly acidophilic (Fig. 2-10). This layer, which is of variable occurrence, represents dead or dying cells. Nuclei are either indistinct or missing and the cytoplasm is agranular. Occasionally, granules of *eleidin* are present. The closely packed cells of this region may be several layers thick.

The *stratum corneum* (Fig. 2-11) is a well-developed layer of closely packed, dead cells in those regions typified by a high degree of *keratinization* (footpads). The remainder of the skin is less keratinized, but this stratum is still present. The cells which are being sloughed comprise a *stratum disjunctum*. Lesser degrees of keratinization or a total absence thereof are characteristic of the entrance and exit of the digestive tube, as well as portions along its length (esophagus, nonglandular portions of the ruminant stomach).

In those stratified squamous epithelia that are either minimally keratinized or nonkeratinized, not all of the aforementioned layers are distinguishable (Fig. 2-12). The basal layer is usually the only distinct layer. The remaining layers are sometimes referred to as *parabasal*, *intermediate* and *superficial*.

Occurrence (*keratinized*): General body surface; buccal cavity; anal region; ruminant forestomach.

Occurrence (*nonkeratinized*): Vestibular region of respiratory system; oral, esophageal and anal portions of digestive system; cornea of eye; conjunctiva; portions of the male and female urogenital systems.

Stratified Cuboidal Epithelium. This

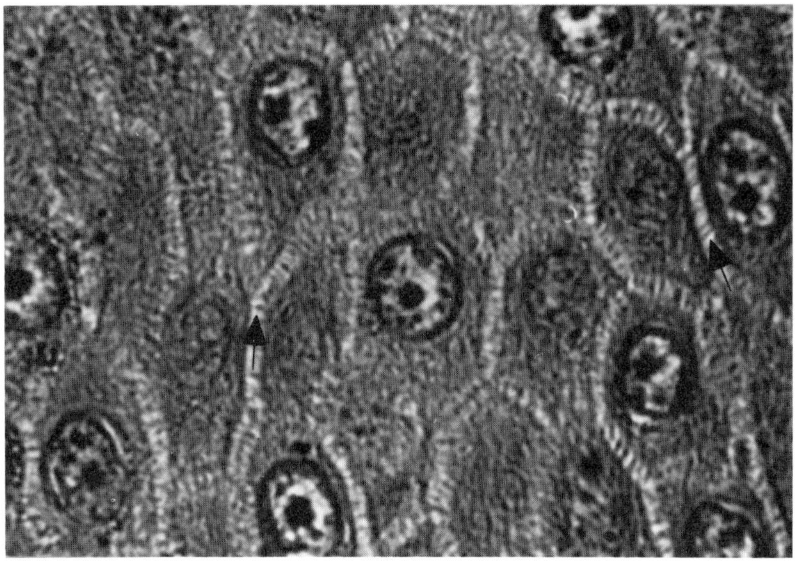

Fig. 2-9. The stratum spinosum of stratified squamous epithelium of the canine muzzle. Spinous processes (*arrows*) are apparent. ×400.

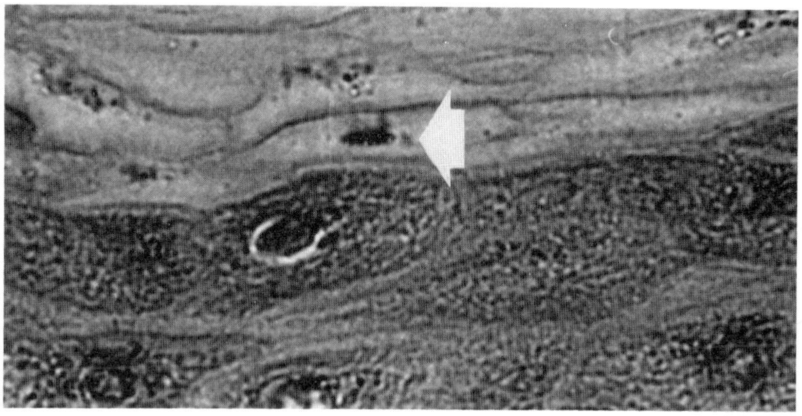

Fig. 2-10. The stratum granulosum (*below arrow*) and stratum lucidum (*at arrow*) of stratified squamous epithelium of the canine muzzle. ×400.

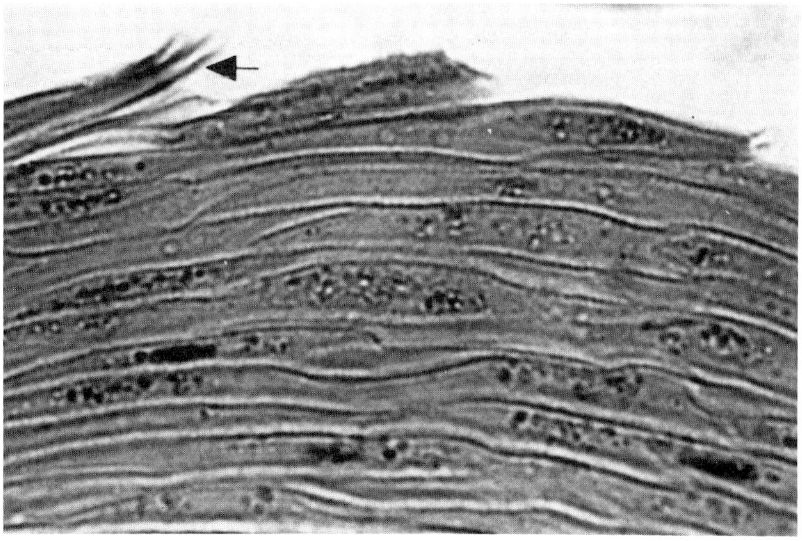

Fig. 2-11. The stratum corneum and stratum disjunctum (*arrow*) of stratified squamous epithelium of the canine muzzle. ×400.

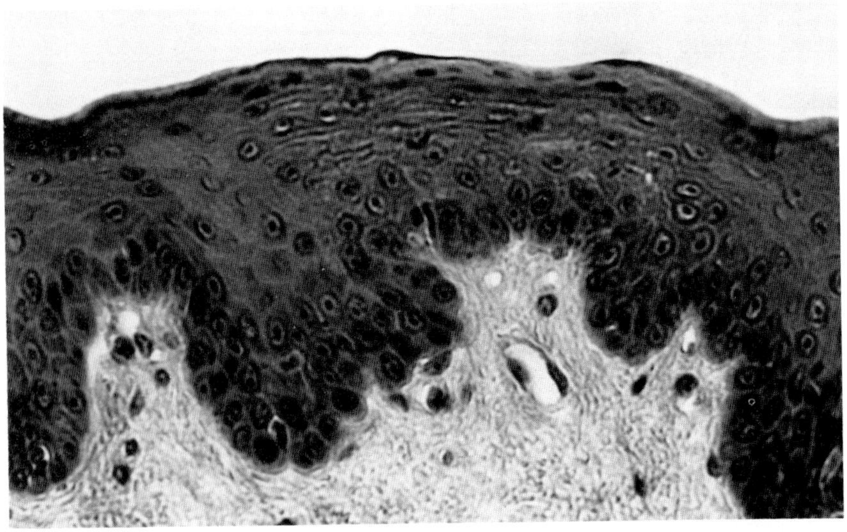

Fig. 2-12. Nonkeratinized stratified squamous epithelium from the feline buccal cavity. ×125.

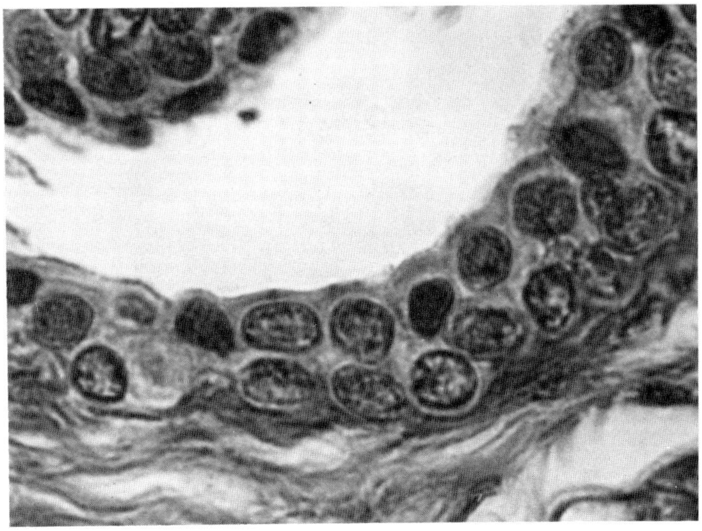

Fig. 2-13. Bistratified cuboidal epithelium of a duct from a feline salivary gland. ×400.

epithelium consists of two layers of cells (Fig. 2-13). The basal layer consists of polygonal cells responsible for the regeneration of lost cells. The superficial or luminal layer is occupied by cuboidal cells. Although this epithelium is characteristic of a few loci, it is frequently encountered in areas of transition from simple to stratified epithelia. Some authors refer to transitional epithelium as stratified cuboidal.

Occurrence: Specific portions of genital system; ducts of various glands, zones of transition between simple and stratified epithelia.

Stratified Columnar Epithelium. This tissue may consist of two or three layers of cells (Fig. 2-14). The basal and luminal cells are sometimes separated from each other by an intermediate cell type. The basal cells are normally cuboidal; the intermediate, polygonal; the apical cells, columnar. This tissue is sometimes difficult to distinguish from pseudostratified epithelium.

Occurrence: Points of transition between columnar or pseudostratified and stratified epithelium; portions of the upper respiratory tract; ducts of some glands.

Transitional Epithelium

Transitional Epithelium. This tissue is normally considered a stratified type. However, a recent study has indicated that it may be pseudostratified. Whichever is the case, it still deserves special attention because of its ability to change shape as a result of the pressure applied on it from the luminal surface. Because it is associated only with the urogenital system, it is sometimes referred to as *urothelium*.

In the relaxed state, it may consist of as many as 6 or 7 layers (Fig. 2-15). The basal cells are very small and assume a polyhedral configuration. The cells of the intermediate region are polyhedral or pear-shaped. The cells at the luminal border are cuboidal and their apical borders bulge into the lumen.

During distention, the thickness of the epithelium is markedly reduced (Fig. 2-16). As few as two or three layers may be apparent. In a state of distention, this tissue is sometimes mistaken for stratified squamous epithelium.

Occurrence: Lining of specific regions of the urinary system.

Glandular Epithelia

General Features and Classification. Although epithelia are primarily lining tissues, a significant function of these tissues is associated with the ability of single cells and populations of cells to produce a variety of products for extracellular use.

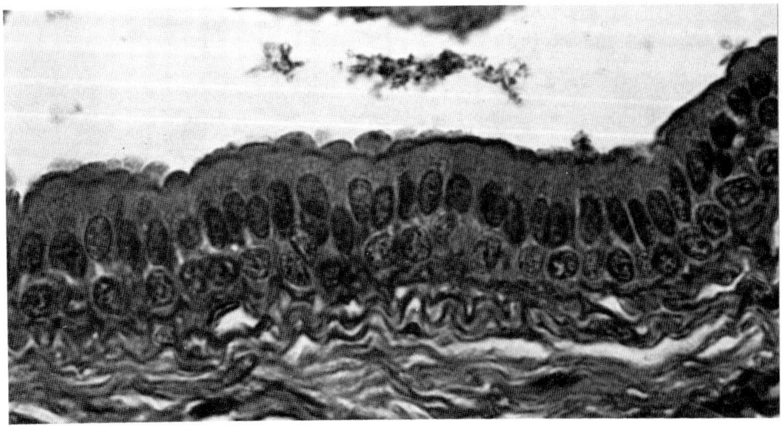

Fig. 2-14. Bistratified columnar epithelium of a duct from a feline salivary gland. ×400.

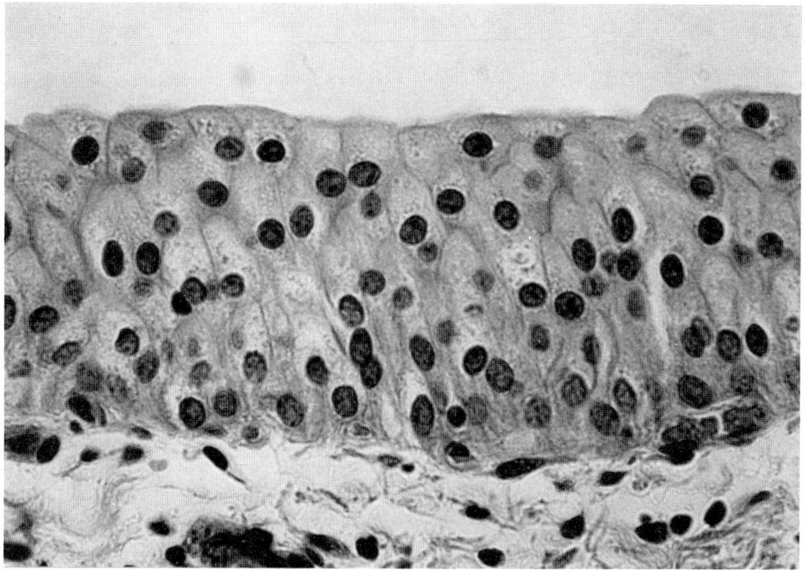

Fig. 2-15. Relaxed transitional epithelium of the bovine bladder. ×160.

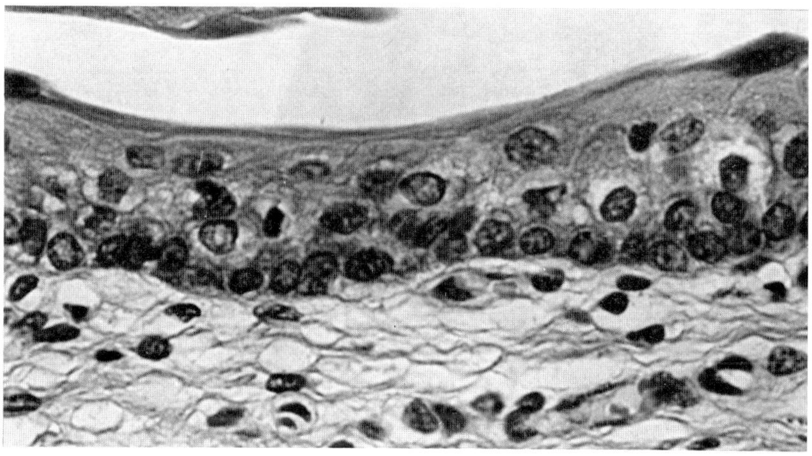

Fig. 2-16. Distended transitional epithelium of the canine bladder. ×160.

Modifications of these surface linings are manifested in a variety of ways to accomplish a diversity of secretory functions. Not only are epithelia modified morphologically to accomplish secretory activity, but there are various mechanisms utilized as well. Also, the relationship of glandular tissue to surrounding tissue is varied. Accordingly, there are numerous ways by which glandular tissue may be classified:

1. Number of cells comprising the gland
   a. Unicellular
   b. Multicellular
2. Relationship to lining and surrounding tissue
   a. Exocrine
   b. Endocrine
3. Configuration of multicellular glands
   a. Simple
   b. Compound
4. Method of elaboration
   a. Apocrine
   b. Merocrine
   c. Holocrine
5. Type of secretory product
   a. Serous
   b. Mucous
   c. Miscellaneous

Since "Man classifies and nature doesn't," there are numerous examples that do not fit perfectly into any one of the classifications. However, an awareness of the organization of glandular tissue through these varied classifications will serve to give insights into this specialized function of epithelial tissues.

Number of Cells in a Gland. Glands are either *unicellular* or *multicellular*.

Unicellular glands are simply specialized cells that are scattered throughout an epithelial lining. Although there are varied modifications, the most common and representative unicellular gland is the goblet cell (Fig. 2-17). It is scattered commonly throughtout the respiratory and digestive systems and occasionally in the urinary system. Until active, it cannot be distinguished from other columnar cells with which it is associated. When activity commences, droplets appear in the cytoplasm and eventually accumulate until the entire apical and middle portion of the cell is filled and swollen with the *premucin* droplets. These impart a foamy and basophilic appearance to the cytoplasm. The remainder of the cytoplasm and nucleus is displaced to the narrow basal region of the cell. Expulsion of the mucoid substances may be explosive or gradual. If explosive, the cell returns to a columnar configuration from which state the process will resume. If gradual, the continuing process does not alter the configuration of the cell.

Multicellular glands are quite diversified. Entire sheets of epithelia may perform a secretory function as in the lining of the glandular stomach. Intraepithelial glands, which are rare, represent accumulations of specialized secretory cells within an epithelial lining (Fig. 2-18). These are found in the lining of the upper respiratory system and male genital system. The greatest diversity of form and function is represented by those multicellular glands that assume an extraepithelial relationship to the epithelial lining. This type of gland represents most of those encountered in the body. Their true relationship to the epithelial lining is sometimes obscured by the morphological complexity they assume and the plane of section during observation. Their relationship to the lining is best understood by examining their developmental process (Fig. 2-19). Specific loci within the epithelial lining retain the potential for mitosis. The mitotic process is directed in such a way that a cord of cells invaginates into the underlying connective tissue space. These cells, however, do *not* actually invade the space but are separated from it by the basement membrane. A tube develops within the cord while the remainder of the cells continue to proliferate and are subsequently converted to secretory cells. The secretory cells as a unit are referred to as an *adenomere*. The tube connecting the adenomere to the epithelial surface is the duct of the gland. In some instances, portions of the duct may also become secretory. Further modifications to this basic scheme for extraepithelial glands will be discussed subsequently.

Relationship to Lining and Surrounding Tissue. In the previous example of the formation of an extraepithelial gland, the persistence of the duct establishes that the gland will be of the *exocrine* variety. The growth of the adenomere and associated ducts is not

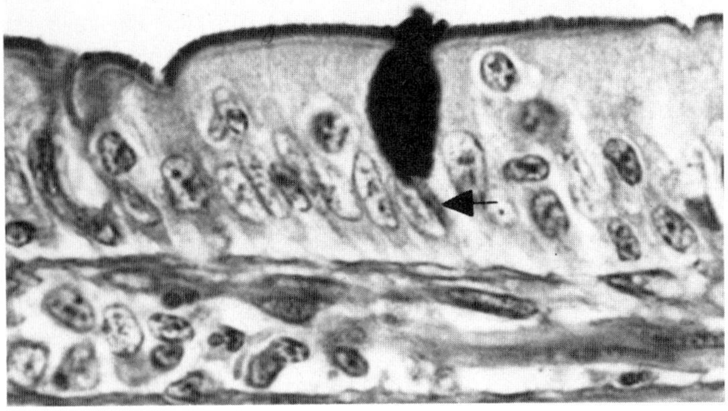

Fig. 2-17. Goblet cell from the feline jejunum. The bulk of the goblet cell (*dark mass*) contains premucin. The nucleus (*arrow*) is displaced basally. Note the extrusion of the secretory product by the merocrine method. ×250 (Alcian blue and PAS).

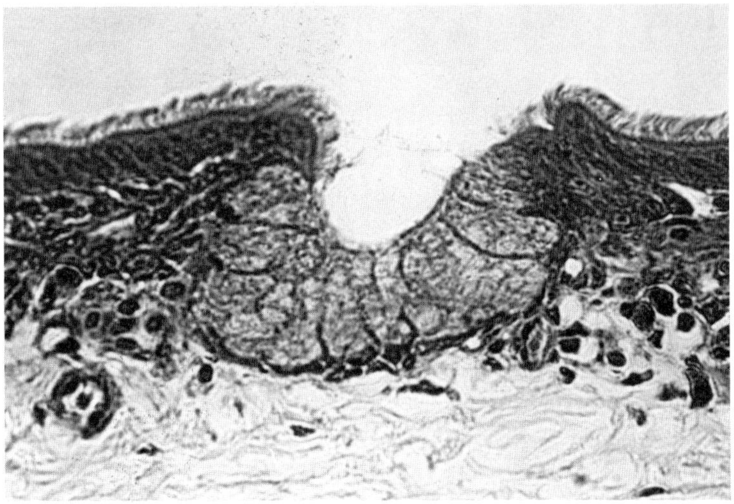

Fig. 2-18. Intraepithelial gland from the avian respiratory mucosa. ×200.

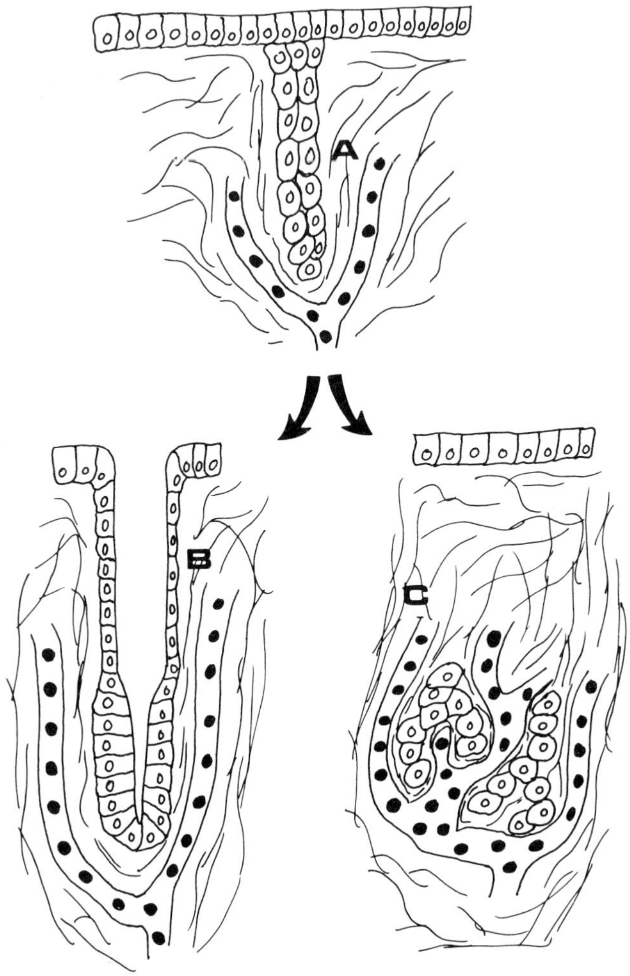

Fig. 2-19. Development of exocrine and endocrine glands. Mitotic activity of the lining cells results in an invagination of the epithelium into the connective tissue (*A*). A duct may persist and terminate in an adenomere (*B*) or the connecting cells may disintegrate and isolate cords or clumps of cells in close association with capillaries (*C*). (Redrawn and modified from Ham, A. H.: *Histology*, 5th ed. J. B. Lippincott Company, Philadelphia, 1965.)

limited to the simple example which has been cited. Rather, very elaborate duct and secretory conformations may develop. Whether a simple or complex arrangement, all these glandular types possess the common characteristic of cellular secretions being deposited into a system of ducts that will eventually open at an epithelial surface.

In contrast to the aforementioned type, some glands lose their connection to an epithelial surface (Fig. 2-19). In such cases, the adenomere does not assume a tubular configuration. Rather, the secretory cells arrange themselves as cords or clumps of cells and deposit their secretory products into the adjacent connective tissue space. These are *endocrine* or ductless glands of the body.

Some glands may be both exocrine and endocrine. The pancreas and liver are examples. These will be described with the endocrine and digestive systems, respectively.

Configuration of Multicellular Glands. Various configurations are assumed by multicellular glands in extraepithelial positions. In a single section of these glands the three-dimensional relationships can only be inferred. The following classification is based on serial sections and three-dimensional reconstructions of them. For this reason diagrams have been used. In the subsequent sections on organology the student should refer back to this classification to appreciate fully the relationship of specific glandular tissue to the organs with which they may be associated. Multicellular exocrine glands may be either *simple* or *compound*. This classification is based upon the simplicity or complexity of the duct system associated with the secretory portions of the gland. The *secretory endpieces* (*adenomeres*) may be *tubular* (a hollow cylinder), *alveolar* (globular or pear-shaped) or *tubuloalveolar* (combination).

In a *simple* gland, the adenomere deposits its products into an unbranched duct. The adenomeres may be ***straight tubular*** as are the intestinal glands (Fig. 2-20), ***coiled tubular*** as are the sweat glands (Fig. 2-21) or *alveolar* (Fig. 2-22). The adenomeres may be branched and still deposit their products into a single duct system. In these instances, they are referred to as *branched tubular* as in the submucosal glands of the intestine (Fig. 2-23) or *branched alveolar* as in the sebaceous glands (Fig. 2-22). The terms *alveolar* and *acinar* are often used synonymously.

In *compound* glands there are numerous subdivisions of the duct system and a variety of adenomeres. They may be *compound tubular* as in some of the salivary glands, *compound acinar* as in the pancreas or *compound tubuloalveolar* as in some of the salivary glands and the mammary gland (Fig. 2-24).

There are numerous examples of simple and compound glands associated with organs or structured as entire organs. These will be described as encountered in subsequent sections.

Method of Elaboration. Not all of the secretory cells of the body elaborate their products in a manner identical to one another. Three secretory methods have been recognized: *merocrine*, *apocrine* and *holocrine*. This classification is based upon the amount the cell actually contributes to the secretory end product.

In the *merocrine* method of elaboration, the cell contributes nothing more than the actual product it has produced. The membrane surrounding the secretory droplet fuses with the plasma membrane and thus opens the product to the extracellular space (Figs. 2-17, 1-35, 1-36). None of the cytoplasmic components along the secretory surface are lost, except the secretory product itself. This method is typical of most of the glands of the body (Fig. 2-25).

In the *apocrine* method of secretion, the secretory product and a portion of the cytoplasm along the secretory surface are lost as the secretory end product. Characteristically, blebs or bulges along the secretory surface may be recognized during this process (Fig. 2-26). The extent of the cytoplasmic contribution in this method has been questioned recently. This method is typical of most of the sweat glands of domestic species, some of the sweat glands of man and some products of the mammary gland.

Two mechanisms are characteristic of the *holocrine* method in which the entire cell comprises the secretory end product. In the genital organs, the germ cells (spermatozoa and ova) are the result of *cytogenic processes* (Fig. 2-27). In hematopoietic organs, various blood cells result from the same process. In the aforementioned instances, however, the cells are secreted intact and as highly specialized products of stem cell activity. In the sebaceous glands, the cells accumulate a lipid secretory product, die

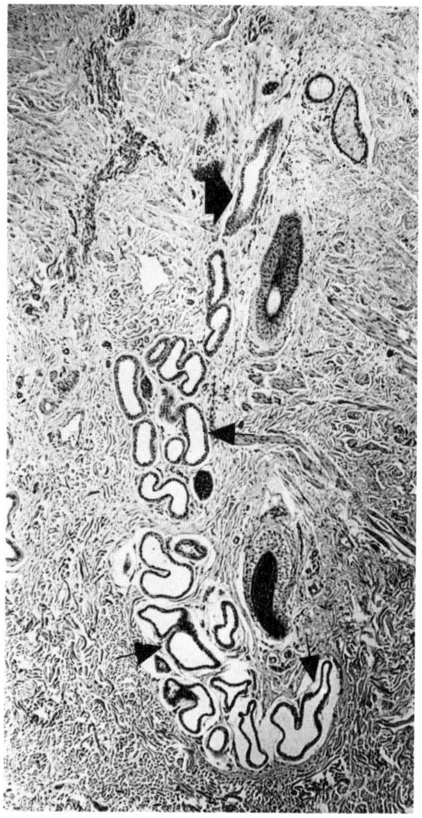

Fig. 2-21. Coiled tubular sweat gland (*small arrows*) from the ovine skin. Its tortuous configuration is responsible for the discontinuities. *Large arrow*, the excretory duct which eventually connects to the surface. ×9.

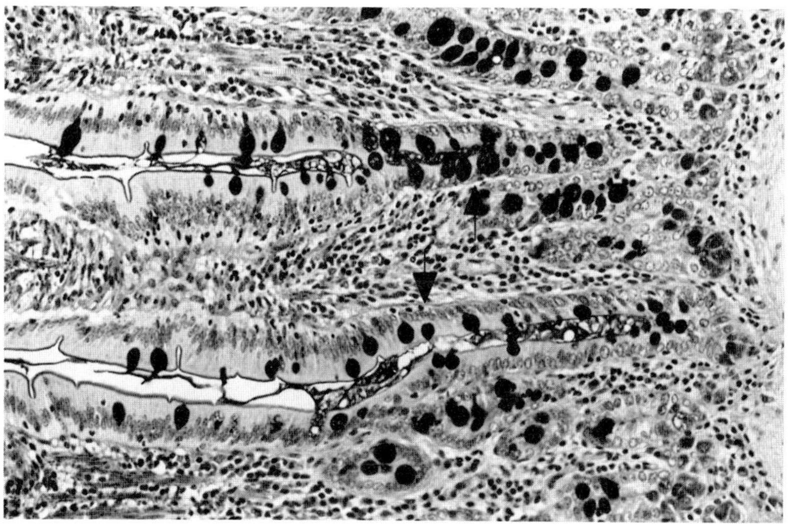

Fig. 2-20. Straight tubular glands (*arrows*) from the equine duodenum. ×40 (Alcian blue and PAS).

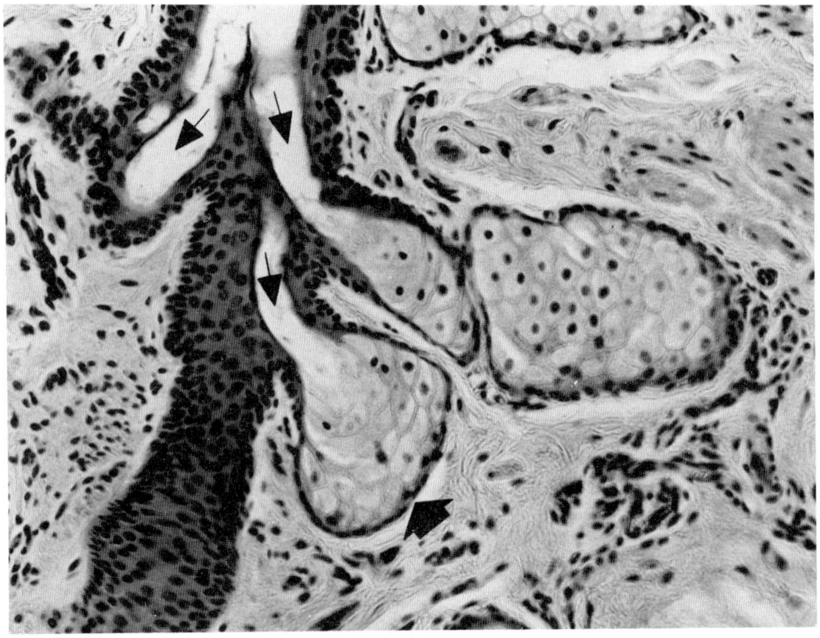

Fig. 2-22. Alveolar gland from ovine skin. This sebaceous gland is a branched alveolar gland. The ducts (*small arrows*) are apparent. One adenomere (*large arrow*) and its associated duct represents the configuration of a simple alveolar gland. ×50.

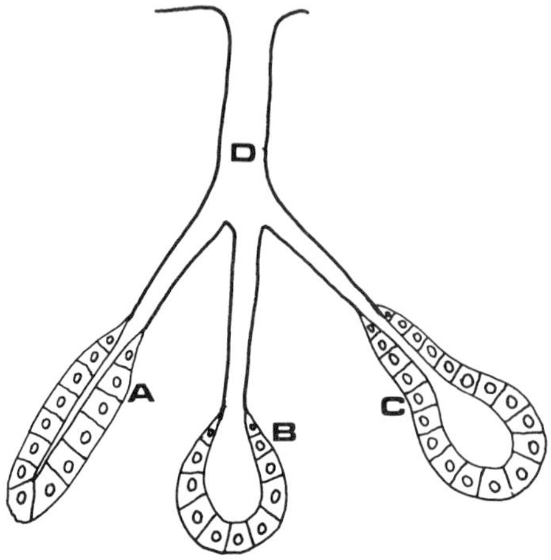

Fig. 2-24. Configuration of compound glands. The branching duct system (*D*) may terminate in tubular (*A*), acinar (*B*) or tubuloalveolar adenomeres (*C*).

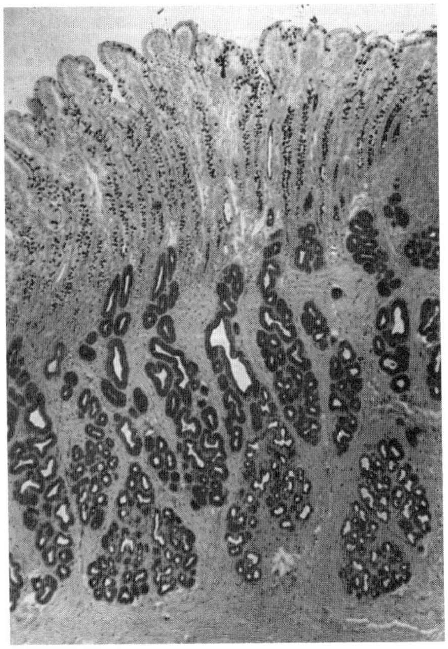

Fig. 2-23. Submucosal glands of the canine duodenum. These branched tubular glands are stained dark. ×8 (Alcian blue and PAS).

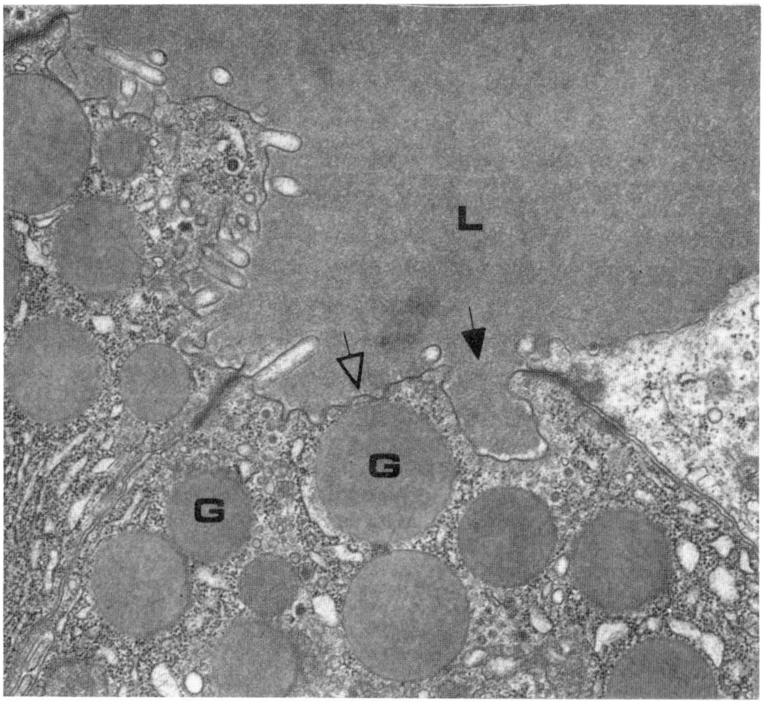

Fig. 2-25. An electron micrograph of the luminal border of pancreatic acinar cells. The lumen (*L*) is filled with secretory material from the zymogen granules (*G*). A granule (*solid arrow*) may have fused with the cell membrane, while another granule (*open arrow*) is about to fuse with the cell membrane. ×22,000. (Figs. 2-5, 2-17 and 2-20 are of merocrine cells also.)

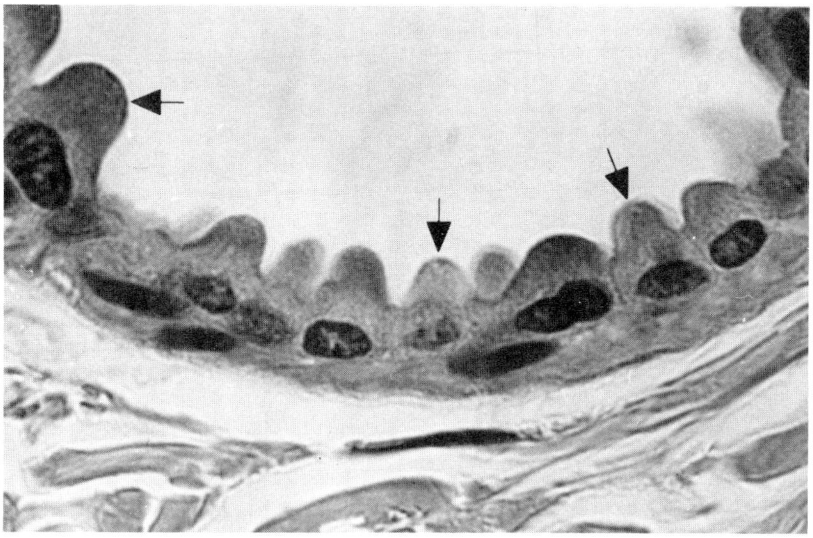

Fig. 2-26. Apocrine tubular sweat gland from the ovine skin. The apical blebs (*arrows*) are indicative of this secretory method. ×500.

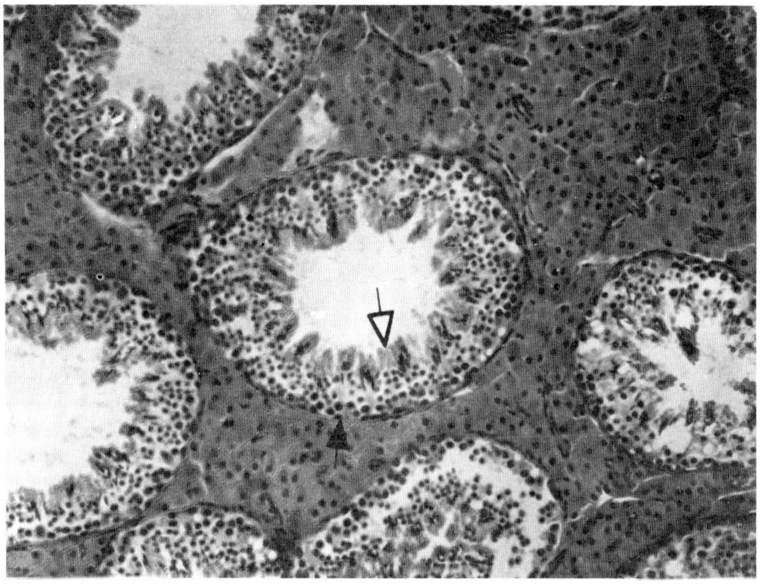

Fig. 2-27. Semininferous tubules of the porcine testis. The germinal cells (*solid arrow*) differentiate into spermatozoa (*open arrow*). These are secreted into the lumen of the tubules. ×40.

and then disintegrate (Fig. 2-28). The original cells plus the secretory product comprise the entire end product. A good supply of stem cells is required for the holocrine type of activity.

Types of Secretory Units. The varied secretory products of the body require that many different cells are involved. Of this vast diversity, two distinct types of secretory cells are recognized: *serous* and *mucous cells*. Besides a cellular morphological basis for recognition, the secretory products of these two cell types are different. The serous cell secretes a clear, watery type of fluid which may contain enzymes, while the mucous cell produces a more viscous fluid which is rich in mucoid materials. Not all secretory cells can be included in this classification. Rather, the cells of many secretory units associated with the digestive, reproductive and respiratory systems conform to this classification. It is espeically applicable to the salivary glands.

In *serous exocrine glands*, the serous cell is the predominant secretory unit. It is a wedge-shaped or pear-shaped cell which may possess a finely granular, acidophilic cytoplasm (Fig. 2-29). A distinct polarity may be apparent; the apical portion of the cell is acidophilic, while the basal portion is basophilic due to the accumulation of ergastoplasm. The rounded nucleus is either central or paracentral in position. The lateral margins of the cells usually are indistinct.

Entire adenomeres may be composed of these cells. These adenomeres may assume a tubular, alveolar or tubuloalveolar configuration.

In *mucous exocrine glands* the predominant secretory unit is the mucous cell. It is a pear-shaped cell with a foamy and basophilic cytoplasm (Fig. 2-30). A marked polarity is apparent; i.e., the hyperchromatic, flattened nucleus is situated against the basal margin of the cell. This cell is similar to the goblet cell described previously.

Entire adenomeres may be composed exclusively of these cells. These units may assume a tubular or alveolar configuration.

Mixed glands may be composed of these two cell types in various arrangements. An entire gland may possess separate serous and mucous adenomeres (Fig. 2-31). Serous and mucous cells may be intermingled with each other and discharge their products on the luminal surface (Fig. 2-32). *Serous demilunes* may be attached to a mucous adenomere (Fig. 2-33). In this instance,

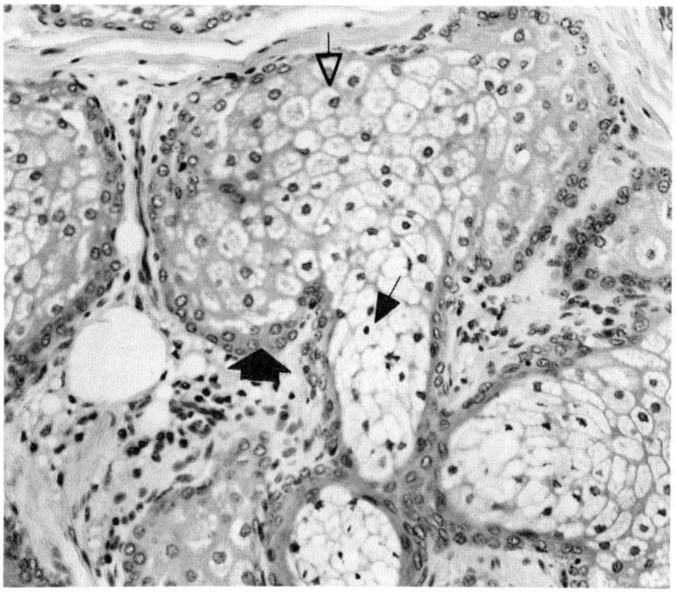

Fig. 2-28. Sebaceous glands from the ovine orbital sinus. The peripheral cells (*large arrow*) are the stem cells for the gland. The cells accumulate lipids (*open arrow*), the nuclei become pyknotic (*dark arrow*) and the cells die. ×50.

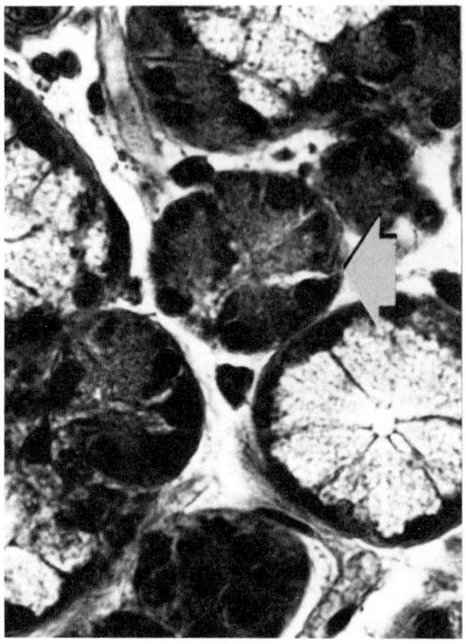

Fig. 2-29. Serous cells of an adenomere from a salivary gland (*arrow*). The cells are pyramidal and the nuclei are round and basal in position. The dark cytoplasm is granular and acidophilic. ×160.

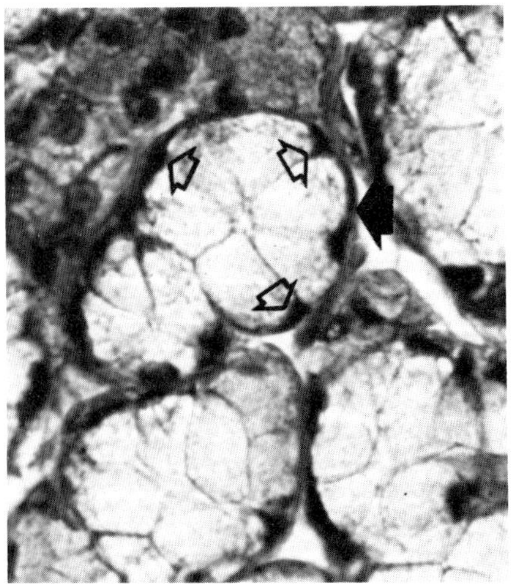

Fig. 2-30. Mucous cells of a mucous adenomere from a salivary gland (*solid arrow*). The cells are pyramidal, the cytoplasm is foamy and the flattened nuclei (*open arrows*) are basally positioned. ×160.

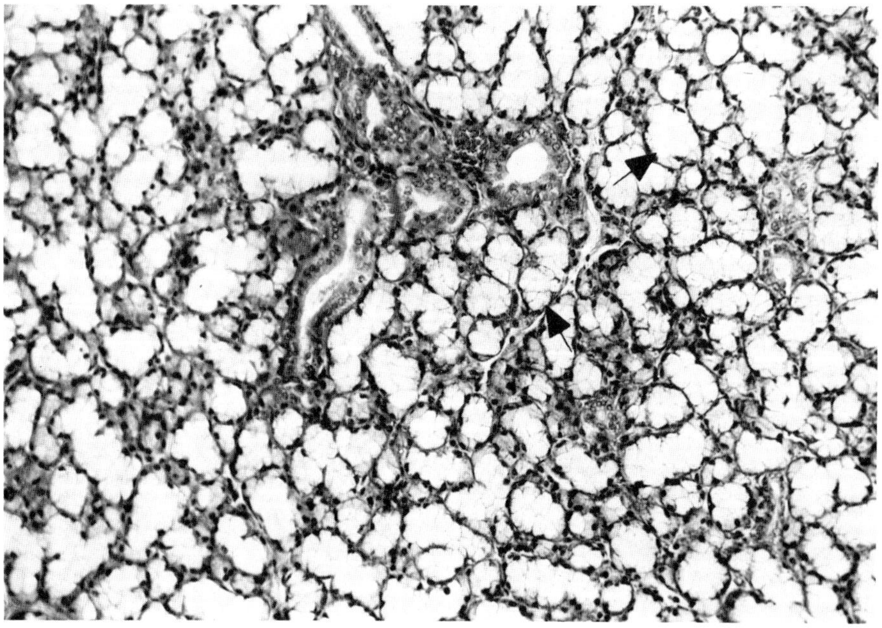

Fig. 2-31. Canine salivary gland. The mucous adenomeres (*arrows*) comprise the bulk of the gland. ×40.

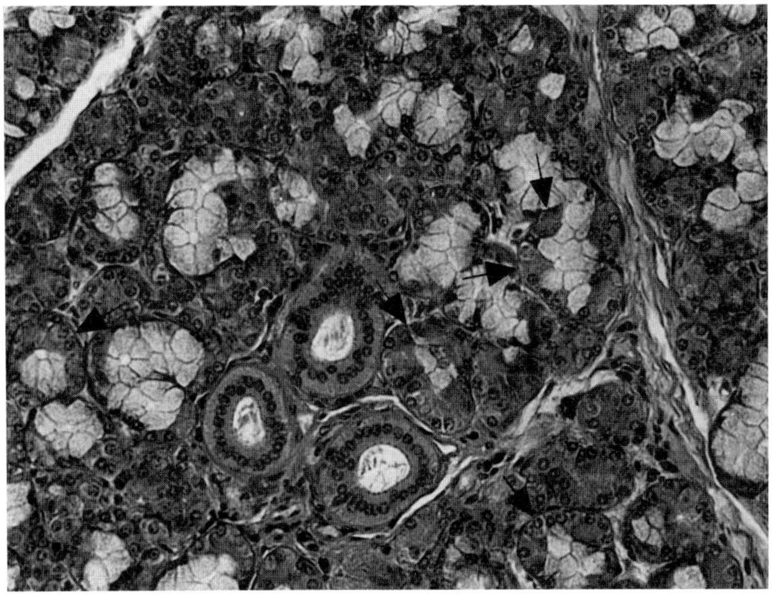

Fig. 2-32. Porcine salivary gland. *Arrows*, areas in which serous cells are intermingled among mucous cells in the adenomeres. ×63.

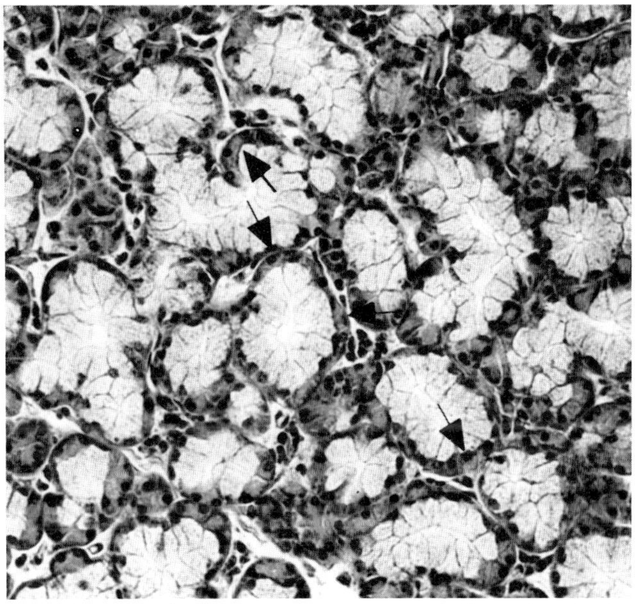

Fig. 2-33. Equine salivary gland. The serous cells (*arrows*) are disposed as demilunes around the mucous adenomeres. ×63.

small canals (*secretory canaliculi*) connect the serous cells with the luminal surface.

Special Epithelia

At certain loci, epithelial tissues are modified to perform highly specialized functions. Among these epithelial tissues are *ciliated epithelium*, *neuroepithelium*, *pigmented epithelium* and *myoepithelium*.

Ciliated Epithelium. Cilia are slender, cytoplasmic processes of the luminal surfaces of cells. Cilia are modified either for movement of materials along a sheet of epithelium or for the facilitation of secretory activity. They are referred to as *kinocilia* and *stereocilia*, respectively.

Kinocilia are highly structured, cytoplasmic processes which are usually associated with cells of pseudostratified columnar or simple columnar epithelia (Fig. 2-5). Isolated cells within the epithelial sheet or the majority of cells within the epithelial sheet may be ciliated. Kinociliated cells are found in the respiratory tract and the male and female genital system.

Stereocilia are long, unstructured, branched, protoplasmic structures from the luminal surface of cells which increase surface area for secretory activity (Fig. 2-34). They occur on the pseudostratified columnar cells of the ductus epididymidis of the male genital system.

Neuroepithelium. Certain cells of epithelial sheets are modified to receive and transmit sensory information. These cells are associated with organs modified to receive optic, olfactory, gustatory, auditory and kinesthetic sensations. Although these cells may transmit information to the central nervous system by different means, they are similar in that all of them perceive stimuli through typical or modified cilia. *Support cells* (*sustentacular cells*) are normally associated with these sensory cells. The hair cells of the spiral organ of the ear and of the semicircular canals are examples of these modified epithelial cells.

Pigmented Epithelium. Various cells of the body typically possess various types of pigments. In one instance, however, an entire sheet of epithelium, the pigmented epithelium of the retina of the eye (Fig. 2-35), is modified to contain large quantities of melanin.

Myoepithelium. *Myoepithelial cells* or *basket cells* are specialized epithelial cells associated with the adenomeres of most exocrine glands of the body. They are spindle cells which surround the secretory endpieces (Fig. 2-36). Although of epithelial origin, they contain myofibrils, are contractile and are responsible for the expression of secretory products into ducts. They are associated with salivary glands, sweat glands, mammary glands and others.

Surface Specializations of Epithelia

Cell to Cell Modifications. The surfaces of epithelial cells are modified variously for different functions. The lateral surfaces are specialized to hold cells together as well as to serve as diffusion barriers.

At the light microscopic level, *terminal bars* are situated near the apical portion of the lateral cell margin. They are not separate entities but are continuous around the periphery of the cell. At the electron microscopic level, terminal bars are *junctional complexes* which are composed of three discrete units (Fig. 2-37). From the apical portion of the cell toward the base, the units are: *tight junction* (*zonula occludens*), *intermediate junction* (*zonula adherens*) and *desmosome* (*macula adherens*).

In a *tight junction* (Fig. 2-37), the outer laminae of the two adjacent cell membranes are fused as one. There is, therefore, an obliteration of the intercellular space. A condensation of the cytoplasm on either side of this junction may be apparent. This type of union between cells forms an effective diffusion barrier between the luminal and intercellular space.

The *intermediate junction* (Fig. 2-37) is characterized by the juxtaposition of two adjacent cell membranes. They are not fused but are separated by a 20-nm space which is filled with a homogeneous material. The

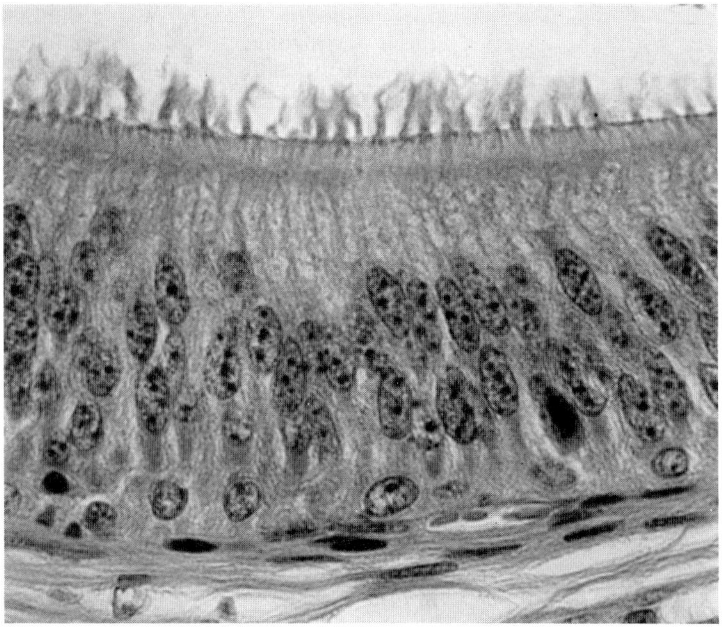

Fig. 2-34. Stereocilia from the equine ductus epididymidis. ×200. (See Fig. 2-50 also.)

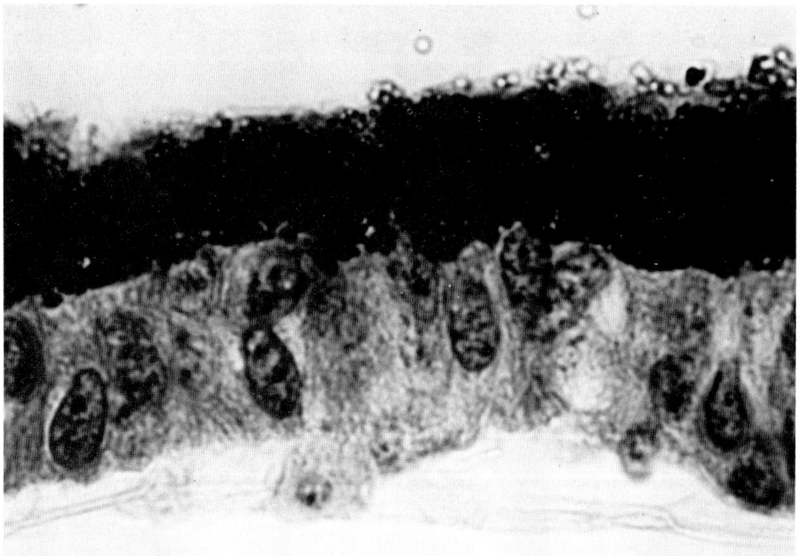

Fig. 2-35. Non-nervous portion of the feline retina. The pigmented epithelium is at the *top* of the micrograph. The pigment granules obscure the nuclei. The columnar cells in the *lower* part of the micrograph comprise a separate layer. ×320.

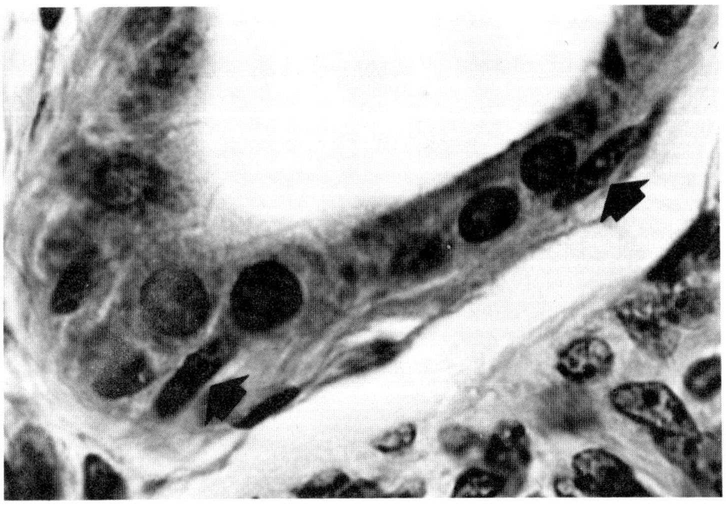

Fig. 2-36. Secretory endpiece of a bovine sweat gland. *Arrows*, myoepithelial cells. ×320.

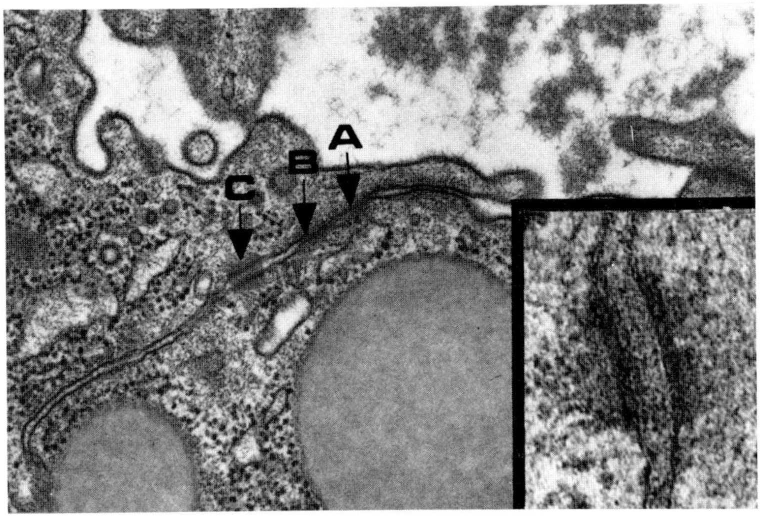

Fig. 2-37. Junctional complex between pancreatic acinar cells. The tight junction (*A*), intermediate junction (*B*) and desmosome (*C*) are indicated. ×41,000. *Inset:* High magnification of a desmosome. ×146,000.

adjacent cytoplasmic condensations contain numerous tonofilaments which are continuous with the terminal web of the cell. The two aforementioned attachments totally encircle the cell.

The *desmosome* (Fig. 2-37) does not totally encircle the cell but is scattered along the cellular margin at discrete locations. Moreover, it is not confined to junctional complexes but may be found scattered along the lateral cell surfaces. The inner margin of each contributing cell membrane is coated by a dense material. Tonofilaments are embedded in this dense material and are obvious in the associated cytoplasmic condensations. A space of 25 nm between adjacent cell membranes is typical and a dense intermediate line may be apparent in this intercellular space. At the lateral margins of the desmosome a tight junction may be present. Although desmosomes vary in structure, the aforestated description is typical.

The remaining 15-nm space between cells is occupied by a cell coat of glycoproteins and carbohydrate-rich substances. These materials, as well as extensive cellular *interdigitations* (Fig. 2-38) and the aforementioned junctional complexes, serve as mechanisms for adhesion.

Basal Border Modifications. The primary modifications associated with the basal border of epithelial cells are: *basal laminae*, ***basal invaginations***, *caveolae* and *pinocytotic vesicles*, and *hemidesmosomes*.

All epithelial tissues, except in a few specific instances, are separated from the underlying or surrounding connective tissue by a boundary layer called the *basement membrane*. It is readily demonstrable with periodic acid-Schiff (PAS) staining or silver impregnation, but it is not observable with routine hematoxylin and eosin staining (Figs. 2-39, 2-40).

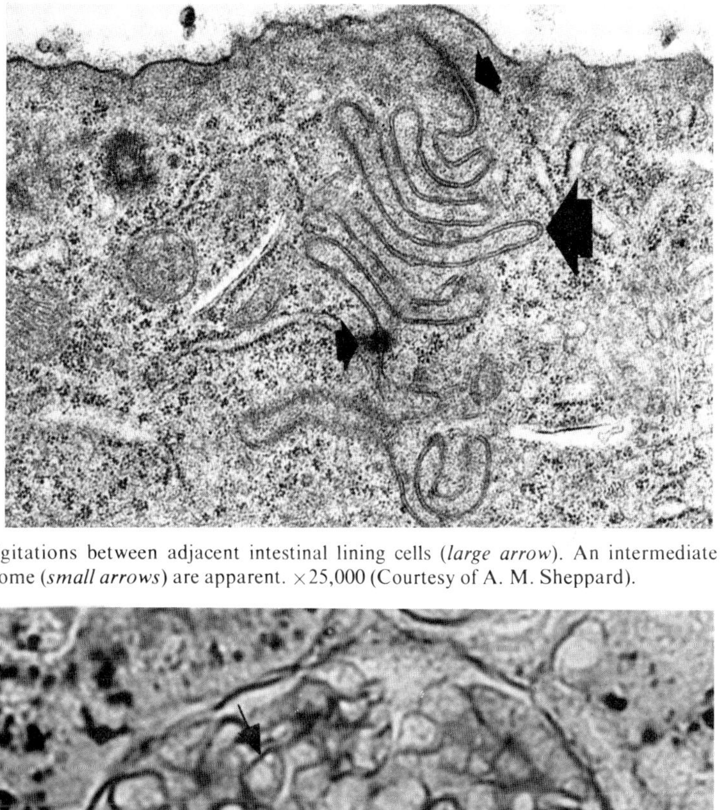

Fig. 2-38. Interdigitations between adjacent intestinal lining cells (*large arrow*). An intermediate junction and desmosome (*small arrows*) are apparent. ×25,000 (Courtesy of A. M. Sheppard).

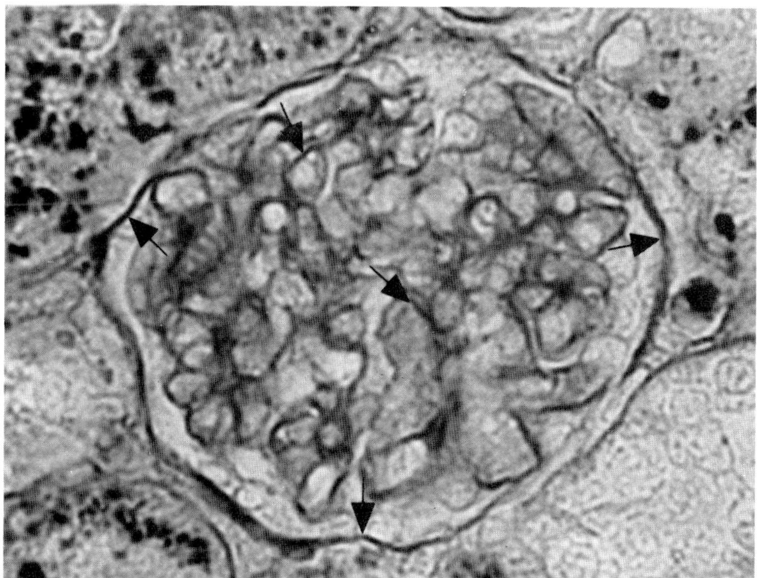

Fig. 2-39. Glomerulus of a kidney stained with PAS. The basement membrane (*arrows*) is clearly defined. Compare with Fig. 2-40. ×250.

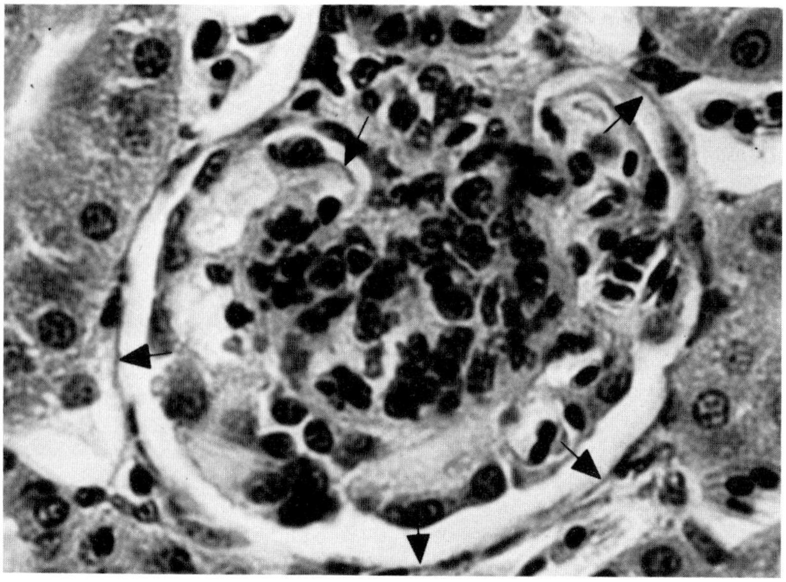

Fig. 2-40. Glomerulus of a kidney stained with hematoxylin and eosin. The cellular limits (*arrows*) are visible, but the basement membrane is not apparent. Compare with Fig. 2-39. ×250.

The ultrastructural detail of the basement membrane has been elucidated with the electron microscope (Fig. 2-41). The light microscopic entity actually includes the basal cell membrane, amorphous cell coat, some dense material and associated connective tissue fibrils. Some dense material (50–70 nm wide) underlies the basal cell membrane and closely follows the contour of this membrane. This dense band of the *basal lamina* is homogeneous and contains a fine feltwork of filaments which project into the underlying connective tissue space as well as into the 40-nm space between the dense band and epithelial cell membrane. This light-staining zone of the basal lamina represents the cell coat.

Although the basal lamina has been considered a condensation product of the connective tissue space, current immunological evidence indicates that it may be of epithelial origin. Whatever its origin, the basal lamina is a structure significant in adhesion and filtration.

The terms basement membrane and basal lamina are not synonymous. One is a light microscopic term, while the other is derived from electron microscopy. Importantly, the basement membrane of light microscopy includes the basal cell membrane, basal lamina (dark and light zones) and associated connective tissue fibers.

The basal cell membranes may be regularly contoured or may possess numerous infoldings (Fig. 2-42). The latter modification is especially apparent in cells involved in transport activities. In either case, small bulblike invaginations of the cell membrane (*caveolae*) exist (Fig. 2-43). These pinch off from the membrane and form *pinocytotic vesicles* (Fig. 2-43). These two structures may represent mechanisms for *endocytotic* and/or *exocytotic* activity.

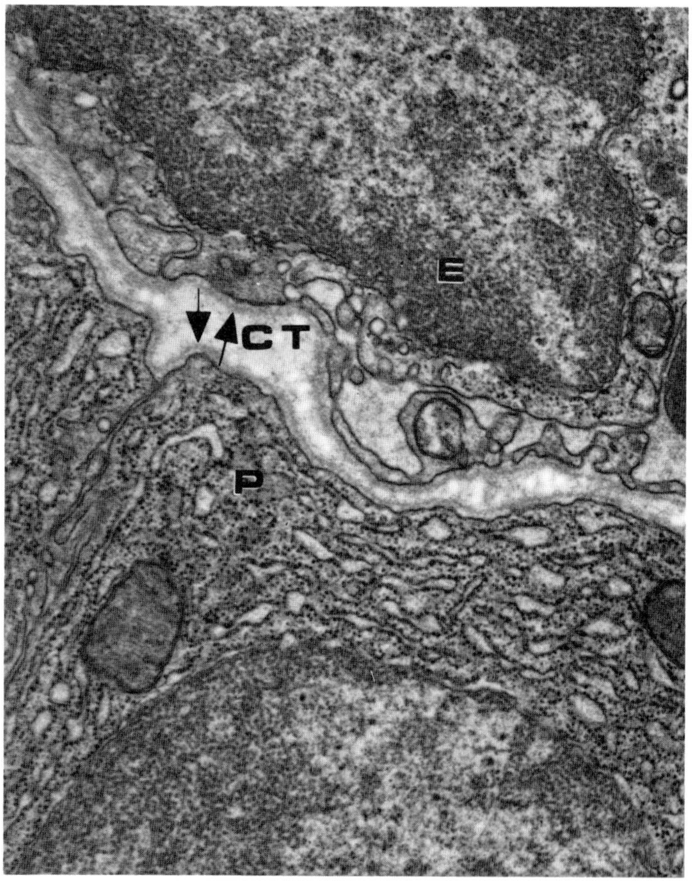

Fig. 2-41. Basal lamina. The endothelial cell (*E*) and pancreatic acinar cell (*P*) are separated from each other by individual basal laminae (*arrows*). These define the limits of the connective tissue space (*CT*). ×25,000.

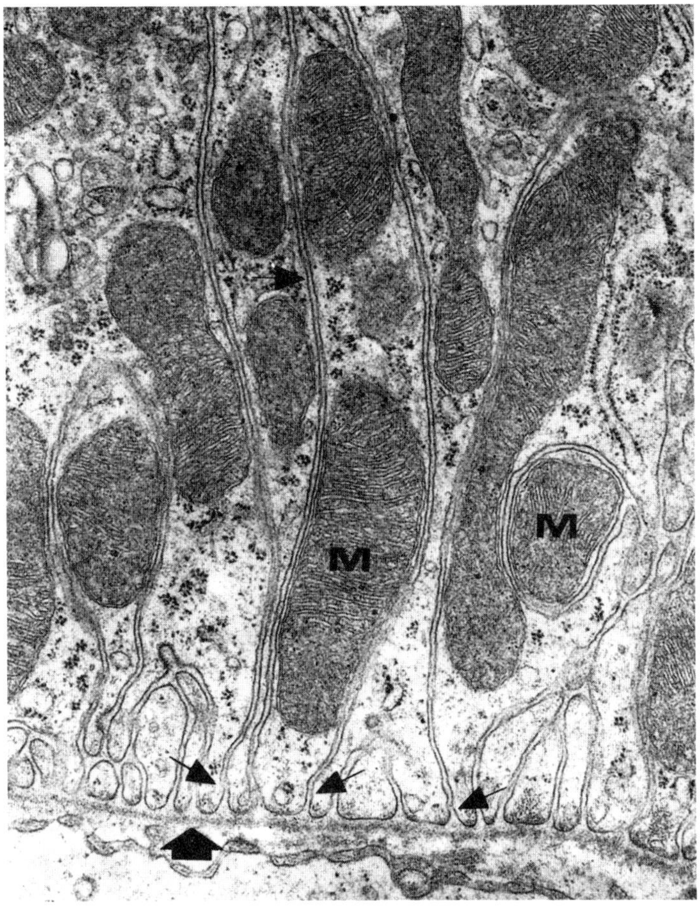

Fig. 2-42. Basal infoldings of a lining cell of a proximal convoluted tubule of a kidney. Mitochondria (*M*) are contained within cytoplasmic portions of a highly folded basal border (*small arrows*). The basal lamina (*large arrow*) is apparent. ×18,000.

Hemidesmosomes (*half-desmosomes*) are sometimes encountered along the basal cell membrane (Fig. 2-44). As the name implies, these structures are identical to one-half of a desmosome, with one exception. Fine filaments traverse the light zone perpendicular to the desmosome and are continuous with the dense zone of the basal lamina.

Apical Border Modifications. The primary apical border modifications of epithelia are: *microvilli*, *caveolae*, *pinocytotic vesicles* and *cilia*.

Microvilli are found on the surfaces of most cells. They are extremely variable in size, distribution and organization. Their prime function is to increase the absorbing surface area of a cell. Microvilli achieve their highest degree of development in epithelia. They are slender, cylindrical cellular processes which are oriented perpendicular to the apical, free or luminal surface.

Microvilli of intestinal epithelial cells are highly ordered structures on the free borders which form a *striated border* or *brush border* (Fig. 2-45). These processes are 1 to 1.5 μm long and approximately 0.1 μm in diameter. They are juxtaposed to each other in a parallel arrangement (Fig. 2-46). The

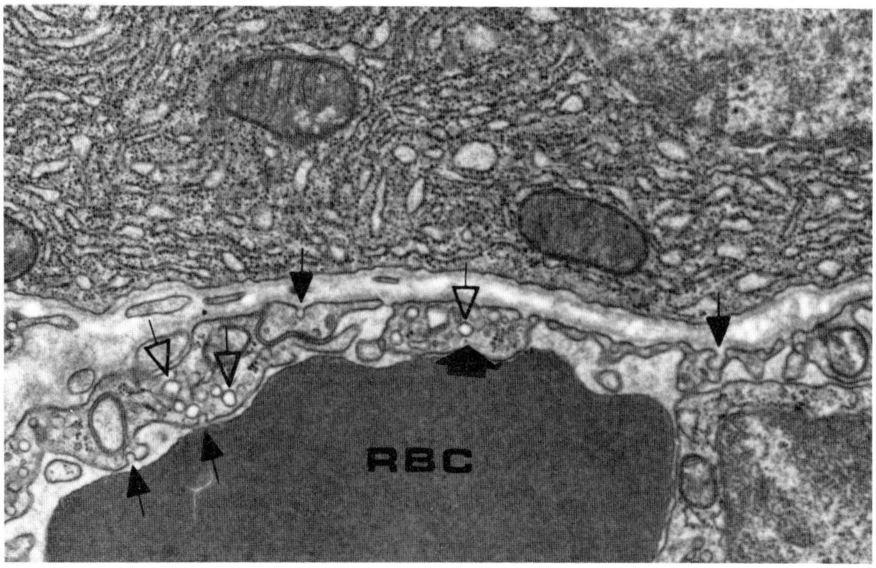

Fig. 2-43. Basal lamina and vesicles. An erythrocyte (*RBC*) is bounded by capillary endothelium (*large solid arrow*). Pinocytotic vesicles (*open arrows*) and caveolae (*solid arrows*) are apparent. Note the basal laminae. ×18,000.

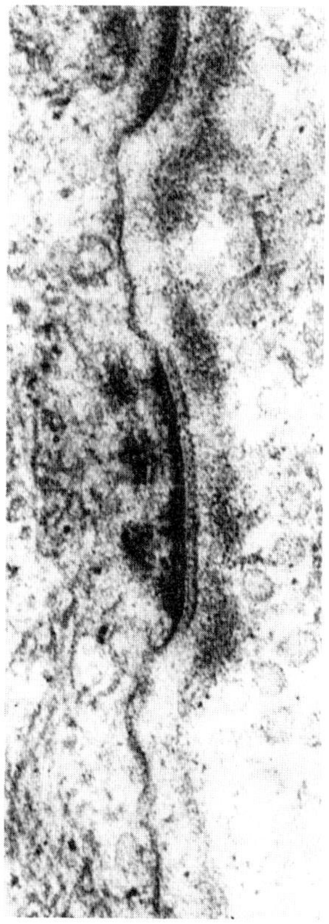

Fig. 2-44. Hemidesmosome along the basal border of an intestinal lining cell of a mouse. ×91,000.

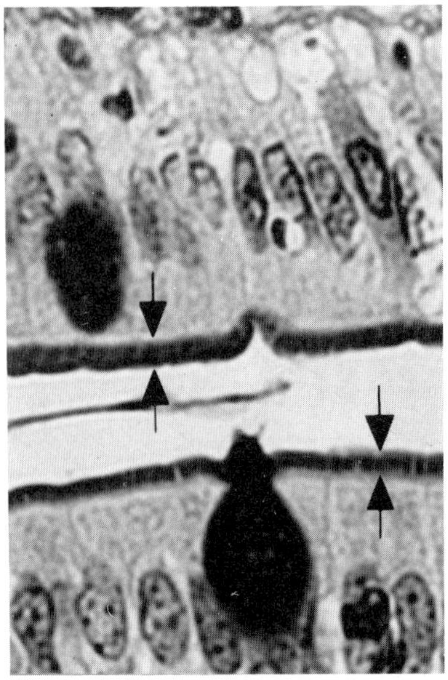

Fig. 2-45. Striated border of lining cells of the equine jejunum (*arrows*). ×250 (Alcian blue and PAS).

cores of the microvilli are composed of cytofilaments which extend down to the ectoplasm in which the terminal web is located. The cytofilaments of the microvilli are connected to those of the terminal web.

Certain lining cells of the kidney also possess a marked development of microvilli on their apical borders. These, however, are not in as orderly an arrangement as those described previously (Fig. 2-47). In the past, this arrangement was referred to as a *brush border*, while the highly ordered array was called a *striated border*. Now these terms are used synonymously, since both represent modifications to increase the cell surface. The surface coat or glycocalyx associated with microvilli is prominent.

Cilia are typical apical modifications of specialized epithelial cells (Figs. 2-5, 2-18, 2-34). These structures, however, are not confined to epithelial cells. *Kinocilia* or motile cellular processes may be as long as 10 μm with a diameter of approximately 0.2 μm (Fig. 2-48). These long, cylindrical and tapered processes contain microtubules embedded within a matrix and are covered by the plasma membrane. A central pair of tubules is surrounded by nine doublets of tubules (Fig. 2-49). These tubular structures are connected by fine cytofilaments. At the point of union between the cilium and the cell, the central pair of tubules terminate above a *basal plate*, while the peripheral pairs of tubules gain another tubule and are converted to nine sets of triplets of the basal body.

Stereocilia do not possess this complex organizational pattern (Fig. 2-50). They may be considered extremely long and branched microvilli.

The *caveolae* and *pinocytotic vesicles* of the apical border are similar in structure and function to those structures associated with the basal border (Fig. 2-43).

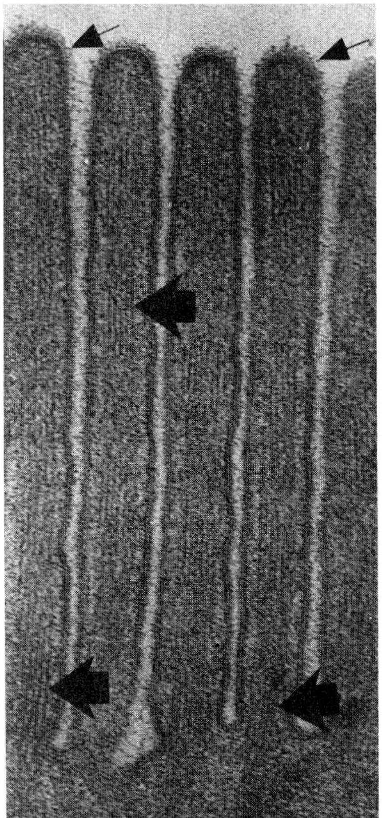

Fig. 2-46. Striated border of an intestinal lining cell of a mouse. The microvilli are in an orderly arrangement, are covered by a glycocalyx (*small arrows*) and contain cytofilaments (*large arrows*). ×70,000.

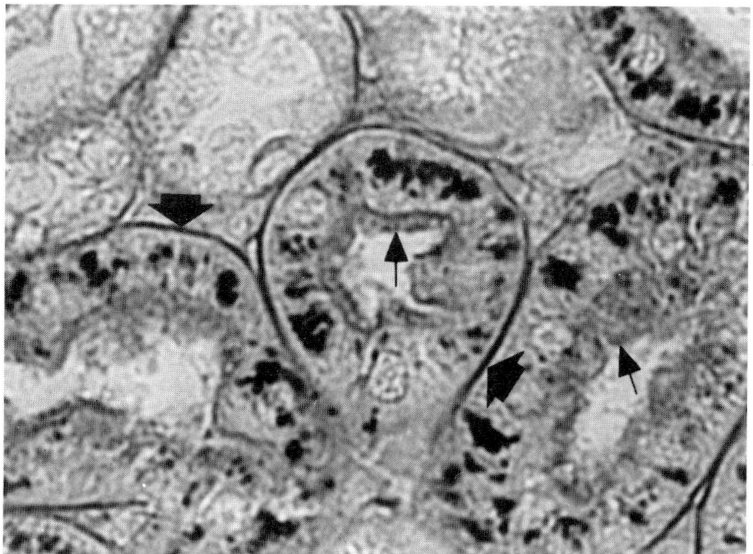

Fig. 2-47. Brush borders of the proximal convoluted tubules of the kidney (*small arrows*). The basement membranes are clearly defined also (*large arrows*). ×250 (toluidine blue and PAS).

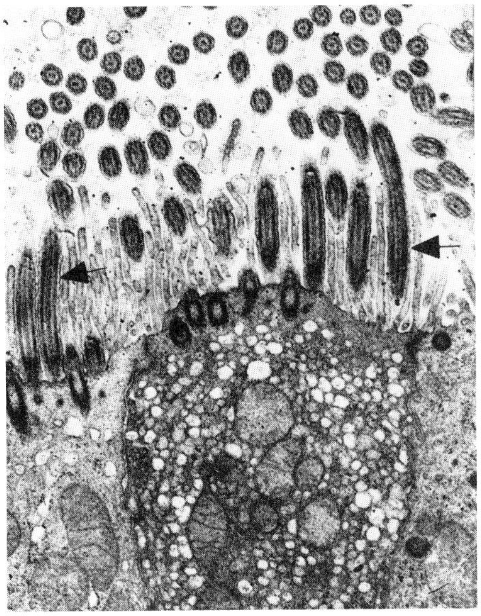

Fig. 2-48. Ciliated cells from the trachea of a mouse. *Arrows*, cilia. ×8,000.

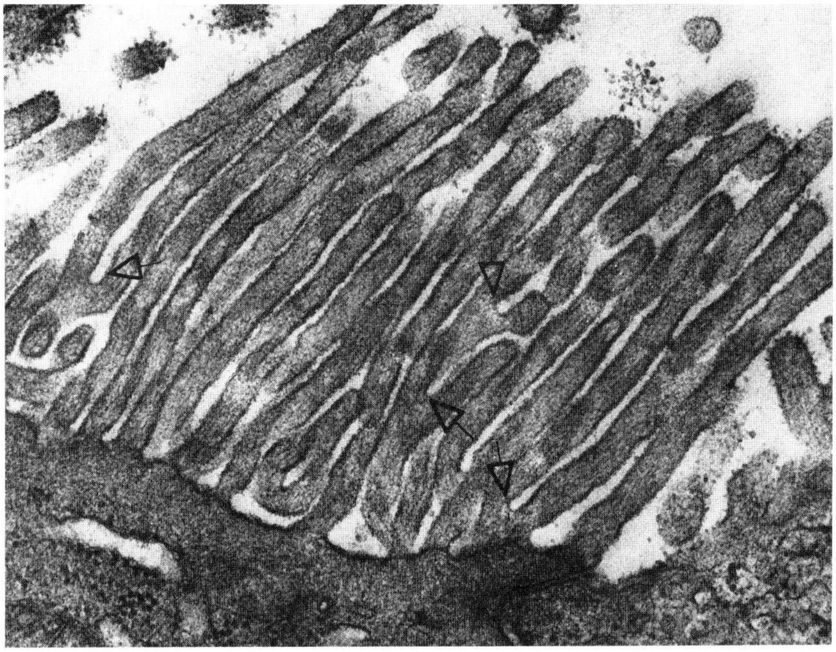

Fig. 2-50. Stereocilia from the trachea of a mouse. Note the branching (*arrows*) and lack of internal organization. ×46,000.

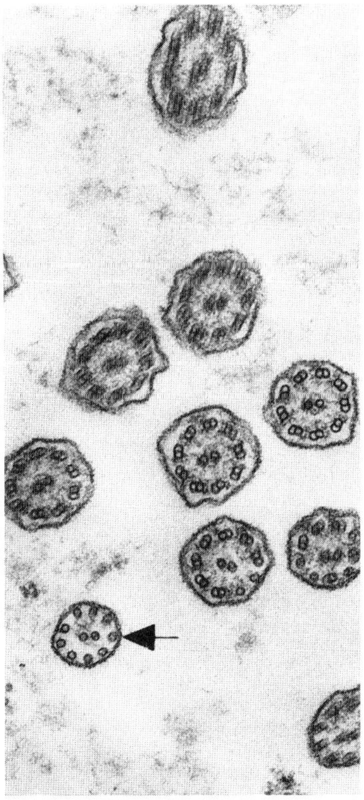

Fig. 2-49. Cross-sections of cilia. The doublets and central pairs are apparent. The configuration of the peripheral microtubules is altered at the tip of the cilia (*arrow*). ×44,000.

References

Epithelium

Brody, I.: The keratinization of epidermal cells of normal guinea pig skin revealed by electron microscopy. J. Ultrastruct. Res. *2:*482, 1959.

Dunn, J. S.: The fine structure of the absorptive epithelial cells of the developing small intestine of the rat. J. Anat. *101:*57, 1967.

Hackemann, M., Grubb, C. and Hill, K. R.: The ultrastructure of normal squamous epithelium of the human cervix uteri. J. Ultrastruct. Res. *22:*443, 1968.

Hicks, R. M.: The fine structure of the transitional epithelium of rat ureter. J. Cell Biol. *26:*25, 1965.

Zelickson, A. S.: *Ultrastructure of Normal and Abnormal Skin.* Lea and Febiger, Philadelphia, 1967.

Glandular Epithelium

Bullough, W. S. and Ebling, F. J.: Cell replacement in the epidermis and sebaceous glands of the mouse. J. Anat. *86:*29, 1952.

Ekholm, R. and Edlund, Y.: Ultrastructure of the human exocrine pancreas. J. Ultrastruct. Res. *2:*453, 1959.

Parks, H. F.: Morphological study of the extrusion of secretory materials by the parotid glands of mouse and rat. J. Ultrastruct. Res. *6:*449, 1962.

Scott, B. L. and Pease, D. C.: Electron microscopy of the salivary and lacrimal glands of the rat. Amer. J. Anat. *104:*115, 1959.

Special Epithelia

Arstila, A. and Wersall, J.: The ultrastructure of the olfactory epithelium of the guinea pig. Acta Otolaryng. Stockholm *64:*187, 1967.

Edwards, E. and Duntley, S.: The pigments and color of living skin. Amer. J. Anat. *65:*1, 1939.

Fitzpatrick, T. B. and Szabo, G.: The melanocyte; cytology and cytochemistry. J. Invest. Derm. *32:*197, 1959.

Frisch, D.: Ultrastructure of mouse olfactory mucosa. Amer. J. Anat. *121:*87, 1967.

Lundquist, P. G., Kimura, R. and Wersall, J.: Ultrastructural organization of the epithelial lining in the endolymphatic duct and sac in the guinea pig. Acta Otolaryng. Stockholm *57:*65, 1963.

Rhodin, J. and Dulhan, T.: Electron microscopy of the tracheal ciliated mucosa in rat. Z. Zellforsch. *44:*345, 1956.

Travill, A. A. and Hill, M. F.: Histochemical demonstration of myoepithelial cell activity. Quart. J. Exp. Physiol. *48:*423, 1963.

Surface Specializations

Barber, V. C. and Boyde, A.: Scanning electron microscopic studies of cilia. Z. Zellforsch. *84:*269, 1968.

Curtis, A. S. G.: Cell contact and adhesion. Biol. Rev. *37:*82, 1962.

Farquhar, M. G. and Palade, G. E.: Junctional complexes in various epithelia. J. Cell Biol. *17:*375, 1963.

Fawcett, D. W.: Physiologically significant specializations of the cell surface. Circulation *26:*1105, 1962.

Fawcett, D. W.: Surface specializations of absorbing cells. J. Histochem. Cytochem. *13:*75, 1965.

Fawcett, D. W. and Porter, K. R.: A study of the fine structure of ciliated epithelia. J. Morph. *94:*221, 1954.

Granger, B. and Baker, R. F.: Electron microscope investigation of the striated border of intestinal epithelium. Anat. Rec. *107:*423, 1950.

Hashimoto, K., Gross, B. G. and Lever, W. F.: Electron microscopic study of apocrine secretion. J. Invest. Derm. *46:*378, 1966.

Ito, S.: The surface coat of enteric microvilli. J. Cell Biol. *27:*475, 1965.

Kelly, D.: Fine structure of desmosomes, hemidesmosomes and an adepidermal globular layer in developing newt epidermis. J. Cell Biol. *28:*51, 1966.

Kurtz, S. M. and Feldman, J. D.: Experimental studies on the formation of the glomerular basement membrane. J. Ultrastruct. Res. *6:*19, 1962.

Pierce, G. B., Jr., Midgley, A. R., Jr. and Sri Ram, J.: The histogenesis of basement membranes. J. Exp. Med. *117:*339, 1963.

Satir, P.: Cilia. Sci. Amer. *204:*61, 1961.

Sorokin, S. D.: Reconstruction of centriole formation and ciliogenesis in mammalian lungs. J. Cell Sci. *3:*207, 1968.

Susi, F. R., Belt, W. D. and Kelly, J. W.: Fine structure of fibrillar complexes associated with the basement membrane in human oral mucosa. J. Cell Biol. *34:*686, 1967.

3 Embryonal and Adult Connective Tissues

General Characteristics

Form and Function. Connective tissues, as one of the four basic tissues of the body, are composed of heterogeneous cell populations and copious amounts of extracellular secretory products. Diverse cells are abundant, but they are not in intimate contact with each other. Rather, they are separated by the fibrous and amorphous components of the connective tissue *matrix*. This matrix is composed of various nonliving fibers secreted by the cells, as well as a *ground substance* which is composed of cellular secretory products (*mucopolysaccharides*). It is variation in the type, distribution and number of cells, as well as variation in the type and quantity of matrix components that permits great latitude in the form and function of the connective tissues.

The peripheral limits of the connective tissues are surrounded by a *basal lamina*, which underlies epithelial tissues and surrounds the endothelial cells of the blood vascular system. Individual cells, such as fat cells, are surrounded by a basal lamina. The occurrence of a basal lamina, therefore, establishes, limits and defines a highly vascularized connective tissue compartment which is separated from other tissues.

Connective tissues, dependent upon the cell population and type of matrix, serve numerous and multiple functions. By virtue of their fibrous components they *connect* one tissue or organ to another. Also, they are the means through which organs are *suspended* from the walls of the body. Various connective tissues *insulate* organs from mechanical damage as well as insulate the body against extremes of heat loss and gain. These tissues are responsible for the form of organs and the body. They are an important line of *defense* because numerous protective cells are part of their cellular population. The connective tissues serve a *nutritive* function as well. Not only do vascular beds have to traverse connective tissues to reach other tissues, but metabolites also move through the connective tissue space to reach individual cells. *Heat regulation*, *water metabolism* and *food storage* are also important functions. In conjunction with other tissues they aid in the *support* and *locomotion* of the body. Some connective tissues also play an important role in *repair* and *regeneration*.

Classification. Three criteria are used primarily for the classification of connective tissues:

1. Predominant cell type or types. 2. Nature of the matrix components. 3. Orderliness of the matrix components.

There are numerous gradations that sometimes make definitive classification difficult. The classification shown in Scheme 3-1, however, is didactically helpful.

Extracellular Components

Fibers. Three types of fibers are characteristic of connective tissues: *collagenous*, *reticular* and *elastic* fibers. They occur in varying quantity, organization and combination in these tissues. These fibers, in combination with the ground substance, impart the varied physical characteristics associated with connective tissues.

These fibers are the *neutral mucosubstances* (*glycoproteins*) of the connective tissues.

Collagenous fibers, the secretory products of *fibroblasts*, are the most numerous of the fibers encountered in connective tissues. In light microscopic sections stained with hematoxylin and eosin (H and E) they appear as pink-staining, wavy bundles of indefinite length with a diameter of between 1 and 12 μm (Fig. 3-1). In most connective tissues they are oriented in random directions; thus, these fibers may be cut in cross-section, longitudinally or diagonally. In stretch preparations their length, thickness and random orientation are more apparent (Fig. 3-2).

With the electon microscope and appropriate staining, a light and dark banding is observed. One light and dark band represents a 64-nm period. This periodicity is repeated along the entire length of the collagenous fiber (Fig. 3-3). The collagenous fibers of both light and electron microscopy are composed of smaller units. The basic unit of collagen is the *tropocollagen* molecule. This macromolecule is composed of three proteins that are entwined about each other in a helical array along their entire 280-nm length. This molecule is synthesized by the cell and secreted into the extracellular environment. Once outside the cell, numerous tropocollagen molecules polymerize into

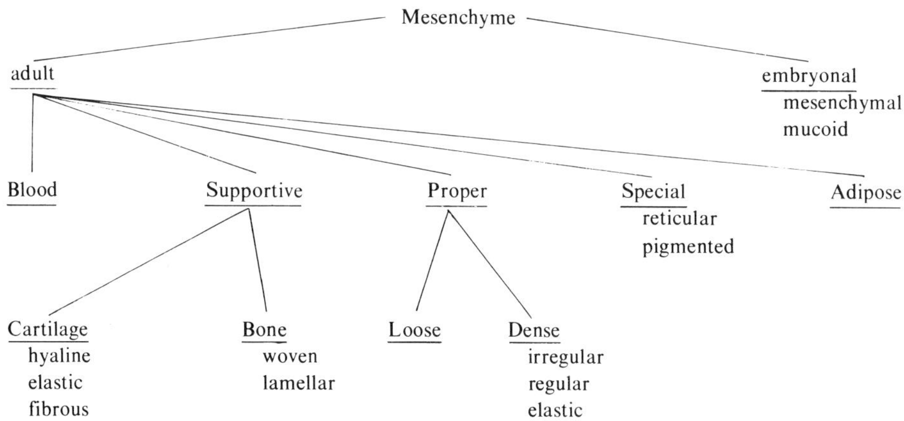

Scheme 3-1.

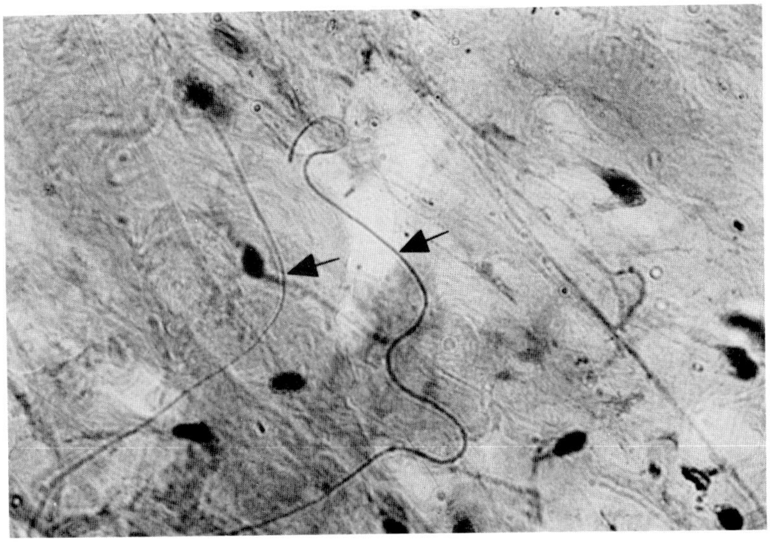

Fig. 3-6. Elastic fibers in a stretch preparation of loose connective tissue. The elastic fibers (*arrows*) are broken and appear wavy. ×160.

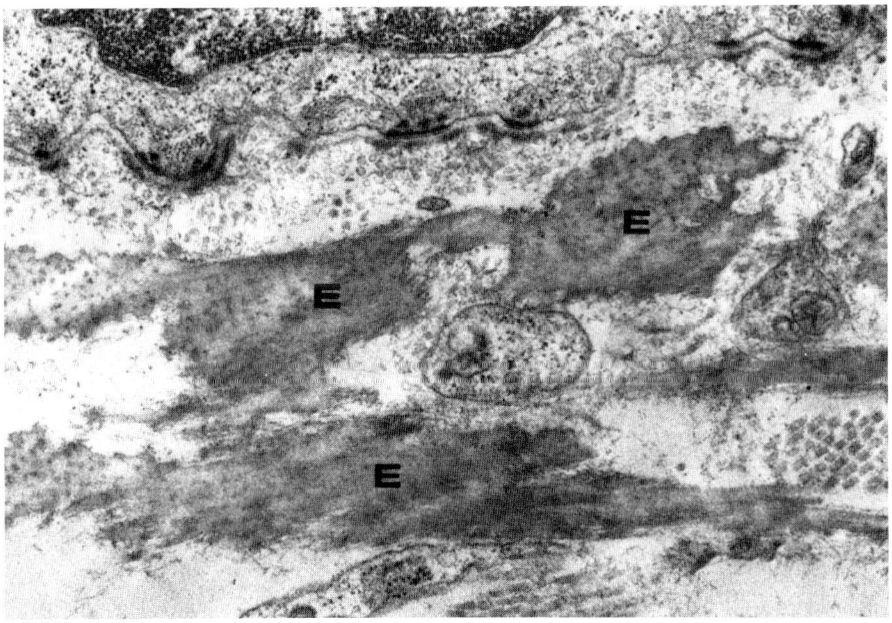

Fig. 3-7. Electron micrograph of elastic fibers. The elastic fibers (*E*) are scattered in the connective tissue space. ×26,000.

rigid as bone. In the latter instance, mineral is added to the matrix.

Resident Cell Population

The cell population of any connective tissue will vary with the tissue, as well as the physiological state of the tissue at the time of observation. Nevertheless, there are some cells of connective tissues that are encountered frequently. These may be referred to as the *resident cell population* and include *mesenchymal cells, primitive reticular cells, fibroblasts, macrophages, pericytes, fat cells* and *mast cells*.

Mesenchymal Cells. The *mesenchymal cell* is the precursor of most connective tissue cells. It is a stellate or spindle cell with a high nuclear to cytoplasmic ratio. It has a large, vesicular nucleus which is rich in euchromatin (Fig. 3-8). The cytoplasm is acidophilic and scant. In most preparations the cytoplasm is indistinguishable from surrounding matrix components. At the ultrastructural level, the predominant cytoplasmic organelle is the polyribosome (Fig. 3-9). The combination of prominent euchromatin and extensive polyribosomes is indicative of the high protein synthesis potential of this cell. The protein produced, however, is for intracellular use initially. Few other organelles are apparent.

Although mesenchymal cells are scattered throughout the connective tissue space, they are sometimes difficult to distinguish. They are most prominent in the perivascular area. These cells, scattered throughout the connective tissue compartment, are probably the primary means through which *metaplasia* occurs.

Primitive Reticular Cells. The *primitive reticular cells* are stellate or spindle cells which are usually in intimate association with reticular fibers. They are similar to mesenchymal cells in that they are capable of differentiating into numerous other cell types. The nucleus is round to oval and vesicular (Fig. 3-10). The cytoplasm is extensive and slightly basophilic. The cytoplasmic processes of these cells are in contact with one another and form a *cellular meshwork* or *reticulum*.

Some differentiated version of the primitive reticular cell probably secretes the reticular fibers with which they are associated. However, they are morphologically indistinguishable.

These cells also differentiate into *phagocytic reticular cells* or *fixed macrophages*. This line of differentiation will be discussed in a subsequent section. This cell is associated with reticular connective tissue.

Fibroblasts. The *fibroblasts*, or fiber-forming cells of connective tissues, are the most frequently encountered cells. As young cells, the fibroblasts are stellate or spindle shaped with long cellular processes. The large oval or round nucleus is vesicular and has a prominent nucleolus (Fig. 3-11). There is an abundance of basophilic cytoplasm. This form of the cell is the active fiber-forming cell, one in which there is an abundance of granular endoplasmic reticulum and a well-developed Golgi apparatus (Fig. 3-12).

The older fibroblasts, sometimes referred to as *fibrocytes*, have a nucleus that has more heterochromatin than its younger counterpart. These spindle cells have scant cytoplasm that, when seen, is acidophilic. They also have a corresponding reduction in their intracellular organelles.

The fibroblast is responsible for the secretion of tropocollagen; thus, it is responsible for collagen production. It is probably responsible for the secretion of the precursors of reticular fibers and elastic fibers as well. This cell also secretes materials that are components of the ground substance.

Macrophages. *Macrophages* are also referred to as *histiocytes* and *clasmatocytes*.

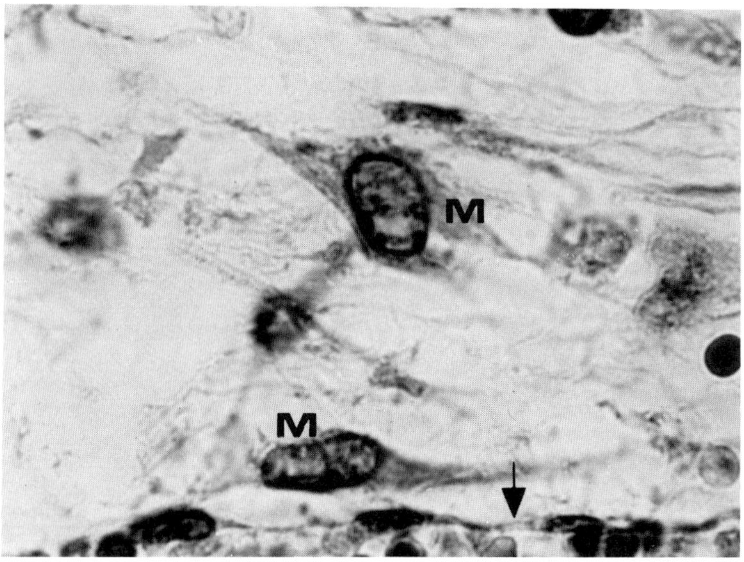

Fig. 3-8. Mesenchymal cells from perivascular space of loose connective tissue. The mesenchymal cells (*M*) are typical and close to a vessel (*arrow*). ×400.

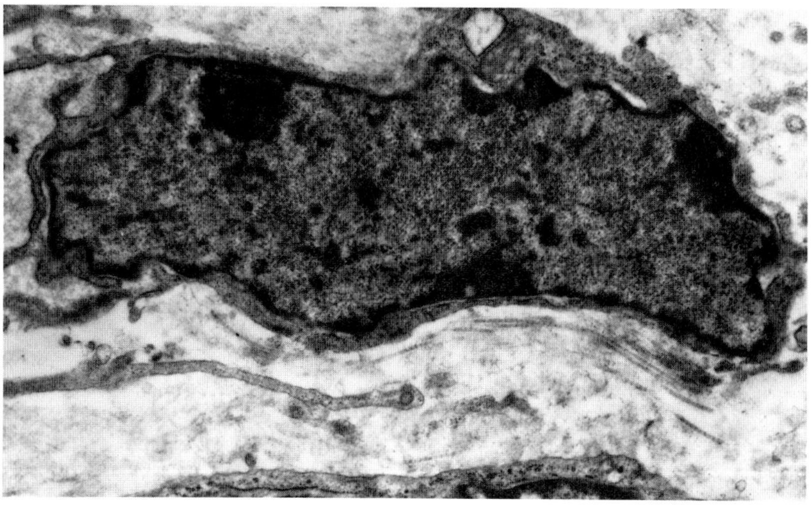

Fig. 3-9. Electron micrograph of a mesenchymal cell. The nuclear/cytoplasmic volume of the cell is great. ×12,000.

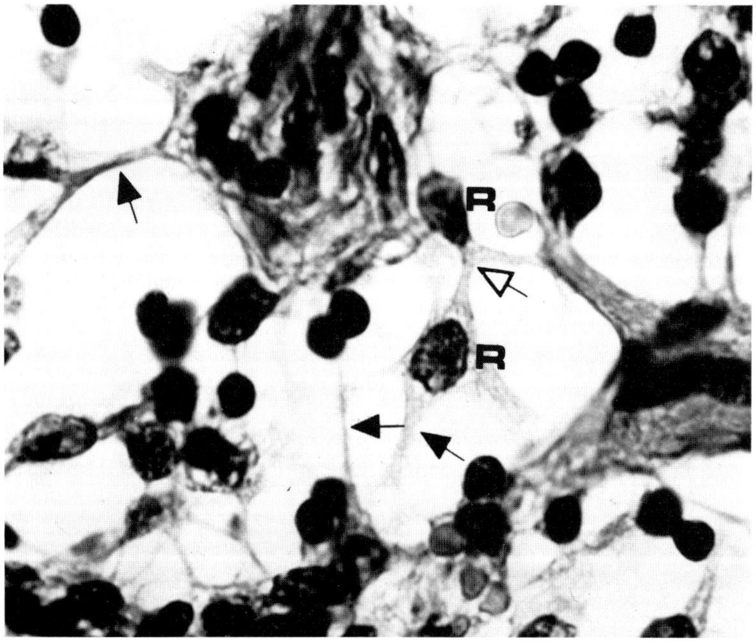

Fig. 3-10. Cells from the medullary region of a lymph node. The reticuloendothelial cells (*R*) extend cytoplasmic processes (*solid arrows*) which form a cellular reticulum. Points of contact between cells (*open arrow*) are sometimes apparent. ×320.

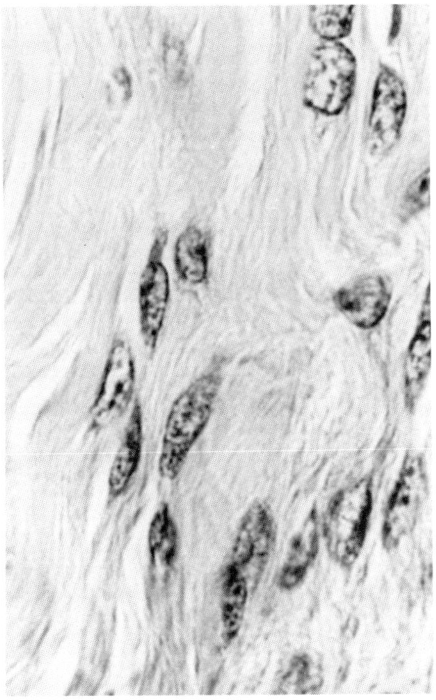

Fig. 3-11. Fibroblasts of loose connective tissue. The cytoplasm is not apparent, while the vesicular nature of the nuclei is apparent. Collagen is randomly oriented throughout the section. ×340.

They are the resident phagocytic cells of the connective tissue compartment. They may be either *fixed* or *wandering*. As fixed cells they are most prominent in the pericapillary space. However, they may also be fixed along the length of a collagenous fiber. When activated by various stimuli they become ***wandering*** or ***amoeboid***.

Macrophages are pleomorphic. They vary from spindle-shaped in the fixed configuration to round or oval with blunt cellular processes in the wandering stage. The nucleus of the macrophage is the key to the identification of this cell (Fig. 3-13). The nucleus is slightly smaller than the fibroblast nucleus and is darker because of the coarse heterochromatic pattern. Lastly, but most importantly, the nucleus is often indented; i.e., it is *bean-shaped* or *kidney-shaped*. Usually, the cell is polarized. The concavity or indentation of the nucleus faces the bulk of the cytoplasm. The basophilic cytoplasm may possess a juxtanuclear pale-staining region.

At the ultrastructural level, the prominent organelles in macrophages are the Golgi apparatus (in the nuclear indentation), rough endoplasmic reticulum and lysosomes (Fig. 3-14). At the light and electron microscopic level, ingested particulate material may be apparent if the cell is active.

There are multiple origins of this cell in the connective tissue compartment. Mesenchymal cells and reticular cells may give rise to this cell. The blood *monocyte* and the macrophage are either closely related or identical cells. Within the confines of the blood vascular system (*intravascular*) this cell is referred to as a monocyte. Once it enters the connective tissue compartment (*extravascular*) it is referred to as a histiocyte or macrophage.

Macrophages are one of the prime cellular agents for defense against the invasion of particulate matter into the body. They are important members of the reticuloendothelial system.

Pericytes. Any cell that occurs around a capillary or small vessel may be a pericyte. Thus, macrophages, mesenchymal cells and fibroblasts, by virtue of their perivascular position, may be referred to as pericytic. However, in a more specific context, the *pericyte* is a specific cell or cell type. *Pericytes* or *cells of Rouget* are in intimate contact with the endothelial lining cells of the small vessel with which they are associated (Fig. 3-15). They are invested with a basal lamina except at a point of contact with the endothelial cell (Fig. 3-16). Some of these cells have been shown to be contractile; thus, they may control the size of the vascular lumen. Others have not been demonstrated as contractile and their function is unknown.

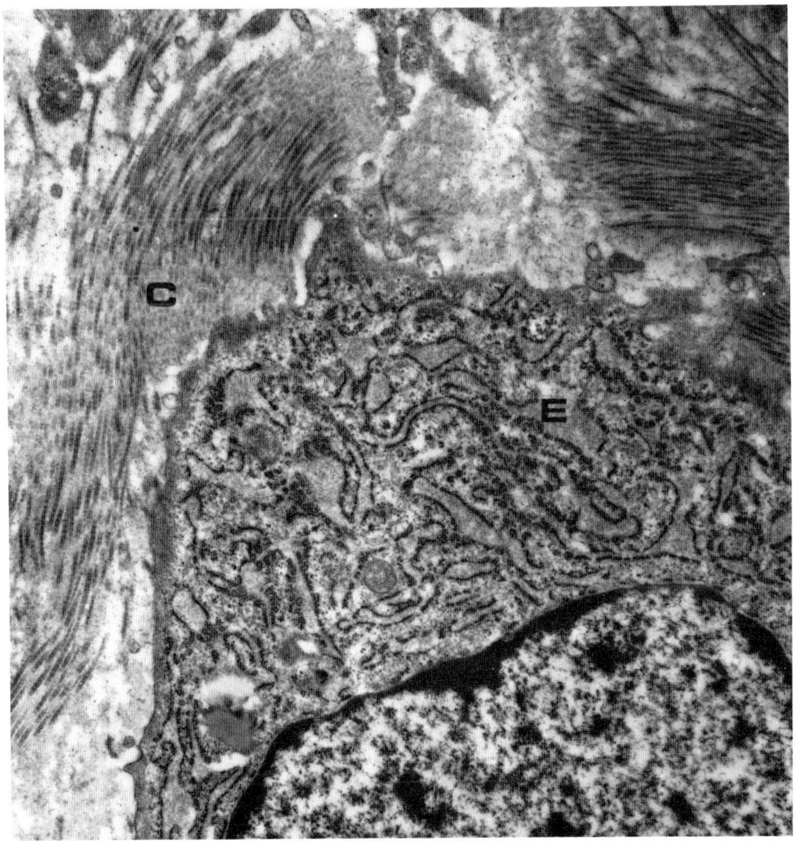

Fig. 3-12. Electron micrograph of a fibroblast. The cell contains extensive quantities of granular endoplasmic reticulum (*E*). Collagen (*C*) occupies the connective tissue space. ×6,000.

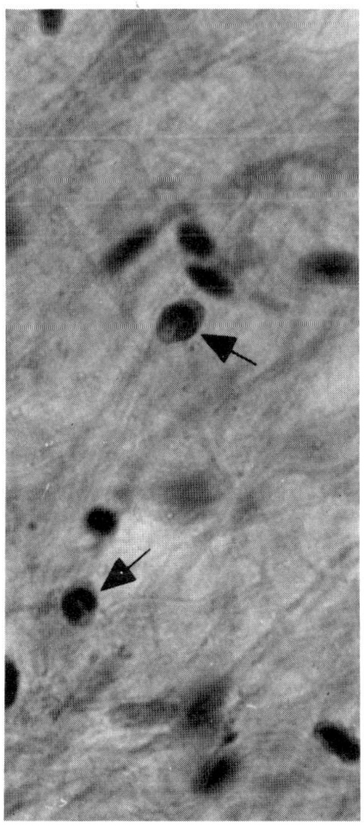

Fig. 3-13. Macrophages in a stretch preparation of loose connective tissue. The nuclei of the macrophages (*arrows*) are typical. The remaining cells are out of the plane of focus. ×100.

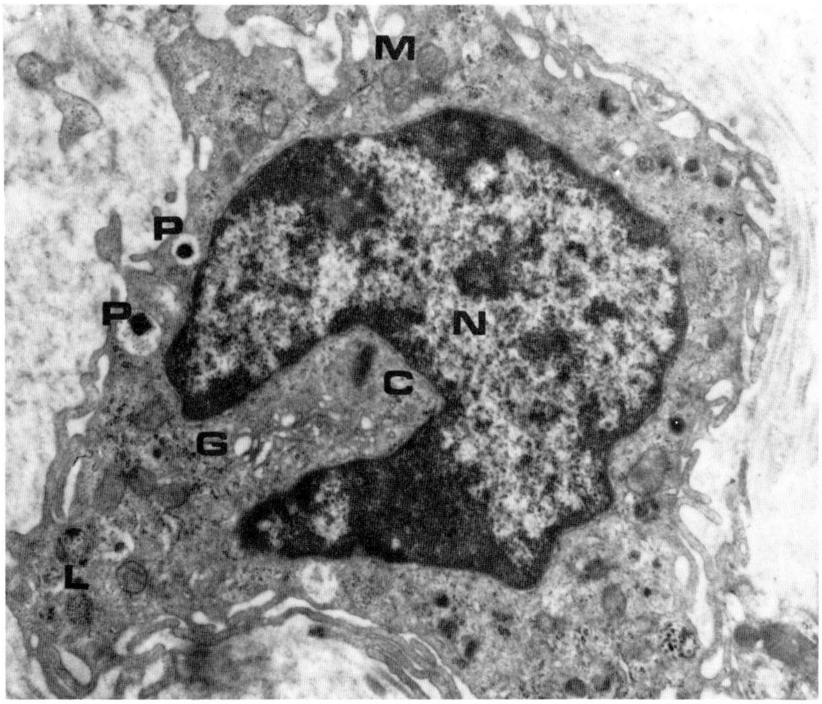

Fig. 3-14. Electron micrograph of a macrophage from loose connective tissue. The horseshoe-shaped nucleus (*N*) is typical. The Golgi apparatus (*G*) is well-developed. One of the centrioles (*C*) is visible. Mitochondria (*M*) are scattered throughout the cell. Phagosomes (*P*) and lysosomes (*L*) are typical features of active macrophages. ×26,000.

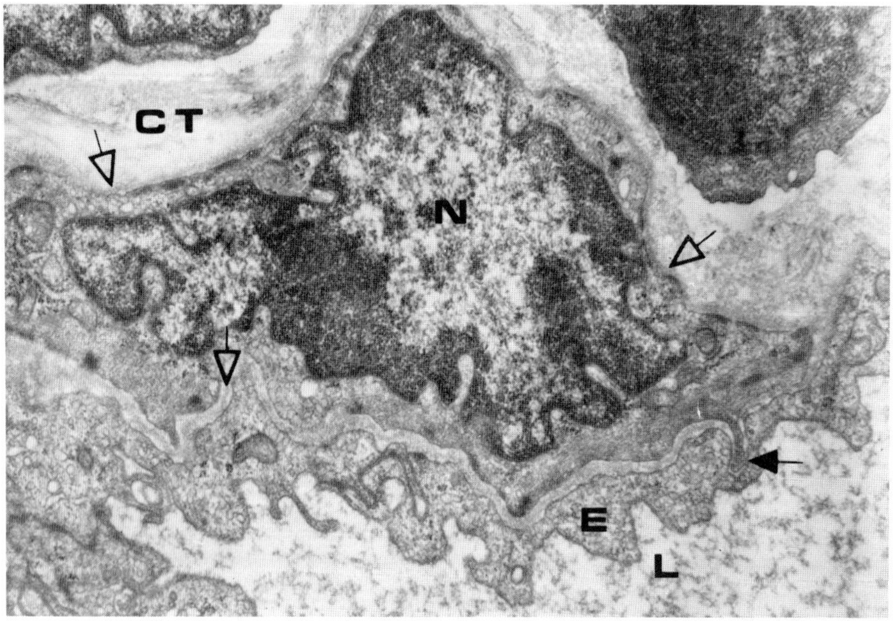

Fig. 3-15. Electron micrograph of a pericyte. The nucleus (*N*) of the pericyte is prominent. The pericyte is in close association with an endothelial cell (*E*) which defines the lumen (*L*) of the capillary. The basal lamina (*open arrows*) surrounds the pericyte and separates it from the connective tissue (*CT*) and the endothelium. The area indicated by the *solid arrow* is enlarged in Fig. 3-16. ×17,000. (Courtesy of G. P. Epling)

Mast Cells. *Mast cells* are sometimes referred to as *tissue basophils*. These cells are of variable occurrence in the connective tissue space but can be found readily along the pathway of small vessels. Usually, these cells occur in small clusters. These cells are of variable size and shape in different species. Generally, they are ovoid cells with a small, pale, ovoid and centrally located nucleus. The prominent feature is the presence of basophilic granules in the cytoplasm (Fig. 3-17). It is not uncommon to find these highly refractile granules surrounding the mast cell. These cells are fragile and rupture readily during preparatory techniques. The granules are also highly water-soluble; thus, they are rarely preserved by routine techniques.

The granules of mast cells contain two substances of medical significance, *heparin* and *histamine*. The mast cells of some species also contain *serotonin*. Heparin is significant as an anticoagulant. *Fibrinogen*, as well as other proteins, escape into the connective tissue. Heparin prevents fibrin formation and thus insures against the possible clotting of this substance in the local environment. Heparin also acts as a *clearing agent* on blood. Through a mechanism that is not understood, heparin is linked with *lipoprotein lipase*. The latter is responsible for clearing fat from blood plasma.

The release of histamine from mast cells is thought to bring about the *anaphylactic response*. This response includes the contraction of smooth muscle as well as the dilation and increased permeability of blood capillaries that results in focal swelling. Serotonin is a vasoconstrictor.

The origin, maintenance and fate of mast cells is not understood. However, it is important that the mast cell is not related to the blood basophil.

Fat Cells. *Fat cells* occur as single entities, as groups of cells or as massive sheets of cells associated with the connective tissues. Although they are associated with the connective tissues, they are not within the connective tissue space. Each cell is surrounded by a basal lamina.

Two types of fat cells are distinguishable, *unilocular* and *multilocular fat cells*. *White* or *unilocular fat cells* have a signet-ring appearance. The bulk of the cell is occupied by a large fat droplet which is rimmed by a thin margin of cytoplasm. The nucleus is displaced to one side of the cell (Fig. 3-18). In certain planes of section, the nucleus will not be apparent. In routine paraffin sections of fat cells, the space occupied by the fat droplet is all that is apparent; the solvents used in the process will have leached out the fat. Special preparation techniques, through the use of freezing and special stains, are required to demonstrate the lipids of fat cells.

In *multilocular* or *brown fat cells*, the pre-

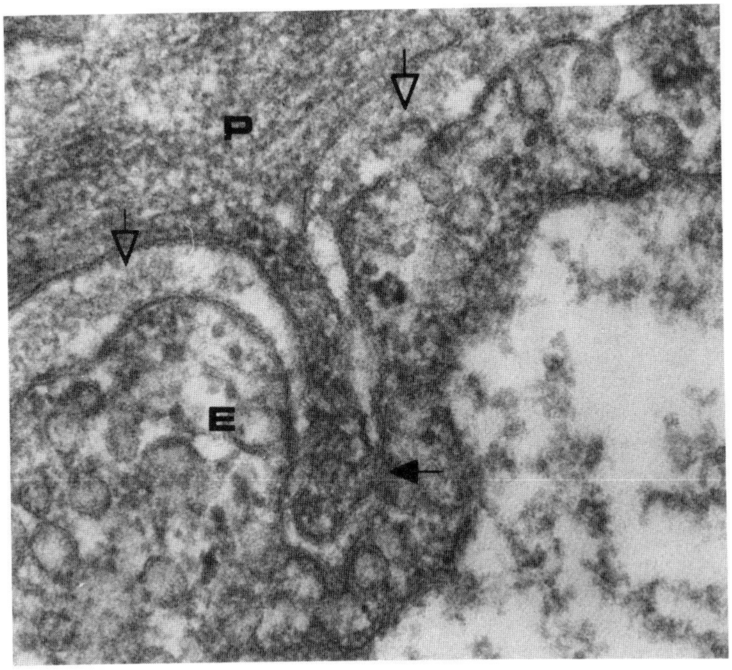

Fig. 3-16. Electron micrograph of the contact between a pericyte and an endothelial cell. The pericyte (*P*) and endothelial cell (*E*) are separated by a basal lamina (*open arrows*) except at a single contact point (*solid arrow*). ×125,000. (Courtesy of G. P. Epling).

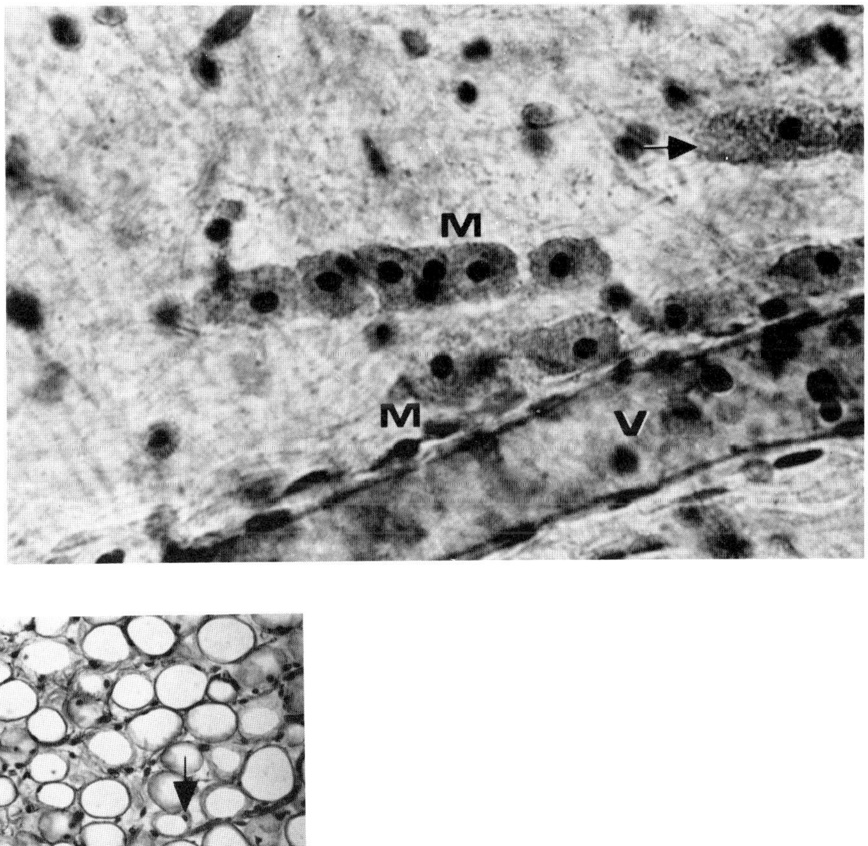

Fig. 3-17. Mast cells in a stretch preparation of loose connective tissue. The mast cells (*M*) are aligned along a blood vessel (*V*). A ruptured mast cell (*arrow*) has extruded its granules into the surrounding environment. ×160.

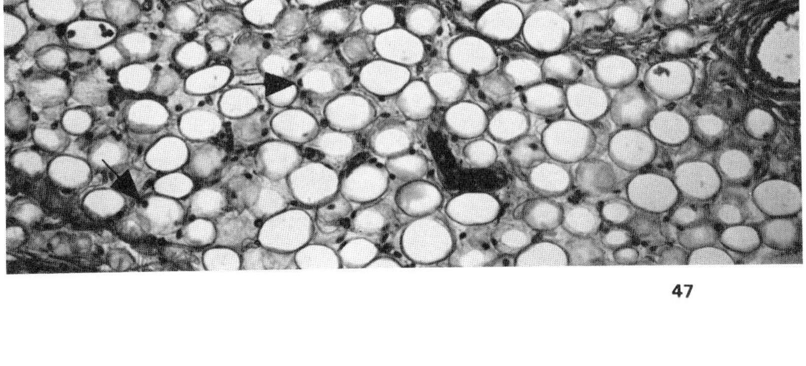

Fig. 3-18. A section of unilocular adipose tissue. *Arrows*, nuclei of those cells in a typical signet-ring configuration. ×40.

dominant feature is numerous small fat droplets. The rounded nucleus is not displaced to one side of the cell but may assume any position (Fig. 3-19). Unless special preparatory precautions are taken, the lipids are lost from this cell as well. The resulting spaces from loss of lipids by routine preparation and scattered cytoplasmic components impart a foamy appearance to these cells.

The lipid droplets of both types of fat cells are not membrane-bound. Rather, they are rimmed by a condensation of the cytoplasm which may contain some cytofilaments.

Both of these cells are important mediators of lipid and water metabolism.

Transient Cell Population

Since the resident cell population can vary with the tissue and its physiological state, it is reasonable to assume that similar conditions will influence the transient cell population. Most of the transient cells are protective and in some areas of connective tissue may be considered residents. However, in most instances their numbers will vary. The ***transient cell population*** includes *plasma cells*, *pigment cells*, *lymphocytes*, *monocytes*, *neutrophils*, *eosinophils* and *basophils*. Only the plasma cell and pigment cell will be discussed here; the blood cells are described in Chapter 7.

Plasma Cells. *Plasma cells* are responsible for the production of antibodies and occur

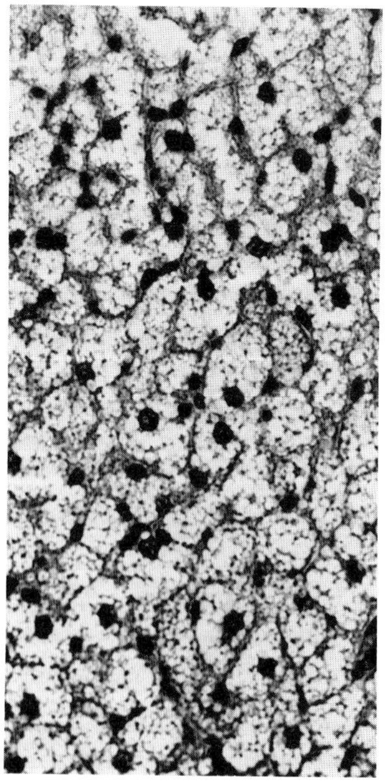

Fig. 3-19. A section of multilocular adipose tissue. Individual locules of fat are apparent within the cells. ×100.

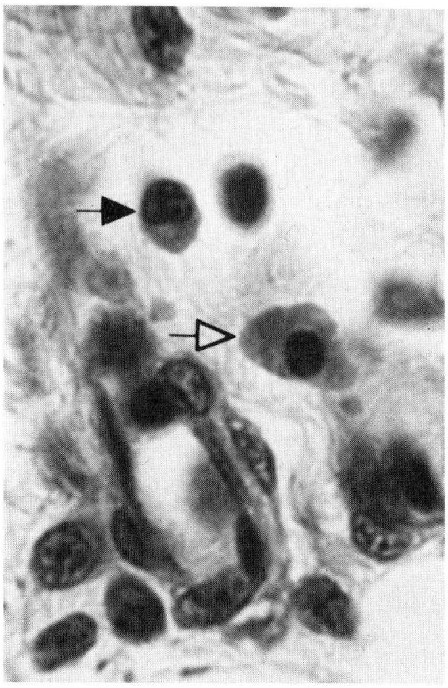

Fig. 3-20. A plasma cell of loose connective tissue. The plasma cell (*solid arrow*) is typical. Note the position of the nucleus and the negative Golgi area. A macrophage (*open arrow*) is also indicated. ×160.

in those areas of connective tissue that are subject to continuous insult. They are especially numerous in the connective tissue of the gastrointestinal, respiratory and urogenital mucous membranes.

The plasma cell is easily demonstrated by routine techniques. It is a rounded cell with a definite polarity. The basophilic cytoplasm contains the eccentrically placed and round nucleus (Fig. 3-20). The nucleus contains extensive heterochromatin which is sometimes arranged as the spokes of a wheel. A juxtanuclear, pale-staining region is often apparent. This region corresponds to the position of the well-developed Golgi apparatus. The basophilia of the cytoplasm is due to the extensive development of rough endoplasmic reticulum and free ribosomes.

Pigment Cells. This is a nondescriptive term for any cell that contains pigment. However, the means by which cells acquire pigment are quite different. *Melanoblasts* are cells derived from ***neural crest ectoderm***. These cells migrate throughout the body and come to reside in various regions—the connective tissue associated with the skin, as well as the iris and choroid of the eye. They possess the potential to produce melanin but do not do so until they have achieved their place of residence. When they begin to synthesize melanin, they are termed *melanocytes* (Fig. 3-21). Melanocytes are able to invade epithelial layers and pass their pigmentation to other cells. These passive recipients of this pigment are termed *melanophores*. Melanocytes rarely occur in the connective tissue compartment. The pigmented cells of this compartment have either passively received the pigment or have phagocytosed the pigment. Thus, they are *melanophores* or *chromatophores*.

A simple histochemical test, the *dihydroxyphenylalanine* (*DOPA*) *reaction*, is used to determine which cells are melanocytes. Only melanocytes are capable of converting DOPA into melanin because of the presence of the enzyme *tyrosinase*.

The primary function of these cells is to protect the body from excessive exposure to ultraviolet radiation. Of interest, melanoblasts and melanocytes can be involved in the formation of rapidly spreading and, therefore, potentially dangerous cancerous growths.

Embryonal Connective Tissues

Mesenchymal Connective Tissue. This typical, unspecialized mesodermal tissue of the embryo is a transitory tissue which disappears rapidly from the developing organism as differentiation occurs (Fig. 3-22). The primary constituent of this tissue is the mesenchymal cell. These stellate or fusiform cells form numerous cellular contacts and give the appearance of a ***cellular reticulum***. Although the intercellular spaces are usually pale-staining and appear devoid of any material, a ground substance of mucopolysaccharides is present. Although fibers are not common in this tissue, it is not unusual to encounter delicate collagenous or

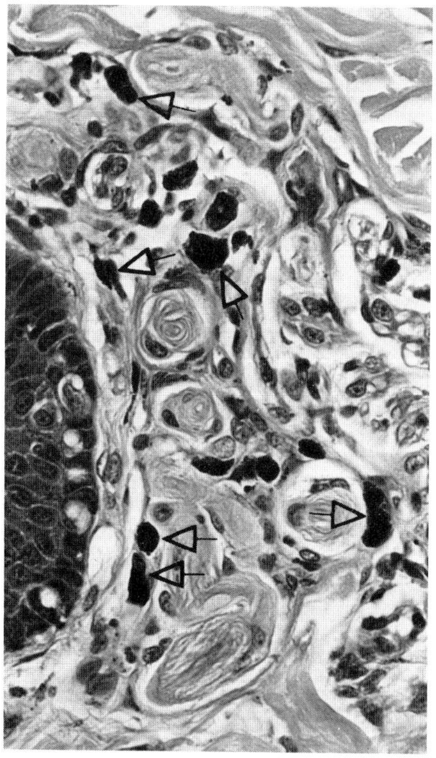

Fig. 3-21. Pigment-bearing cells. The pigment-bearing cells (*arrows*) are visible in the dermis. ×100.

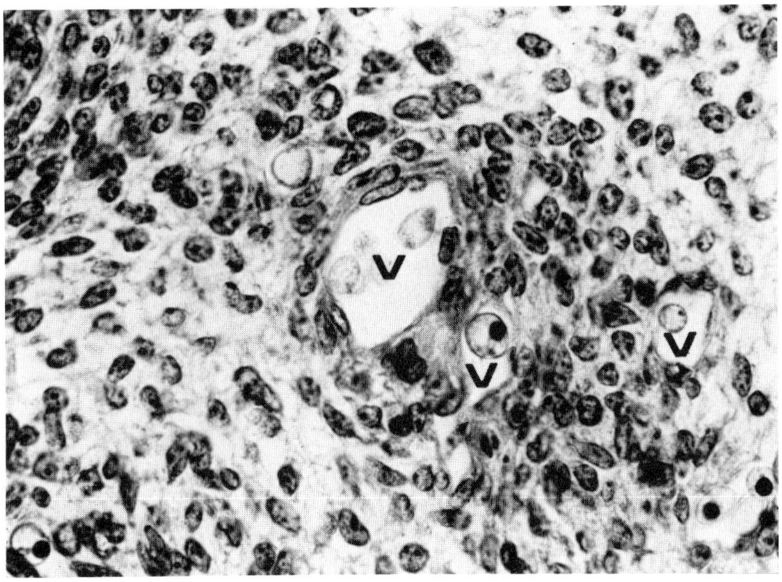

Fig. 3-22. Mesenchymal connective tissue from the limb bud of a hamster. Vessels (*V*) are scattered among the mesenchymal cells. ×160.

reticular fibrils close to cells that are differentiating into fibroblasts.

This tissue is derived from mesoderm. Most importantly, this tissue is the precursor for other tissues, such as *proper* and *special connective tissues*, *cartilage*, *bone*, *blood* and *muscle*.

In the adult, the mesenchymal connective tissue is reduced to isolated and scattered foci of mesenchymal cells in those tissues derived from it.

Mucous Connective Tissue. This connective tissue is a more advanced stage of the one described previously. It is the characteristic connective tissue of the umbilical cord (but it is not confined to it), wherein it is referred to as *Wharton's jelly* (Fig. 3-23). It consists of a cellular reticulum of *fibroblasts* and a few scattered *mesenchymal cells*. The matrix is composed of mucin and contains delicate collagenous fibers. With proper fixation the ground substance will appear granular.

In the developing embryo, this connective tissue occurs in the subepidermal regions as well as the umbilical cord. In the adult it is usually the transitory tissue deposited during the repair of supportive tissues. Also, it is found normally in the comb and wattles of gallinaceous birds. It also occurs in specific portions of the lamina propria of the ruminant omasum.

Proper Connective Tissues

Areolar Connective Tissue. This tissue is often referred to as *loose* or *ordinary* connective tissue. It is the most ubiquitous of the connective tissues. It is composed of a loose array of randomly oriented *collagenous*, *reticular* and *elastic fibers*. Collagenous fibers, however, are the predominant extracellular formed elements. All of the cells previously described, except the primitive reticular cell, may be found in this tissue. Normally, the predominant cell type is the fibroblast or fibrocyte (approximately 90 per cent). The prevalent ground substance component is hyaluronic acid; however, some chondroitin sulfate and dermatan sulfate are also present. This combination of matrix components imparts a soft, pliable and elastic quality to the tissue.

The accompanying photomicrograph of a stretch preparation of subcutis serves as an example of loose connective tissue (Fig. 3-24). Within the ground substance, collagenous and elastic fibers are apparent in random orientation. Reticular fibers are present but require special staining techniques for their demonstration. Numerous vessels and scattered fat cells are present. At higher magnification, all the cells mentioned should be encountered.

In section, loose connective tissue assumes a different appearance (Fig. 3-25). Nevertheless, the interlacing and randomly oriented bundles of fibers with cells scattered between is typical. In this instance the primary cell population consists of fibroblasts. Examination at higher magnification will reveal the other cells.

In a section of loose connective tissue associated with the upper digestive tract a very different appearing tissue is observed (Fig. 3-26). Although the fibers and fibroblasts are present, the predominant feature is the presence of defensive cells—lymphocytes, plasma cells and macrophages. This appearance is typical in this and similar regions that are subjected to constant insult. The previous example of this tissue (Fig. 3-25) would appear similar in response to an insult.

Morphological features:

1. A fine network of collagenous, reticular and elastic fibers loosely arranged in random array.
2. The predominance of collagenous fibers and fibroblasts.
3. The large number of cells and few fibrous components.
4. The variation of cellular constituents with location and physiology.

Occurrence: Subepithelial connective tissue, mesenteries, between muscles and nerves, components of most organs.

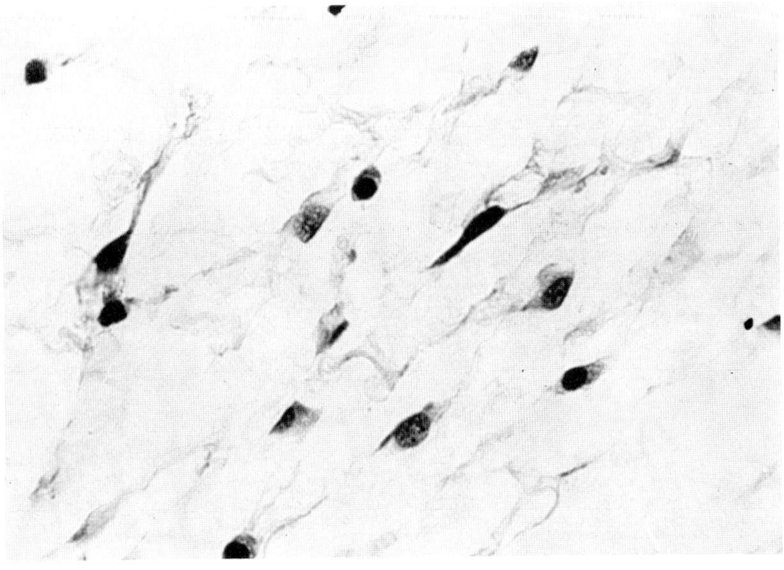

Fig. 3-23. Mucous connective tissue from the ovine umbilical cord. ×160.

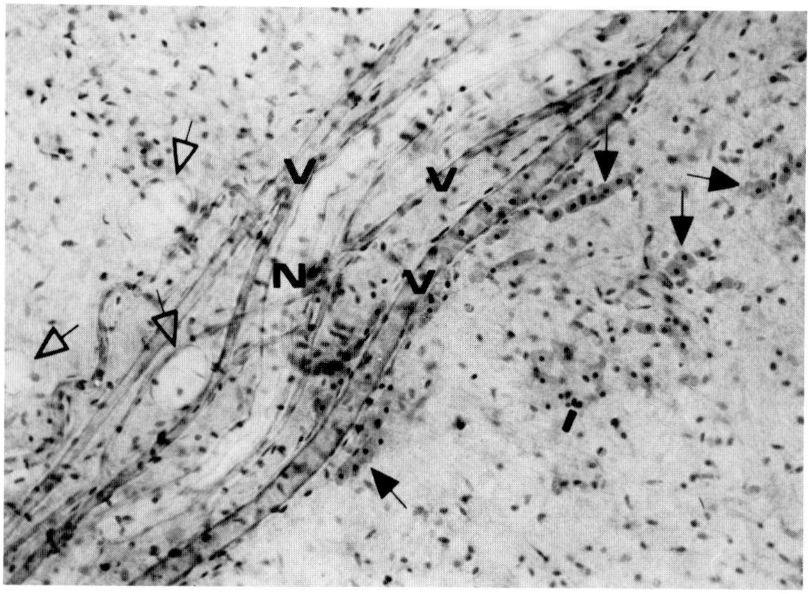

Fig. 3-24. Stretch preparation of loose connective tissue. Vessels (*V*) and a nerve (*N*) traverse the tissue. Mast cells (*solid arrows*), a macrophage (*bar*) and fat cells (*open arrows*) are present. ×40.

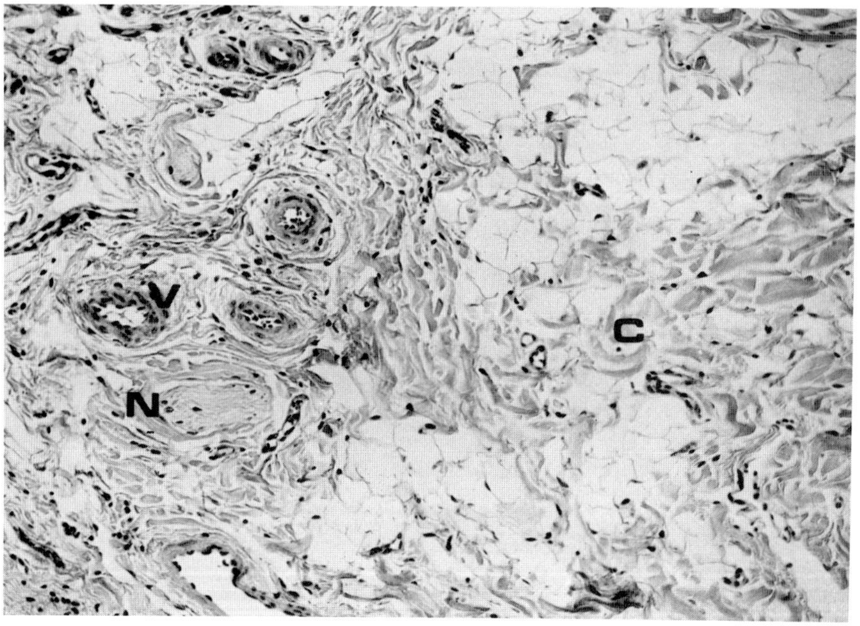

Fig. 3-25. Section of loose connective tissue. Collagen (*C*), nerves (*N*) and blood vessels (*V*) are scattered throughout the tissue as well as fibroblasts and fat cells. ×40.

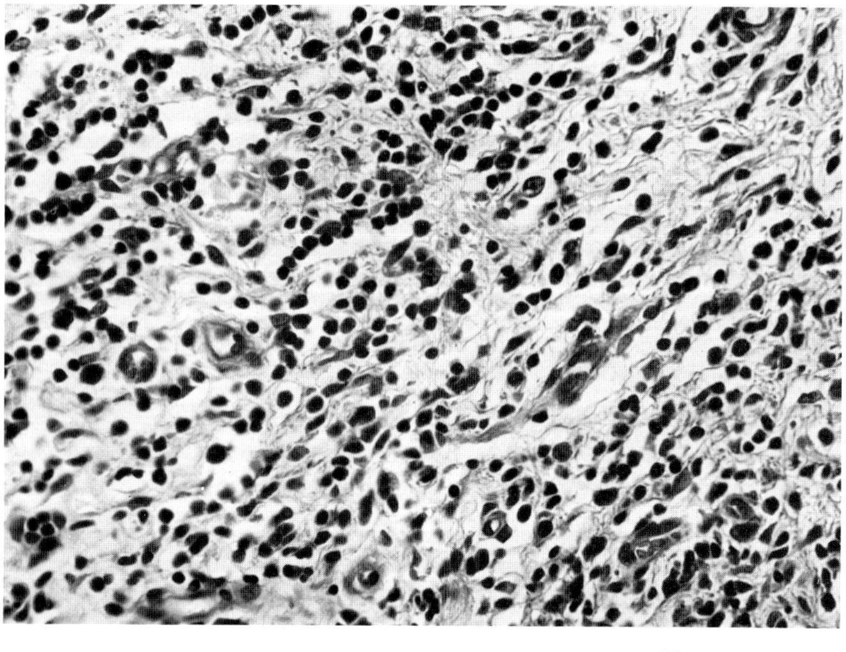

Fig. 3-26. Section of loose connective tissue from the upper digestive tract. The basic components are similar to those of Fig. 3-25. However, the presence of lymphocytes imparts a hypercellular appearance to the tissue. ×100.

Dense White Fibrous Connective Tissue—Irregular. This connective tissue, most often abbreviated as *DWFCT*, is closely related to areolar connective tissue. Admittedly, there are gradations between the two extremes of loose and dense. Primarily, DWFCT differs quantitatively from loose connective tissue.

In section (Fig. 3-27), thick, wavy collagenous fibers predominate. Reticular and elastic fibers, however, are also present. The same cells encountered or potentially present in loose connective tissue are also present or potentially so in this tissue. Normally, however, there are fewer cells in this tissue.

Morphological features:

1. A coarse network of collagenous fibers with some reticular and elastic fibers.
2. The reduced number of cells and increased number of fibers when compared to loose connective tissue.

Occurrence: Subepidermal connective tissue, capsules of organs.

Dense White Fibrous Connective Tissue—Regular. The significant feature of this connective tissue is the orderly, parallel orientation of collagenous fibers (Fig. 3-28). Although distinct bundles of fibers are present, they do not appear as such in routine preparations. Rather, the fibers (with H and E) form a relatively homogeneous pink-staining background. The fibrocytes seem to delimit the extent of individual bundles. The nuclei of these cells vary from oval to thin and elongated. They are dark-staining. Although present, it is rare that the thin processes of the cytoplasm will be distinct. The nuclei and fibers may appear wavy. Although other cell types may be present normally, they are extremely rare.

This connective tissue is the predominant type that forms *tendons* and *ligaments*. However, individual bundles of these highly organized fibers are held together by loose connective tissue. Also, the few blood vessels and nerves observed are surrounded by loose connective tissue. The ordered collagenous fiber arrangement resists the great amount of strain applied to tendons and ligaments.

The varied and reduced vascularity of this tissue at different foci accounts for the variable regenerative ability. It is not avascular. Once damaged, revascularization from loose connective tissue occurs sufficiently to bring about good repair.

Diagnostic features:

1. Very few cells, mostly fibrocytes.
2. Predominance of heavy collagenous fibers which appear as a relatively homogeneous background matrix between cells.
3. Longitudinal arrangement of fibrocytes.
4. Cells and fibers may appear wavy.
5. Collagen stains a light pink with H and E.

Occurrence: Tendons (attachments of muscle to bone), ligaments (attachments of bone to bone), aponeuroses (thin, sheetlike tendons).

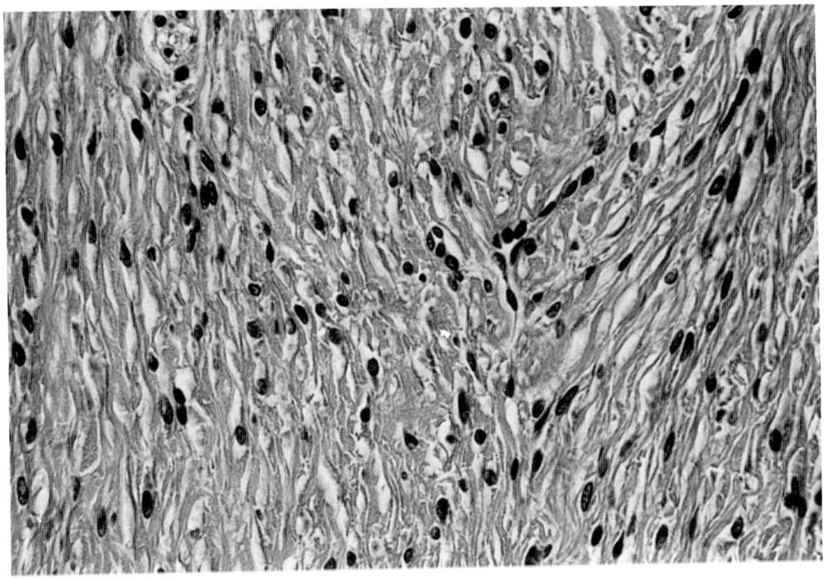

Fig. 3-27. A section of DWFCT, irregularly arranged, from tunica albuginea of the canine testis. Collagenous fibers and fibroblasts are the predominant elements. ×100.

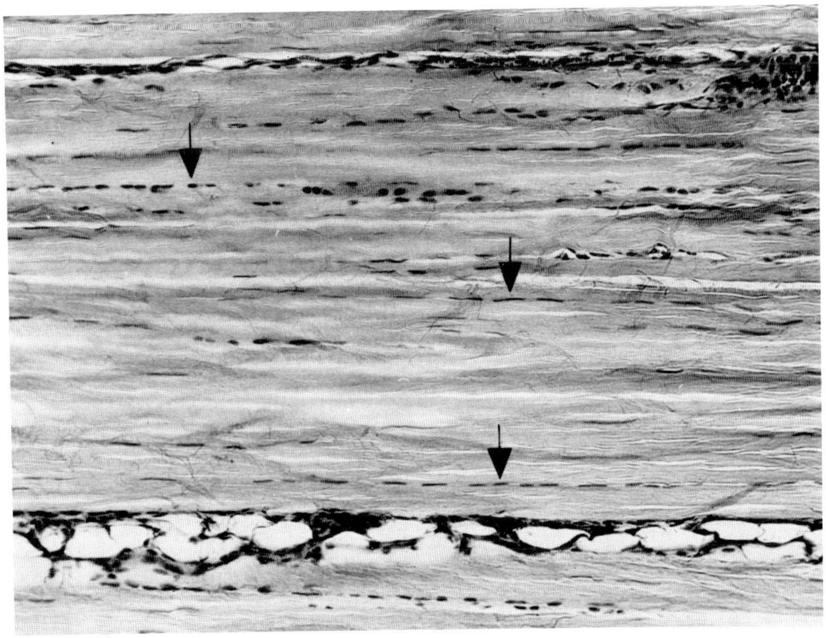

Fig. 3-28. A section of DWFCT, regularly arranged. The arrangement of the fibrocytes (*arrows*) in this tendon is typical. ×40.

Elastic Connective Tissue. This type of connective tissue is a basic modification of the type previously discussed. The predominant fiber type is the elastic fiber, while the predominant cell type is the fibroblast (Fig. 3-29). The fibers are larger than collagenous fibers and branch and anastomose with each other. Individual elastic fibers are surrounded by areolar connective tissue. The elastic fibers are quite ordered as evidenced by the orderliness of the fibroblasts. Without careful examination, this tissue is easily confused with DWFCT. Upon careful examination, however, the presence of bright pink-staining fibers (with H and E) is a good distinguishing characteristic. With special staining, the elastic fibers are readily apparent (Fig. 3-30).

In cross-section, care must be taken to distinguish the extrafibrillar position of the nuclei (Fig. 3-31) of the fibroblasts. Otherwise, this tissue could be mistaken for others we will encounter later. Note also the large cross-sectional area of the fibers.

This tissue is of limited but important occurrence. It is extensively modified in the walls of arteries, wherein it forms a very resilient complex with smooth muscle.

Diagnostic features:

1. Predominance of elastic fibers in parallel and branched array.

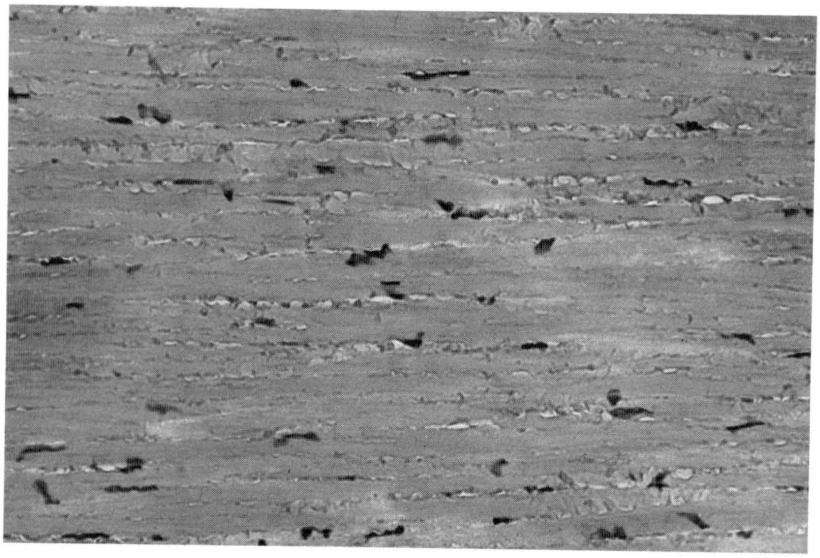

Fig. 3-29. A longitudinal section of elastic connective tissue from the nuchal ligament. ×100.

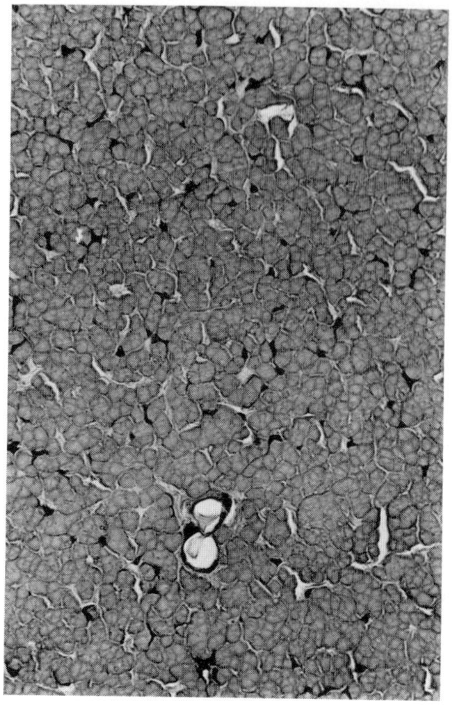

Fig. 3-31. Cross-section of elastic connective tissue. ×80.

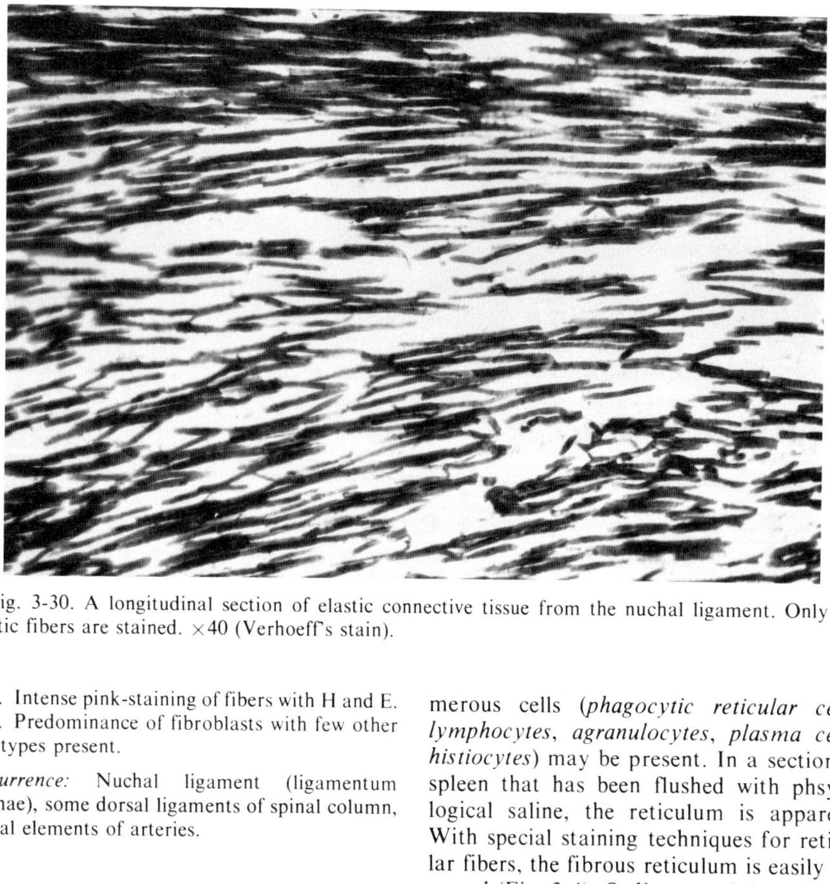

Fig. 3-30. A longitudinal section of elastic connective tissue from the nuchal ligament. Only the elastic fibers are stained. ×40 (Verhoeff's stain).

2. Intense pink-staining of fibers with H and E.
3. Predominance of fibroblasts with few other cell types present.

Occurrence: Nuchal ligament (ligamentum nuchae), some dorsal ligaments of spinal column, mural elements of arteries.

Special Connective Tissues

Reticular Connective Tissue. The predominant fiber in this tissue is the reticular fiber. The fibrous network is complemented by a cellular reticulum of primitive reticular cells. Since this type of tissue is associated with *cytogenic organs* (*cell-producing*), careful examination is required to observe the cellular and fibrous reticulum through the mass of other cells normally present. Numerous cells (*phagocytic reticular cells*, *lymphocytes*, *agranulocytes*, *plasma cells*, *histiocytes*) may be present. In a section of spleen that has been flushed with phsyiological saline, the reticulum is apparent. With special staining techniques for reticular fibers, the fibrous reticulum is easily observed (Fig. 3-4). Ordinary staining will not definitively demonstrate this tissue; however, the association with certain cell types is a good key to its identification.

Reticular fibers also constitute the finer interstitial connective tissue of some parenchymatous organs. In this instance, the defensive cells will be absent or of an occurrence similar to that expected of areolar connective tissue. In these areas the predominant cell is the fibroblast.

Diagnostic Features:
1. A fine reticulum of fibers and cells; the fibers are argyrophilic.
2. Usually associated with cytogenic organs that produce defensive cells.

Occurrence: Stroma (fibrous support) of lymphatic and hematopoietic organs; finer interstitial connective tissue of some organs.

Pigmented Connective Tissue. This tissue is areolar connective tissue in which pigment-containing cells occur (Fig. 3-21). It is of limited but significant occurrence.

Diagnostic feature: occurrence of pigment-bearing cells.

Occurrence: Iris and choroid coat; connective tissue associated with pigmented skin.

Special Tissue

Adipose Tissue. Adipose tissue has been considered a special connective tissue. However, the occurrence of a basal lamina around each cell is inconsistent with the concept of the basal lamina and its relationship to the connective tissue space. The exact relationship of adipose tissue to connective tissue needs further clarification.

This tissue may consist of multilocular or unilocular fat cells. It may occur as vast sheets of fat cells or as isolated populations of fat cells. Each fat cell is surrounded by reticular fibers which are continuous with the associated areolar connective tissue. Numerous vessels are scattered throughout this tissue, which may be composed of brown or white fat cells or a mixture of both. In sections the cells may appear hexagonal (Figs. 3-18, 3-24).

Diagnostic features:

1. High density of closely packed fat cells.
2. White adipose tissue, unless specifically stained, appears as a loose fibrous network.
3. Brown fat appears as a mass of foamy cells.

Occurrence: White fat is scattered throughout the soma; brown fat is found in rodents and hibernating animals in the region of the pectoral girdle and at various other foci in other mammals.

References

Extracellular Components

Bensley, S. H.: On the presence, properties and distribution of the intercellular ground substance of loose connective tissue. Anat. Rec. *60:*93, 1934.

Chain, E. and Duthie, E. S.: Identity of hyaluronidase and the spreading factor. Brit. J. Exp. Path. *21:*234, 1940.

Fahrenback, W. H., Sandberg, L. B., and Cleary, E. G.: Ultrastructural studies on early elastogenesis. Anat. Rec. *155:*563, 1966.

Greenlee, T. K., Jr., Ross, R. and Hartman, J. L.: The fine structure of elastic fibers. J. Cell Biol. *30:*59, 1966.

Hodge, A. J. and Petruska, J. A.: Recent studies with the electron microscope on ordered aggregates of the tropocollagen macromolecules. In *Aspects of Protein Structure*. Academic Press, New York, p. 239, 1964.

Lillie, R. D.: Histochemistry of connective tissues. Lab. Invest. *1:*30, 1952.

Mancini, R. E.: Connective tissue and serum proteins. Int. Rev. Cytol. *14:*193, 1963.

Petruska, J. A. and Hodge, A. J.: A subunit model for the tropocollagen macromolecule. Proc. Nat. Acad. Sci. USA *51:*871, 1964.

Cellular Components

Chapman, J. A., Gough, J. and Elves, M. W.: An electron microscopic study of the *in vitro* transformation of human leucocytes. II. Transformation to macrophages. J. Cell Sci. *2:*371, 1967.

Cohn, Z. A., Fedorko, M. E. and Hirsch, J. G: The *in vivo* differentiation of mononuclear phagocytes. IV. The ultrastructure of macrophage differentiation in the peritoneal cavity and in culture. J. Exp. Med. *123:*747, 1966.

Cohn, Z. A., Fedorko, M. E. and Hirsch, J. G.: The *in vivo* differentiation of mononuclear phagocytes. V. The formation of macrophage lysosomes. J. Exp. Med. *123:*757, 1966.

Downey, H.: The development of histiocytes and macrophages from lymphocytes. J. Lab. Clin. Med. *45:* 499, 1955.

Fawcett, D. W.: An experimental study of mast cell degranulation and regeneration. Anat. Rec. *121:*29, 1955.

Hayward, J. S., Lyman, C. P. and Taylor, C. R.: The possible role of brown fat as a source of heat during arousal from hibernation. Ann. N. Y. Acad. Sci. *131:*441, 1965.

Kolouch, F., Jr.: The lymphocyte in acute inflammation. Amer. J. Path. *15:*413, 1939.

Litt, M.: Eosinophils and antigen-antibody reaction. Ann. N. Y. Acad. Sci. *116:*964, 1964.

Maximow, A. A.: The morphology of the mesenchymal reactions. Arch. Pat. Lab. Med. *4:*557, 1927.

Movat, H. Z. and Fernando, N. V. P.: The fine structure of connective tissue. I. The fibroblast. Exp. Molec. Path. *1:*509, 1962.

Movat, H. Z. and Fernando, N. V. P.: The fine structure of connective tissue. II. The plasma cell. Exp. Molec. Path. *1:*535, 1962.

Padawer, J. (ed.): Mast cells and basophils. Ann. N. Y. Acad. Sci. *103:*1, 1963.

Sheldon, H., Hellenberg, C. H. and Winegard, A. I.: Observations on the morphology of adipose tissue. Diabetes *11:*378, 1962.

Smith, R. E. and Hock, R. J.: Brown fat: thermogenic effector of arousal in hibernation. Science *140:*199, 1963.

Taliaferro, W. H.: The cellular basis for immunity. Ann. Rev. Microbiol. *3:*159, 1949.

Weinstock, A. and Albright, J. T.: The fine structure of mast cells in normal human gingiva. J. Ultrastruct. Res. *17:*245, 1967.

4 Supportive Tissues—Cartilage

General Characteristics

Form and Function. Cartilage is a specialized connective tissue which consists of a few cells embedded within an amorphous, gel-like substance. In a manner similar to the activity of fibroblasts in other connective tissues, the cells of cartilage secrete various substances and become embedded in their own secretory products. However, these secretory products impart a firm but resilient quality to the matrix. These qualities suit cartilage to its functional role in *weight-bearing, movement* and *organ integrity*.

Cartilage does not have primitive mesenchymal cells scattered throughout it. Rather, the mesenchymal cells from which it arises, as well as those that allow growth, are located at the periphery of the cartilage in a membrane referred to as the *perichondrium*. These cells differentiate into *chondroblasts*, the cartilage-forming cells of the body. At a different stage in their life cycle, chondroblasts are referred to as *chondrocytes*.

The chondroblastic line of differentiation is the means by which new cartilage is deposited upon pre-existing cartilage. This type of growth is called *appositional* growth. Once growth has occurred and the chondroblasts have become embedded in their own products, growth does not cease. Chondroblasts are capable of dividing within the confines of their *lacunae*. This mitotic activity from within causes expansion of the resilient matrix. This type of growth is *interstitial*. Most cartilage utilizes both mechanisms for growth.

Cartilage is an avascular tissue. Although large blood vessels pass through cartilage, there are no capillaries which directly supply the nutritional needs of this tissue. All metabolites must diffuse from the periphery to the cells in the depths of the tissue. The porosity of the matrix, therefore, is an important factor in maintaining the tissue. With age this task becomes more difficult. The natural fate of cartilage is to become mineralized. This increases the problem of percolation of metabolites through the matrix. The older cells die, the tissue is removed by phagocytic cells and bone is deposited in its place.

Cartilage is the primary support tissue of the fetus. It provides good support for the body and affords an easy mechanism for growth. It is not, however, limited to the fetus. Its primary locations in the adult are the *articular surfaces of bones, upper respiratory passages* and *larynx*, and the *pinna of the ear*.

The repair of cartilage is not readily mediated even though there is a good supply of mesenchymal cells. Normally, the repair process proceeds through fibrous connective tissue which later may be converted into cartilage or replaced by bone. Fibrocartilage repair offers special problems because this tissue lacks a perichondrium.

Classification. Three types of cartilage are recognized and readily distinguished from each other: *hyaline, elastic* and *fibrous*.

Matrix Components

Fibers. The predominant fiber of cartilage is the fine collagenous fiber. In hyaline cartilage, these fibers are scattered in a random pattern throughout the matrix. In routine preparations they are rarely observed because their index of refraction is similar to that of the ground substance.

In fibrocartilage, however, the collagenous fibers are easily observed because they are the primary constituents of the cartilage. The amount of ground substance is greatly reduced.

The fibers of elastic cartilage include both collagenous and elastic fibers. Elastic fibers are readily visualized with normal preparatory techniques, as well as by special staining procedures.

Ground Substance. The principal constituents of the ground substance are the *acid mucopolysaccharides*. These repeating units of *monosaccharides* (acetylglucosamine, glucuronate) are sulfated. These are the *chondroitin sulfates* which are conjugated to proteins. These sulfated substances strongly attract basic dyes and are responsible for the basophilia that characterizes some cartilage matrices. However, this basophilia is not homogeneous. Moreover, some matrices are acidophilic. These differences in the staining of cartilage ground substance imply either an uneven distribution, a masking or a total absence of sulfates in various regions of the matrix.

Types of Cartilage

Hyaline Cartilage. Grossly, hyaline cartilage has a white, glassy appearance; thus the name (*hyalos* (Gr.), glass). In section this avascular tissue is separated from the surrounding tissue by the *perichondrium* (Fig. 4-1), which is analogous to the capsule of other organs. The perichondrium consists of a *fibrous* and a *cellular* portion. The fibrous portion is dense white fibrous connective tissue (DWFCT) which may blend insensibly with the surrounding connective tissue. Unless artifactual separation of the connective tissue occurs, the peripheral limits of the perichondrium are difficult to define. The cellular portion contains *mesenchymal cells* which give rise to fibroblasts of the fibrous perichondrium as well as to chondroblasts (Fig. 4-2). The cellular portion will be prominent in young growing cartilage only.

In young cartilage a definite gradation from *mesenchymal cells* to *chondroblasts* to *chondrocytes* is observed (Fig. 4-3). As mesenchymal cells differentiate into chondroblasts, these cells deposit matrix components and surround themselves in their own secretory products. As a result a small *lacuna* (lake) is formed. The cells reside within these spaces without any contact with other cells or the surface. Although the lacunae of cartilage may be devoid of cells in some sections, this is an artifact of sectioning. The lacunae, as well as the cells within them, are flattened with their long axis parallel to the surface. The matrix of this region is generally acidophilic.

Maturation of the chondroblasts into

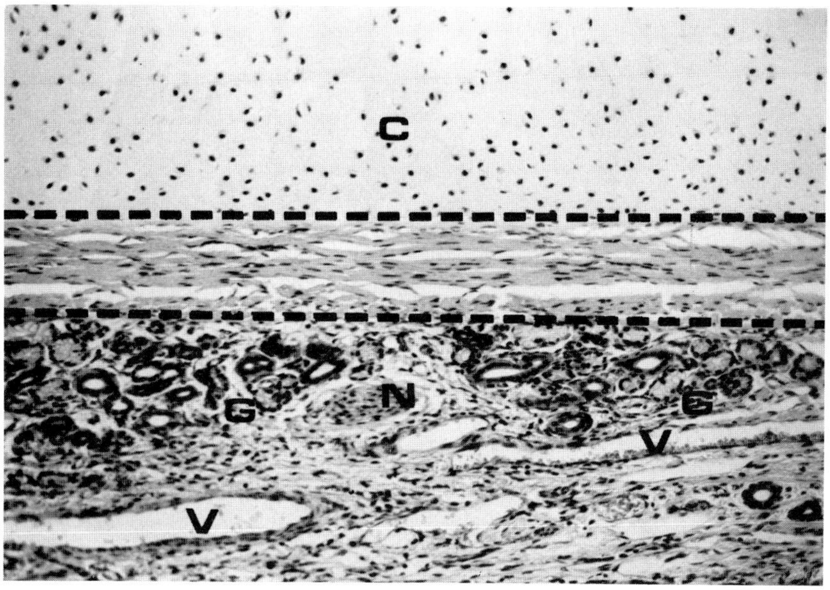

Fig. 4-1. Cartilage and associated tissue from an ovine nasal turbinate. The cartilage (*C*) is surrounded by a perichondrium (within *dashed lines*). The peripheral loose connective tissue (below perichondrium) contains nerves (*N*), glands (*G*) and vessels (*V*). ×40. All light micrographs are the original magnifications. All electron micrographs are the final magnifications.

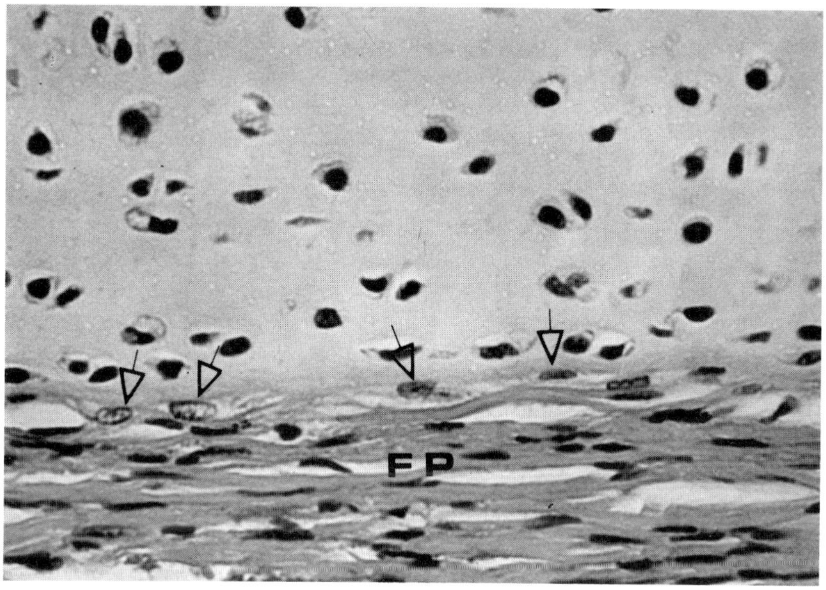

Fig. 4-2. Perichondrium of cartilage. The fibrous perichondrium (*FP*) consists of collagenous fibers and fibroblasts. The cellular perichondrium consists of mesenchymal cells (*arrows*) ×160.

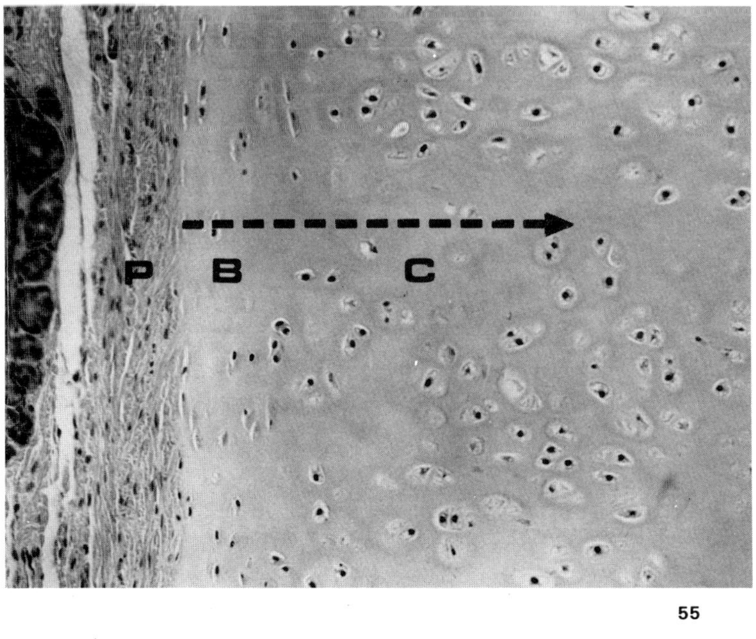

Fig. 4-3. Growing cartilage from the feline larynx. The perichondrium (*P*) is peripheral to the chondroblastic layer (*B*). Enlargement of chondroblasts and differentiation into chondrocytes (*C*) is apparent. *Dashed arrow*, progression of differentiation. ×40.

chondrocytes is accompanied by a cellular hypertrophy, an enlargement of the lacunae and a change in lacunar shape to an ovoid or angular configuration (Fig. 4-4). Chondrocytes are also clustered as *isogenous groups* or *cell nests*. These cell nests represent the daughter cells of a single chondrocyte that underwent mitosis during the growth process. Further, these nests indicate that interstitial growth has been accomplished.

Chondrocytes appear as smooth-surfaced cells that are withdrawn away from the lacunar margins (Fig. 4-5). In fact, with the electron microscope the numerous processes of these cells are seen in intimate contact with the lacunar margins (Fig. 4-6).

The lacunar margin of individual chondrocytes or isogenous groups are more basophilic than other portions of the matrix. This marked basophilia delimits the *capsule* or *territorial matrix* of these cells, while the lighter area of basophilia marks the *interterritorial matrix*. The marked basophilia of the territorial matrix is attributable to numerous sulfate groups on mucopolysaccharides and probably represents the active contribution of chondrocytes to the maintenance of its matrix.

In some instances hyaline cartilage is devoid of a perichondrium. This is typical of the hyaline cartilage of the articular surfaces (Fig. 4-7). Growth and/or replacement of cartilage in these locations is accomplished by the interstitial mechanism only.

Diagnostic features:

1. Few cells embedded within a gel-like matrix which appears afibrillar.
2. Limits of the tissue are usually well marked by a perichondrium.
3. The matrix generally stains with basic dyes.

Occurrence: Most bone-forming sites of the fetus and neonatal animal; articular cartilages; airways of the respiratory tree; support structures of nose and larynx.

Elastic Cartilage. Grossly, this tissue is yellow and is more resilient than hyaline cartilage due to the content of elastic fibers. Other than the presence of elastic fibers, this tissue is identical to hyaline cartilage. In some foci, more isogenous groups than those characteristic of hyaline cartilage may be apparent.

The elastic fibers are demonstrable with hematoxylin and eosin as pink-staining fibers scattered throughout the matrix (Fig. 4-8). They are more easily demonstrated with special staining techniques (Fig. 4-9).

Diagnostic features:

1. Identical to hyaline cartilage, except for the presence of elastic fibers.
2. Isogenous groups may be more frequently observed.

Occurrence: External ear (pinna); external auditory canal; eustachian tube; parts of the laryngeal cartilages; epiglottic cartilage.

Fibrous Cartilage. This tissue is also called *fibrocartilage* and is of limited occurrence

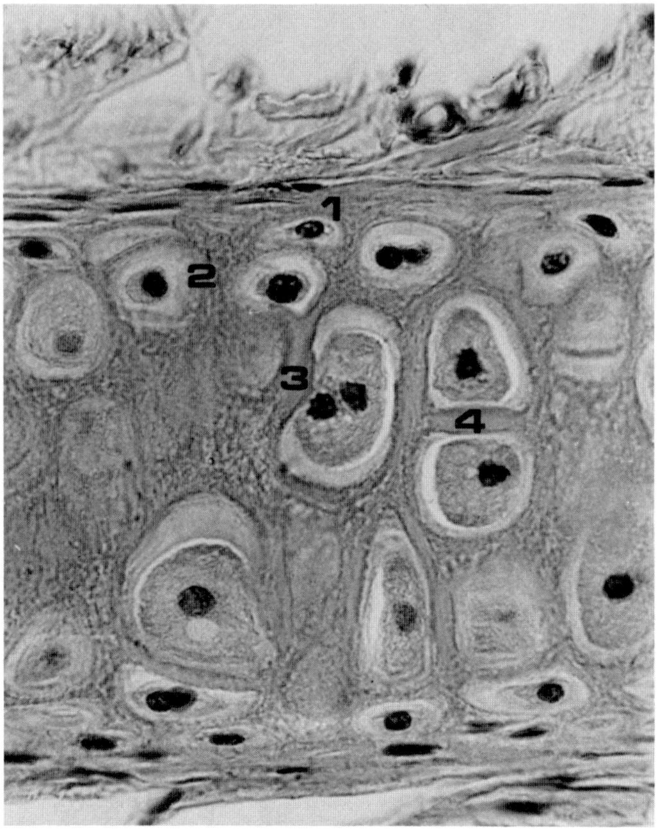

Fig. 4-4. Young elastic cartilage of the porcine pinna. Chondroblasts (*1*) enlarge as chondrocytes (*2*), divide (*3*) and form isogenous groups (*4*). ×160.

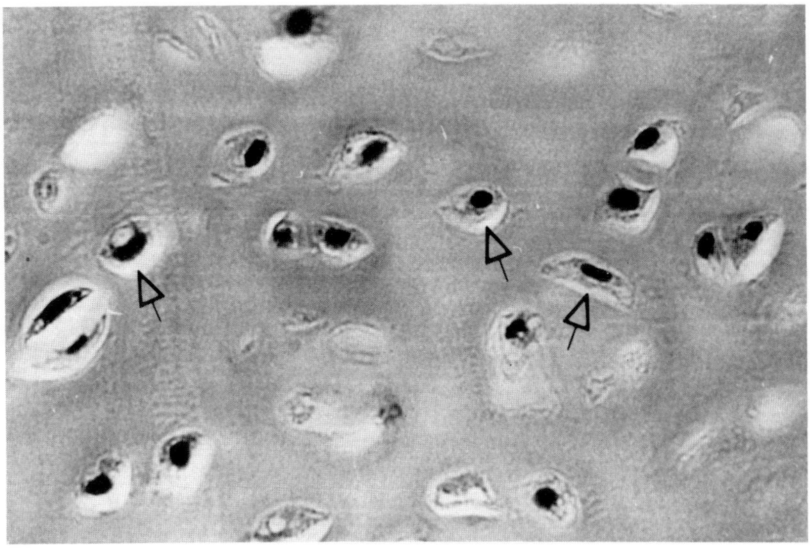

Fig. 4-5. Mature chondrocytes as single cells and cell nests. The cellular limits are withdrawn from the lacunar margins (*arrows*). ×100.

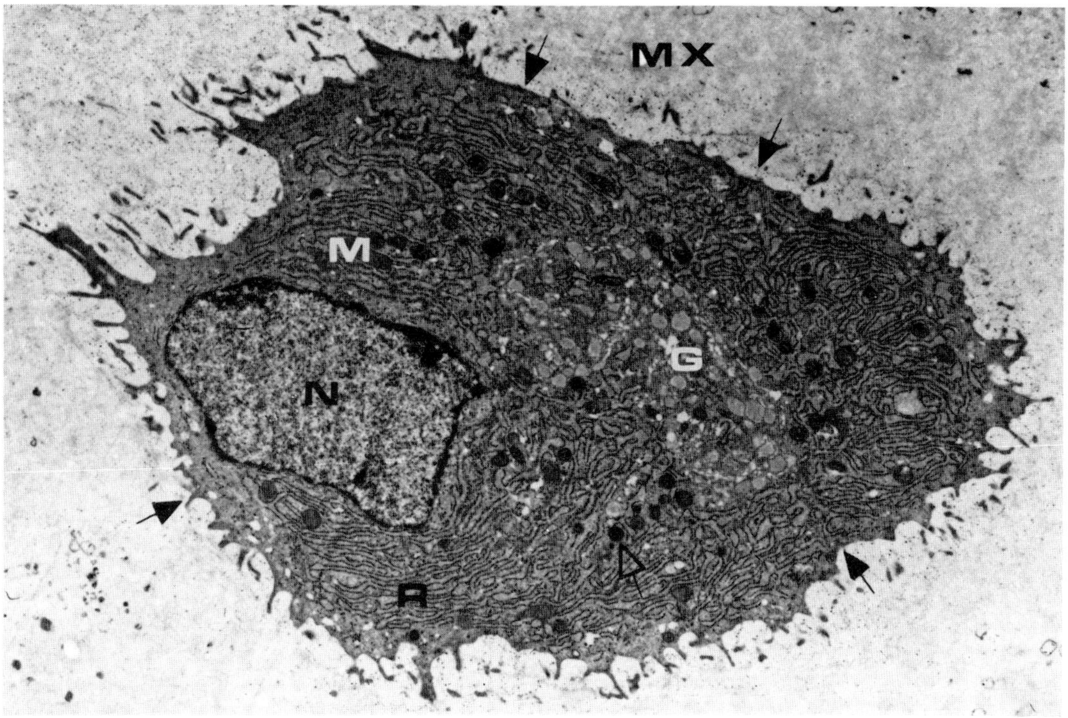

Fig. 4-6. Electron micrograph of a chondrocyte. The nucleus (*N*) is vesicular. The cytoplasm has an extensive Golgi apparatus (*G*) and granular endoplasmic reticulum (*R*). Mitochondria (*M*) and dense bodies (*open arrow*) are also present. The interface (*solid arrows*) between the cell and matrix (*MX*) is very close. The lacunar space of light microscopy is probably artifact. ×5,000.

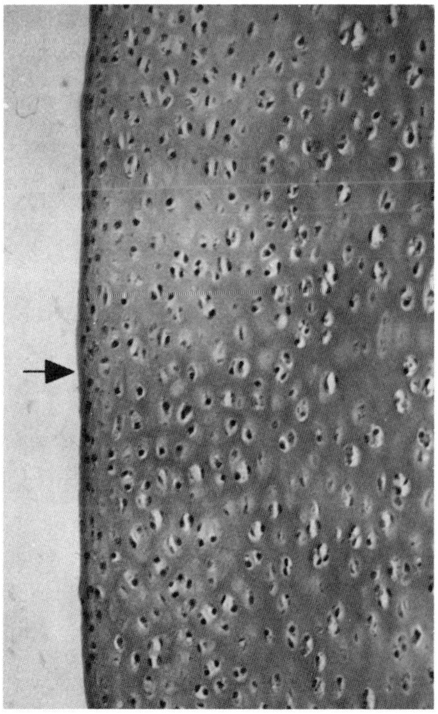

Fig. 4-7. Articular cartilage. The articular surface (*arrow*) is devoid of a perichondrium. ×38.

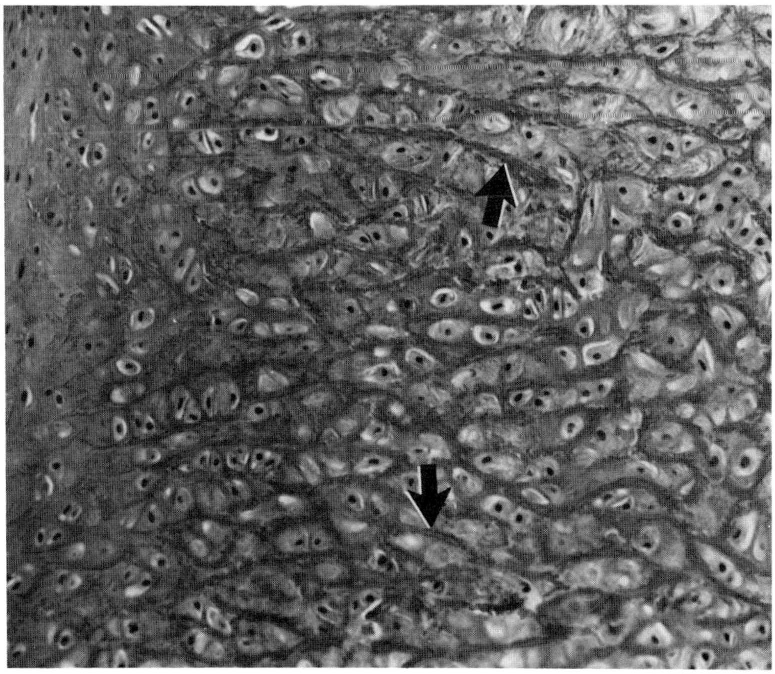

Fig. 4-8. Elastic cartilage from the bovine epiglottis. The elastic fibers (*arrows*) are predominant features between the chondrocytes. ×40.

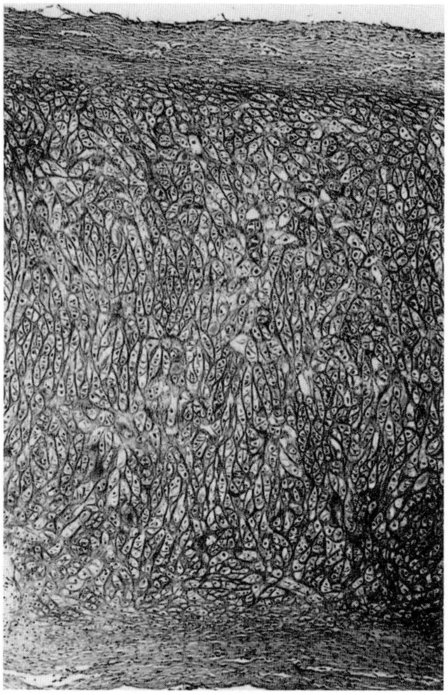

Fig. 4-9. Elastic cartilage with a special stain. The elastic fibers are stained black. ×13 (Verhoeff's stain).

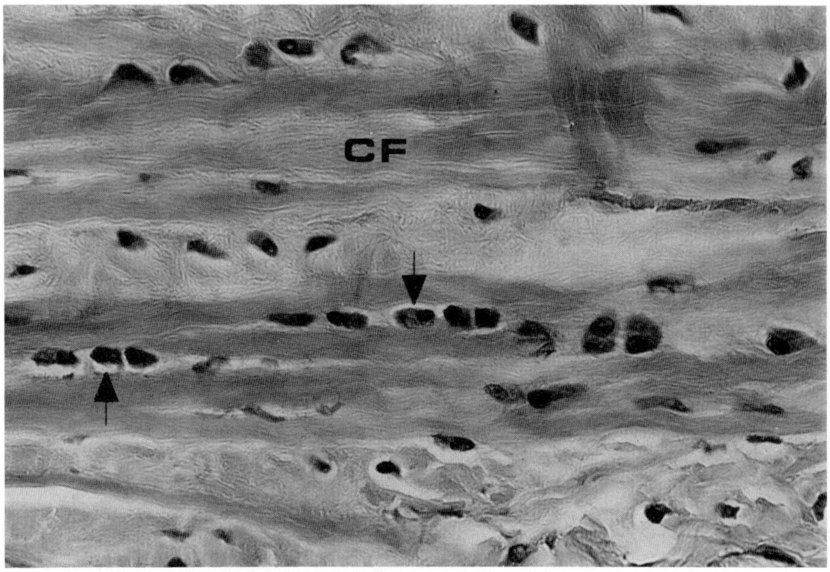

Fig. 4-10. Fibrocartilage. The collagenous fibers (*CF*) are predominant. Chondrocytes and their lacunae (*arrows*) are spaced between the collagen. ×100.

in the body. Although of limited occurrence, it imparts additional strength to cartilage and DWFCT.

Fibrocartilage is an intermediate form between DWFCT and cartilage. Since visible collagenous fibers predominate, it may be considered a modified DWFCT.

Large collagenous *fascicles* (bundles) are oriented in an orderly array and are separated by isolated portions of cartilage (Fig. 4-10). The chondrocytes, located between the fascicles, secrete diminutive quantities of territorial matrix materials.

The classical appearance of this tissue is the *herringbone* configuration (Fig. 4-11) in which collagenous bundles are oriented to each other in the form of a V. Typically, however, the orientation of the fibers may not appear as orderly as that (Fig. 4-12).

Fibrocartilage is usually located at points of transition between DWFCT and cartilage and between DWFCT and bone. It imparts additional strength to these points of transition and/or attachment.

The lack of a definitive perichondrium creates repair problems for this tissue.

Diagnostic features:

1. Predominance of coarse collagenous bundles in parallel and/or V-shaped orientation.
2. Presence of chondrocytes and limited amounts of matrix material between the bundles.

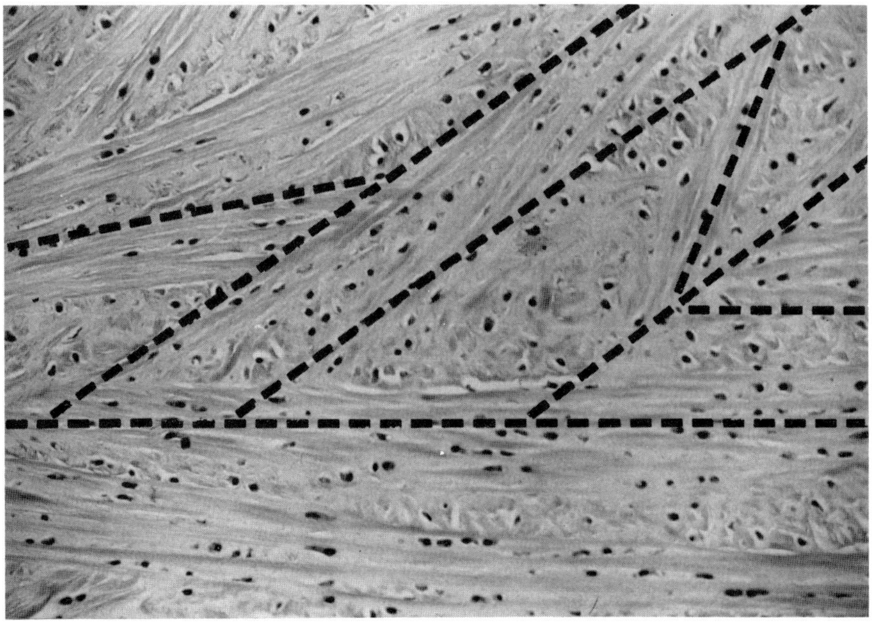

Fig. 4-11. Fibrocartilage from a meniscus. The herringbone configuration (*dashed lines*) is readily apparent. ×40.

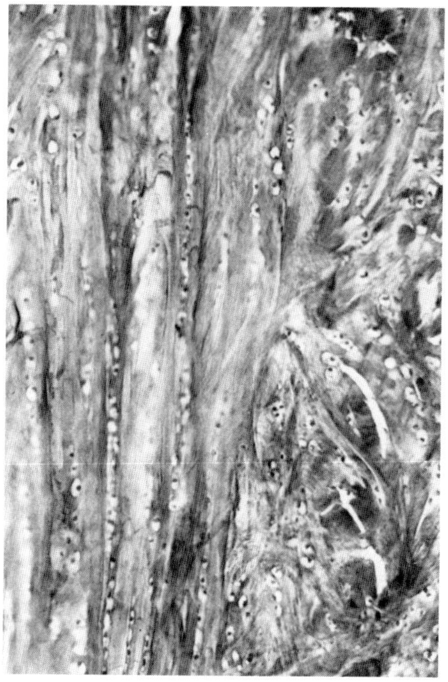

Fig. 4-12. Fibrocartilage. The herringbone configuration is not as apparent as in the previous micrograph. ×39 (Verhoeff's stain).

Occurrence: Intervertebral disks; attachments of certain tendons and ligaments to bone; menisci.

References

Amprino, R.: On the incorporation of radiosulfate in the cartilage. Experientia *11*:65, 1955.

Cameron, D. A. and Robinson, R. A.: Electron microscopy of epiphyseal and articular cartilage matrix in the femur of the newborn infant. J. Bone Joint Surg. *40*:163, 1958.

Godman, G. C. and Lane, N.: On the site of sulfation in the chondrocyte. J. Cell Biol. *21*:353, 1964.

Godman, G. C. and Porter, K. R.: Chondrogenesis studies with the electron microscope. J. Biophys. Biochem. Cytol. *8*:719, 1960.

Kuettner, K. E., Soble, L. W., Ray, R. D., Croxen, R. L., Passovoy, M. and Eisenstein, R.: Lysozyme in epiphyseal cartilage. II. The effect of egg white lysozyme on mouse embryonic femurs in organ cultures. J. Cell Biol. *44*:329, 1970.

Maroudas, A.: Distribution and diffusion of solutes in articular cartilage. Biophys. J. *10*:365, 1970.

Palfrey, A. J. and Davies, D. V.: The fine structure of chondrocytes. J. Anat. *100*:213, 1966.

Pritchard, J. J.: A cytological and histochemical study of bone and cartilage formation in the rat. J. Anat. *86*:259, 1952.

Sheldon, H. and Robinson, R. A.: Studies on cartilage. I. Electron microscope observations on normal rabbit ear cartilage. J. Biophys. Biochem. Cytol. *4*:401, 1958.

Spycher, M. A., Moor, H. and Ruettner, J. R.: Electron microscopic investigations on aging and osteoarthritic human articular cartilage. II. The fine structure of freeze-etched aging hip joint cartilage. Z. Zellforsch. *98*:512, 1969.

Svajger, A.: Chondrogenesis in the external ear of the rat. Z. Anat. Entwicklungsgesch. *131*:236, 1970.

5 Supportive Tissues—Bone

General Characteristics

Form and Function. Bone is a very specialized connective tissue which consists of a few cells embedded within a gel-like substance which becomes mineralized to varying degrees. The method of secretion and the manner in which the cells become embedded in the matrix are similar to those phenomena observed in cartilage. Although the fibrous and ground substance components of bone are similar to those of cartilage (collagen and acid mucopolysaccharides), the mineral phase of the matrix makes bone distinct from the other connective tissues. This mineral component consists of *amorphous calcium phosphate* and the *hydroxyapatite crystal*.

Three other characteristics significantly distinguish bone from cartilage. Whereas cartilage cells are embedded within a matrix without contact with each other or the surface, bone cells (*osteocytes*) are in contact with each other through cellular processes located in small canals (*canaliculi*) in the matrix. The cellular processes are not only a means through which coordinated activity may be mediated, but they and the canalicular space are significant in transport mechanisms through bone. Since materials diffuse less readily through mineralized matrices (as in mineralized cartilage), the significance of this canalicular system to bone viability cannot be overemphasized.

Whereas cartilage is avascular, bone is an extremely vascular tissue. Numerous blood vessels are scattered throughout bone. The cells of bone are rarely more than 2 mm from a supply of blood vessels.

Ossification, or the formation of bone, occurs in two distinct but related steps. The *osteoblasts* (bone-forming cells) secrete the *osteoid* (collagen and ground substance) which then undergoes *mineralization*. This mineralized matrix, unlike the normal cartilaginous matrix, is minimally expandable. Bone, therefore, is unable to grow by the interstitial mechanism. Appositional growth is the only mechanism by which bone can grow. This requires a copious supply of *stem cells* or *osteoprogenitor cells*.

The stem cells of bone are located in covering membranes called the *periosteum* and *endosteum*. The periosteum consists of a *fibrous* and *cellular layer* and is similar to the perichondrium. The endosteum is functionally similar to the periosteum but does not have a well-developed fibrous layer. A cellular layer is present, but the cells form a less definitive lining than the periosteum. Whereas the periosteum surrounds the outside or growing peripheral limits of bone, the endosteum lines the inside of bone and is intimately associated with the vessels that traverse the bone. Because of the periosteal and endosteal relationships to bone, all surfaces of bone (except some in old age) are covered by cells.

Besides its obvious function in the support and locomotion of the body, bone satisfies some very important metabolic requirements by virtue of its labile nature. Once formed, the mineral of bone is not irreversibly lost to the body. Rather, it may be removed by very distinct mechanisms. It functions, therefore, as an important dynamic store of calcium and phosphate. Calcium is significant in numerous metabolic activities (cardiac irritability, muscle contraction, enzyme activation and others), while phosphorus is the basis for a phosphate-based metabolism involving the production of energy-rich adenosine triphosphate.

Classification. As a tissue, bone may be organized in numerous and varied configurations. Despite this great diversity, there are just two types of bone, *woven* and *mature*.

Matrix Components

Fibers. The fibrous component of bone is the typical fine collagenous fiber. Unlike most of the other connective tissues, the collagen of bone may be organized into highly ordered arrays. In *mature bone* this organization pattern is manifested as layers of collagenous fibers deposited upon each other in a helical pattern; each layer of a helix is oriented at a different angle to the previous layer. This pattern of collagen deposition imparts a lamellar appearance to mature bone (*lamellar bone*) which is especially apparent with polarizing microscopy.

The collagenous fibers of *woven* (*immature*) *bone* are not as organized. Accordingly, the lamellar appearance, as well as the ordered appearance with polarizing microscopy, is lacking.

Ground Substance. The ground substance of bone is similar to that of cartilage. The acid mucopolysaccharide content of bone, however, is less than that of hyaline cartilage. The ground substance, therefore, usually is acidophilic. The mucopolysaccharides are conjugated to proteins. Numerous cross-linkages between the mucosubstances and collagen (glycoprotein) impart a rigidity to the ground substance.

Unmineralized ground substance is referred to as *osteoid*. These substances, including collagen, comprise the organic phase of the matrix.

Matrix. The amount of organic material in bone remains relatively constant throughout life. It usually comprises about 35 per cent per unit volume. The remaining percentage, up to 65 per cent, is occupied by the mineral phase of bone. Bone mineral is not deposited maximally at the time osteoid is formed. Rather, there is a gradual deposition which begins with about 50 per cent of the maximum mineral load. Gradually, 100 per cent mineralization is achieved. The addition of mineral is at the expense of water in the matrix. Maximally mineralized bone contains less water than minimally mineralized bone. Although there are differences in the amount of mineral in bone, normal bone should contain about 65 per cent mineral per unit volume. Any deviation from this value may be indicative of an abnormality.

The *hydroxyapatite crystal* is the predominant form of bone mineral. This is a complex lattice structure consisting of calcium, phosphorus and hydroxyl ions. The molecular formula for this crystalline structure is $Ca_{10}(PO_4)_6(OH)_2$. Although the formula $Ca_5(PO_4)_3OH$ is also correct, the spatial arrangement of the crystal cannot be satisfied with the latter. Numerous cations (Mg^{++}, Mn^{++}, Na^+ and others) and anions (lactate, citrate, carbonate, Cl^-, F^-) may be substituted into the crystalline structure, as well as being complexed to the surface of the molecule.

Amorphous calcium phosphate also occurs in variable quantities in bone mineral. The exact significance of its occurrence is not understood but is currently the object of intensive research.

The histological study of bone may be approached by examination of either *demineralized* or *mineralized* (ground) sections. Demineralization is accomplished by two primary means, *chelation* or *acid hydrolysis*. Through this approach, sectioning is facilitated. The tissue section thus prepared consists of osteoid (bone from which mineral has been removed). Good cytological detail is retained. The use of mineralized samples, however, complements the information available from sections that have been demineralized. Mineralized samples are usually cut with a diamond-tipped saw blade or ground on an abrasive material. Through special staining techniques, information concerning the quality and quantity of the mineral phase is available. Both approaches will be presented in this discussion.

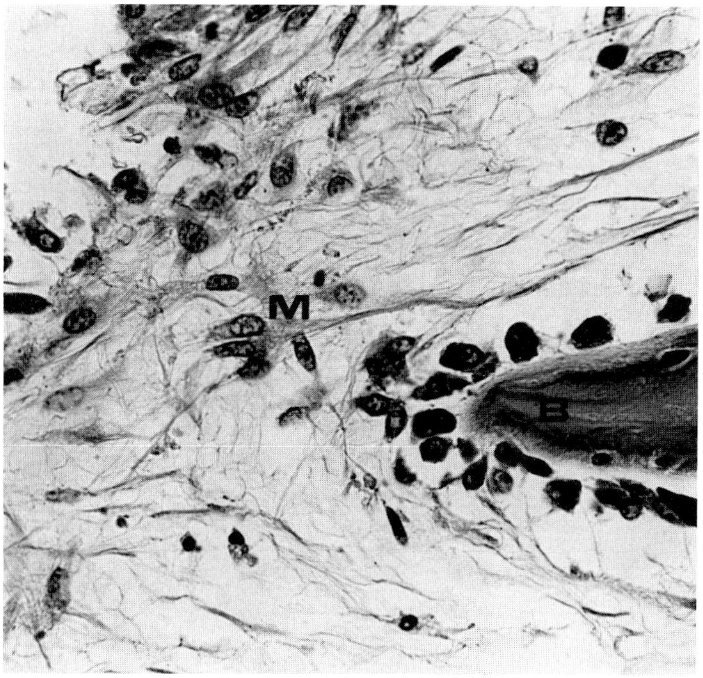

Fig. 5-1. Stem cells of bone. A spicule of bone (*B*) is surrounded by bone cells. Mesenchymal cells (*M*) are located peripheral to these. ×100. All light micrographs are the original magnifications. All electron micrographs are the final magnifications.

Cellular Components

Stem Cell. The *stem cell* or *mesenchymal cell* associated with bone is typical. It is located in the periosteum or endosteum and is the "back-up" cell of those that are in contact with the bone surface (Fig. 5-1). During differentiation, the mesenchymal cell gives rise to an *osteoprogenitor cell*. This is a cell that is biochemically and cytochemically different from the mesenchymal cell. It is, in essence, committed to become a bone cell. Mesenchymal cells undergo mitosis and commit *one* of the daughter cells to the differentiation of bone cells. In this way, the mesenchymal cell population as well as the bone cell population is maintained. This is the typical mode of operation of all stem cells.

Osteoblasts. These cells are the bone-forming cells of the body. They are responsible for the secretion of tropocollagen and acid mucosubstances. Most importantly, they are also the storage cells of the mineral used in mineralization. This mineral is stored in mitochondria and is released upon some activation signal.

Osteoblasts cover most bone surfaces. During periods of inactivity these cells assume a spindle shape (Fig. 5-2). The cytoplasm is weakly basophilic and surrounds a single oval or round nucleus. During periods of activity the cells hypertrophy and become polarized (Fig. 5-3). The single nucleus, with a prominent nucleolus, is displaced to the end of the cell away from the bone surface. The cytoplasm is moderately basophilic due to the high content of ribosomal ribonucleic acid. A well-developed Golgi apparatus and numerous mitochondria are characteristic.

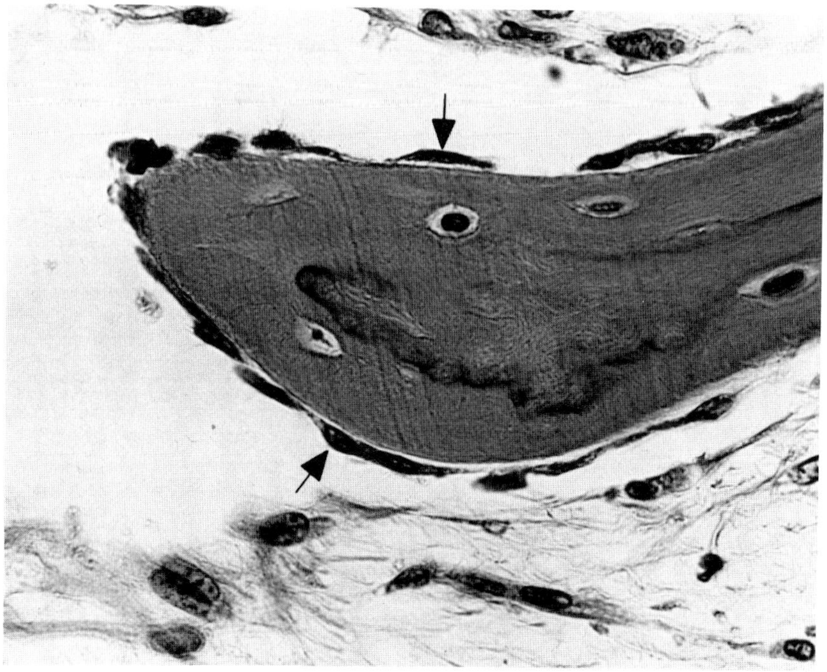

Fig. 5-2. Inactive lining cells. The spindle-shaped lining cells (*arrows*) are osteoblasts. ×160.

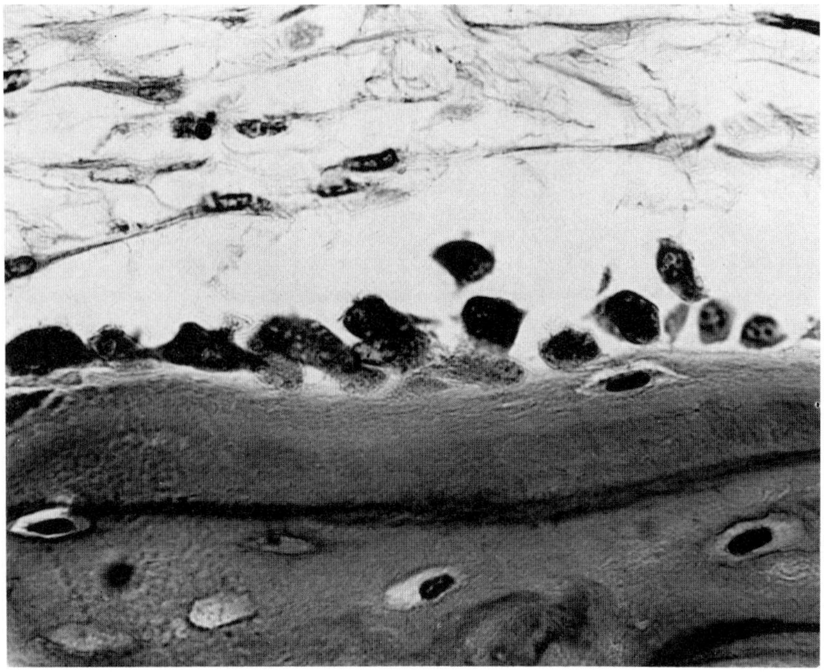

Fig. 5-3. Active lining cells. The lining cells are cuboidal and active. Compare with Fig. 5-2. ×160.

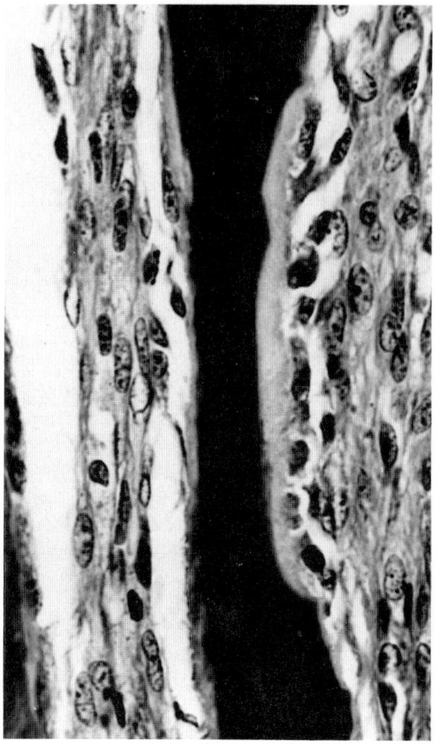

Fig. 5-4. Osteoid seam in a demineralized section of bone. The light-staining region is osteoid seam. ×140.

The activity of osteoblasts along a bone-forming surface is well-synchronized. The cells produce approximately 2 μm^3 of osteoid per day. This osteoid accumulates, layer upon layer, until a definitive *osteoid seam* is apparent which is approximately 10–15 μm thick. This osteoid seam, which has never been mineralized, is a lighter pink (hematoxylin and eosin stain) than the osteoid which has been mineralized (Fig. 5-4). The osteoid seam is set apart from the remaining osteoid by a dark-staining *reversal line*, the region from which mineralization of the osteoid seam will progress. With mineralized sections and special staining techniques, the osteoid seam is apparent; however, cellular detail is not preserved (Fig. 5-5).

As the osteoblasts secrete their products and retreat before the advancing front of osteoid, a few of the cells (about 1 of 10) become embedded in their own secretory products. At this point the osteoblasts are called osteocytes.

Osteocytes. *Osteocytes* are osteoblasts that have become embedded in their own secretory products. Osteocytes are sometimes observed shortly after they have become embedded in the osteoid seam. These cells are referred to as *osteoid osteocytes* (Fig. 5-6). Once the interstitial substance becomes mineralized, these cells are simply referred to as osteocytes.

With the light microscope, the osteocytes appear similar to osteoblasts. How-

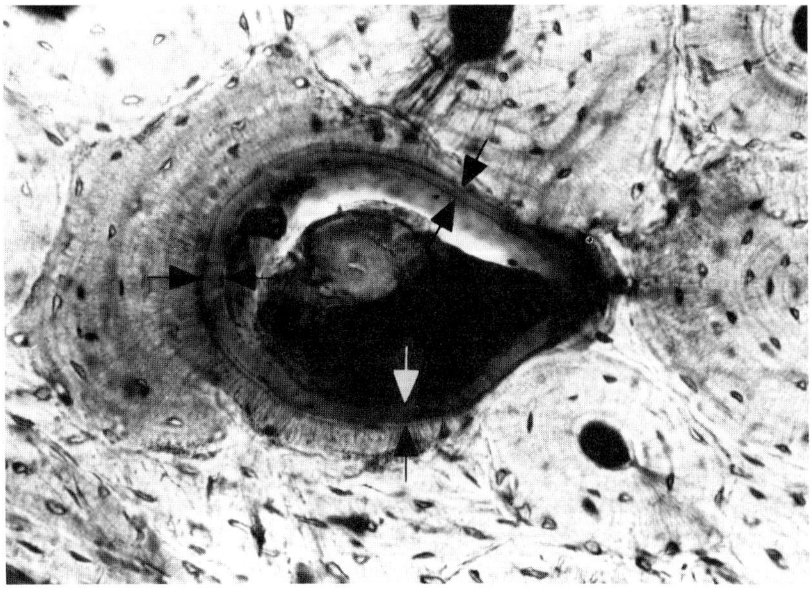

Fig. 5-5. Osteoid seam in a mineralized sample of bone. The *arrows* delimit the osteoid seam. ×25 (ground bone section).

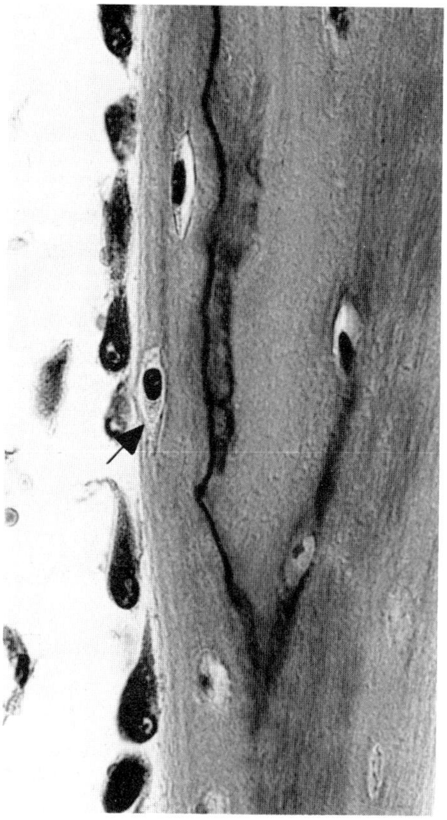

Fig. 5-6. An osteoblast has just been incorporated into the bone as an osteoid osteocyte (*arrow*). ×160.

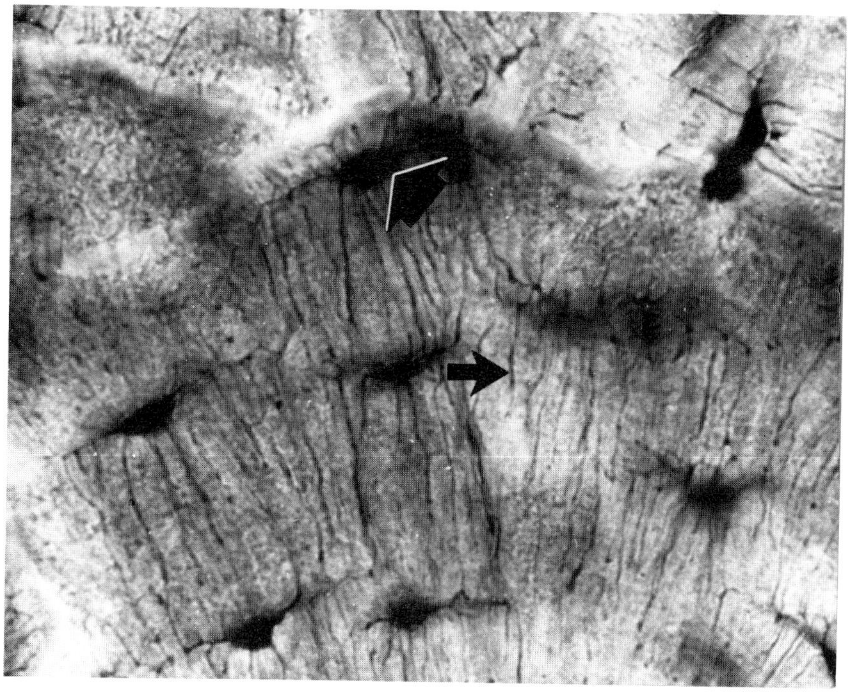

Fig. 5-7. The canalicular system of bone. Osteocytic lacunae (*large arrow*) are continuous with canaliculi (*small arrow*). ×200 (ground bone section).

ever, cellular processes are more prominent and the cytoplasm is either weakly basophilic or acidophilic. The osteocyte is a less active form of the osteoblast. The *lacunae*, and the cell as well, may vary from round to lenticular depending upon the type of bone in which they reside. As a result of fixation, osteocytes will be retracted away from the lacunar surface. Occasionally, lacunae may appear empty; this is the artifactual result of sectioning. However, empty lacunae may also indicate pathological changes in bone.

Although the cellular processes of osteocytes are not readily seen at the light microscopic level, the *canaliculi* are easily observed in mineralized sections (Fig. 5-7). These canaliculi form an extensive communicative network between osteocytes and the cells on the bone surface (Fig. 5-8). Each canaliculus is occupied by a cellular process of an osteocyte.

The osteocytes, once the "forgotten cells of bone," are significant in the maintenance of bone matrix. Moreover, they are responsible for the removal of bone mineral from the perilacunar region for the homeostatic maintenance of serum calcium levels. This process is referred to as *osteolysis*.

Osteoclasts. *Osteoclasts* are multinucleated giant cells of the body which are re-

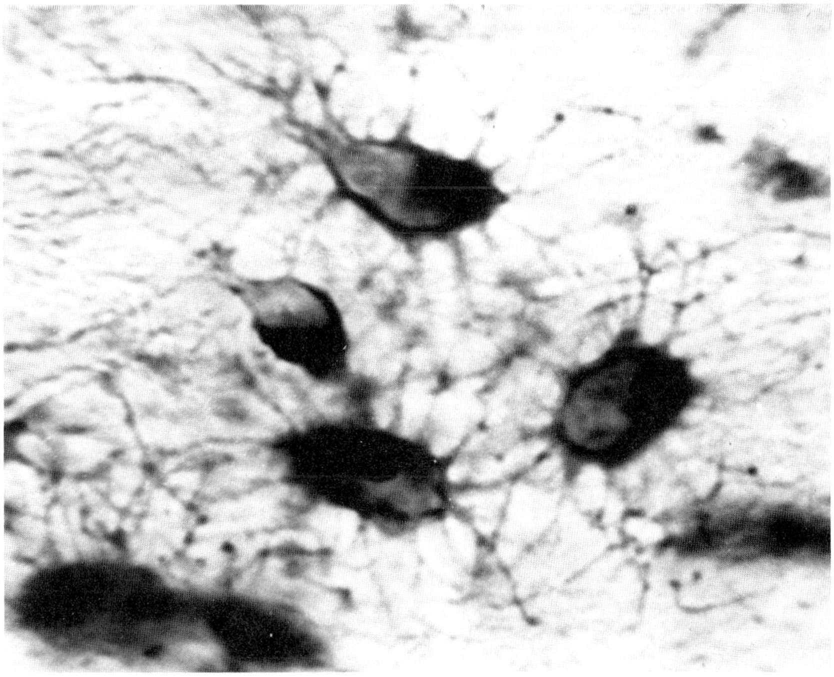

Fig. 5-8. The canalicular system of bone. The extensive canalicular system contains osteocytic processes of adjacent cells which are in contact with each other. ×320 (ground bone section).

sponsible for the removal of bone. These cells possess the cellular mechanisms necessary for the dissolution of bone mineral as well as the digestion of the organic matrix. The process of bone removal mediated by osteoclasts is termed *osteoclasia.*

These cells have few to numerous nuclei contained within a foamy and acidophilic cytoplasm (Fig. 5-9). The cell is polarized; the nuclei are displaced to the cellular border away from the bone. The cellular border adjacent to the bone is composed of numerous cellular processes—a *brush border* (Fig. 5-10).

Osteoclasts reside on the surfaces of bones in concavities called *Howship's lacunae* (Fig. 5-11). They may be artifactually separated from the surface by sectioning. Osteoclasts may be observed along a bone surface in which bone deposition is occurring (Fig. 5-12), or an entire surface may be occupied by osteoclasts. In this instance, the continuity of Howship's lacunae forms a *resorption space* (Fig. 5-13). Even with the absence of the cells, the serrated edges of the Howship's lacunae are sufficient evidence that bone resorption is occurring.

Osteoclasts may arise from mesenchymal cells, from histiocytes or by the fusion of osteoblasts. Osteoclastic nuclei, however, do not divide. A source of the multinucleation may be the incorporation of osteocytic cells as the osteoclasts move through the bone matrix.

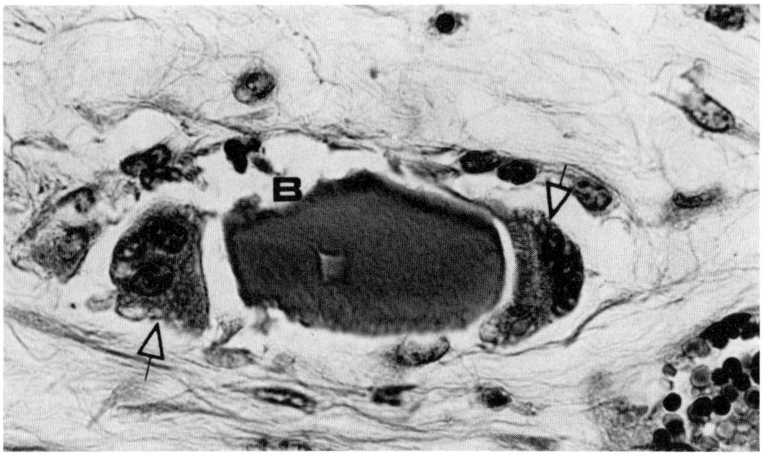

Fig. 5-9. A spicule of bone (*B*) is being removed by osteoclasts (*arrows*). ×160.

Types of Bone

Woven Bone. This type of bone is often referred to as *immature bone* or *coarsely bundled bone*, as well as *woven bone*. It is very cellular and the lacunae are very large and round (Fig. 5-14). The lacunae and their contained cells are dispersed randomly throughout the matrix. Bundles of collagenous fibers are arranged in a haphazard pattern; thus, there is no regular birefringent pattern with polarizing microscopy. The organic matrix is basophilic, stains unevenly and holds less mineral than mature bone.

Immature bone is the first bone that forms in ossification centers of the fetus and the primary spongiosa of developing adolescent bones. It is also the first bone that forms at the site of fracture repair. Certain types of bone tumors are characterized by this type of bone. Normally, it occurs in alveolar bone associated with teeth and at points of attachment of ligaments and tendons to bone.

Lamellar Bone. This bone is also referred to as *mature bone*. It comprises the bulk of the adult skeleton. The lacunae, and thus the cells of this bone, are more lenticular than in immature bone (Fig. 5-15). Also, they are dispersed in an orderly fashion throughout the matrix in a pattern that re-

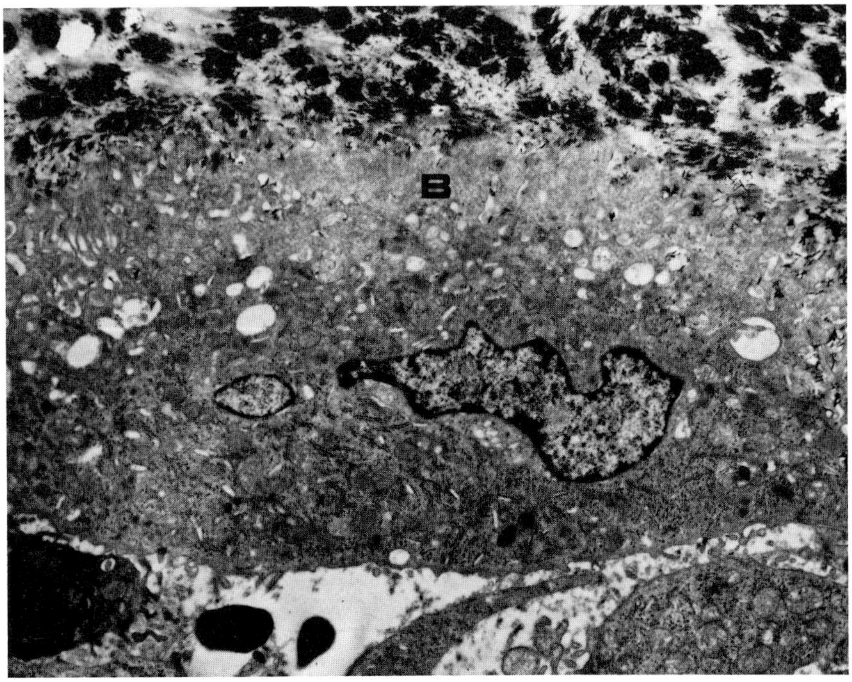

Fig. 5-10. An electron micrograph of an osteoclast. The cell is multinucleated and polarized. The brush border (*B*) is in contact with the bone surface. ×5,000.

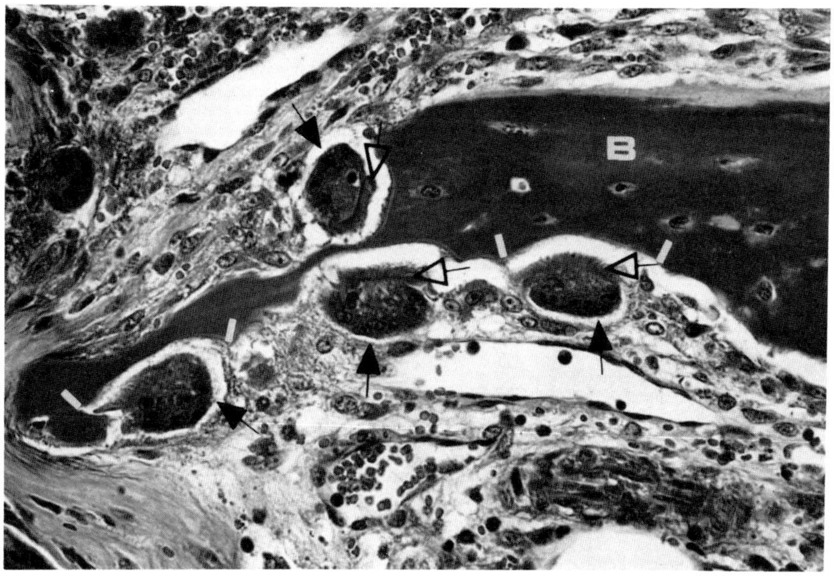

Fig. 5-11. A spicule of bone (*B*) is being remodeled by numerous osteoclasts (*solid arrows*). The boundaries of Howship's lacunae are indicated by *white bars*. Note the brush borders (*open arrows*). ×100 (Masson's trichrome).

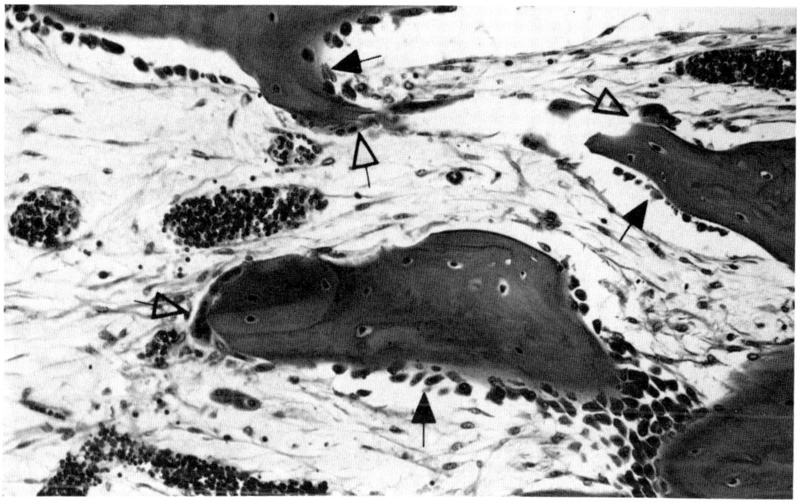

Fig. 5-12. Simultaneous deposition and removal of bone. Osteoblastic activity (*solid arrows*) and osteoclastic activity (*open arrows*) are occurring at the same time. ×40.

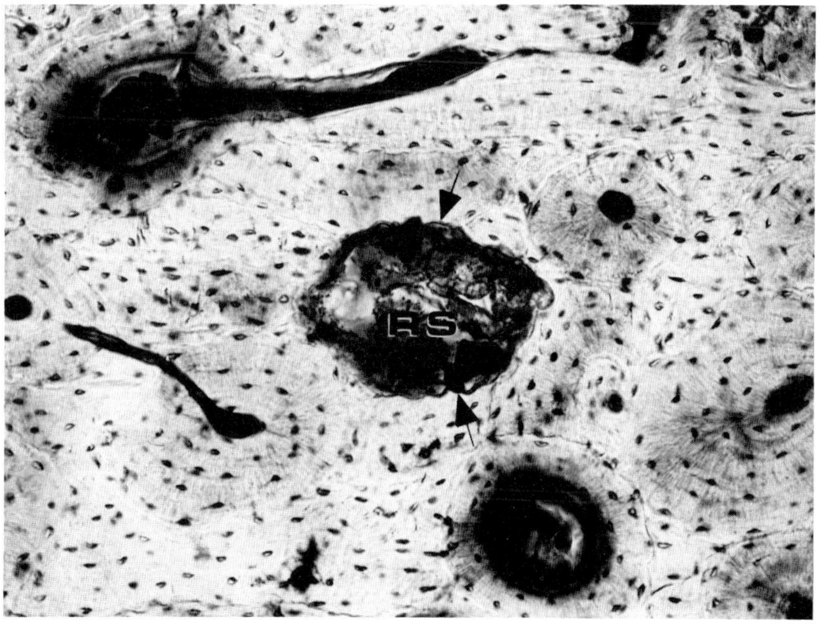

Fig. 5-13. A resorption in bone. The resorption space (*RS*) is recognized by the Howship's lacunae (*arrows*). ×40 (ground bone section).

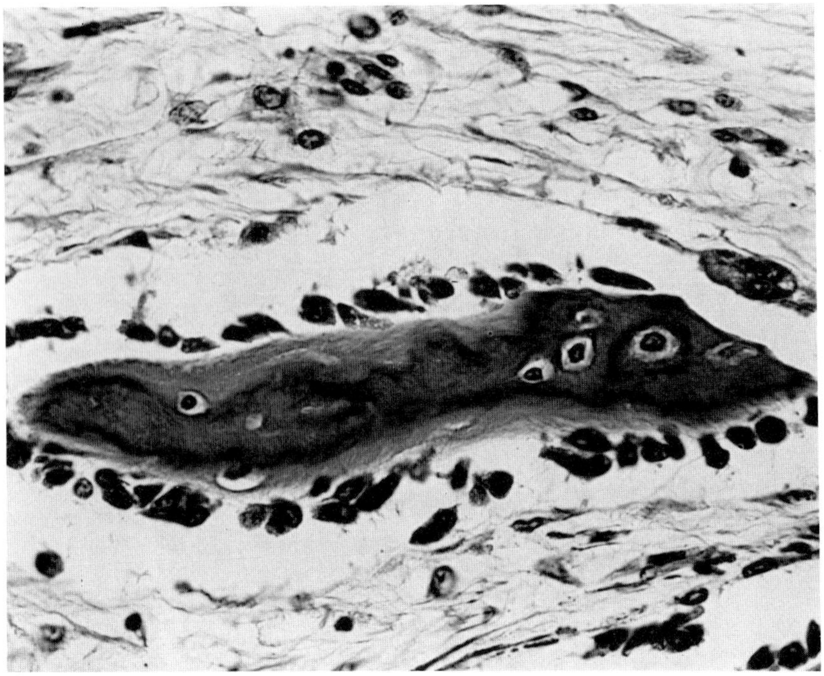

Fig. 5-14. Woven bone in the developing bovine mandible. ×100.

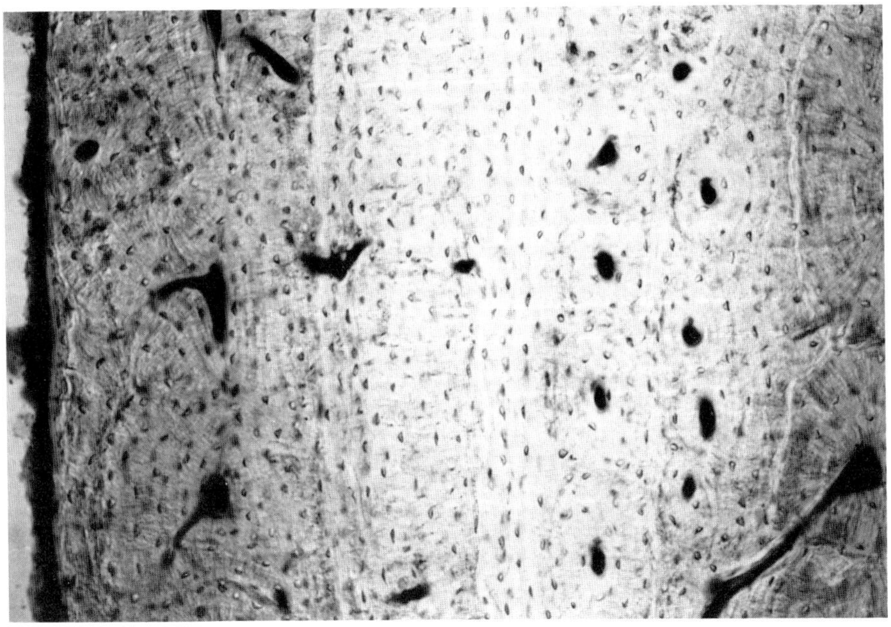

Fig. 5-15. Lamellar bone. The lamellar nature of the bone is indicated by the ordered disposition of the osteocyte lacunae. ×40 (ground bone section).

flects the ordered, lamellar arrangement of the collagen. The collagenous fibers are deposited in helical array at varying angles in successive lamellae; thus, a very ordered pattern of birefringence is apparent with polarizing microscopy. The demineralized organic matrix of mature bone stains lightly and evenly and is acidophilic.

Configurations of Bone

Cancellous Bone. Cancellous bone is that bone that is arranged into *spicules* or *trabeculae*. These spicules may be either *woven bone* or *mature bone*. In the adult skeleton they are most probably composed of mature bone.

The diagnostic feature of cancellous bone is that there is more interosseous space than there is bone (Fig. 5-16). There are, however, numerous gradations of this type of configuration (Fig. 5-17).

Compact Bone. Compact bone represents the extreme in amount of bone formation. Characteristically, there is more bone than interosseous space (Fig. 5-18). In this configuration, there are gradations also. Compact bone may be organized into *laminae* (*lamellae*) or *osteons* (*Haversian systems*).

Organization of Bone

Lamellae of Bone. This organizational pattern is typical of the bone-forming activity of the *periosteum* and portions of the *endosteum*. Successive *lamellae* or *laminae* of mature bone are deposited in extensive sheets of bone which are referred to as the *outer circumferential lamellae* or *periosteal lamellae* (Fig. 5-19). The endosteum associated with the marrow cavity also gives rise to laminae or lamellae of bone. This bone constitutes the *inner circumferential lamellae* or *endosteal lamellae* (Fig. 5-20). These inner lamellae may be continued on trabeculae of bone comprising the cancellous bone of the marrow cavity.

Osteonal Bone. Osteonal bone is the bone that comprises *osteons* or *Haversian systems*. It is disposed in concentric laminae or sheets around an *osteonal canal* or *Haversian canal* (Fig. 5-21). The peripheral limits of the osteonal bone are marked by a *reversal line* or *cement line*. The osteonal canal contains blood vessels as well as cells of the endosteum.

Osteons may abut each other or may be separated by segments of *interstitial bone*. These are remnants of osteons or circumferential lamellar bone (Fig. 5-22). Osteons may also be isolated within circumferential bone.

Osteons are referred to by some as the *structural units of bone*. In their simpliest form they are long cylinders with a hollow

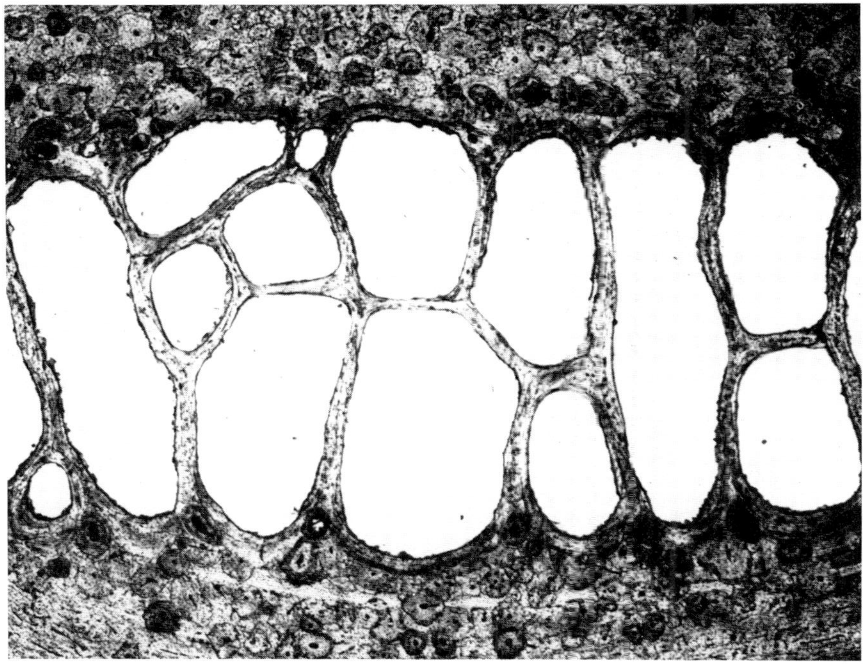

Fig. 5-16. Cancellous bone of the marrow cavity of a rib ×10 (ground bone section).

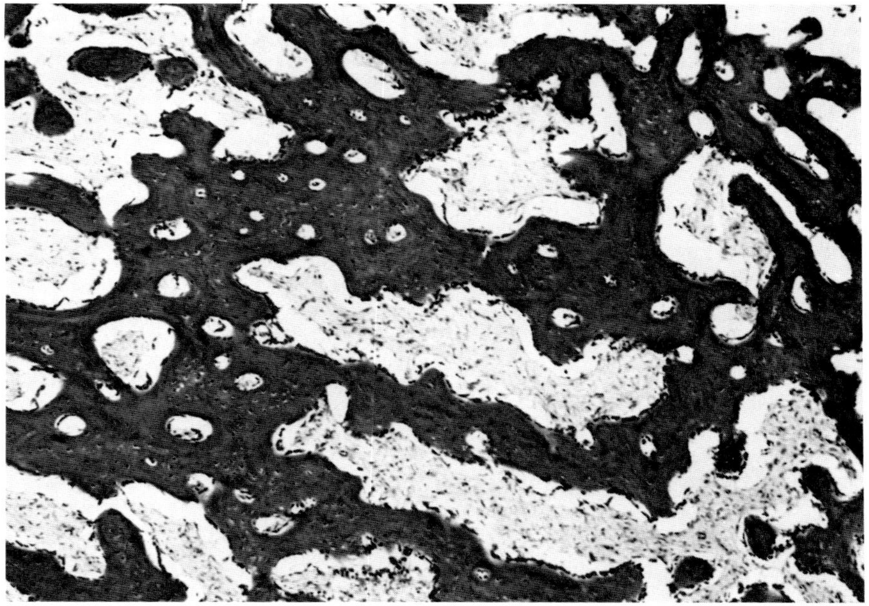

Fig. 5-17. Dense cancellous bone. The interosseous space is reduced and the amount of bone is increased. ×16.

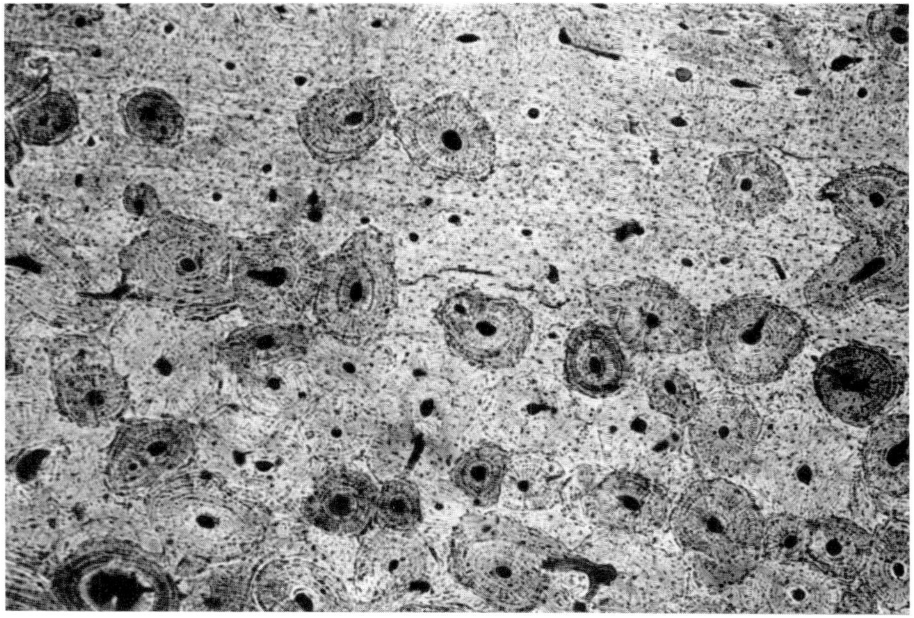

Fig. 5-18. Compact bone. The interosseous space is greatly reduced. The bone is comprised of portions of outer circumferential bone, interstitial bone and osteons. ×16 (ground bone section).

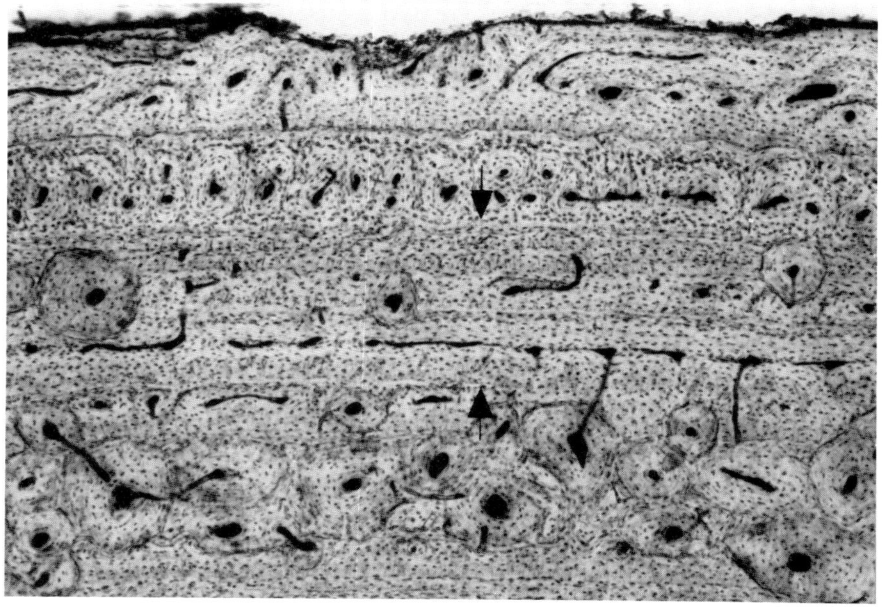

Fig. 5-19. Outer circumferential lamellar bone. The lamellae of this bone are between the *arrows*. They are alternated with layers of primary osteons. The outer circumferential lamellar bone may also assume a configuration indicated in Fig. 5-20. ×16 (ground bone section).

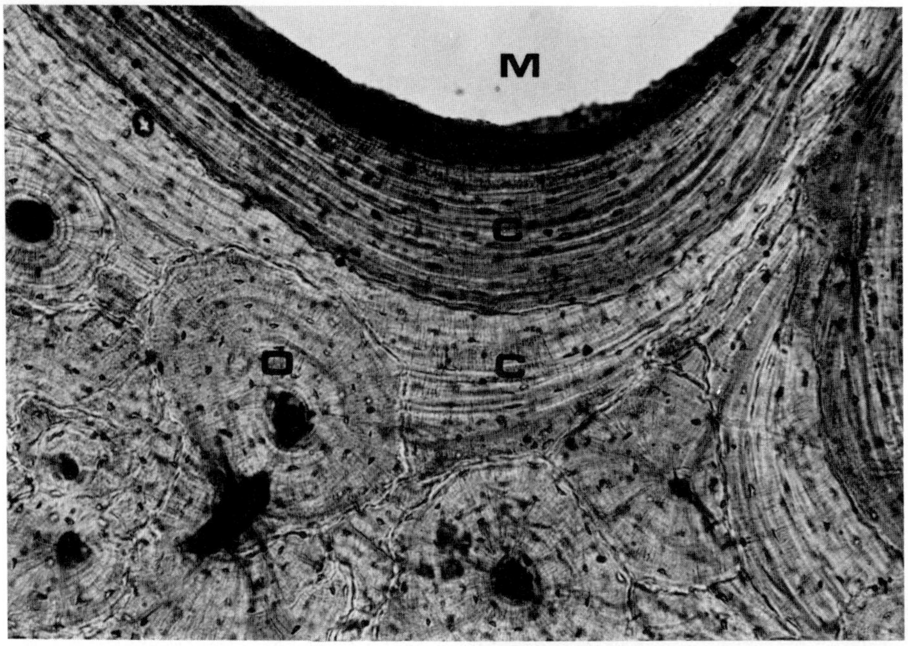

Fig. 5-20. Inner circumferential bone. The marrow cavity (*M*) is bordered by inner circumferential bone (*C*). One osteon (*O*) is formed partially within these lamellae as a result of remodeling. ×40 (ground bone section).

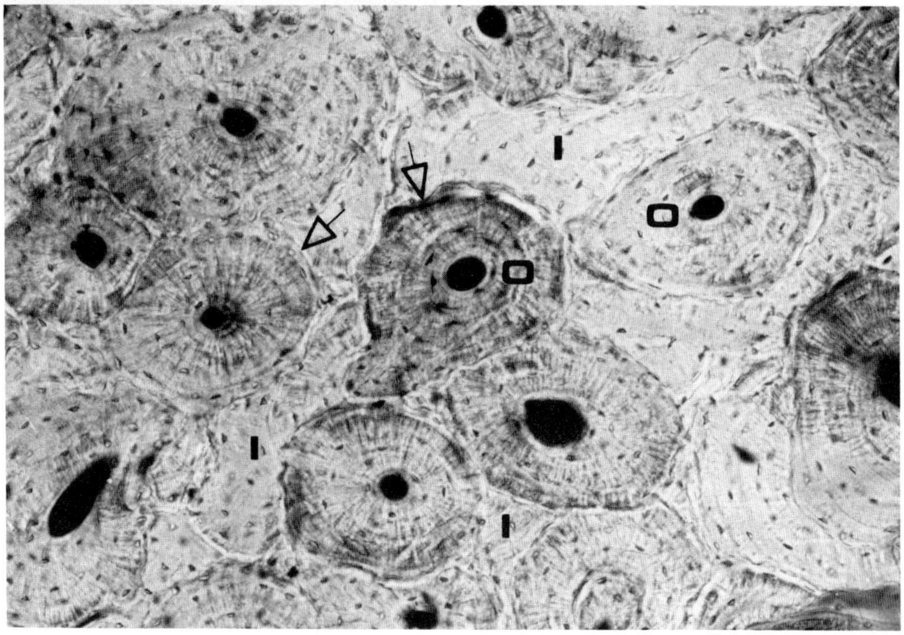

Fig. 5-21. Osteons. I, interstitial bone; *O*, osteonal bone. The osteonal canals are dark. The limits of the osteons (*arrows*) are the reversal lines. ×40 (ground bone section).

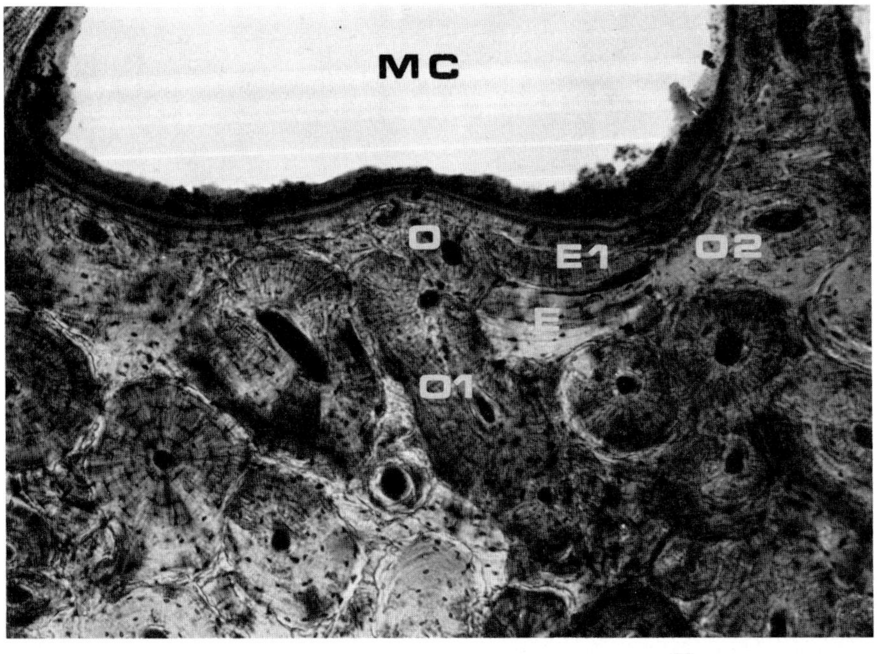

Fig. 5-22. Secondary osteons and interstitial bone. The marrow cavity (*MC*) is bordered by remnants of the inner circumferential bone (*E1*) which is interrupted by an osteon (*O*). Osteons (*O1* and *O2*) also interrupt the endosteal bone (*E*). Compare this figure with Figs. 5-20 and 5-21. ×25 (ground bone section).

cavity, the osteonal canal, in their center. In actuality, they may be extensively branched. They are usually found in those areas where bone is subjected to great stress. Thus, they may be likened to bundles of reinforcing rods in concrete.

The blood vessels of bone, whether associated with circumferential lamellae or osteons, were entrapped during developmental stages. These vessels are connected with vessels at the periosteal or endosteal surface through large *Volkmann's canals*. Osteonal vessels freely communicate with each other through *communicating canals* (Fig. 5-23). Thus, the internal vascular supply is extensively anastomotic and is in communication with endosteal and/or periosteal vessels. The three-dimensional relationship of all these elements is important to keep in mind.

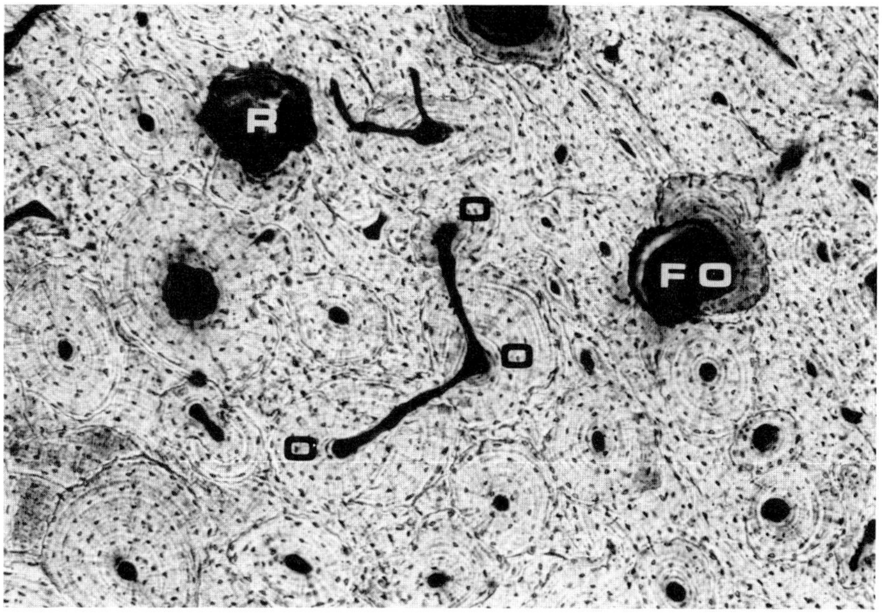

Fig. 5-23. Communicating canals. The osteonal canals of three osteons (*O*) are connected by communicating canals. A resorption space (*R*) and a filling osteon (*FO*) are also present. ×25 (ground bone section).

Dynamicity of Bone

Internal Remodeling. Contrary to popular opinion, bone is not a dead, unchanging tissue. Actually, although the gross morphology of a bone does not change appreciably throughout life, many changes occur within bone. The process by which bones change their internal characteristics without altering gross morphology is termed *internal remodeling*. Not only does bone change internally, but it leaves a record of past and current events because of the nature of the matrix. These alterations in the organization of bone may be used as valuable insights into the normal or abnormal state of bone.

Osteons may be developed in various ways. Once developed, however, they may be altered appreciably in response to somatic calcium needs, stress or numerous other factors. Stem cells within the osteonal canal can differentiate into osteoclasts and begin resorption of osteons (Fig. 5-24). All or part of the osteons may be removed. At some later date the osteons may begin to refill by osteoblastic activity (Fig. 5-25). Remnants of the older osteons may become interstitial bone. The rate of refilling can be determined by administering therapeutic dosages of tetracyclines (broad-spectrum antibiotics) at timed intervals and by examining the labeled and mineralized sections with fluorescence microscopy.

The homeostatic maintenance of the skeletal volume is achieved through the balanced activity of osteoblasts and osteoclasts. In time of calcium need or other stress, a net calcium loss from the skeleton is achieved through the balance of activity favoring the osteoclasts. In times of refilling or growth, the activity favors the osteoblasts.

Laminae of inner and outer circumferential bone may be turned over in a similar manner.

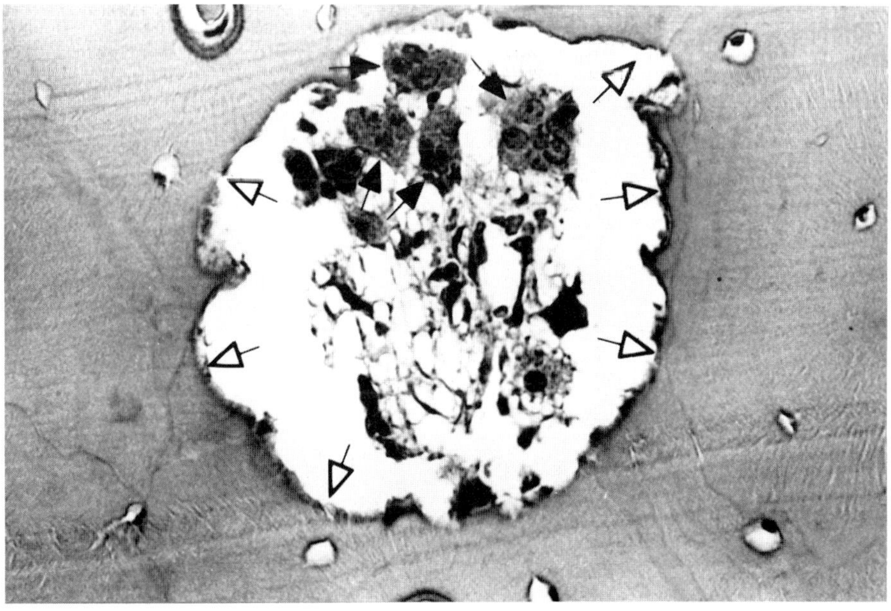

Fig. 5-24. Resorption space. The border of the resorption space is serrated by Howship's lacunae (*open arrows*). Osteoclasts (*solid arrows*) have been displaced from the lacunae by the preparation techniques. ×125.

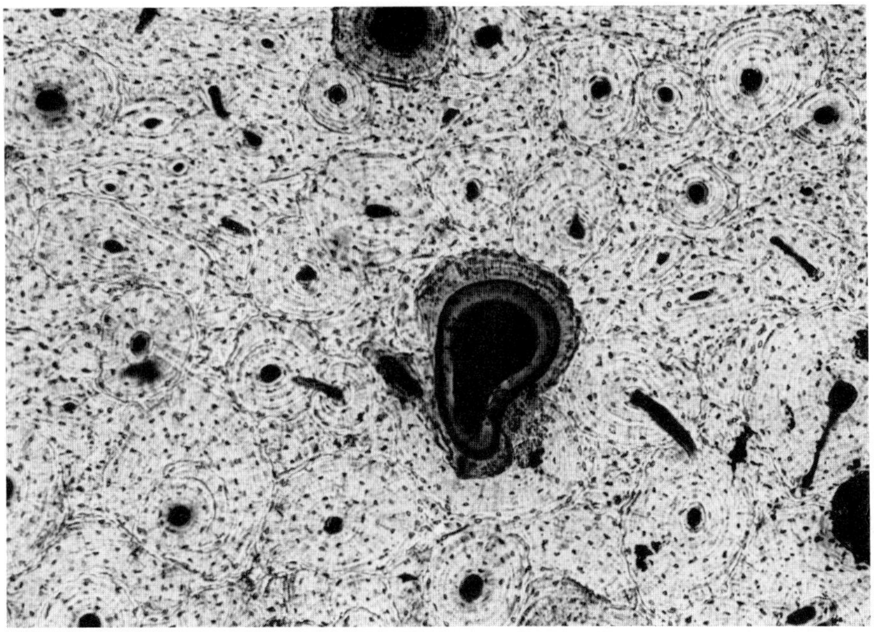

Fig. 5-25. Refilling osteon. One osteon is actively refilling. Compare the morphology with that of Fig. 5-5. The osteon at the top of the micrograph is immature and inactive. The remaining osteons are mature. ×25 (ground bone section).

References

Amprino, R. and Engstrom, A.: Studies on x-ray absorption and diffraction of bone tissue. Acta Anat. *15:* 1, 1952.

Ascenzi, R., Bonucci, E. and Bocciarelli, D. S.: An electron microscope study on primary periosteal bone. J. Ultrastruct. Res. *18:*605, 1967.

Belanger, L. F., Robichon, J., Migicovsky, B. B., Copp, D. H. and Vincent, J.: Resorption without osteoclasts (osteolysis). In *Mechanisms of Hard Tissue Destruction*, edited by R. F. Sognnaes. AAAS, Washington, D. C., 1963.

Cohen, J. and Harris, W. H.: The three dimensional anatomy of Haversian systems. J. Bone Joint Surg. *40A:*419, 1958.

Cooper, R. R., Milgram, J. W. and Robinson, R. A.: Morphology of the osteon: An electron microscopic study. J. Bone Joint Surg. *48A:*1239, 1966.

Gonzales, F. and Karnovsky, M. J.: Electron microscopy of osteoclasts in healing fractures of rat bone. J. Biophys. Biochem. Cytol. *9:*299, 1961.

Heller-Steinberg, M.: Ground substance, bone salts, and cellular activity in bone formation and destruction. Amer. J. Anat. *89:*347, 1951.

Hobdell, M. H. and Boyde, A.: Microradiography and scanning electron microscopy of bone sections. Z. Zellforsch. *94:*487, 1969.

Martin, J. H. and Matthew, J. L.: Mitochondrial granules in chondrocytes, osteoblasts and osteocytes. Clin. Orthop. *68:*273, 1970.

6 Osteogenesis

Methods of Ossification

General Characteristics. Osteogenic processes, beginning in the embryo and continuing throughout the life of the animal, are mediated through the secretory activity of osteoblasts. These cells deposit a mucopolysaccharide-protein and collagenous matrix which subsequently becomes mineralized. Although the actual cellular mechanism of bone deposition is the same in all osteogenic processes, the differentiation of mesenchymal cells into osteoblasts normally occurs in two different microenvironments. For this reason, two types of normal ossification processes are recognized, *intramembranous* and *endochondral*. The quality and appearance of the bone in both instances are identical; however, the primary association of osseous material with other tissues in the different environments greatly alters the appearance of the developing osseous organ.

In *intramembranous ossification*, the differentiation of osteoblasts occurs in an environment in which some mesenchymal cells have previously differentiated into fibroblasts. The presence of fibers and cells (mesenchymal and fibroblastic) imparts a fibrocellular or membranous quality to the microenvironment. The *de novo* formation of bone under these conditions, therefore, appears to occur in a minimally supported membranous environment.

In *endochondral ossification*, the differentiation of osteoblasts occurs in an environment in which cartilage has already been deposited. Foci of perivascular mesenchymal cells within certain areas of the cartilaginous tissue give rise to the osteoblasts. Bone deposition, as described previously, takes place. However, the cartilage is used as a temporary support or scaffold upon which bone is deposited. The cartilage is not transformed into bone but is eventually replaced by bone.

Occasionally, bone formation occurs in foci not normally occupied by osseous tissues. This *metaplastic ossification* may be observed in cicatrices, lymphatic organs and numerous other organs. Although the environment is different from the two described previously, the mesenchymal cell differentiation and resulting osteoblastic activity are the same.

Although the cellular mechanism of normal ossification is the same, it functions quite differently in the growing animal. Intramembranous ossification is responsible for the attainment of the definitive shape of those bones that are not preformed in cartilage. This includes longitudinal and latitudinal growth of a limited number of bones of the body. Endochondral ossification is responsible for the longitudinal growth of the bones of the body. Endochondral ossification, however, does not occur alone. The latitudinal or transverse growth of these bones is mediated through intramembranous ossification. Both of these ossification processes, prior to adulthood, are responsible for the *modeling* of bones or the attainment of the definitive, recognizable gross structure.

After the initial deposition of bone in a membranous or cartilaginous environment, subsequent bone formation occurs on preexisting bone surfaces by appositional growth. Continued deposition naturally leads to bone growth. The modeling of bones, however, is the combined result of osteoblastic and osteoclastic activity. The balance of these combined activities favors the deposition of bone during periods of growth.

Although osteogenic processes most noticeably occur during adolescence, they are not confined to this period. The deposition and removal of bone, without any significant alteration of the gross form of the structure, occur throughout life. This *remodeling* process complements the adolescent modeling of bones. Throughout the remainder of life, bone formative and resorptive phenomena are maintained in a homeostatic balance. Any disruption to this balance during the pre- and/or postnatal period can result in serious metabolic bone disorders.

Intramembranous Ossification. This process begins in areas occupied by mesenchyme, the packing tissue of the embryo. The bones destined to form, either totally or partially in this manner, are the bones of the skull, mandible and clavicle, which are not weight-bearing structures.

Initially, the regions in which bone is to be formed are occupied by mesenchymal cells embedded within a homogeneous, fluid ground substance. The subsequent development of a *fibrocellular* tissue is brought about by the differentiation of some *fibroblasts* from mesenchymal cells (Fig. 6-1). The ability to distinguish one of these cells from the other is difficult. Generally, however, mesenchymal cells are larger and more pale-staining than their more differentiated counterparts, fibroblasts. *Collagenous fibers* are randomly scattered among the numerous *stellate cells*, which include fibroblasts and mesenchymal cells. Many of these cells are destined to become *osteoprogenitor cells*; i.e., cells that will give rise to osteoblasts.

The next recognizable step in the differentiation process is the recognition of osteoblasts (Fig. 6-2). These cells stain quite darkly and are basophilic. During active secretion of their products they assume a cuboidal configuration. However, during periods of nonactivity they assume a spindle-shaped configuration. Although bone matrix is not always visible during early stages of differentiation, subsequent secretory activity by these cells will produce bone. Thus, these areas represent ossification centers in their early stages of development.

Progressive development and differentiation produces recognizable spicules of bone (Fig. 6-3). A fibrocellular connective tissue with numerous blood vessels surrounds the developing bone. As osteoblasts deposit bone appositionally, some cells remain entrapped in their own secretory products. Osteoblastic cells that become entrapped are then referred to as osteocytes. The bone being deposited in these ossification centers is the *woven* type. The large lacunae and the nonlamellar arrangement of the osteocytes are typical of this type of bone.

The development of bone in any ossification center involves the activity of *osteoblasts* and *osteoclasts* (Fig. 6-4). The osteoblasts may be in different states of activity. Osteoclasts are present at foci where bone is being removed. The differential activities of these cells, osteoblasts and osteoclasts,

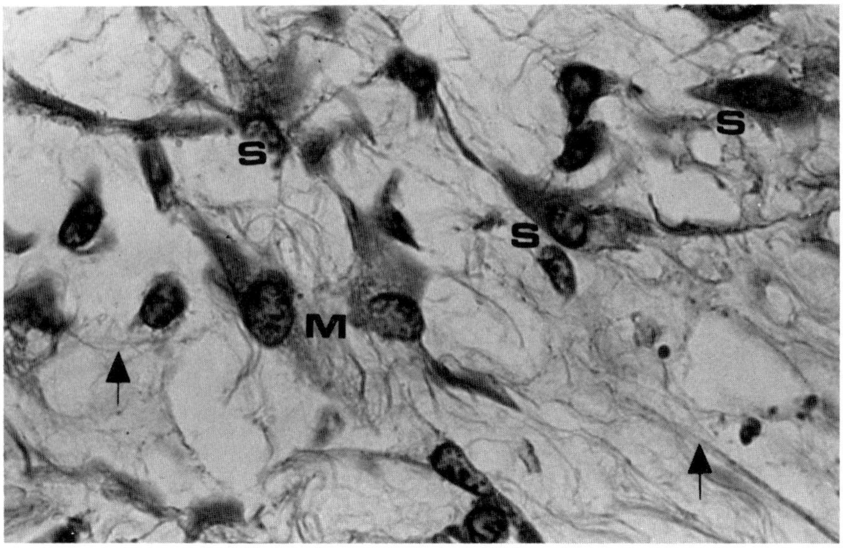

Fig. 6-1. Early cellular differentiation in intramembranous ossification (bovine fetal jaw). Mesenchymal cells (*M*), stellate cells (*S*) and collagenous fibers (*arrows*) are identifiable. ×160. All light micrographs are the original magnifications. All electron micrographs are the final magnifications.

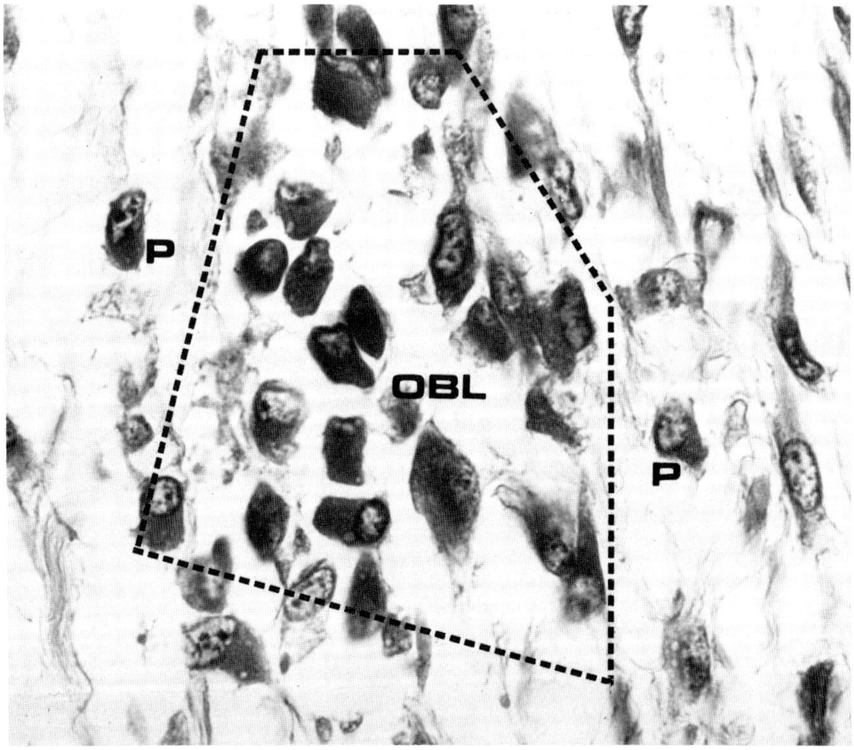

Fig. 6-2. Differentiation of osteoblasts in intramembranous ossification (bovine fetal jaw). The *outlined area* represents an ossification center which contains osteoblasts (*OBL*). The light-staining cells at the periphery are osteoprogenitor cells (*P*). The surrounding tissue is similar to that of Fig. 6-1. ×160.

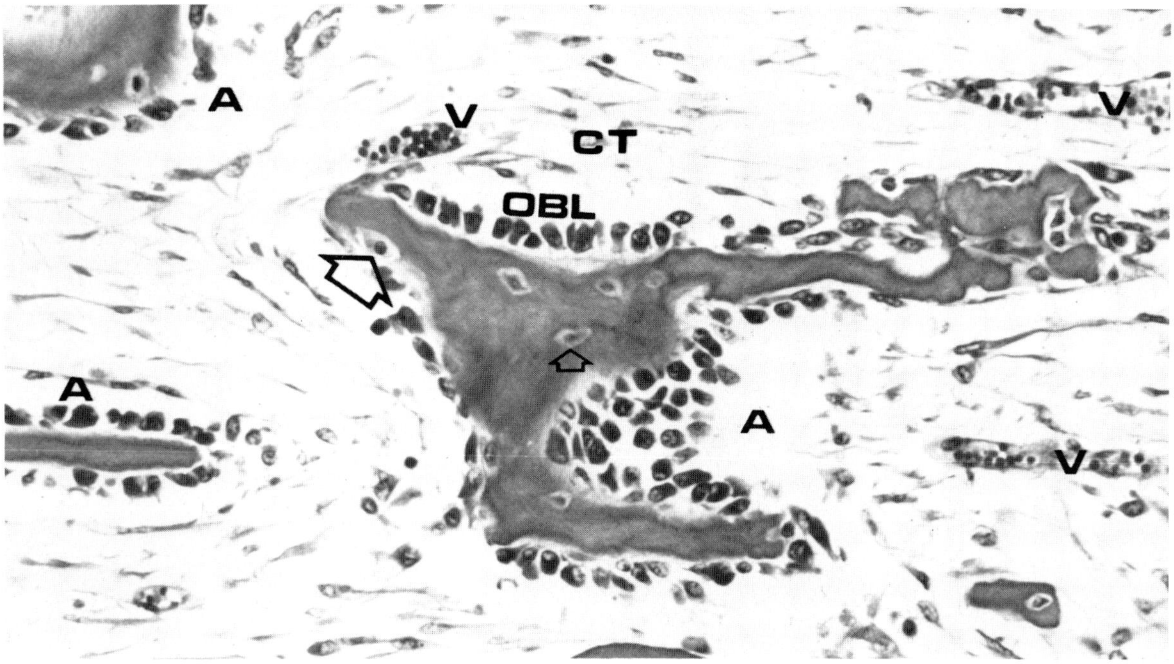

Fig. 6-3. The appearance of bone in the ossification center (bovine fetal jaw). A spicule of bone is contained within a fibrocellular connective tissue (*CT*) which contains numerous blood vessels (*V*). The connective tissue is artifactually separated from the bone (*A*). Osteoblastic cells (*OBL*) become entrapped in bone (*large arrow*) and are eventually recognized as typical osteocytes (*small arrow*). ×63.

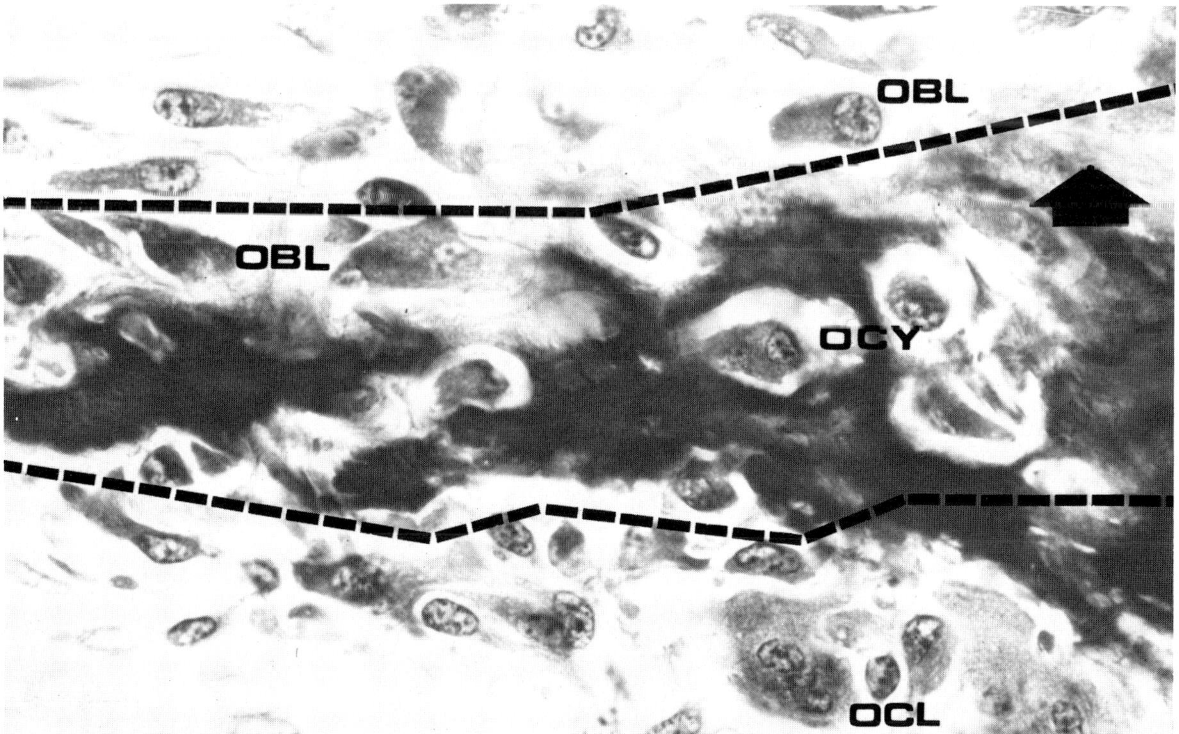

Fig. 6-4. Progressive development and activity of the ossification center (bovine fetal jaw). The osteoblasts (*OBL*) on the upper portion of the spicule are active, whereas those on the lower portion are inactive. Osteoclasts (*OCL*) are present also. If the same activity were to progress beyond the stage depicted, the spicule would be altered as outlined and appear to move upward (*arrow*). Osteocytes (*OCY*) are randomly oriented in this immature bone. ×160.

account for the movement of the bone spicules through the connective tissue space. The bone being deposited is also *woven*, *fibrous* or *immature bone*.

The progressive growth of the ossification center (Fig. 6-5) leads to the development of cancellous bone. Further growth (Fig. 6-6) produces a more densely arranged cancellous bone in which *osteons* may be apparent. Subsequent filling of the interosseous spaces would lead to the formation of compact bone.

Endochondral Ossification. The development of bone by this process involves, initially, the differentiation of cartilage. Subsequently, the simultaneous formation and removal of cartilage is accompanied by the formation of bone. This process, occurring in most of the bones of the body, is responsible for the elongation of osseous organs.

In those areas of the body in which bone is to develop by this method, a *mesenchymal cell condensation* is observed (Fig. 6-7). These cells will eventually differentiate into cartilage cells and will initiate the formation of the *cartilaginous model* of the developing bone. The cells of the model are

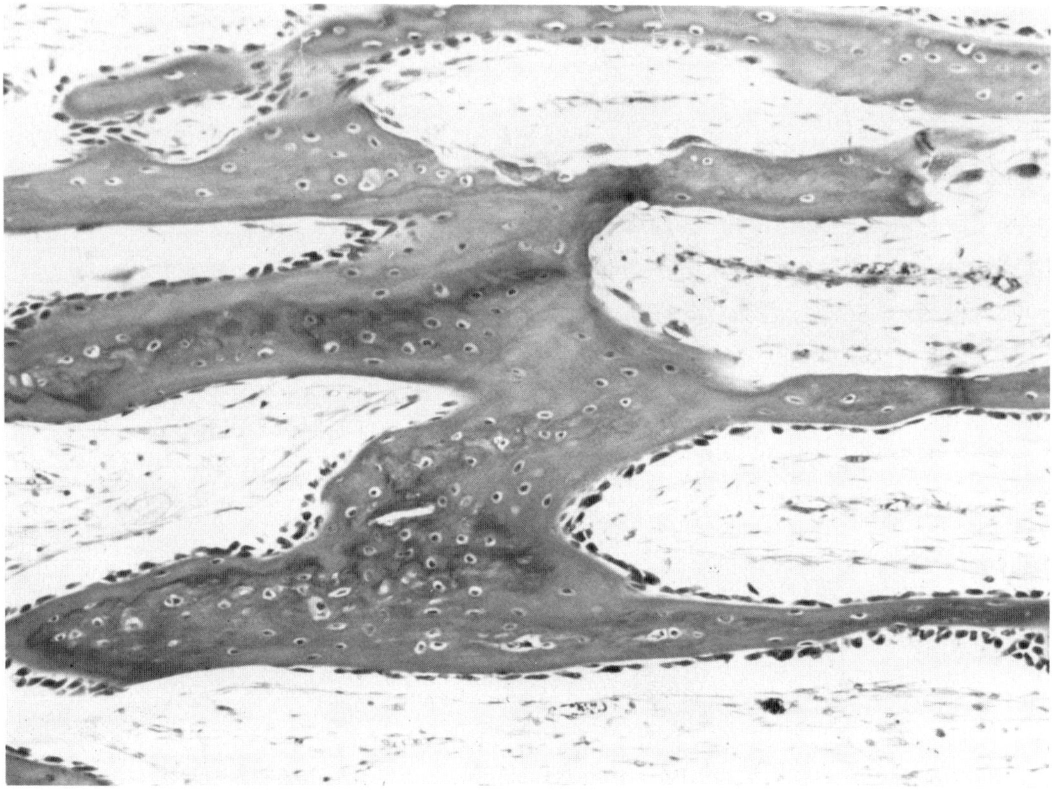

Fig. 6-5. Progressive growth of the ossification center (bovine fetal jaw). The union of spicules occurs and cancellous bone continues to develop. ×63.

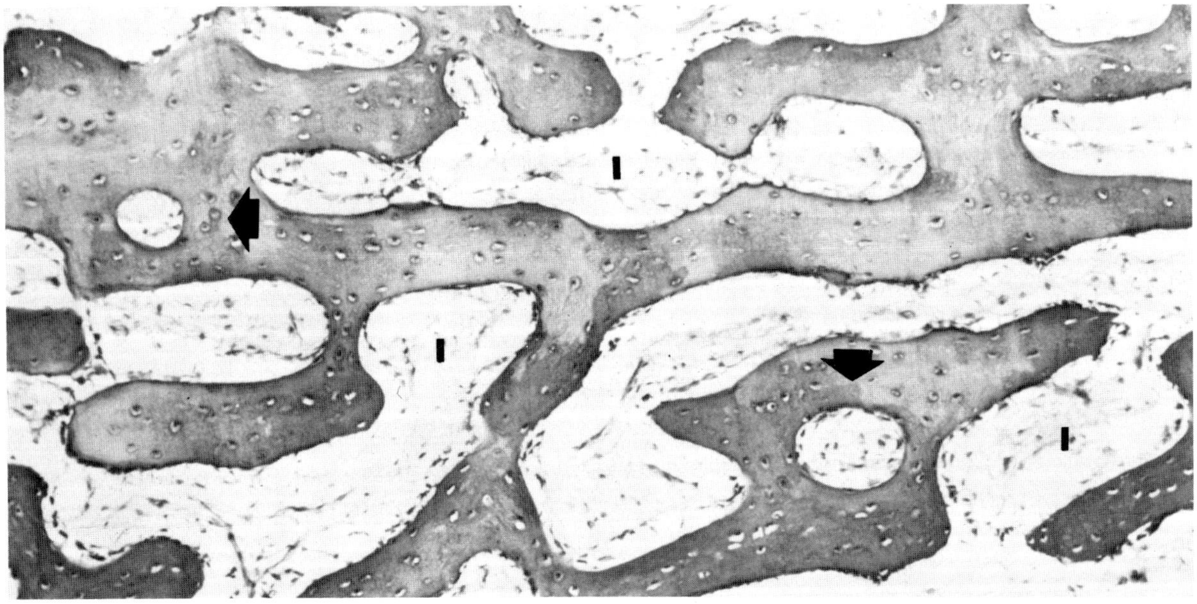

Fig. 6-6. Reduction of interosseous space in the ossification center (bovine fetal jaw). The interosseous space (*I*) is being replaced by bone, and osteons (*arrows*) are forming. ×63.

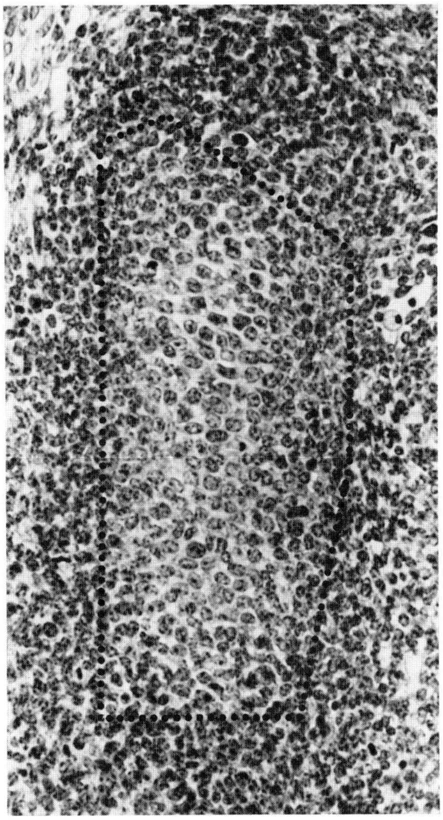

Fig. 6-7. Mesenchymal condensation in the early stages of bone formation (hamster humerus). The condensation is outlined and a perichondrium will differentiate peripheral to the condensation. ×60 (periodic acid-Schiff).

surrounded by layers of mesenchymal cells which form a *perichondrium*. The peripheral portions of the perichondrium will differentiate into fibrous components, whereas the cells adjacent to the developing chondrocytes will remain undifferentiated.

By both *appositonal* and *interstitial* growth mechanisms, the cartilage model will elongate as well as thicken (Fig. 6-8). By the time this is achieved, the cells in the central portion will have matured and hypertrophy of these cells will be apparent.

Progressive hypertrophy of these cells eventually leads to mineralization of the cartilage matrix (Fig. 6-9). Cut off from their diffusing nutritive supply, the chondrocytes die. Cavities develop within this zone of mineralized cartilage by dissolution of the cartilaginous matrix. At the same time, the perichondrium in the mid-diaphyseal region is invaded with blood vessels and some of the undifferentiated cells of this membrane begin to differentiate into osteoblasts; thus, the perichondrium is converted to a *periosteum*. A *periosteal collar* or *sleeve* of bone is then formed. *Osteoprogenitor cells*, *osteoblasts* and *blood vessels* then invade the disintegrating mineralized cartilaginous matrix as a *periosteal bud*, and bone cells begin to deposit their osseous products on remnants and spicules of mineralized cartilage. There is, however, a continuity of bone between the periosteal collar and that which is being deposited on the mineralized cartilaginous matrix. This is early development of the *diaphyseal ossification center*. In those bones that develop from a single ossification center, the sequence of events as described proceeds proximad and distad from the diaphyseal center. This, of course, is accompanied by the continued appositional and interstitial addition of cartilage until the definitive shape and size of the bone is achieved. During this process, the amount of cartilage is progressively diminished until it is eventually reduced to the articular surfaces.

In other bones, however, *secondary ossification centers* develop in the *proximal* and/or *distal epiphyses*. The sequence of events that occurs in these centers is identical with those described for the diaphyseal center. In these types of developing bones, the growing cartilage is confined to a definitive *growth plate* or *epiphyseal plate* (Fig. 6-10).

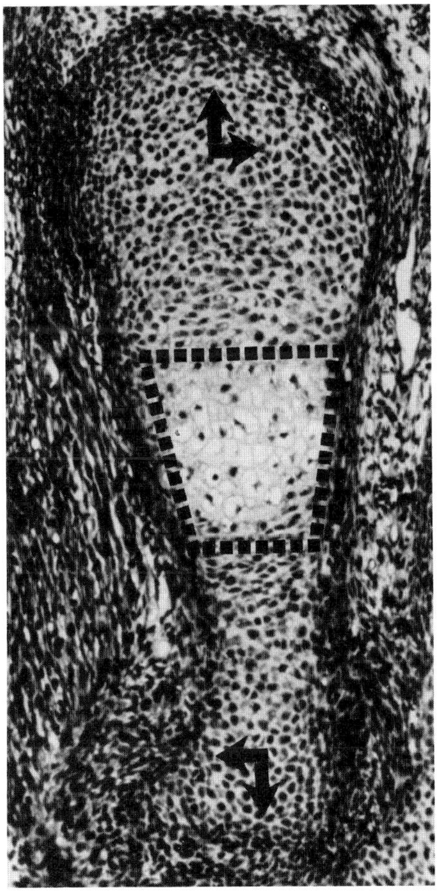

Fig. 6-8. Differentiation of cartilage in the primary ossification center (hamster phalanx). The hypertrophied cells of the primary ossification center are apparent (*outlined area*). The mesenchymal cells will continue to grow in the directions indicated (*arrows*). ×34.

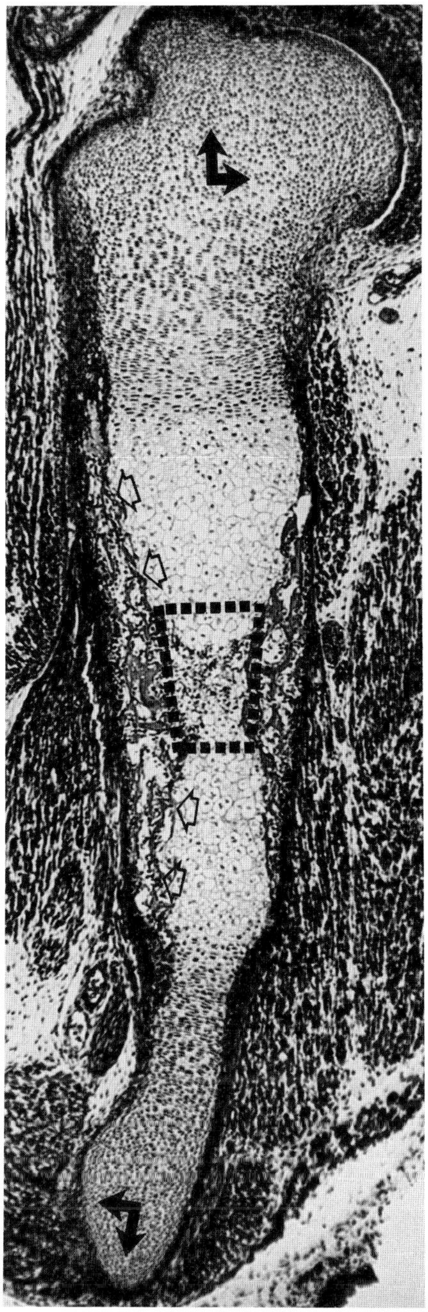

Fig. 6-9. Progressive development of the primary ossification center (hamster humerus). *Outlined area*, primary ossification center. Periosteal collar bone develops (*open arrows*). The bone continues to grow in the directions indicated (solid arrows). ×7.

In Fig. 6-10, the *proximal epiphyseal* and *diaphyseal ossification centers* are apparent. The epiphyseal center is bounded by the *articular cartilage* and the *growth plate*. Bone spicules and marrow elements

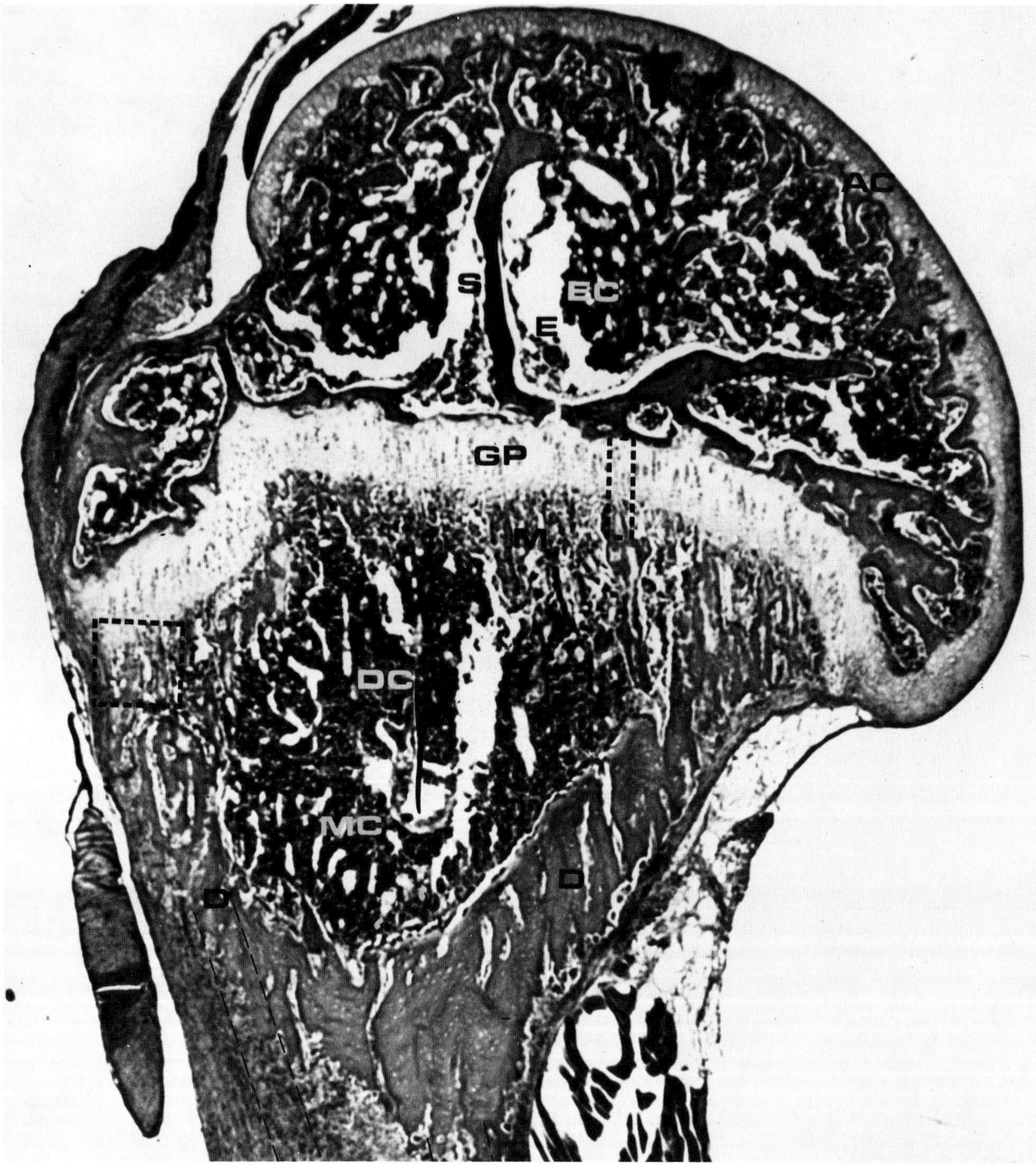

Fig. 6-10. The proximal head of the growing humerus of a gerbil. The growth plate (*GP*) separates the diaphyseal ossification center (*DC*) from the epiphyseal ossification center (*EC*). The diaphyseal bone (*D*) is joined to the growth plate by the metaphyseal bone (*M*). Articular cartilage (*AC*), marrow cavity (*MC*), marrow elements of the epiphyseal center (*E*) and bone spicules (*S*) are indicated. Since this is a parasagittal section the *dashed lines* represent the extension of the shaft. The *square area* is enlarged in Fig. 11; the *rectangular area* is enlarged in Fig. 12. ×6.

are present in the epiphyseal center. Cartilaginous growth on the epiphyseal side of the growth plate has ceased. Cartilage and bone growth on the *metaphyseal* side of the plate, however, is still active. The trabeculae of the metaphysis join the *diaphyseal bone* and connect the shaft to the plate. The diaphyseal center has been sufficiently remodeled to form a large marrow cavity.

The area of junction between the articular cartilage, growth plate, trabeculae of the metaphysis and spicules of the diaphysis is shown in Fig. 6-11. The remnants of mineralized cartilage are present in the metaphyseal trabeculae and are surrounded by temporary bone. Bone that has been deposited by *intramembranous mechanisms* from the periosteum, however, is devoid of cartilage. The fibrous and cellular zones of the *periosteum* are apparent.

Fig. 6-12 is an enlargement of the growth plate showing the relationship of the plate to the epiphyseal bone and the metaphysis. The epiphyseal bone is no longer being deposited via endochondral mechanisms; simple appositional deposition of bone on bone is occurring. The epiphyseal bone is joined to the growth plate via a direct abutment with the zone of *resting cartilage*. Through interstitial mechanisms, the zone of *proliferating cartilage* is the means by which chondrocytes are added to replace

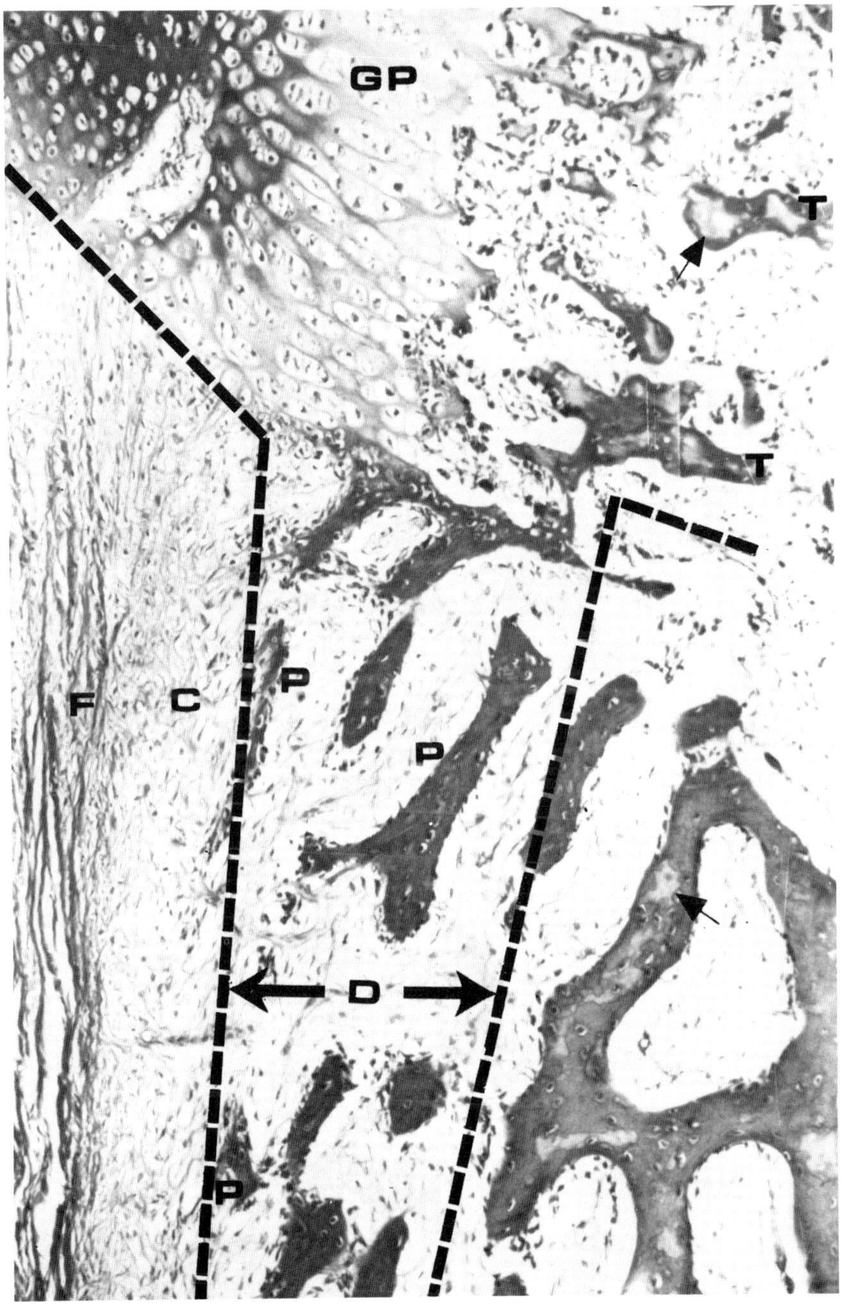

Fig. 6-11. The articular cartilage is continuous with the growth plate (*GP*) in the upper left portion of the micrograph. The diaphysis (*D*) contains bone (*P*) from the periosteum and is continuous with the temporary bone (*T*) deposited at the growth plate. Areas of calcified cartilage (*arrows*) are contained within spicules of the temporary bone. The fibrous (*F*) and cellular (*C*) portions of the periosteum are indicated. ×25.

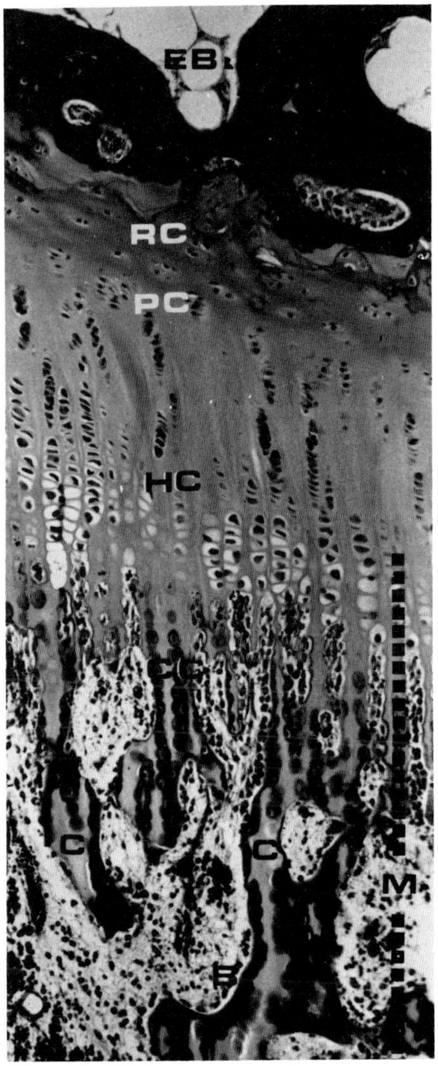

Fig. 6-12. The growth plate of a deer humerus. The epiphyseal bone (*EB*) is not growing by the endochondral mechanism. The reserve cartilage (*RC*), proliferating cartilage (*PC*), hypertrophied cartilage (*HC*) and mineralized cartilage (*CC*) are indicated. Bone (*B*) is deposited on remnants of mineralized cartilage (*C*) within the metaphysis (*M* and *dashed line*). ×21.

those that are lost through this growth process. Note the columnar and parallel arrangement of these cells. The zone of *hypertrophy* contains cells in various stages of maturation. The addition of cells, as well as the enlargement of cells in this zone, moves the epiphyseal bone further from any fixed point in the diaphysis. Cytological changes within the *hypertrophic chondrocytes* bring about a mineralization of the matrix. In a manner similar to the periosteal bud invasion during early development of the ossification center, the matrix disintegrates; vessels with accompanying osteoprogenitor cells invade this area and deposition of bone takes place on the spicules and remnants of *mineralized cartilage* (Figs. 6-13, 6-14). These events occur in the metaphyseal region.

Mineralized cartilage persists for some time until it is replaced by bone. The *primary spongiosa* consists of mineralized cartilage and bone. Eventually, the remodeling process will remove all of the mineralized cartilage and woven bone. These will be replaced by the lamellar bone of the *secondary spongiosa*.

The aforementioned sequence of events continues until the proliferative zone ceases its activity. At this time the other sequences proceed until the joint becomes totally replaced by bone.

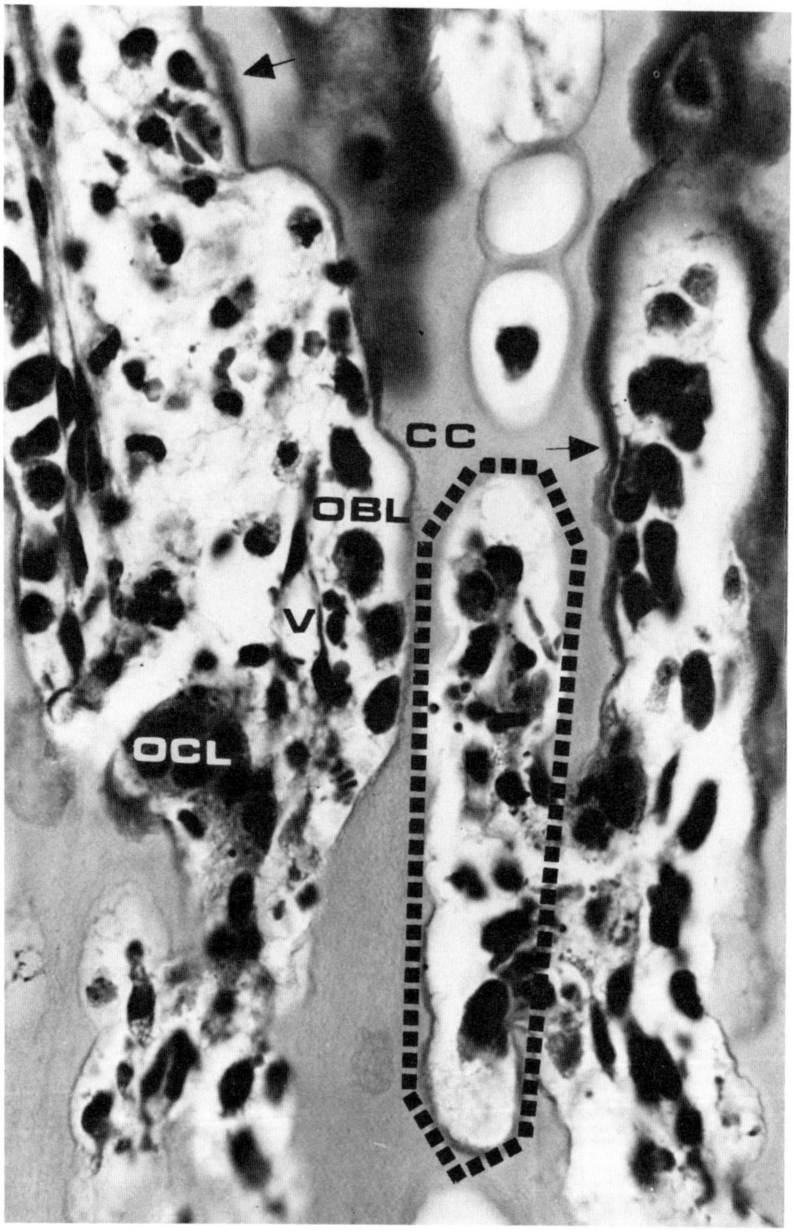

Fig. 6-14. Osseous replacement in the zone of mineralized cartilage. The disintegration of the mineralized cartilaginous matrix (*CC*) is indicated by the confluence of lacunae (*outlined*) which have been invaded by vessels (*V*) and numerous perivascular cells. Osteoblasts (*OBL*) and osteoclasts (*OCL*) are active. Bone (*arrows*) is being deposited on remnants of mineralized cartilage. ×160.

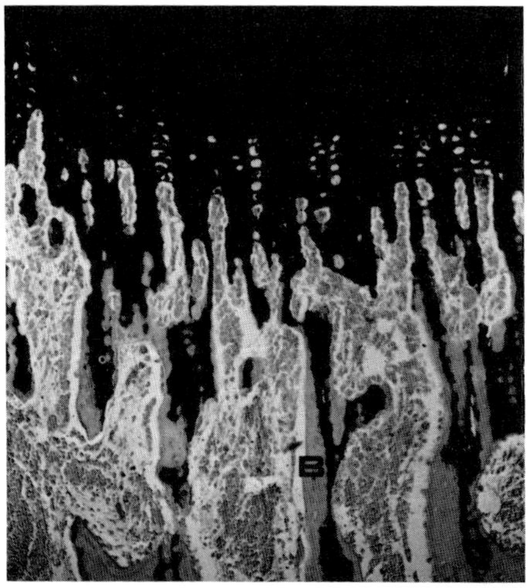

Fig. 6-13. The extent of the cartilage (*black*) beyond the growth plate is apparent. Bone (*B*) is deposited on spicules of mineralized cartilage. ×18 (aldehyde fuchsin).

References

Anderson, C. E. and Parker, J.: Electron microscopy of the epiphyseal cartilage plate. Clin. Orthop. *58*:225, 1968.

Bassett, A. L.: Current concepts of bone formation. J. Bone Joint Surg. *44A*:1217, 1962.

Bonucci, E.: Fine structure of early cartilage calcification. J. Ultrastruct. Res. *20*:33, 1967.

Brookes, M.: Cortical vascularization and growth in foetal trabecular bones. J. Anat. *97*:597, 1963.

Clark, E. R. and Clark, E. L.: Microscopic observations on new formation of cartilage and bone in the living animal. Amer. J. Anat. *70*:167, 1942.

Kuettner, K. E., Sobel, L. W., Ray, R. D., Croxen, R. L., Passovoy, M. and Eisenstein, R.: Lysozyme in epiphyseal cartilage. J. Cell Biol. *44*:329, 1970.

Matthews, J. L., Martin, J. H., Lynn, J. A. and Collins, E. J.: Calcium incorporation in the developing cartilaginous epiphysis. Calc. Tiss. Res. *1*:330, 1968.

Schenk, R. K. Spiro, D. and Wiener, J.: Cartilage resorption in the tibial epiphyseal plate of growing rats. J. Cell Biol. *34*:275, 1967.

Schenk, R. K. Wiener, J. and Spiro, D.: Fine structural aspects of vascular invasion of the tibial epiphyseal plate of growing rats. Acta. Anat. *69*:1, 1968.

Scherft, J. P.: The ultrastructure of the organic matrix of calcified cartilage and bone in embryonic mouse radii. J. Ultrastruct. Res. *23*:333, 1968.

7 Blood—Adult Formed Elements

General Characteristics

Form and Function. Blood may be considered a special type of connective tissue which consists of a large volume of fluid matrix and numerous formed elements. A fibrous component is also present during blood clotting when *fibrinogen* is converted to *fibrin*. Blood and its transudative components as tissue fluid are probably the most ubiquitous of the connective tissues.

The fluid phase (*plasma*) consists of approximately 90 per cent water and about 10 per cent solids. The solids include:

1. Protein: albuminoids, globulins, fibrinogen.
2. Inorganic substances: sodium, calcium, potassium, phosphorus and others.
3. Organic substances: urea, uric acid, amino acids, lipids, carbohydrates and others.
4. Hormones, antibodies, enzymes.

All materials that pass to or from the cells through the connective tissue compartment may occur as components of the liquid phase of the blood. This includes materials occurring normally as well as abnormally (bacteria, toxins, etc.). Also, the blood is often used as the carrier medium for many chemotherapeutic materials.

Upon removal of *fibrinogen* as *fibrin*, the remaining fluid is termed *serum*.

Suspended within the plasma are varied cells and/or fragments of cells. These formed elements serve numerous functions within the *intravascular space*, as well as within the *extravascular space*.

The functions of blood are numerous and varied. The *transport* of oxygen and carbon dioxide is an important complement to pulmonary and cellular respiration. All food substances must pass through the blood; thus, *nutrition* is of considerable importance. An *excretory* function is obvious through the removal of metabolic waste products. The *maintenance of the water content* of the body is accomplished through a balance between the blood-vascular system, tissue fluid space and lymphatics. Besides the necessity of fluids for the transport of various materials, the water content of the body is an important medium for *heat regulation*. Also, the transport of hormones gives the blood a *regulatory* function. The blood is also an important *protective device* for the body through its cells and various suspended materials (antibodies, antitoxins, etc.).

Classification of Formed Elements. The formed elements of the blood include cells and/or fragments of cells which may be classified accordingly:

- Erythrocytes
- Leukocytes
  - Agranulocytes
    - Lymphocytes
    - Monocytes
  - Granulocytes
    - Neutrophils (heterophils)
    - Eosinophils
    - Basophils
- Platelets and thrombocytes

Mammalian blood contains all of the previously mentioned elements except thrombocytes. Platelets are often referred to as thrombocytes, but in avian species the thrombocyte is a cell. In mammalian species the platelet is a cell fragment.

Of the cells that occur in the blood, there are numerous species differences concerning size, number and specific characteristics. Table 7-1 represents normal values for cellular elements contained in the blood of various domestic and laboratory species. There may be some differences between reported and observed values, since ranges are not reported here.

The staining properties for the subsequently described cells are done so in terms of the use of Wright's or Giemsa stain.

Mammalian Formed Elements

Erythrocytes. The *erythrocytes* are also referred to as *red blood cells* (*RBC*), *red blood corpuscles* and *rubricytes*. The RBC is an anucleated, biconcave disk which is round in most mammalian species. It is, however, oval in the members of the Camelidae (camel, dromedary, llama and alpaca). The diameter range is 3.5–7.4 μm in different species.

In smear preparations the biconcavity is readily apparent because of the differential light transmission from the periphery to the central part of the corpuscle (Fig. 7-1). However, if care is not taken with the preparation solutions, the RBC's may swell in hypotonic media or shrink in hypertonic media. All cells respond in this manner to varying tonicity, but it is most easily demonstrated in the RBC.

In sections stained by routine procedures,

Table 7-1
Corpuscular Values of Selected Species

Species	RBC[a]	WBC[b]	Per Cent Distribution L[c]	M	N	E	B	T[d]
Horse	6.9	10.3	38	4	54	4	1	
Ox	6.3	7.9	64	10	21	5	1	160
Sheep	8.1	7.4	48	6	42	4	1	350
Goat	13.9	8.9	48	5	45	1.5	1	2500
Pig	7.4	17.1	47	8	41	2.5	1	
Dog	6.2	12.6	25	8	57	10	1	620
Cat	8.4	13.8	32	6	57	5	1	232
Rabbit	5.6	7.9	42	9	43	2	4	500
Rat	8.5	11.5	70	5	22	2	1	532
Guinea pig	5.6	10.8	45	8	42	5	1	500
Domestic fowl	2.8	16.6	64	6	26	2	2	27.6

[a] RBC, $10^6/mm^3$.
[b] WBC, $10^3/mm^3$.
[c] L, lymphocytes; M, monocytes; N, neutrophils; E, eosinophils; B, basophils; N (domestic fowl), heterophils; T, platelets (mammals), thrombocytes (domestic fowl).
[d] T, $10^3/mm^3$.

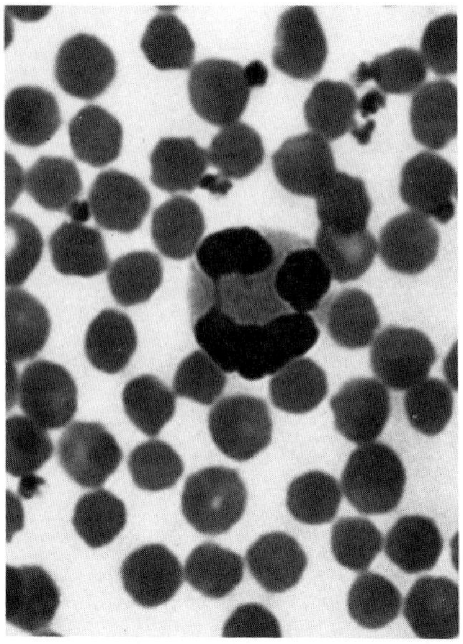

Fig. 7-1. Bovine red blood corpuscles and a neutrophil. ×400. All light micrographs are the original magnifications. All electron micrographs are the final magnifications.

the RBC's will stain pink. Within the capillary beds, larger vessels and even as extravasated blood, RBC's may become stacked one upon the other in a typical *rouleaux* formation. Rouleaux formation, however, is species-specific. This formation is indicative of the manner by which they move through the smallest blood vessels (capillaries). The occurrence of RBC's outside the vascular bed is usually an artifact of preparation techniques.

The RBC is uniquely modified to perform its primary function, carrying oxygen to the tissues in the form of *oxyhemoglobin* and carrying some carbon dioxide away from the tissues in the form of *carboxyhemoglobin*. Most of the cellular organelles (nucleus, Golgi, mitochondria, etc.) are lost and the bulk of the cell is composed of *hemoglobin*. The structural modification as a biconcave disk also facilitates the movement of this entity through the capillary bed.

Although the mature mammalian RBC is anucleated, it begins its life as a typical nucleated cell. During the differentiation process most of the organelles are lost. Sometimes, however, immature cells containing remnants of ribosomal material gain access to the peripheral circulation. These cells, characterized by a diffuse cytoplasmic basophilia, are referred to as *reticulocytes*. They normally occur in small percentages in the peripheral blood; in large numbers, they may be indicative of an abnormal condition. Similarly, remnants of the nucleus (Howell-Jolly bodies) may also occur in mature erythrocytes.

The shape, size and number of the erythrocytes may vary. These parameters may be indicative of an abnormality. The erythrocytes may not have the normal shape (*poikilocythemia*). They may be of varying sizes (*anisocytosis*) with cells larger than normal (*macrocytes*) or cells smaller than normal (*microcytes*). Also, there may be an increase (*polycythemia*) or a decrease (*oligocythemia*) in cell number.

The constant size of red blood cells in normal conditions, as well as their presence in most tissue sections, gives the microscopist a "built-in micrometer." Although there may be some shrinkage or swelling associated with the tissue processing, as well as species differences, the RBC's are generally about 5–6 μm in diameter.

The life-span of an erythrocyte is approximately 120 days in man. The life-span of these cells is shorter in other mammals. At the termination of their life-span certain cells of the reticuloendothelial system within the liver, spleen and bone marrow phagocytose the RBC's. The resulting brown pigment, ***hemosiderin***, may be found normally in these organs. Hemosiderin is an iron-containing pigment resulting from the breakdown of hemoglobin. Since the body is incapable of storing iron, hemosiderin may be important in the reutilization of iron for the synthesis of hemoglobin. How it is related to the synthesis of new hemoglobin, however, is unknown.

Non-iron-containing pigments, ***bilirubin*** and *biliverdin*, are also formed during the degradation of hemoglobin. These, however, are dissolved in the blood and removed by the liver; they then become part of the bile.

Granulocytes. The granulocytes are those *white blood cells* or *leukocytes* of the blood that contain specific granules and have lobed nuclei. These are the *neutrophils*, *eosinophils* and *basophils*.

The *neutrophil*, *heterophil* or *polymorphonuclear leukocyte* (*PMN*) is the most frequently encountered granulocyte. The cell is about twice the size of the RBC (9–12 μm) and is characterized by a segmented nucleus which may have from 3 to 5 lobes connected by a fine strand of nucleoplasm (Fig. 7-1). The granules, usually described as neutrophilic, may vary from light pink to purple depending upon the stain used; thus, the term *heterophil*. In some species (rabbit, guinea pig) these particles stain with acid dyes and the cells are usually referrred to as *pseudoeosinophils*. In some cases, due to preparatory techniques, the particles may not be apparent.

Electron microscopic examination and cytochemical studies have confirmed that these specific granules are lysosomes. Thus, the primary function of the neutrophil is phagocytosis of various particles, bacteria and other microorganisms. This activity is especially apparent in acute local inflammation during which time great numbers of these cells are present in the connective tissue.

The *eosinophil* or *acidophil* is the next most frequently encountered granulocyte. Its diameter is approximately 12–14 μm. Usually, the nucleus is bilobed, but it may be polymorphic (Fig. 7-2). Characteristically, the acidophilic granules are the distinguishing feature. They are uniform within a cell, but they do vary from species to species (Fig. 7-3). They are especially large in equids. These granules also are lysosomes (Fig. 7-4).

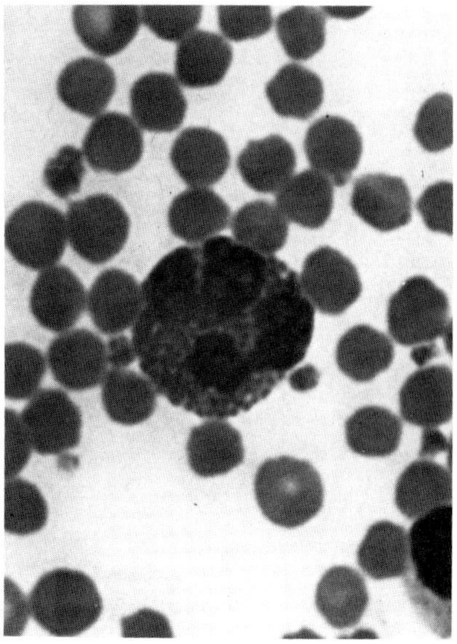

Fig. 7-2. Bovine eosinophil. ×400.

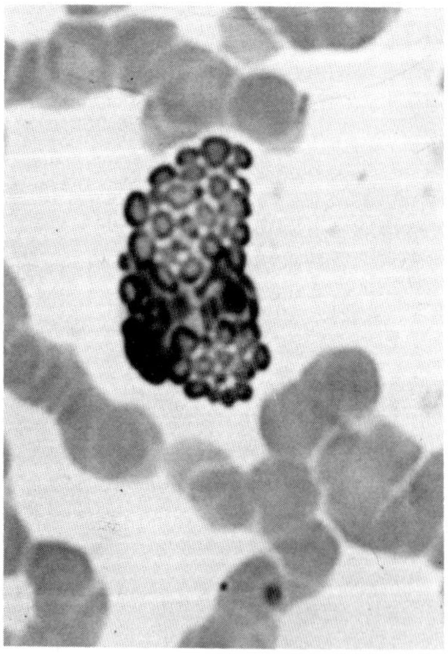

Fig. 7-3. Equine eosinophil. ×400.

These cells increase in number during allergic reactions and parasitic infections, while their numbers may be reduced in response to adrenocorticosteroids. Their primary function is phagocytosis but to a lesser degree than that of the neutrophil.

The *basophil* or *basophilic leukocyte* is the least numerous of the granulocytes. It is about the same size as the neutrophil (9–12 μm). The nucleus is bilobed, although more lobes may be present. The granules are round, coarse and variable in size (Fig. 7-5). They stain much darker than the nucleus and may partially obscure it. These granules are basophilic and metachromatic.

The function of these cells is obscure. They rarely increase in number in pathological conditions. There is some evidence, however, that they are responsible for the elaboration of histamines and heparin in circulating blood.

Agranulocytes. The *agranulocytes* are those white blood cells that do not contain specific granules. Moreover, their nuclei are usually round. These include the *lymphocytes* and *monocytes*.

The *lymphocytes* are usually the most frequently encountered white blood cells. They are characterized by a high nuclear/cytoplasmic ratio (Fig. 7-6). The nucleus is usually round and of sufficient density to obscure the nucleolus. A slight indentation of the nucleus may also be seen. The clear, basophilic cytoplasm may contain some nonspecific, azurophilic granules. Their occurrence, however, is variable. Generally, the nucleus is outlined by a peripherally condensed heterochromatin which readily diffracts light through the minimally granulated cytoplasm. The predominant cytoplasmic organelles are ribosomes, polyribosomes and rough endoplasmic reticulum. The Golgi apparatus and mitochondria are scant.

Lymphocytes vary appreciably in size. *Small lymphocytes* have a diameter of 5–10 μm and are the predominant lymphocytes in the circulating blood. *Medium-sized lymphocytes* range from 10–18 μm. The medium-sized lymphocytes are sometimes difficult to distinguish from monocytes. *Large lymphocytes* typically occur in extravascular tissues such as lymphatic tissue.

The functions of lymphocytes have not been clearly defined. They have been implicated in antibody production and are reactive cells in inflammation and delayed hypersensitivity. There is some evidence that small lymphocytes may be responsible for the development of clones of plasma cells.

The life-span of lymphocytes may vary from hours to years.

Monocytes are consistently the largest of the blood vascular elements. They range from 16–25 μm in diameter. The nucleus is kidney-shaped or bean-shaped, but it may be round as well as trilobed (Fig. 7-7). The nuclear chromatin is lighter and more reticular than the lymphocytic nuclear material. With appropriate staining, the cytoplasm is generally gray. The even distribution of clear granules imparts a ground-glass appearance to the cytoplasm. Scattered azurophilic granules are responsible for this staining quality. The nuclear configuration is an excellent and quite definitive diagnostic feature.

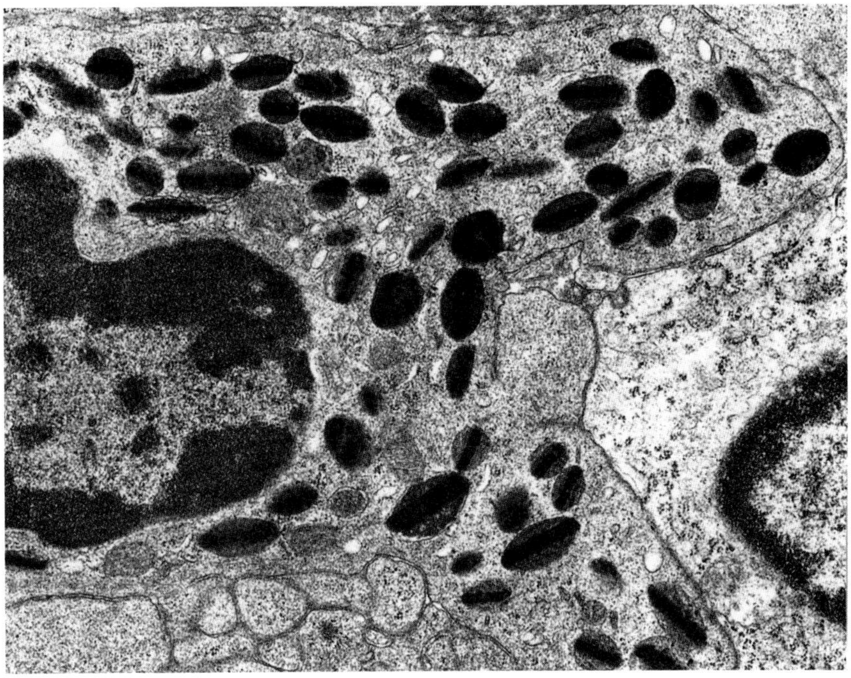

Fig. 7-4. An electron micrograph of an eosinophil. The dark bodies are the specific granules or lysosomes of this cell. ×17,000. (Courtesy of A. M. Sheppard)

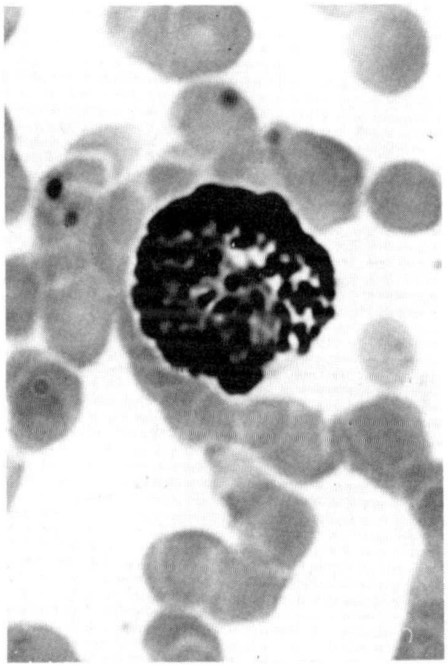

Fig. 7-5. Equine basophil. ×400.

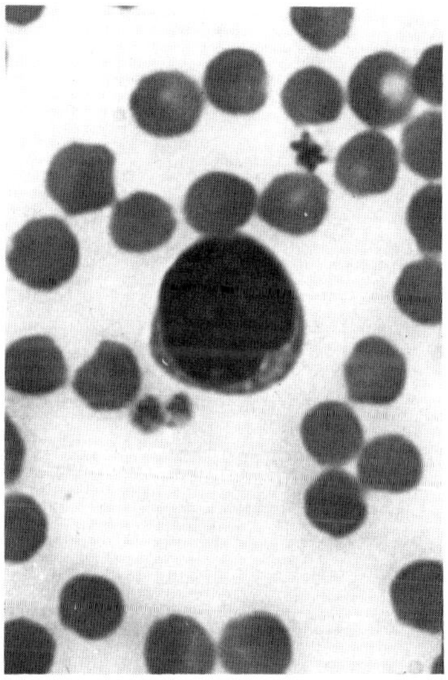

Fig. 7-6. Bovine lymphocyte. ×400.

Monocytes are phagocytic cells that are difficult to distinguish from macrophages once they have gained access to the extravascular space.

Platelets. *Blood platelets* are small protoplasmic disks which are about 2–4 μm in diameter (Fig. 7-8). They are actually cytoplasmic fragments of a large cell, the *megakaryocyte*. The platelets are membrane-bound, round to oval fragments that contain a central, basophilic region (*chromomere*) and a pale, homogeneous peripheral zone (*hyalomere*). The chromomere contains

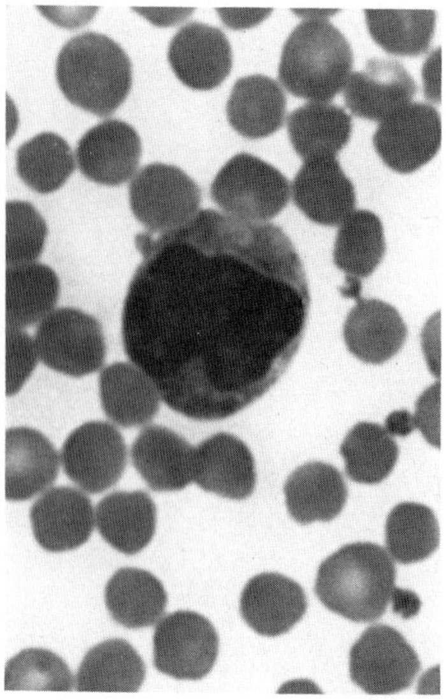

Fig. 7-7. Bovine monocyte. ×400.

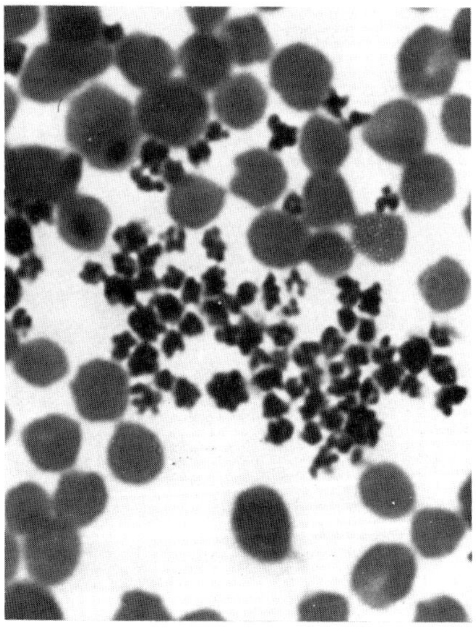

Fig. 7-8. Bovine blood platelets. ×400.

mitochondria, endoplasmic reticular profiles and granules. The hyalomere may contain some glycogen, but it is usually characterized by a homogeneous cytoplasmic matrix. A nucleus is not present.

Platelets are functionally significant in hemostasis. They may form a *white thrombus* by adhering to the walls of injured vessels. They are also responsible for the production of an enzyme, *thromboplastin*. Thromboplastin activates the conversion of *prothrombin* to *thrombin*. Thrombin then converts *fibrinogen* into *fibrin*. They are, therefore, significantly involved in the complex clotting mechanism. Platelets probably also secrete *serotonin*, a *vasoconstrictor*.

Mammalian platelets are often referred to as thrombocytes.

Avian Formed Elements

Erythrocytes. The normal mature erythrocytes of avian blood are oval cells with oval nuclei (Fig. 7-9). These cells range from 10–13 μm long and from 6–7 μm wide. The elongated nucleus is about one-half of the dimensions of the cell. Nuclear heterochromatin may appear uniformly distributed in an oval nucleus. In a contracted nucleus, the heterochromatin may assume a more dense configuration. A nucleolus is not present. The cytoplasm may vary from orange-pink to red with routine blood stains. Numerous artifactual changes may alter the configuration and staining affinity of these cells. Erythrocytes of fishes and amphibians are morphologically similar to those of birds.

Granulocytes. The *granulocytes* of birds are the *heterophils*, *eosinophils* and *basophils*.

The *heterophil* of birds is the equivalent of the neutrophil in other species. The term heterophil is applied to these cells because of the great diversity of staining reaction in various classes of vertebrates. Even in mammalian domestic species this could be appropriately applied.

The heterophil has a diameter of 6–9 μm. Despite its amoeboid properties, it is usually seen as a round cell in blood smears. The multilobed nucleus may have as many as 5 lobes and the heterochromatin is coarsely clumped. The distinguishing feature is the presence of brightly stained, eosinophilic rods with a fusiform configuration (Fig. 7-10). These specific inclusions are randomly scattered throughout the cell. They are easily dissolved in aqueous media and all that may remain is a red-stained *central body* or *vacuole*. As a result of this dissolution, the normally clear cytoplasm usually becomes acidophilic. Under these conditions the heterophils are easily confused with eosinophils.

The avian *eosinophil* has a diameter between 5 and 9 μm. It has a multilobed nucleus with coarsely clumped heterochromatin. The cytoplasm, although usually obscured by tightly packed granules, stains a pale clear blue (Fig. 7-11). This characteristic is of diagnostic significance in distinguishing eosinophils from heterophils in which the rods have been partially dissolved. The granules of some eosinophils may appear as homogeneous bodies. In larger cells, the granules appear to be composed of three or four subunits which are combined in such a manner that a vacuity or clear space appears in the center of the complex. The eosinophilic granule is more refractive than that of the heterophil.

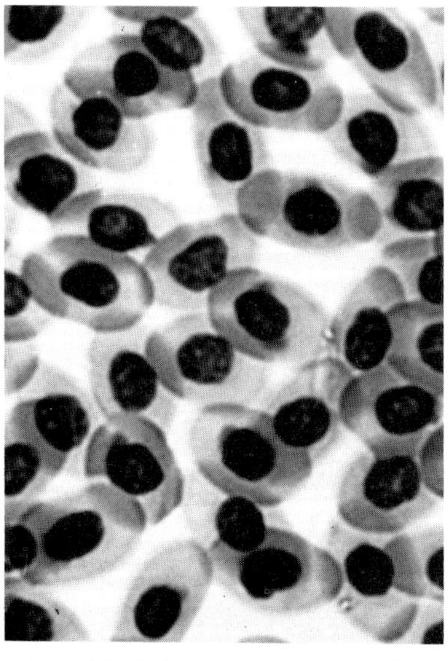

Fig. 7-9. Avian erythrocytes. ×400.

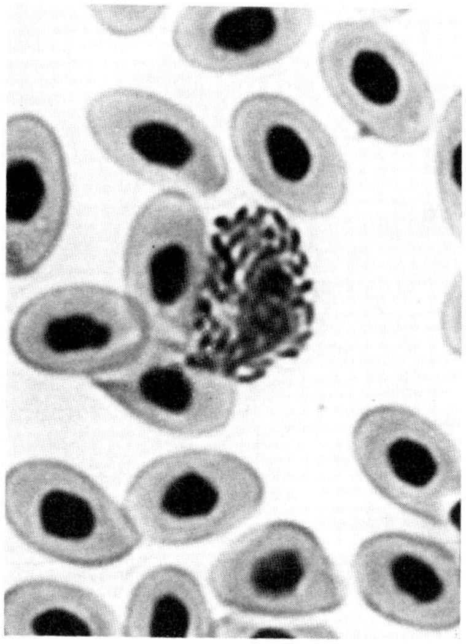

Fig. 7-10. Avian heterophil. ×400.

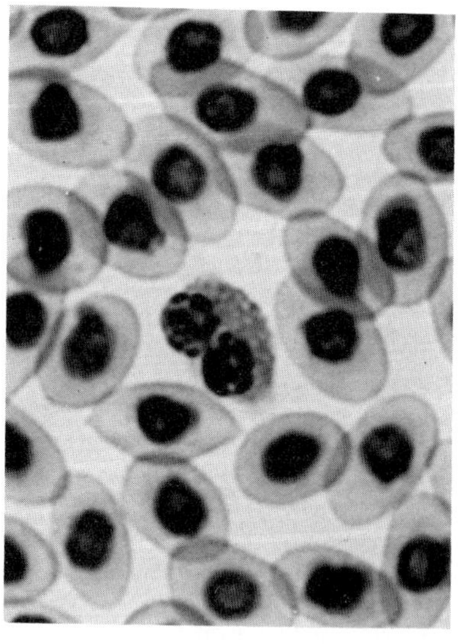

Fig. 7-11. Avian eosinophil. ×400.

The *basophil* of birds is similar to that of mammalian species. These cells are more numerous in avian blood.

Agranulocytes. The *agranulocytes* of avian blood are the *lymphocytes* and *monocytes*. Although the relationship of the *thrombocyte* to the agranulocytic and erythrocytic series has not been clarified, the thrombocyte will be discussed with the agranulocytes.

The avian *lymphocyte* approximates the range of sizes reported for the comparable mammalian cell. Small, medium and large lymphocytes have been described. The cell is generally round with an even contour (Fig. 7-12). Cytoplasmic blebs, however, may be apparent. The nucleus is usually centrally located, but some cells may be polarized. Coarsely clumped heterochromatin is characteristic of this structure. Also, the nuclear/cytoplasmic ratio is high. A sharp indentation in the nucleus may also be apparent. Cytoplasmic characteristics are quite variable. The cytoplasm may stain faintly and be quite homogeneous, or it may stain intensely and be flocculated with basophilic material. The flocculation may be fine and slightly reticulated or heavy and coarsely reticulated. Some magenta-staining granules may be evident.

The avian *monocyte* is the largest cell of the mature elements of the agranulocytic series. Usually, the average lymphocyte diameter approximates the diameter of the monocyte nucleus. Although the monocyte is usually round, numerous other configurations attest to its amoeboid characteristics (Fig. 7-13). The nuclear/cytoplasmic ratio is smaller than that of the lymphocyte. The bean-shaped or kidney-shaped nucleus contains a fine reticulum of heterochromatin. The area of the cytoplasm associated with the nuclear indentation is characteristic for the monocytes. This juxtanuclear area contains orange granules or it may be tinged orange. The ground-glass appearance of the cytoplasm, azurophilic granules and the juxtanuclear characteristics are diagnostic features for the monocyte.

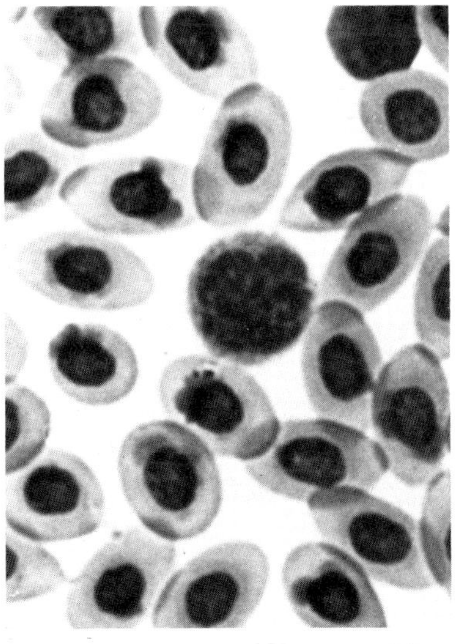

Fig. 7-12. Avian lymphocyte. ×400.

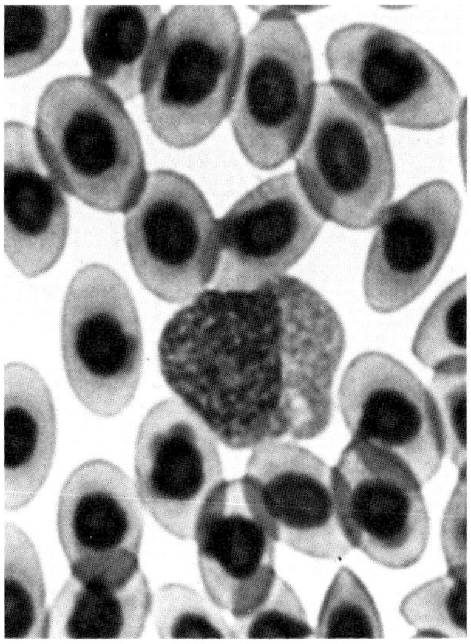

Fig. 7-13. Avian monocyte. ×400.

The *thrombocytes* of birds and other submammalian vertebrates are nucleated cells. These cells are somewhat smaller than erythrocytes and have average dimensions of 5 by 9 μm. The centrally located, elongated nucleus is coarsely granular with heterochromatin (Fig. 7-14). The cytoplasm is finely reticulated and basophilic and may contain a number of azurophilic, specific granules.

Besides functioning in hemostasis in a manner similar to mammalian platelets, the avian thrombocytes have been shown to be *trephocytic* and *phagocytic*.

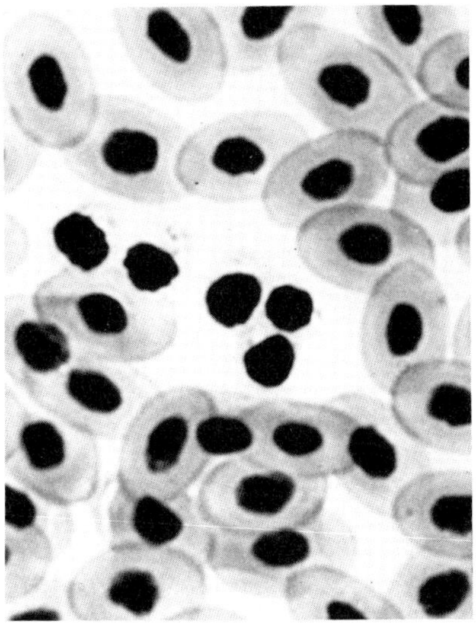

Fig. 7-14. Avian thrombocytes. ×400.

References

Erythrocytes

Baker, R. F.: Ultrastructure of red blood cells. Fed. Proc. *26*:1785, 1967.

Hevesy, G. and Ottesen, J.: Life-cycle of the red corpuscle of the hen. Nature *156*:534, 1945.

Koehler, J. K.: Freeze-etching observations on nucleated erythrocytes with special reference to the nuclear and plasma membranes. Z. Zellforsch. *85*:1, 1968.

Granulocytes

Archer, G. T. and Hirsch, J. C.: Motion picture studies of degranulation of horse eosinophils during phagocytosis. J. Exp. Med. *118*:287, 1963.

Dolowy, W. C., Cornet, J. and Henson, D.: Particles in leukocytes of normal human beings after negative staining in electron microscopy. Nature *209*:1358, 1966.

Franklin, D. A.: Electron microscopic study of human basophils. *29*:878, 1967.

Hamre, C. J.: Origin and differentiation of heterophil, eosinophil and basophil leucocytes of chickens. Anat. Rec. *112*:339, 1952.

Hersch, I. G. and Cohn, Z. A.: Degranulation of polymorphonuclear leucocytes following phagocytosis of microorganisms. J. Exp. Med. *112*:1005, 1960.

Miller, F., DeHarven, E. and Palade, G. E.. The structure of eosinophil leukocyte granules in rodents and in man. J. Cell Biol. *31*:349, 1966.

Natt, M. P. and Herrick, C. A.: Variation in the shape of the rodlike granule of the chicken heterophil leucocyte and its possible significance. Poult. Sci. *33*:828, 1954.

Agranulocytes

Elves, M. W.: *The Lymphocytes*. Lloyd Luke Ltd., London, 1966.

Fiore-Donati, L. and Hanna, M. G., Jr.: *Lymphatic Tissue and Germinal Centers in Immune Response*. Plenum, New York, 1969.

Gowans, J. L.: The life history of lymphocytes. Brit. Med. Bull. *15*:50, 1959.

Gowans, J. L.: The immunological activities of lymphocytes. Progr. Allerg. *9*:1, 1965.

Hoshino, T., Takeda, M., Abe, K. and Ito, T.: Early development of thymic lymphocytes in mice, studied by light and electron microscopy. Anat. Rec. *164*:47, 1969.

Movat, H. Z. and Fernando, N. V. P.: The fine structure of the lymphoid tissue during antibody formation. Exp. Molec. Path. *4*:155, 1965.

Tompkins, E. H.: The monocyte. Ann. N. Y. Acad. Sci. *59*:732, 1955.

Platelets and Thrombocytes

Behnke, O.: Electron microscopic observations on the membrane systems of the rat blood platelet. Anat. Rec. *158*:121, 1967.

Carlson, H. C., Sweeney, P. R. and Tokaryk, J. M.. Demonstration of phagocytic and trephocytic activities of chicken thrombocytes by microscopy and vital staining techniques. Avian Dis. *12*:700, 1968.

Clarke, J. A., Hawkey, C. and Salisbury, A. J.: Surface ultrastructure of platelets and thrombocytes. Nature *223*:401, 1969.

Rodman, N. F. and Mason, R. G.: Platelet-platelet interaction: Relationship to hemostasis and thrombosis. Fed. Proc. *26*:95, 1967.

Simpson, C. F.: Ultrastructural features of the turkey thrombocyte and lymphocyte. Poult. Sci. *47*:848, 1968.

Comparative Hematology

Afonsky, D.: Blood picture in normal dogs. Amer. J. Physiol. *180*:456, 1955.

Ferguson, L. C., Irwin, M. R. and Beach, B. A.: On variation in the blood cells of healthy cattle. J. Infect. Dis. *76*:24, 1945.

Holman, H. H.: A negative correlation between size and number of the erythrocytes of cows, sheep, goats and horses. J. Path. Bact. *64*:379, 1952.

Lucas, A. M.: A discussion of synonymy in avian and mammalian hematological nomenclature. Amer. J. Vet. Res. *20*:887, 1959.

Wintrobe, M. M., Shumacker, H. B., Jr. and Schmidt, W. J.: Values for number, size and hemoglobin content of erythrocytes in normal dogs, rabbits and rats. Amer. J. Physiol. *114*:502, 1936.

8 Muscular Tissue

General Characteristics

Form and Function. The structural element of muscular tissue is the *muscle cell* or *muscle fiber*. Unlike the connective tissue fiber which is noncellular and the nerve fiber which is a cellular process, the term *fiber*, in this context, refers to an entire cell. Although all cells possess the ability to contract to one degree or another, *contractility* in muscle fibers is an especially well-developed characteristic.

Muscle comprises the majority of the "flesh" (*sarcos*, Gr., flesh) or "meat" of an organism. It is also a primary mural (wall) element of tubular organs.

Muscle fibers are elongated cells which may be uninucleated or multinucleated. They are enclosed by a *sarcolemma* (*the combined plasmalemma* and *basal lamina*) and *fine reticular fibers*. The *sarcoplasm*, or cytoplasm, contains typical organelles as well as contractile elements. These *contractile elements* are myofilaments composed of the proteins, *actin* and *myosin*. The *myofilaments* are grouped as *myofibrils*. The organization of the contractile elements is different in the various types of muscular tissue.

The characteristic property of muscle, contractility, is translated into the development of tension upon stimulation. This tension is the means by which work is accomplished. The work may be locomotion, expression of secretions from glands, movement of blood through the cardiovascular system, movement of materials through the digestive system and a host of related functions.

Functionally, muscle may be *voluntary* or *involuntary*. Structurally, it may be *smooth* (*nonstriated*) or *striated*. Through the combination of these characteristics, the following classification is derived:

1. Smooth muscle: nonstriated, involuntary.
2. Skeletal muscle: striated, voluntary.
3. Cardiac muscle: striated, involuntary.

Types of Muscular Tissue

Smooth Muscle. Smooth muscle fibers are elongated, spindle-shaped cells with finely tapered ends. The central region in which the nucleus is located is the widest part of the cell. These cells may be as short as 20 μm as mural elements of a small tubule or as long as 0.5 mm in the wall of a gravid uterus. Although the fibers are as described, this appearance is not always apparent in a single section. Often the cytoplasmic portions of the cells are tightly packed and appear to blend as a homogeneous mass (Fig. 8-1). The elongated, cylindrical nucleus is rounded at the ends and contains a fine chromatin network. Clumped heterochromatin may be apparent along the inner nuclear membrane. Two to several nucleoli may be apparent. The nuclei may be twisted and wrinkled or assume a helical configuration. This may be indicative of active contraction at the time of fixation or a passive distortion due to agonal changes. The nucleus, together with a bright, homogeneous, acidophilic cytoplasm is the key to identification.

The appearance of these cells varies with the plane of section. In longitudinal section, they appear as described previously. Because of their shape, however, not all nuclei will be included in any given section. Only those cells that have been sectioned through their thickest profiles will have nuclei apparent. These cells are staggered; the thickest portion of one is adjacent to the tapered portion of another. The appearance of nuclei reflects this staggering.

In cross-section, the cells are round to oval (Fig. 8-2). The nuclei are round and centrally located or slightly eccentric in position. Again, the nuclei are not seen in all cells sectioned as a result of the staggered relationship.

Smooth muscle fibers are intimately associated with fine reticular fibers. These fibers, although they wrap around the cells, are not in contact with the muscle fibers. Each muscle fiber is surrounded by a polysaccharide-rich basal lamina in which reticular fibers may be embedded. Bundles of muscle fibers may be intimately associated with connective tissue as in the corium. In

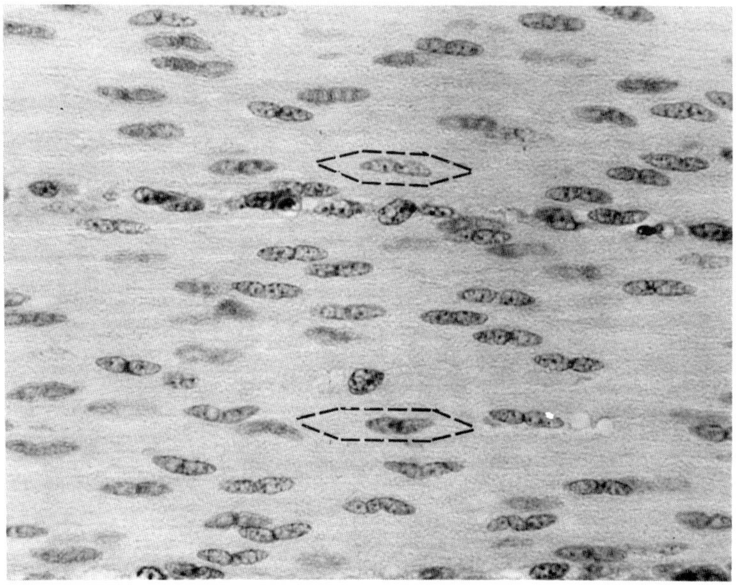

Fig. 8-1. Longitudinal section of smooth muscle. *Dashed lines*, approximate cellular limits. ×160. All light micrographs are the original magnifications. All electron micrographs are the final magnifications.

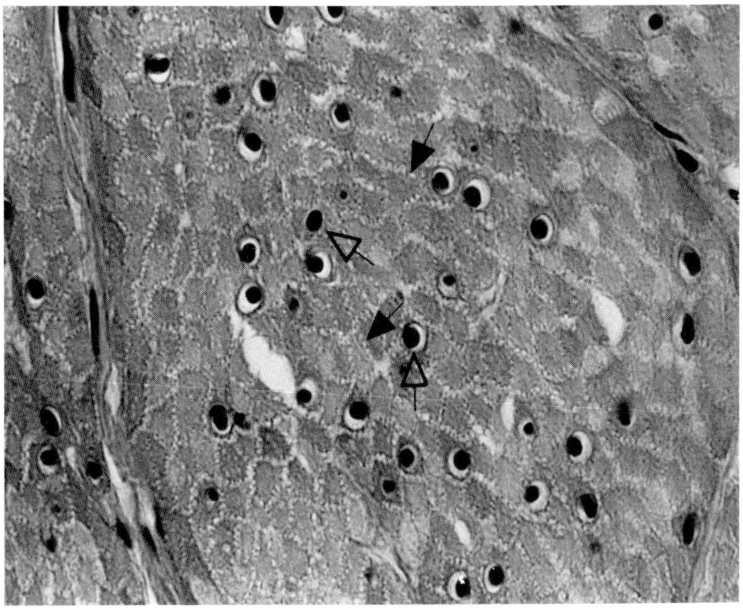

Fig. 8-2. Cross-section of smooth muscle. The nuclei (*open arrows*) and the cellular limits (*solid arrows*) are apparent. ×160.

other areas, the muscle cells are arranged in extensive sheets, a few to many layers thick. In these instances, the finer reticular fibers are eventually continuous with the connective tissue surrounding the entire sheet. These sheets are often arranged so that the muscle fibers of one sheet are at right angles to the muscle fibers of another. In cross-section through a tubular organ, such as the gut, one sheet (circularly oriented and inner) is longitudinally sectioned. The adjacent sheet (longitudinal and outer), at 90° to the other, is cross-sectioned (Fig. 8-3). Naturally, in longitudinal section of an organ the reverse occurs.

At the electron microscopic level, the smooth muscle cell reflects its light microscopic appearance (Fig. 8-4). The nucleus is elongated and finely granular with peripherally clumped heterochromatin. The organelles are confined to the perinuclear regions of the cell, especially at the poles of the nucleus. Mitochondria, rough endoplasmic reticulum, free ribosomes and a small Golgi apparatus are present. The remainder of the cytoplasm is occupied by parallel but discontinuous bundles of myofilaments. Along the plasma membrane are numerous caveolae and pinocytotic vesicles. The basal lamina is broken in specific areas at which points the plasma membranes are tightly attached to each other in a *fascia occludens* (similar to the *zonula occludens* of epithelial tissues). These regions or *nexi* are probably areas of low electrical resistance which facilitate the spreading of excitation from one cell to another.

Functionally, smooth muscle is slow to contract. This may be accounted for by the lack of individual fiber innervation and the necessity of excitation to spread through nexi. The sustained contraction of smooth muscle, however, is resistant to fatigue. The smooth muscle of tubular organs is responsible for the size of lumina as well as the tone of the walls. Also, smooth muscle is responsible for the movement of materials through the lumina of tubular organs.

Smooth muscle is capable of repair and regeneration. However, extensive injury to smooth muscle results in replacement by irregular dense white fibrous connective tissue (DWFCT) as *scar tissue* (*cicatrix*).

Re-examine sections of regular DWFCT in longitudinal and cross-sections and note the differences between it and smooth muscle.

Morphological Features of Smooth Muscle:

1. A homogeneous, brightly acidophilic cytoplasm.
2. Elongated nuclei with a fine chromatin network.
3. Nuclei may be smooth-surfaced, wrinkled, twisted or helical.
4. Cells are tightly packed and cellular boundaries are indistinct.

Skeletal Muscle. The skeletal muscle fiber is an elongated cell which is slightly tapered or blunt at the ends. Although there is great variability in length, most muscle fibers are between 1 and 40 mm. They vary from 10–100 μm in diameter. Two conspicuous features are immediately apparent. These cells are multinucleated and striated (Fig. 8-5). The oval nuclei have moderately abundant quantities of peripherally clumped heterochromatin. The nuclei are located at the periphery of the cells. Some nuclei will appear to be centrally located. This, however, is usually an artifact of sectioning; i.e., the section may be close to the sarcolemma above or below the observation plane.

The cross-striations, or dark and light bands, are oriented perpendicular to the long axis of the muscle fiber. Upon higher magnification the regularity of the banding is resolved (Fig. 8-6). The lighter *I bands* separate the darker *A bands*. Contained within the I bands are dense lines, the *Z lines*. A *sarcomere*, the *unit of muscular contraction*, includes the myofilaments contained between two adjacent Z lines.

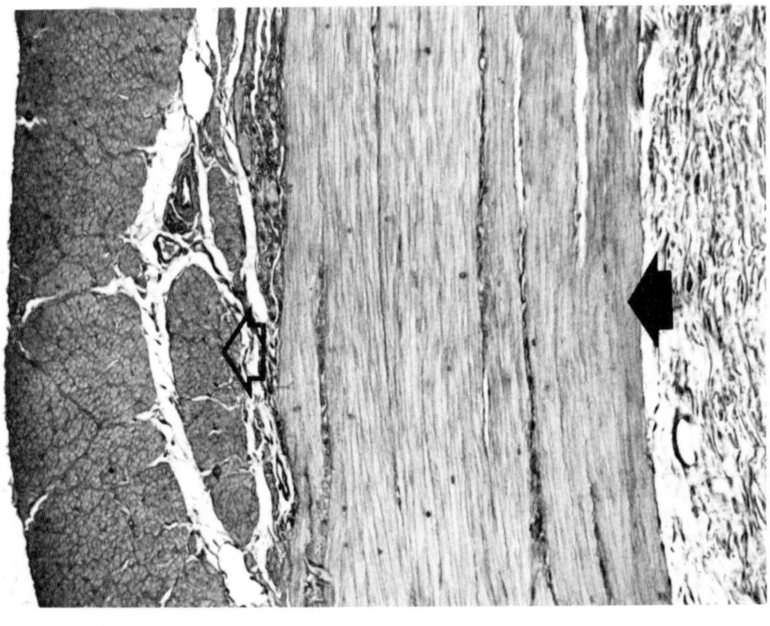

Fig. 8-3. Tunica muscularis of the wall of the gastrointestinal tract. The inner circular muscle (*solid arrow*) is longitudinally sectioned; the outer circular muscle (*open arrow*) is cross-sectioned. ×40.

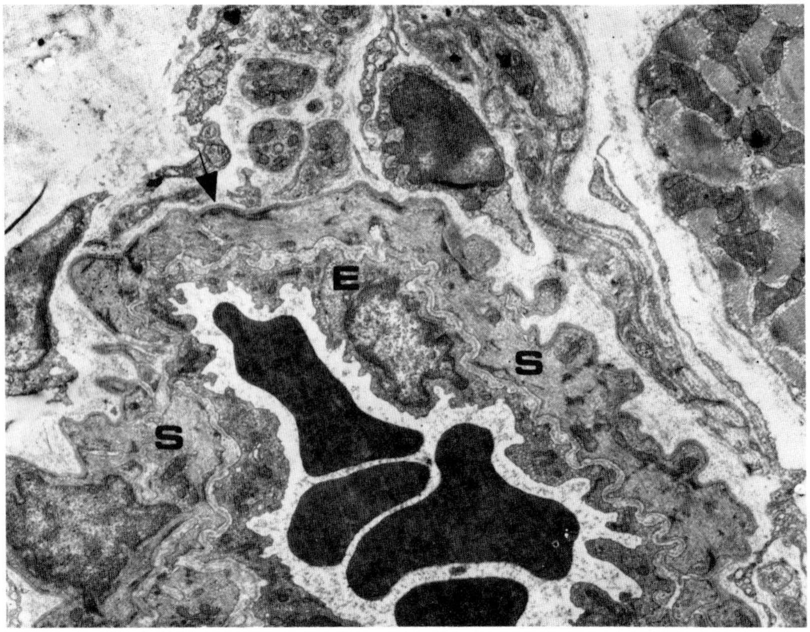

Fig. 8-4. Electron micrograph of a smooth muscle cell of an arteriole. The smooth muscle cell (*S*) surrounds the endothelial cell (*E*). The periphery of the smooth muscle cell is adjacent to a basal lamina (*arrow*). ×14,000. (Courtesy of G. P. Epling)

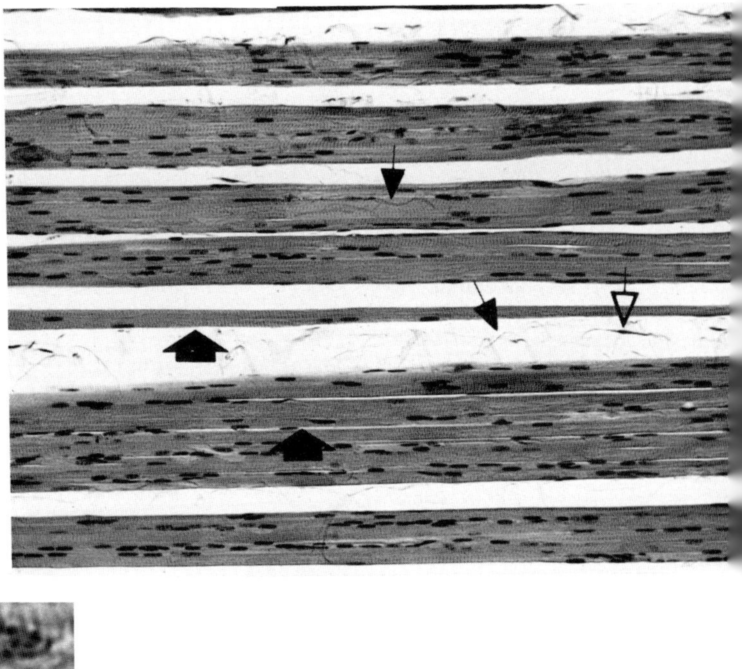

Fig. 8-5. Longitudinal section of skeletal muscle. Individual muscle fibers (*large arrows*) are striated and multinucleated. Compare muscle fiber size with that of connective tissue cells (*open arrow*). Endomyseal connective tissue (*solid arrows*) surrounds the muscle fibers. ×40.

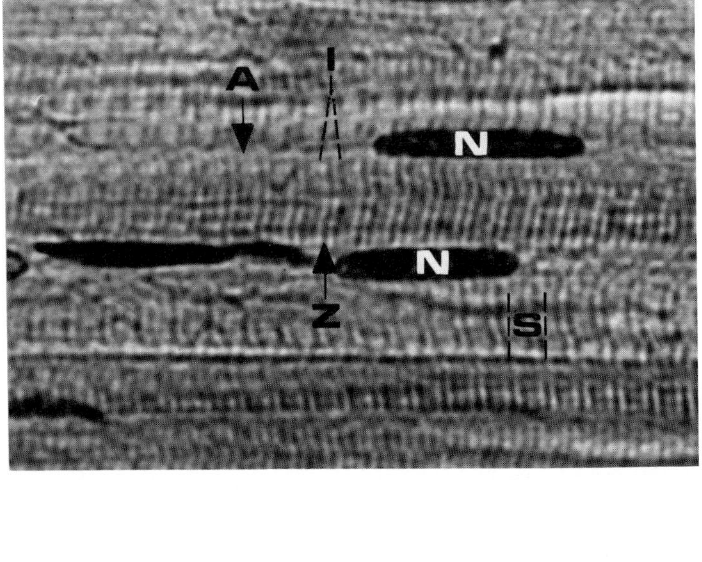

Fig. 8-6. Striations of skeletal muscle. The nuclei (*N*), A band (*A*), I band (*I*) and Z lines (*Z*) are indicated. The sarcomeres of individual myofibrils are registered in such a way as to be visible at the light microscopic level (*S*). ×400.

Individual muscle fibers are oriented in an unbranched, parallel array and are separated from one another by loose connective tissue which contains blood vessels and nerves. Naturally, a basal lamina separates the connective tissue compartment from the associated muscle fibers.

In cross-section, the peripheral relationship of the nuclei to the muscle fibers is more readily observed (Fig. 8-7). Also, the myofibrils are seen as clumps (*Cohnheim's fields*) of acidophilic dots.

The detailed morphology of a sarcomere has been clarified with the electron microscope (Fig. 8-8). One sarcomere extends between two adjacent Z lines in a myofibril and includes one-half of the I bands on either side of the A band. The only myofilaments contained within the I bands are the thin actin filaments. The A band, however, contains both the thin actin filaments and the thick myosin filaments. The actin filaments do not extend uninterruptedly from the Z line through the A band. Rather, there are two separate actin filaments extending from each Z line through the A band. The gap between their ends within the A band is the H band. Upon contraction, the I band is shortened, the H band is obliterated and a dense M line is formed in the space previously occupied by the H band (Fig. 8-9). Contraction, therefore, is a sliding of actin myofilaments over the fixed myosin filaments with a resultant shortening of the component I bands of the sarcomere.

Mitochondria are abundant between the myofibrils. An extensive tubular and vesicular network of smooth endoplasmic reticulum (*sarcoplasmic reticulum*) is also located between these myofibrils (Fig. 8-9). These smooth profiles are in close proximity to tubular invaginations of the plasmalemma. These invaginations are referred to as the *transverse sarcotubular system* (Fig. 8-9).

Skeletal muscle fibers are capable of limited repair; however, extensive trauma to the fibers results in their replacement at the site of injury with fibrous connective tissue originating from the perimuscular space.

Morphological features of skeletal muscle:

1. Large muscle fibers are unbranched and parallel to each other.
2. Peripherally located nuclei.
3. Very distinct striations.
4. Minimal amounts of connective tissue around the individual fibers.

Cardiac Muscle. This tissue is very similar

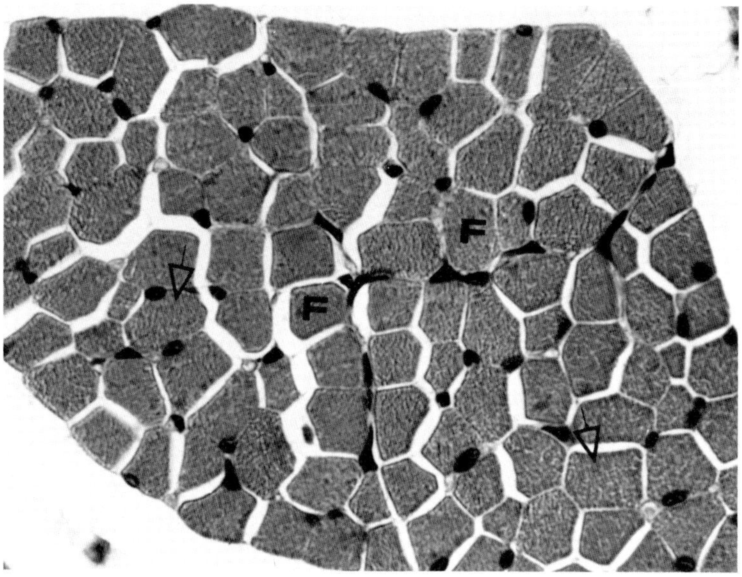

Fig. 8-7. Cross-section of skeletal muscle. The fibers (*F*) are grouped in bundles. The grouping of myofibrils as Cohnheim's areas (*arrows*) are apparent. Note the peripheral position of nuclei. ×160.

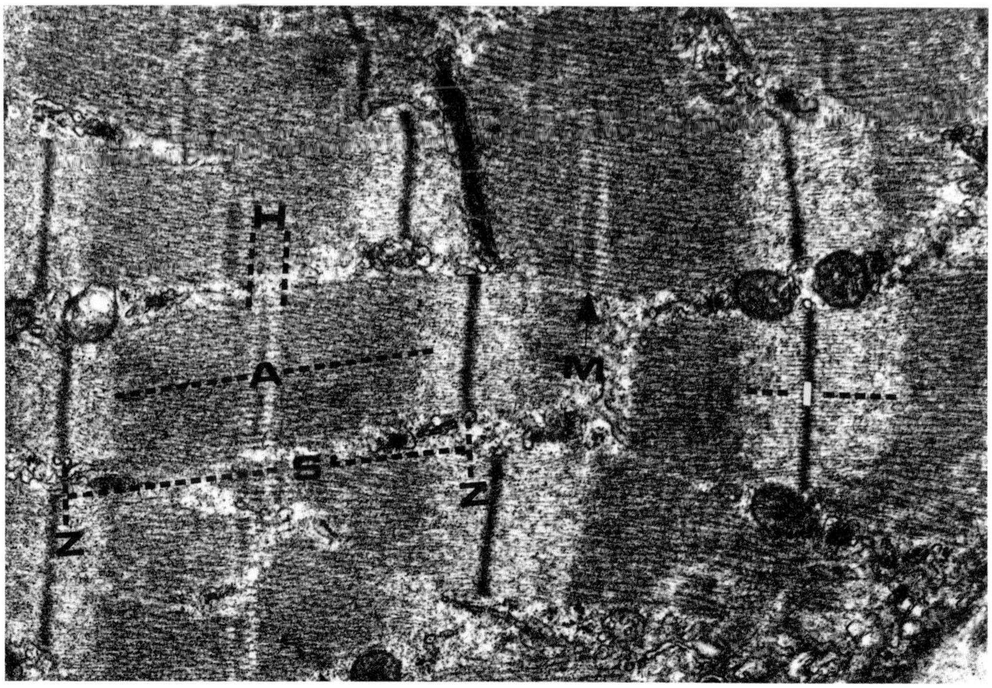

Fig. 8-8. Electron micrograph of partially relaxed skeletal muscle. The sarcomere (*S*), A bands (*A*), I bands (*I*), H bands (*H*), Z lines (*Z*) and M lines (*M*) are indicated. ×26,000.

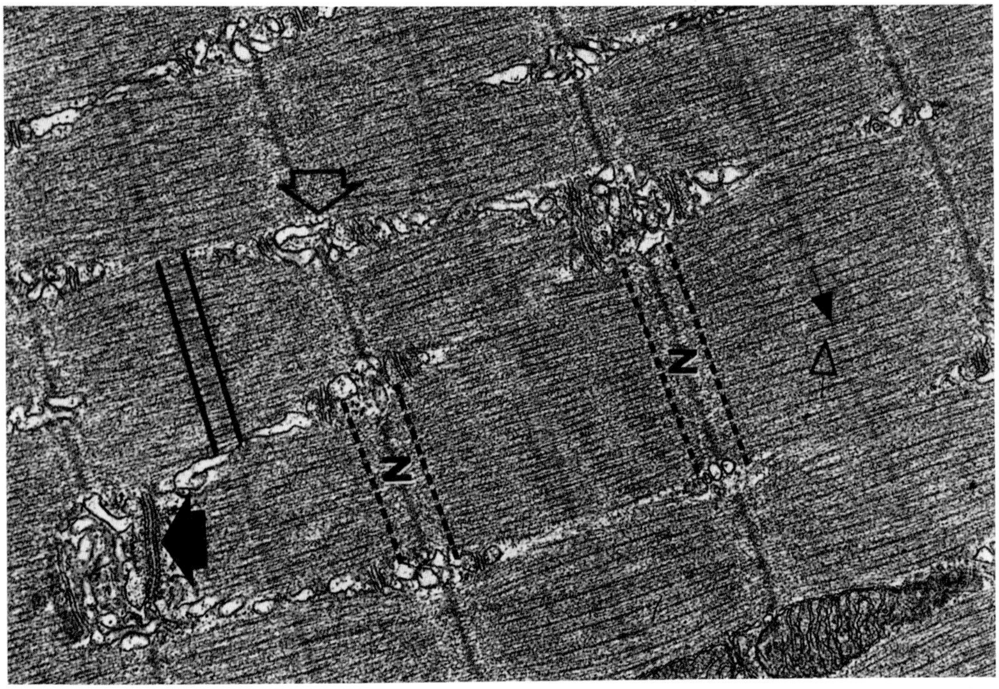

Fig. 8-9. Electron micrograph of partially contracted skeletal muscle. The Z line (Z) is contained within the reduced I band (*dashed line*). A thick myosin filament traverses the M line (*small solid arrow*). Thin actin filaments (*small open arrow*) are apparent. The limits of the H band (*solid lines*) are indicated. The sarcoplasmic reticulum (*large open arrow*) and the transverse sarcotubular system (*large solid arrow*) are apparent at the level of Z lines. ×26,000.

to skeletal muscle. Both are striated; however, cardiac muscle is involuntary. Only those features characteristic of cardiac muscle will be presented here. If a specific characteristic is omitted, the student is to assume that it is similar to skeletal muscle.

There are six morphological features of cardiac muscle that are quite distinct and are aids in identification. The cardiac muscle fibers are branched. In any given section, longitudinally, transversely and obliquely sectioned fibers may be present (Fig. 8-10). The connective tissue surrounding each muscle fiber is more prominent here than in skeletal muscle.

The nuclei of cardiac muscle cells are centrally located and surrounded by a pale-staining cytoplasmic region— a *perinuclear halo* (Fig. 8-11). The sarcoplasm contains myofilaments which are arranged in a manner previously described. Bundles of myofilaments, however, reflect the branching of the muscle fibers. Moreover, the striations that are readily apparent in skeletal muscle are not as prominent in cardiac muscle.

Lastly, distinct darkly stained bands are scattered throughout cardiac muscle. These darkly stained bands are oriented perpendicular to the long axis of the muscle fiber. Moreover, these *intercalated disks* appear as stepwise striations because Z bands are not always in register with each other (Fig. 8-12). The intercalated disks actually are end-to-end points of contact and adhe-

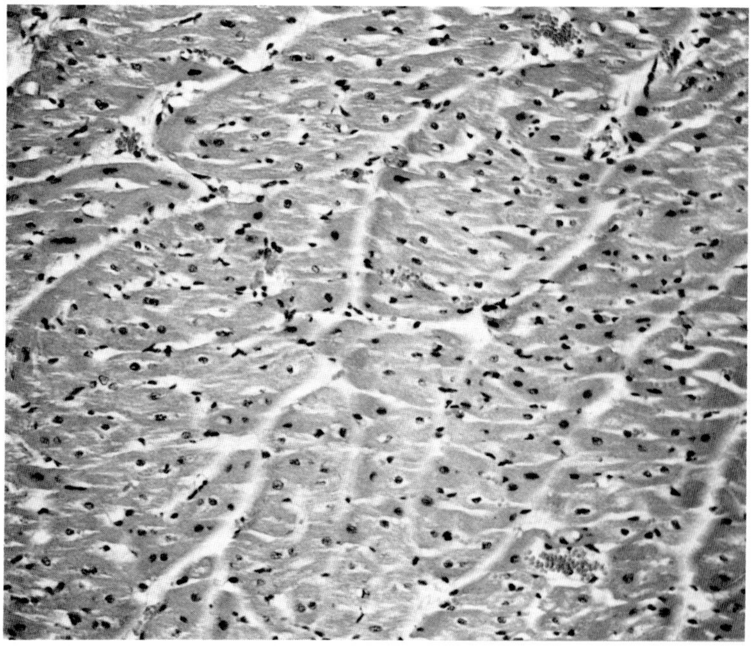

Fig. 8-10. Section of cardiac muscle. ×40.

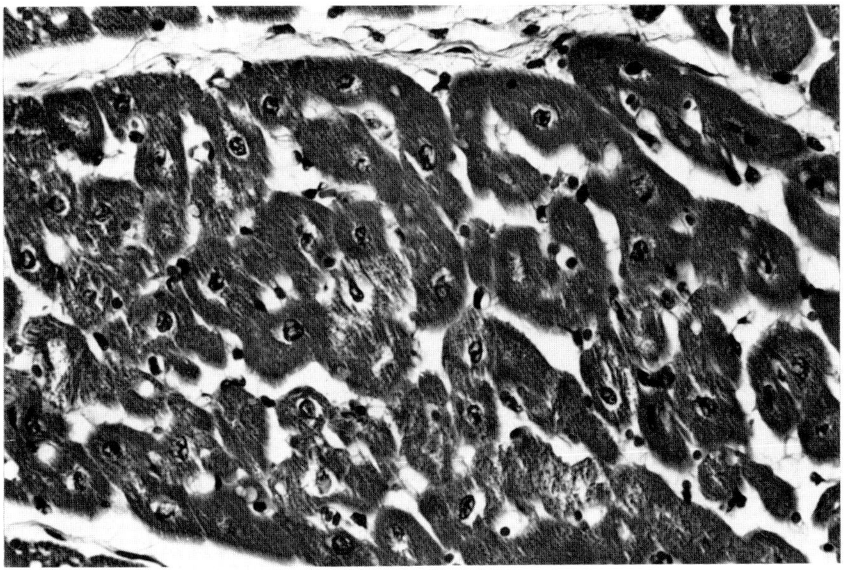

Fig. 8-11. Section of cardiac muscle. The central location of the nuclei and perinuclear halos is apparent. ×100.

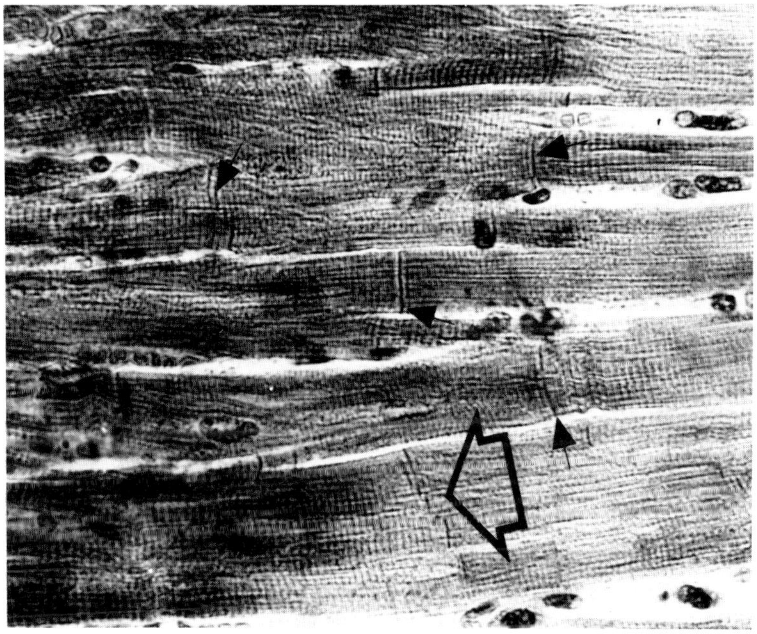

Fig. 8-12. Intercalated disks of cardiac muscle. The disks (*solid arrows*) delimit the boundaries of adjacent muscle cells. They may appear as straight boundaries or have a stepwise appearance (*large open arrow*). ×160.

sion between adjacent cardiac muscle cells. Although various types of junctional complexes comprise the intercalated disks, the most commonly encountered ones are desmosomes (Fig. 8-13). Tight junctions are also present. The myofilaments of sarcomeres embed in the intracellular dense areas associated with the desmosomes. Besides intercellular contact and adhesion, the tight junctions of the intercalated disks may represent areas of increased electrical conductivity which may facilitate the passage of impulses from one cell to another. *Fasciae occludentes*, long tight junctions, occur on the lateral margins of their interdigitations.

Cardiac muscle fibers are incapable of undergoing repair or regeneration. Following trauma these fibers are replaced by fibrous connective tissue from the surrounding connective tissue.

Purkinje Fibers. *Purkinje fibers* are specialized cardiac muscle cells which are modified as impulse-conducting cells (Fig. 8-14). These fibers conduct impulses from the A-V node through the interventricular septum to the ventricles.

In cross-section the Purkinje fibers are much larger than typical cardiac muscle cells (Fig. 8-15). Also, the Purkinje fibers have an abundant pale-staining, acidophilic sarcoplasm which is rich in glycogen. Myofibrils are few and, when present, are usually located peripherally. Nuclei are centrally located.

In longitudinal section these fibers appear as swollen cardiac muscle cells with scattered myofibrils. These fibers are joined to cardiac muscle cells by intercalated disks (Fig. 8-16).

References

Smooth Muscle

Garamvolgyi, N., Vizi, E. S. and Knoll, J.: The regular occurrence of thick filaments in stretched mammalian smooth muscle. J. Ultrastruct. Res. *34*:135, 1971.

Lane, B. P.: Alterations in cytological detail of intestinal smooth muscle cells in various stages of contraction. J. Cell Biol. *27*:199, 1965.

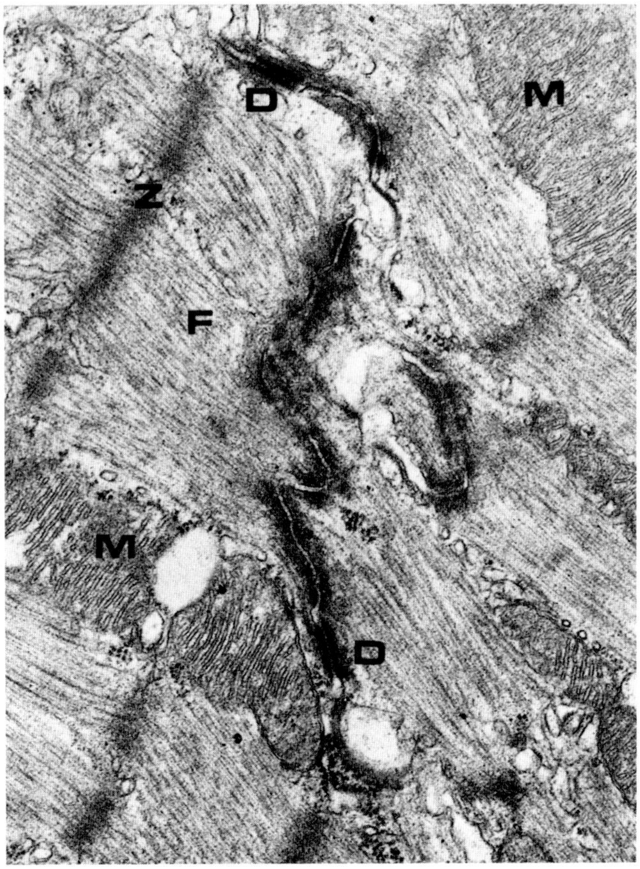

Fig. 8-13. Electron micrograph of an intercalated disk. The tortuous path of the disk is apparent. Desmosomes (*D*) are the dominant type of fusion mechanisms. Mitochondria (*M*) and Z lines (*Z*) are indicated. Myofilaments (*F*) extend into the cytoplasmic densities adjacent to the intercalated disk. ×26, 000.

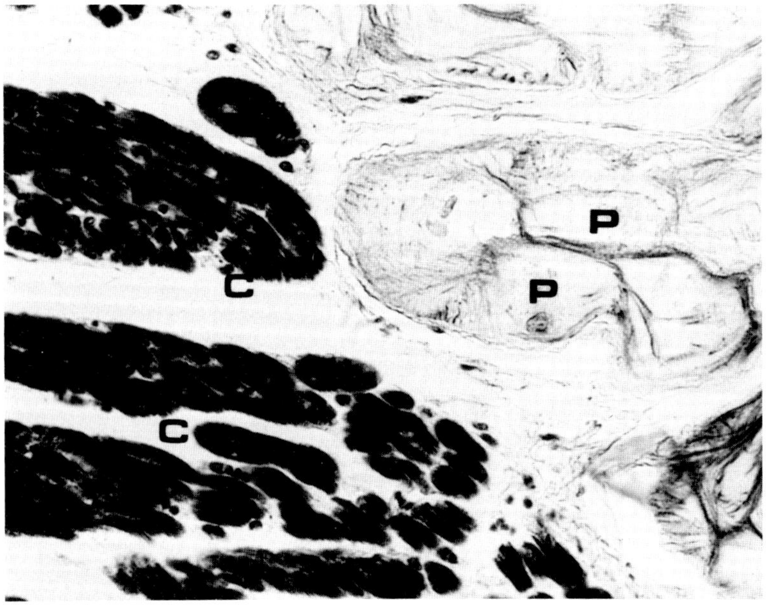

Fig. 8-14. Cardiac muscle cells and Purkinje fibers. The Purkinje fibers (*P*) are larger than cardiac muscle cells (*C*). ×100 (phosphotungstic acid-hematoxylin (PTAH)).

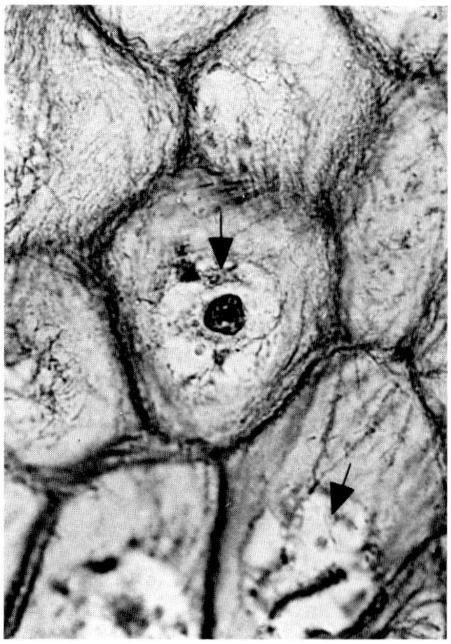

Fig. 8-15. Cross-section of Purkinje fibers. Note the perinuclear halos (*arrows*) and the paucity of myofibrils. ×160 (PTAH).

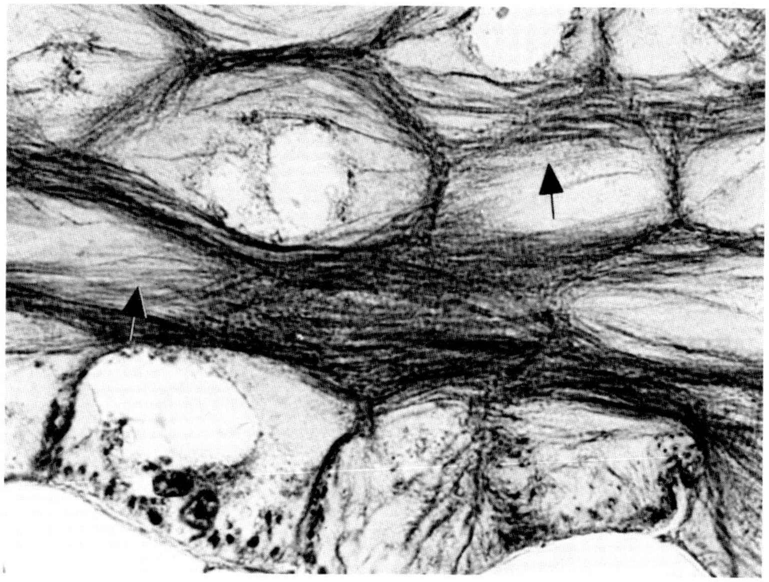

Fig. 8-16. Longitudinal and oblique sections of Purkinje fibers. The myofibrils, which are distributed peripherally, are apparent (*arrows*). ×160 (PTAH).

Osvaldo-Decima, L.: Smooth muscle in the ovary of the rat and monkey. J. Ultrastruct. Res. *29*:218, 1970.

Skeletal Muscle

Franzini-Armstrong, C. and Porter, K. R.: The Z disc of skeletal muscle. Z. Zellforsch. *61*:661, 1964.

Hanson, J. and Huxley, H. E.: Structural basis of the cross-striations in muscle. Nature *172*:530, 1953.

Huxley, H. E.: The contraction of muscle. Sci. Amer. *199*:67, 1958.

Jones, J. K., Cohen, C., Szent-Gyorgyi, A. G. and Longley, W.: Paramyosin: Molecular length and assembly. Science *163*:1196, 1969.

Knappeis, G. G. and Carlsen, F.: The ultrastructure of the M line in skeletal muscle. J. Cell Biol. *38*:202, 1968.

Peachey, L. D.: The sarcoplasmic reticulum and transverse tubules of the frog's sartorius. J. Cell Biol. *25*:209, 1965.

Shafia, S. A., Gorycki, M., Goldstone, L. and Milhorat, A. T.: The fine structure of fiber types in normal human muscle. Anat. Rec. *156*:283, 1966.

Cardiac Muscle

Johnson, E. A. and Sommer, J. R.: A strand of cardiac muscle. Its ultrastructure and the electrophysiological implication of its geometry. J. Cell Biol. *33*:103, 1967.

Rhodin, J. A., Missier, P. and Reid, L. C.: The structure of the specialized impulse-conducting system of the steer-heart. Circulation *24*:349, 1961.

Simpson, F. O. and Oertelis, S. J.: Relationship of the sarcoplasmic reticulum to the sarcolemma in sheep cardiac muscle. Nature *189*:758, 1961.

Spiro, D.: The ultrastructure of heart muscle. Trans. N. Y. Acad. Sci. *24*:879, 1962.

9 Nervous Tissue

General Characteristics

Form and Function. Classically, the study of nervous tissue is integrated with a study of the various organs that comprise the nervous system. This chapter, however, presents the basic histological components of nervous tissue upon which a study of organology is predicated. The organology of the nervous system is presented separately (Chapter 12).

Nervous tissue is distributed throughout the soma and is intimately associated with most of the tissues and organs of the body. The anatomical unit of nervous tissue is the *neuron*. Although there are numerous types of neurons, their primary function is to receive stimuli from the internal (*interoception*) and external (*exteroception*) environment. The subsequent transmission of signals throughout the body or the specific transmission of information to effector organs of the body are also integral parts of their functional significance.

The well-developed cytoplasmic characteristics of *irritability* and *conductivity* uniquely suit them to their task. Moreover, their well-developed cellular processes ensure contact with most parts of the body. These processes are the anatomical bases for the transmission of information throughout the soma. Intimate contact between neurons and cellular processes is achieved through functional regions called *synapses*.

Neurons are intimately associated with other cell types called *neuroglia*. These cells are responsible for the protection, nutrition and structural integrity of nervous tissue. Neurons also may be intimately associated with other cells of the basic tissues.

Although the elements of nervous tissue are few, numerous modifications to neurons and the structural relationships among them allow for a great diversity in the organization of the nervous system.

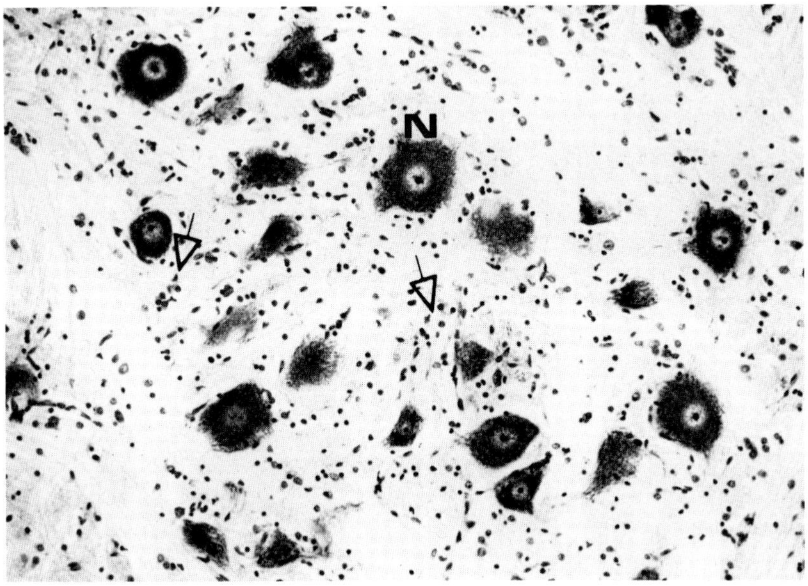

Fig. 9-1. Nervous tissue from the brain stem of a pig. The neurons (*N*) are distributed among numerous neuroglial cells (*arrows*). ×40. All light micrographs are the original magnifications. All election micrographs are the final magnifications.

Cellular Components

Neurons. The *neuron* or *nerve cell* has a cell body, *perikaryon*, and numerous cellular processes of varying length (Fig. 9-1). These cellular processes are the *axon* and *dendrites*. On the basis of the number of cellular processes, neurons may be *unipolar*, *bipolar* or *multipolar*. There is no single description that encompasses all neurons. There is great variety manifested in their size, shape, number and length of cellular processes, as well as their location and distribution. Notwithstanding this great diversity, the following description applies to most neurons to one degree or another.

Although usually large, the perikaryon may vary from 4–135 μm in diameter. Accordingly, the cytoplasmic volume may be as small as in certain cells of the cerebral cortex or as large as in pseudounipolar neurons of craniospinal ganglia. The large, round nucleus is usually centrally located and contains large quantities of euchromatin. It is, therefore, vesicular. A prominent nucleolus is present.

The cytoplasm is basophilic and granular. Abundant granular inclusions are the basophilic *Nissl bodies* (Fig. 9-2). They are scattered throughout the endoplasmic portions of the perikaryon and the dendrites. They are not present in the axon. A clear area, the *axon hillock*, clearly delimits the origin of the axon because of the absence of the Nissl bodies (*tigroid granules*). Nissl substance is quite labile. Upon injury to the cell this material breaks up and diffuses throughout the cytoplasm. Subsequently, the material dissolves (*chromatolysis*).

Typical organelles are present; however, mitochondria and the Golgi apparatus are not extensively developed. *Neurofibrils* and *neurotubules* (microtubules) are well-developed and occur throughout the perikaryon and cellular processes.

Although each neuron possesses one axon, various numbers of dendrites may be present. On this basis various types of neurons have been described: *Golgi type I*, *Golgi type II*, *multipolar*, *bipolar* and *unipolar*. *Golgi type I* neurons have numerous dendrites and a very long axon. These axons typically contribute to peripheral nerves. *Golgi type II* neurons are usually stellate cells with numerous dendrites and a short axon. These are present in the cerebral and cerebellar cortex as well as in the retina. *Multipolar* neurons have numerous cellular processes. These cells are the most common type. *Bipolar* neurons have one dendrite and one axon which are located at opposite poles of the cell. They are confined to areas of special sensation. *True unipolar* neurons have only an axon and are confined in distribution to the developing nervous system. In *pseudounipolar* neurons, the axon and dendrite are fused and then separate some distance from the perikaryon. These are typical neurons of the cranial and spinal ganglia.

Neuroglia. *Neuroglial cells* are those elements responsible for the protection and nutrition of neurons as well as the maintenance of the structural integrity of the nervous tissue. One very specialized function of these cells is the formation of myelin sheaths.

The neuroglia may be subdivided on the basis of the association of these cells with the central or peripheral nervous systems. The *central glia* includes *oligodendrogliocytes*, *astrocytes*, *microgliocytes*, *Müller cells* and *ependymal cells*. The *peripheral glia* includes *amphicytes* and *Schwann cells*.

Since routine staining techniques do not readily demonstrate neuroglial cells and their protoplasmic processes, the routine identification of these cells is usually based on nuclear morphology.

The *oligodendrogliocytes* of the central glia are the most numerous of the neuroglial elements (Fig. 9-3). These cells are characterized by a small, oval or round nucleus which contains a fair amount of heterochromatin. The nucleus, however, may vary from large and pale to small and dark. Generally, this nucleus is smaller and more round than that of the astrocyte. The oligodendrogliocyte contains scant amounts of cytoplasm and few cellular processes. These cells are interdigitated between nerve cell processes and nerve cell bodies. Also, they are intimately associated with the capillaries of the vascular bed.

Oligodendrogliocytes are responsible for myelination of nerve cell processes within the central nervous system.

The *astrocytes* are the next most frequently encountered neuroglial cells of the central nervous system (Fig. 9-3). Astrocytes or spider cells are divided into two different types, *fibrous* and *protoplasmic*. The major difference between these cell types is that one has more cytoplasm than the other. The fibrous type is abundant in the white matter and the protoplasmic type is common in the gray matter. Both have a large, round or oval nucleus which is usually quite pale. Chromatin granules are fine but may be clumped next to the inner nuclear membrane.

The astrocytic processes support blood vessels and, in conjunction with the structures associated with the capillaries, contribute to the blood-brain barrier. Under certain conditions, astrocytes may become phagocytic cells.

The typical phagocytes of the central nervous system, however, are the *microgliocytes* (Fig. 9-3). These cells are scattered throughout the central nervous system and are characterized by a scant cytoplasm which contains an elongated, dark nucleus with evenly distributed chromatin. The cytoplasm is characterized by numerous, short, cellular processes.

Müller cells are neuroglial elements associated with the neurons that comprise the retina.

Ependymal cells are neuroglial elements that line the neural canal (Fig. 9-4). Because of the nature of the embryological origin of the nervous tissue, a tube is formed which is lined with epithelium that may vary from squamous to columnar. The epithelial lining

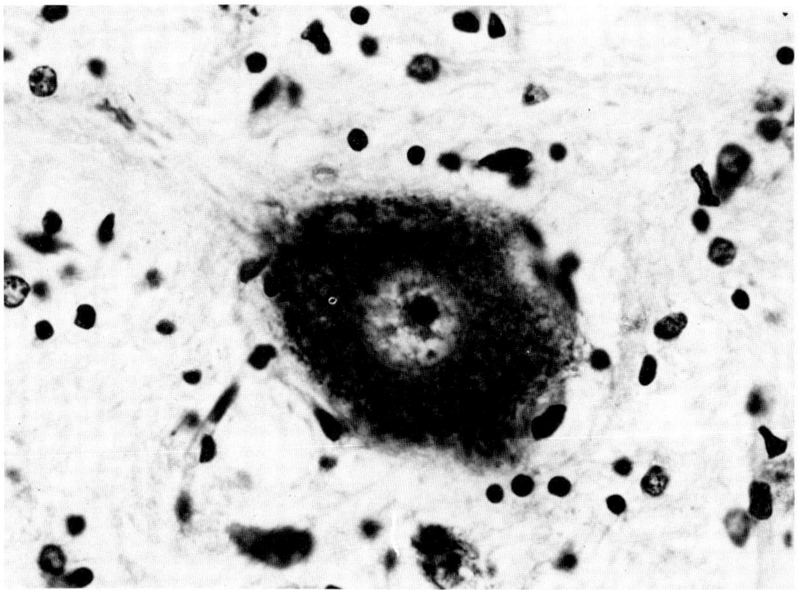

Fig. 9-2. Nissl substance of a neuron. The Nissl substance is the dark material in the cytoplasm. ×160.

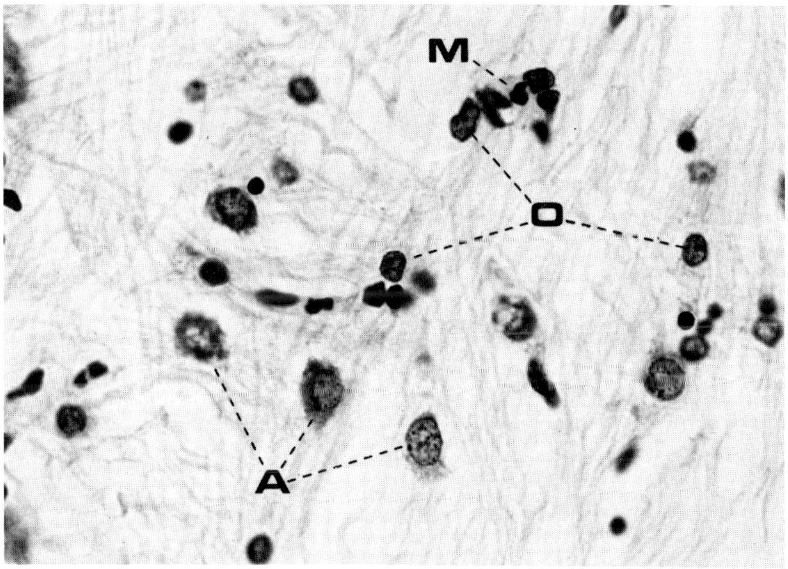

Fig. 9-3. Neurogliocytes from the brain stem of a pig. The oligodendrogliocytes (*O*), astrocytes (*A*) and microgliocytes (*M*) are indicated. ×160.

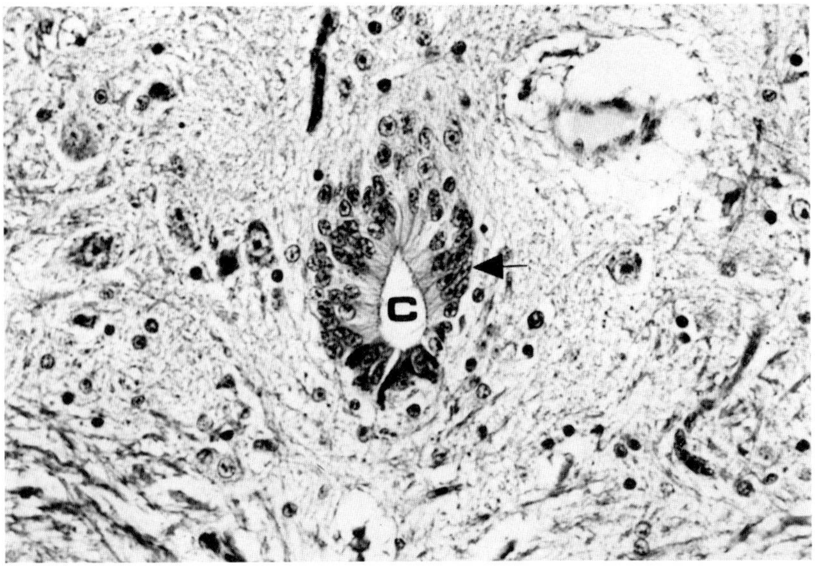

Fig. 9-4. Ependymal cells of the spinal canal of a bird. The spinal canal (*C*) is lined by a layer of columnar cells (*arrow*). ×100. (Note: The section is oblique and the epithelium appears pseudostratified.)

is retained in the adult and is observed as the lining of the central canal of the spinal cord and the four ventricles of the brain. This lining is especially prominent and modified in areas where the *choroid plexuses* are formed. Embryonic ependyma are ciliated cells of a low cuboidal or low columnar configuration. The latter is retained in the adult; occasionally, islands of cilia may be observed projecting from the brushlike luminal border. These cells have large, pale nuclei with one or more nucleoli. The basal borders, in the adult, reside on a basement membrane and are separated from the nervous tissue. In younger animals, however, the basal modifications are quite complex and cellular processes may extend through the mantle layer of the developing nervous tissue.

The *amphicytes* (*satellite cells, capsule cells*) of the peripheral glia are those neuroglial cells that surround the neurons of ganglia (Fig. 9-5). Although the capsule that they form is confined to the perikaryon, it is probably continuous with the sheath of Schwann. Amphicytes are probably closely related to oligodendrogliocytes.

Schwann cells of the peripheral glia are associated with nerve cell fibers (Fig. 9-6). They surround these fibers and are responsible for the formation of myelin. These cells, also, are probably closely related to oligodendrogliocytes.

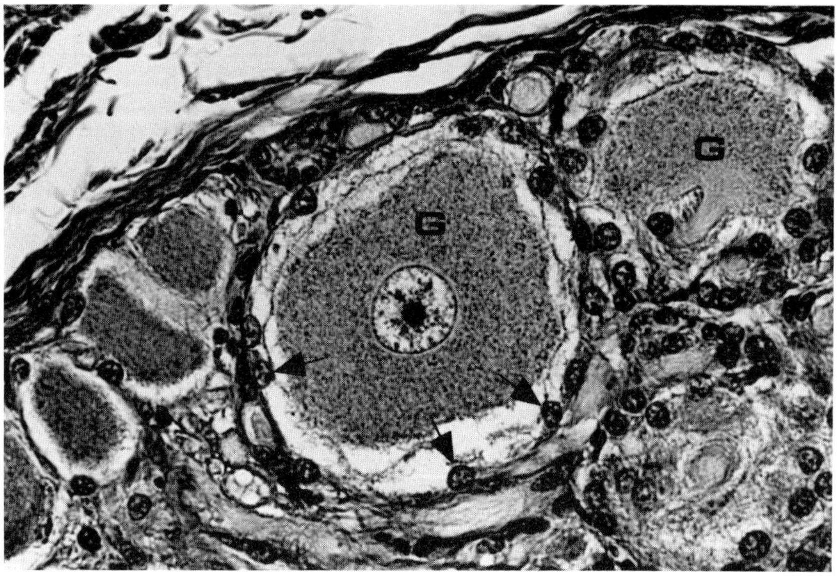

Fig. 9-5. Amphicytes associated with ganglion cells. The amphicytes (*arrows*) surround the ganglion cells (*G*). They have been separated from the ganglion cells artifactually by processing. ×125.

Nerve Cell Processes

Although nerve cell processes are an integral part of the structure and function of neurons, they warrant separate treatment because of 1) their unique relationships with neuroglial cells and 2) the uniqueness of their spatial arrangement.

Nerve cell processes, especially axons and their sheaths, are usually referred to as nerve fibers. All nerve fibers are covered by some sheaths. In the central nervous system the fibers may be covered by the glial cells with which they are intimately associated, or they may be covered by *myelin* produced by the oligodendrogliocytes. In the peripheral nervous system they are covered by a Schwann cell which may or may not form a myelin sheath. Throughout the entire nervous system, therefore, two basic types of nerve cell processes are recognized on the basis of the nature of their involvement, *unmyelinated* and *myelinated*, with neuroglial elements.

Unmyelinated Fibers. *Unmyelinated fibers*, or the *fibers of Remak*, are small fibers that are either unmyelinated or are invested only be a trace of myelin. Such fibers are enfolded by the cytoplasm of the Schwann cell (Fig. 9-7). The *axoplasm* and *axolemma* of the fiber, however, are separated from the Schwann cell by the plasmalemma of this cell. One Schwann cell may enfold many nerve cell fibers.

Myelinated Fibers. These nerve fibers are the largest and most rapidly conducting fibers in the body. The myelin functions in a manner similar to the insulator on an electrical conductor. The oligodendrogliocytes and the Schwann cells are responsible for the formation of myelin. Although their methods and end products are slightly different, the result is that the nerve fiber is invested with a sheath of myelin.

In the peripheral nervous system the *axis*

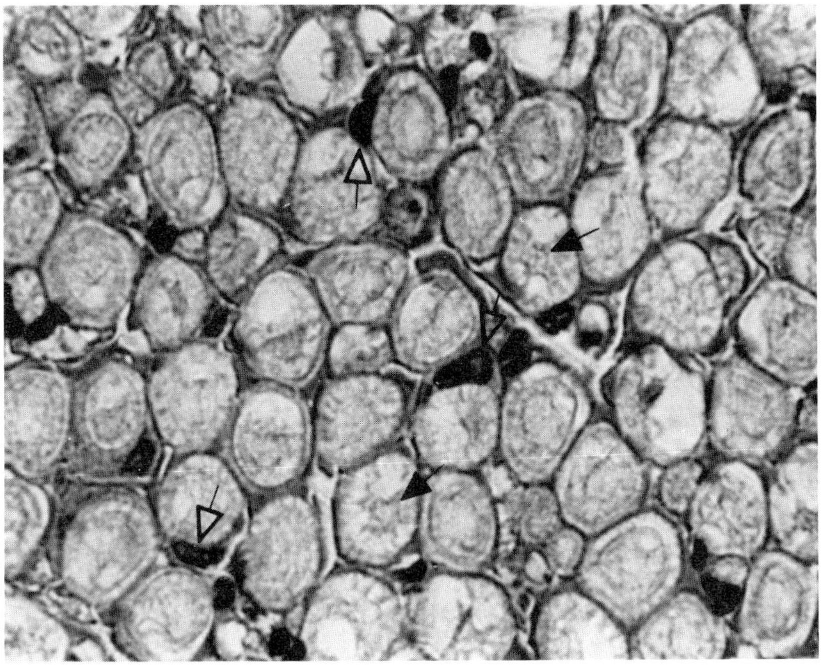

Fig. 9-6. A cross-section of peripheral nerve fibers. The Schwann cells (*open arrows*) surround the nerve cell process. The axoplasm (*solid arrows*) is surrounded by neurokeratin. ×160.

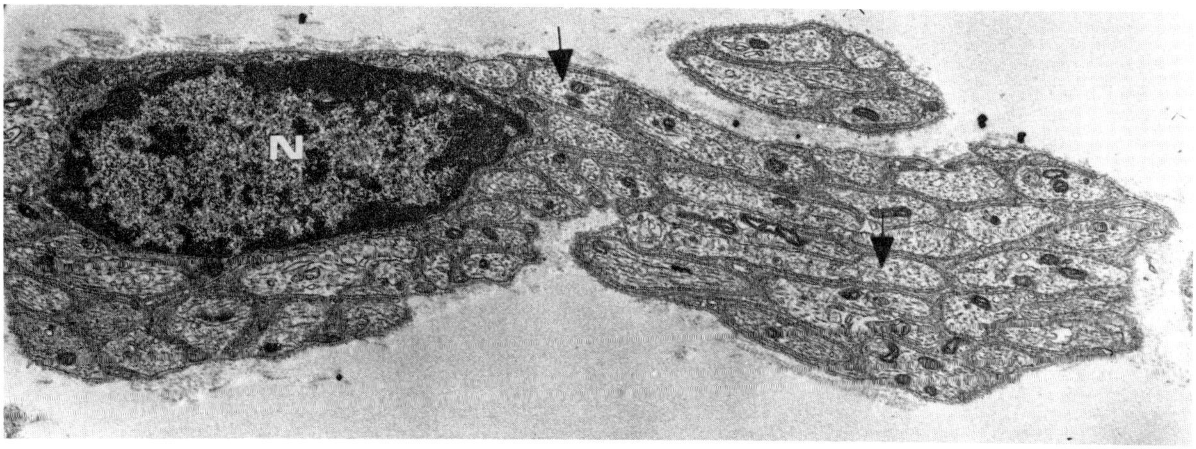

Fig. 9-7. An electron micrograph of unmyelinated nerve fibers. The Schwann cell nucleus (*N*) is the predominant structure of the cell. Numerous nerve fibers (*arrows*) are present in the region of the cytoplasm. ×20,000.

cylinder or nerve cell process contains axoplasm and is limited by a cell membrane, the *axolemma* (Fig. 9-6). The space adjacent to the axis cylinder is occupied by the myelin sheath. In routine preparations, however, the removal of lipids seriously alters the appearance of these membranous whorls. All that remains is the nonlipid component of the myelin sheath, *neurokeratin*. Fingerlike projections of neurokeratin appear as the spokes of a wheel. Peripheral to the remnants of the myelin sheath are the cells responsible for its formation, Schwann cells (Figs. 9-8, 9-9). These cells have a large, vesicular nucleus in which chromatin is clumped peripherally. The cytoplasmic, circumscribing remnants of Schwann cells are referred to as the ***neurolemma*** or the ***sheath of Schwann***.

A single Schwann cell does not invest a nerve cell process along its entire length. Rather, the cell and associated myelin sheath extend a certain distance at which point another Schwann cell and associated myelin sheath are encountered. These breaks in continuity are referred to as *nodes of Ranvier* (Fig. 9-10). One Schwann cell covers the nerve cell process between two nodes. The nodes appear as constrictions along the nerve fiber at which point the myelin configuration stops, but the processes of the Schwann cell continue to contact the axolemma. Although the myelin sheath stops at the node, the axis cylinder continues through the nodal region uninterruptedly.

Synapses

The *synapse* is the point at which nerve cell processes are in contact with each other and nerve cell bodies. Although there are extensive variations at these sites of junction, the following description is applicable to most of them. The synapse is responsible for the transmission of an impulse between cells (transneuronal) and is the means by which nerves communicate with each other.

Ultrastructural studies have shown that

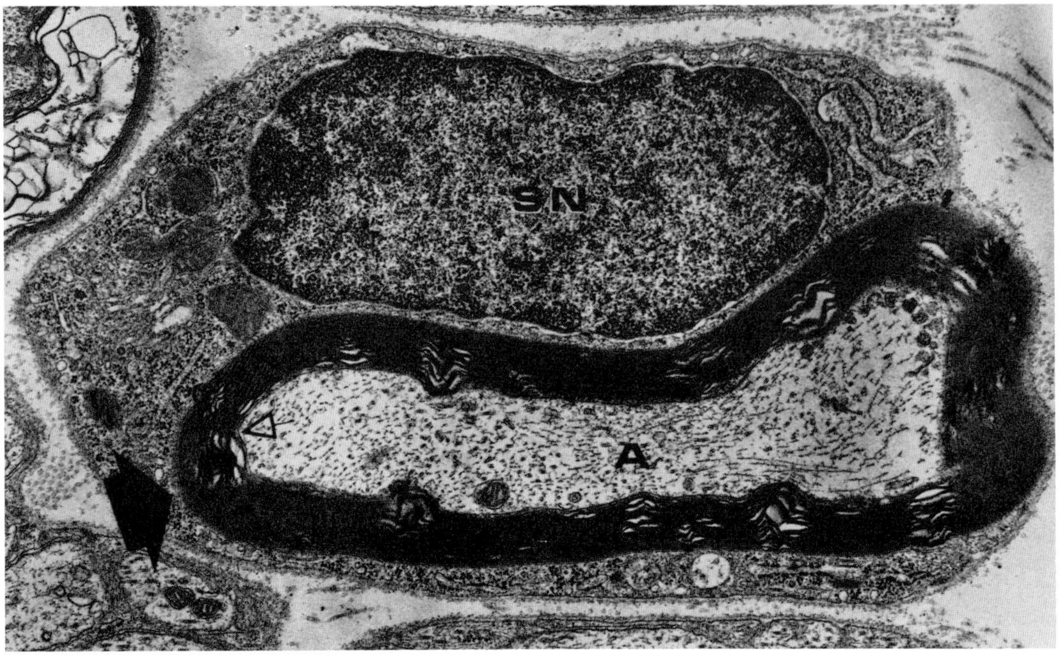

Fig. 9-8. An electron micrograph of a myelinated nerve fiber. The Schwann cell nucleus (*SN*) is above the nerve fiber. The axoplasm (*A*) is surrounded by an axolemma (*open arrow*) and a myelin sheath (*large arrow*). ×17,000.

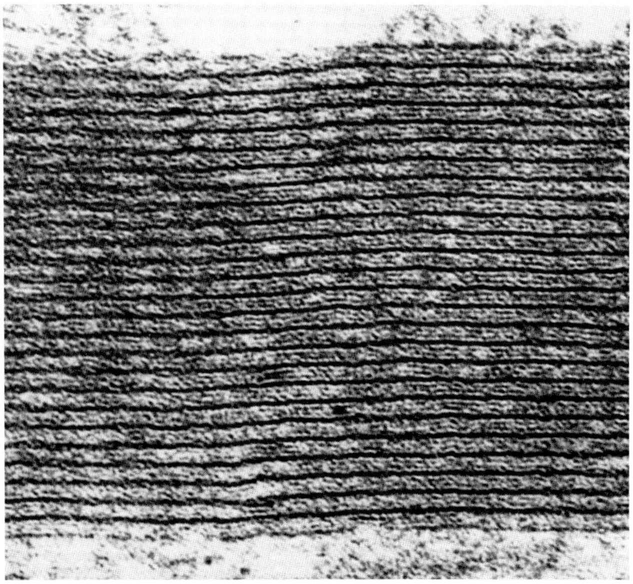

Fig. 9-9. An electron micrograph of myelin. The dark, major period lines and light, interperiod lines are visible. ×154,000.

the synapse is formed by *presynaptic* and *postsynaptic* portions that are separated by a *cleft* which varies from 6 to 20 nm (Fig. 9-11). The presynaptic portion of the axis cylinder expands into bulblike processes *endbulbs*, *endfeet* or *boutons*. Nerve cells and their processes, however, communicate with each other through various types of synapses. *Axosomatic synapses* involve the axon of one nerve and the perikaryon of another. *Axoaxonic synapses* involve the axons of two nerve cells. *Axodentritic synapses* are variable, but they involve the axon of one cell and the dendrite of another. Within the endbulbs are numerous mitochondria, some microtubules (neurotubules) and neurofibrils, as well as *synaptic vesicles*. The synaptic vesicles are approximately 50 nm in diameter and contain the neurotransmitter substance, *acetylcholine*. Dense core vesicles, approximately 100 nm in diameter, contain the *catecholamine*, *norepinephrine*.

The presynaptic and postsynaptic membranes are thickened, while the cleft is traversed by fine filaments. Fine filaments are also associated with the postsynaptic membrane as a *subsynaptic web*.

References

Cellular Components

Bodian, D: The generalized vertebrate neuron. Science *137*:323, 1962.

Bondareff, W. and Hyden, H.: Submicroscopic structure of single neurons isolated from rabbit lateral vestibular nucleus. J. Ultrastruct. Res. *26*:399, 1964.

Fogelson, M. H., Gonates, N. K., Rorke, L. B. and Spiro, A.: Oligodendroglial lamellar inclusions. Arch. Neurol. *19*:150, 1968.

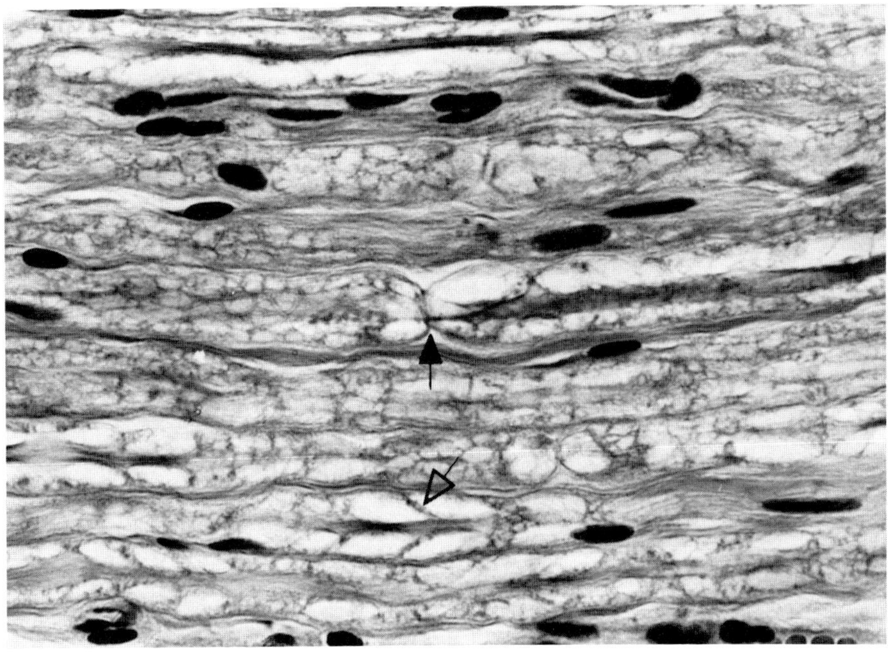

Fig. 9-10. A longitudinal section of nerve fibers. A node of Ranvier (*solid arrow*) and a cleft of Schmidt-Lanterman (*open arrow*) are visible. ×160.

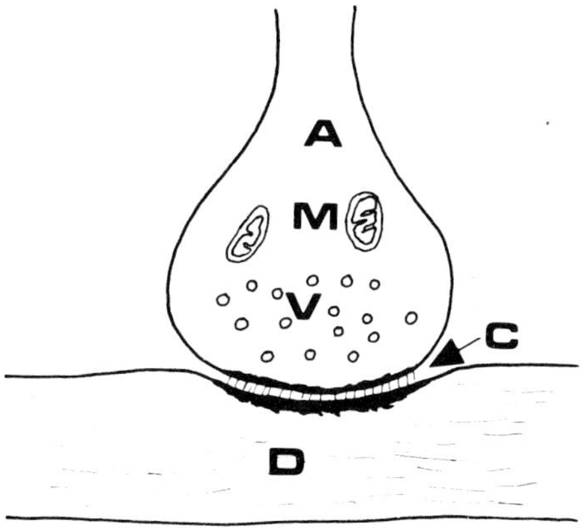

Fig. 9-11. An axodendritic synapse. The end-bulb of the axon (*A*) contains mitochondria (*M*) and synaptic vesicles (*V*). The axon is the presynaptic portion of the synapse. The dendritic (*D*) or postsynaptic membrane and the axonal membrane are thickened. They are separated by a cleft (*C*) which is traversed by fine filaments.

Hamberger, A., Hansson, H. and Sjostrand, F.: Surface structure of isolated neurons. J. Cell Biol. *47*:319, 1970.

Luse, S. A.: Ultrastructure of reactive and neoplastic astrocytes. Lab. Invest. *7*:401, 1958.

Palay, S. L. and Palade, G. E.: The fine structure of neurons. J. Biophys. Biochem. Cytol. *1*:69, 1955.

Sandborn, E. B.: Electron microscopy of the neuron membrane systems and filaments. Canad. J. Physiol. Pharmacol. *44*:329, 1966.

Vaughn, J. E.: An electron microscopic analysis of gliogenesis in rat optic nerve. Z. Zellforsch. *94*:293, 1969.

Nerve Cell Processes

Bischoff, A. and Moor, H.: Ultrastructural differences between the myelin sheaths of peripheral nerve fibers and CNS white matter. Z. Zellforsch. *81*:303, 1967.

Cravioto, H.: The role of Schwann cells in the development of human peripheral nerves. J. Ultrastruct. Res. *12*:634, 1965.

Napolitano, L. M. and Scallen, T. J.: Observations on the fine structure of peripheral nerve myelin. Anat. Rec. *163*:1, 1969.

Peters, A.: Observations on the connections between myelin sheaths and glial cells in the optic nerves of young rats. J. Anat. *98*:125, 1964.

Uzman, B. G. and Nogueira-Graf, G.: Electron microscope studies of the formation of nodes of Ranvier in mouse sciatic nerves. J. Biophys. Biochem. Cytol. *3*:589, 1957.

Synapses

DeRobertis, E. D. P.: Ultrastructure and cytochemistry of the synaptic region. Science *156*:907, 1967.

Gobel, S. and Dubner, R.: Axo-axonic synapses in the main sensory trigeminal nucleus. Experientia *24*:1250, 1968.

Jones, D. G.: The morphology of the contact region of vertebrate synaptosomes. Z. Zellforsch. *95*:263, 1969.

Priedkalns, J. and Oksche, A.: Ultrastructure of synaptic terminals in nucleus infundibularis and nucleus supraopticus of *Passer domesticus*. Z. Zellforsch. *98*:135, 1969.

Takeno, K., Nishio, A. and Yanagiya, I.: Bound acetylcholine in the nerve ending particles. J. Neurochem. *16*:47, 1969.

SECTION 3 □ COMPARATIVE ORGANOLOGY

10 Organization of Organs

Organization of Tubular Organs

Form and Function. All of the organs of the body are formed by a combination of one or more of the basic tissues. Besides the specific cellular differences that may characterize an organ, the amount, types and distribution of various tissues are diagnostic features.

Most tubular organs consists of four concentric layers which are called *tunics* (Fig. 10-1). These are, from the luminal surface to the periphery: the *tunica mucosa, tunica submucosa, tunica muscularis* and the *tunica adventitia* or *tunica serosa*. All of the tunics may be present, one or more may be reduced or eliminated, or one or more may be modified to meet specific local needs. These variations, in conjunction with other factors, permit identification of an organ.

The tunica mucosa is the innermost or luminal coat and consists of four layers: *lamina epithelialis, lamina membrana propria, lamina propria mucosae* and the *lamina muscularis mucosae* (Fig. 10-2).

The *lamina epithelialis* is the epithelial layer of an organ. It may consist of one or more types of epithelial cells as per the specific function of an organ or portion of an organ. It is a consistent lamina of this tunic.

The *lamina membrana propria* is the basement membrane. It is present, as has been discussed previously, as a constant separation between connective tissue and epithelial tissues.

The *lamina propria mucosae* is the connective tissue which underlies the epithelial layer. It is usually areolar and/or reticular connective tissue. Small vessels, nerves and infoldings of the lamina epithelialis mucosae occupy this space. The connective tissue of this space may contain large numbers of protective cells either free or as lymph nodules. Besides a defensive function, this layer is the means by which the epithelium is nourished and controlled.

The *lamina muscularis mucosae* is one or more layers of smooth muscle cells. An inner circular and an outer longitudinal layer may be present.

This lamina is of variable occurrence.

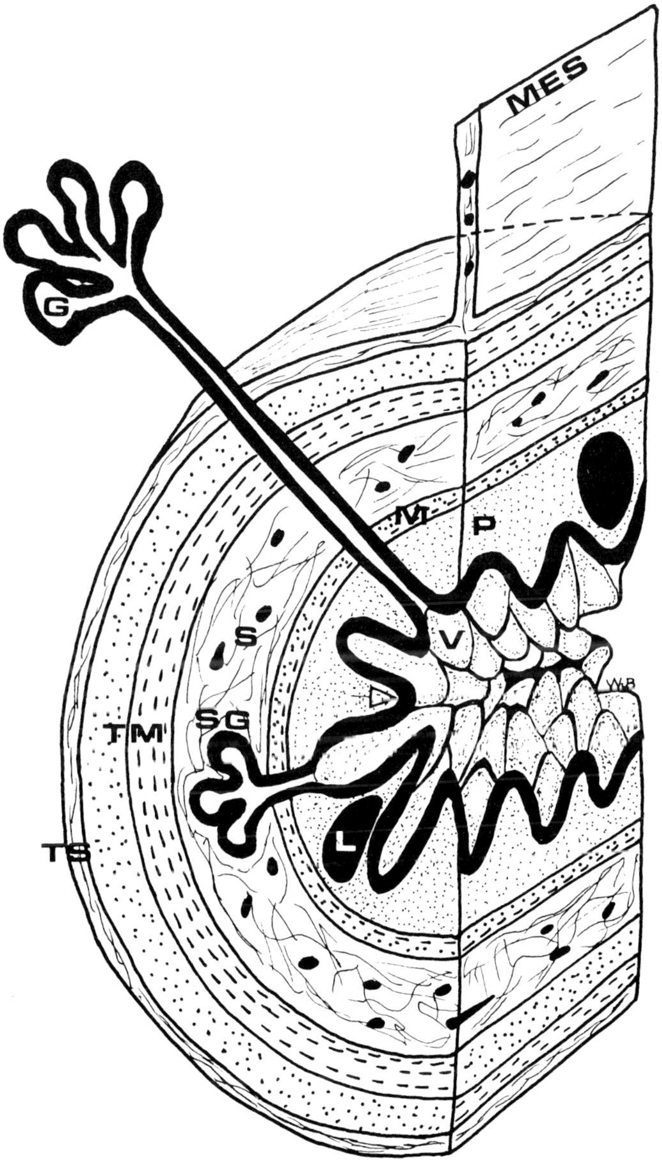

Fig. 10-1. Diagram of a typical tubular organ. The lamina epithelialis mucosae (*arrow*) is underlaid by the lamina propria mucosae (*P*). They are separated by a basement membrane. The lamina muscularis mucosae (*M*) may consist of longitudinally and circularly oriented smooth muscle. The tunica submucosa (*S*) may contain submucosal glands (*SG*) and lymphatic nodules (*L*). The tunica muscularis (*TM*) consists of two lamina of smooth muscle and is bounded peripherally by a tunica serosa (*TS*) or tunica adventitia. The tunica serosa is continued as the mesentery (*MES*) of the organ. Digestive glands (*G*) located some distance from the organ are continuous with the lamina epithelialis mucosae. Other tissue elements of the wall of the gut may contribute to the glands as well. All light micrographs are the original magnifications.

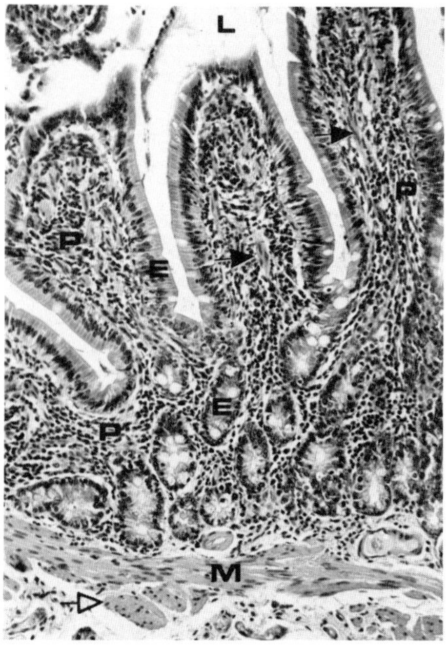

Fig. 10-2. Tunica mucosa of the equine duodenum. The lamina epithelialis (*E*) is adjacent to the lumen (*L*) and invaginates into the lamina propria mucosae (*P*). The lamina propria mucosae is very cellular. The lamina muscularis mucosae (*M*) consists of an inner circular and outer longitudinal layer (*open arrow*). Extensions of the lamina muscularis mucosae (*solid arrows*) are apparent within the projections of the tunica mucosa. ×29.

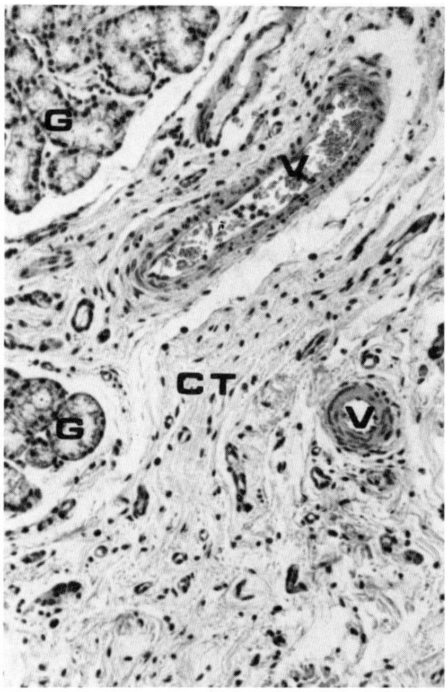

Fig. 10-3. Tunica submucosa of the equine duodenum. This region consists of blood vessels (*V*), nerves and lymphatics. Submucosal glands (*G*) and lymph nodules may be present. The connective tissue (*CT*) is areolar. ×34.

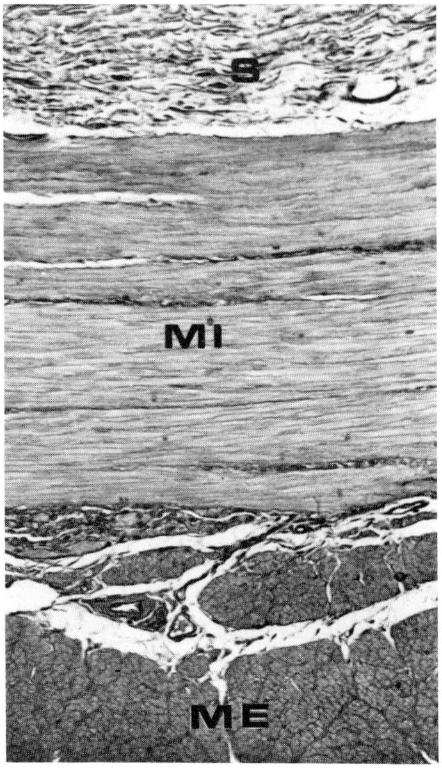

Fig. 10-4. Tunica muscularis of the feline stomach. The tunica muscularis is peripheral to the tunica submucosa (*S*). The tunica muscularis consists of an internal circular layer (*MI*) and an external longitudinal layer (*ME*). ×40.

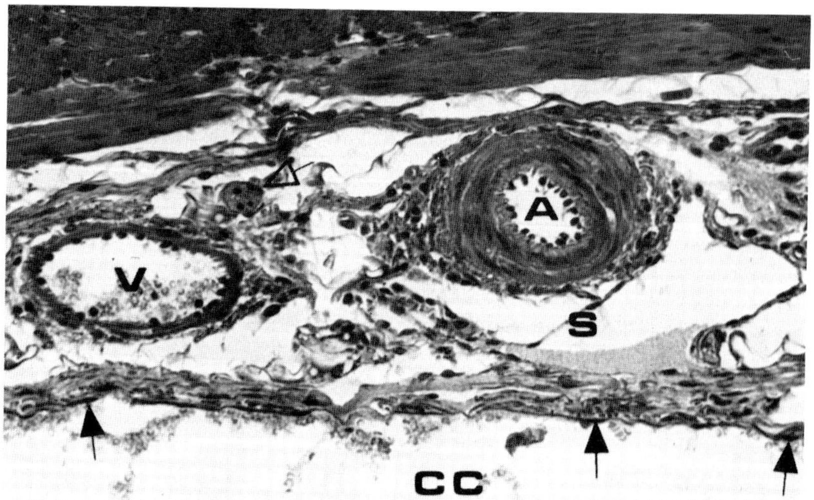

Fig. 10-5. Tunica serosa of the stomach. This tunic is peripheral to the tunica muscularis. The subserosal connective tissue (*S*) is areolar. It contains vessels (*A*, *V*) and nerves (*open arrow*). The mesothelium (*solid arrows*) covers the tunic and separates the organ from the coelomic cavity (*CC*). Connective tissue is closely associated with the mesothelium. The separations in the tissue are artifacts of sectioning. ×63.

When present it serves as a means by which local mobility of organs is achieved. Also, it serves to express secretory products from the glands which may invaginate into the lamina propria mucosae. When present, it serves as a sharp line of demarcation between the connective tissue of the lamina propria mucosae and the tunica submucosa. When absent, these two connective tissue spaces blend together insensibly.

The *tunica submucosa* consists of areolar connective tissue which is more coarsely arranged than the connective tissue of the lamina propria mucosae (Fig. 10-3). Large blood vessels, nerves, nerve plexi and autonomic ganglia are present. In some organs, glands may be present also. This tunic permits motility of the tunica mucosa. In the absence of a lamina muscularis mucosae, the lamina propria mucosae and the tunica submucosa are usually referred to simply as the lamina propria mucosae or lamina propria-submucosa.

The *tunica muscularis* is usually well-developed and consists of two layers of muscle (Fig. 10-4). In some organs, however, it may be absent. Although these layers usually consist of smooth muscle, in some instances they may be comprised of skeletal muscle. The most common arrangement of this tunic is a division into inner circular and outer longitudinal layers. Although described as circular and longitudinal, the inner layer is disposed in a tighter helical pattern than the outer, more loosely oriented helix. Vascular and neural plexi and autonomic ganglia usually separate the two layers. This tunic is responsible for the tone of the organ, size of the lumen and the movement of materials through the hollow organ.

The *tunica adventitia* is a collection of loose connective tissue over the periphery of an organ. Blood vessels, nerves, ganglia and adipose tissue may occur within this tunic. Organs that are intimately associated with the coelomic cavities are surrounded by a layer of mesothelium. In these cases, the most peripheral tunic is referred to as the *tunica serosa* (Fig. 10-5). It is composed, therefore, of mesothelium and connective tissue. It is through the tunica adventitia and/or tunica serosa that the vascular, lymphatic and nerve supplies gain access to an organ. Further, these tunics are responsible for the suspension of organs either through the union of the tunica adventitia with surrounding connective tissue or by the reflection of mesothelium and associated connective tissue as mesenteries.

Although there are numerous variations of this scheme, this organization is basic to tubular organs.

Organization of Parenchymatous Organs

Form and Function. The solid or parenchymatous organs of the body are also composed of a combination of one or more of the basic tissues. Their organizational pattern is somewhat different from that described for tubular or hollow organs.

The components of solid organs may be divided into two definitive subgroups. The *parenchyma* is the specific functional component of a specific organ, while the *stroma* includes those tissues (connective tissue, vasculature, nerves, lymphatics) that metabolically and/or structurally support as well as control the parenchyma.

In its greatest simplicity, the following scheme is applicable to these organs whether they are muscle, nerve trunks or glands (Fig. 10-6). Small groups of parenchyma are surrounded by a fine meshwork of areolar or reticular connective tissue in which vessels and nerves are located. Small groups of parenchyma may be grouped as a unit and surrounded by a more coarse areolar connective tissue, or the connective tissue of these small groups may be continuous with coarse areolar connective tissue *trabeculae*. In either case, the connective tissue is progressively more dense and is continuous with the dense white fibrous connective tissue of the capsule. This type of connective tissue continuity affords structural support and facilitates the entry and/ or exit of vessels and nerves. This scheme or minor variation thereof typify the organization of solid organs.

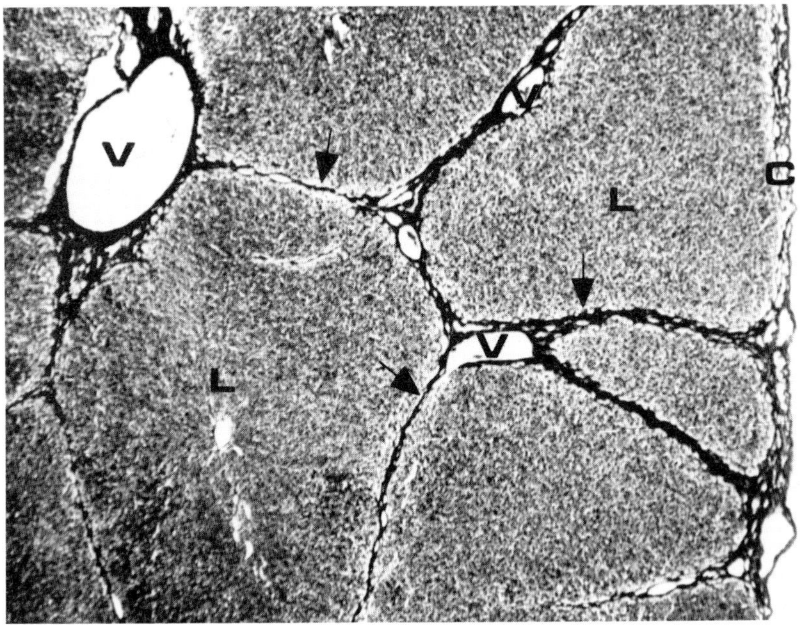

Fig. 10-6. The organization of a solid organ (liver). The connective tissue of the capsule (*C*) is continuous with large trabeculae (*arrows*) which subdivide the organ. Fine connective tissue extends into lobules (*L*). Large vessels (*V*) are located in the trabeculae. ×10 (Snook's reticulum stain).

Mucous and Serous Membranes

Membranes as Simple Organs. *Mucous membranes* include some or all of the components of the tunica mucosa. These membranes are kept moist by secretions from cells within the lamina epithelialis and/or from glands located within the lamina propria mucosae. The lamina epithelialis mucosae may consist of stratified squamous, cuboidal, columnar or pseudostratified columnar epithelium.

A mucous membrane consisting of stratified squamous epithelium typically occurs in the digestive and reproductive systems (Fig. 10-7). Mucous membranes lined by

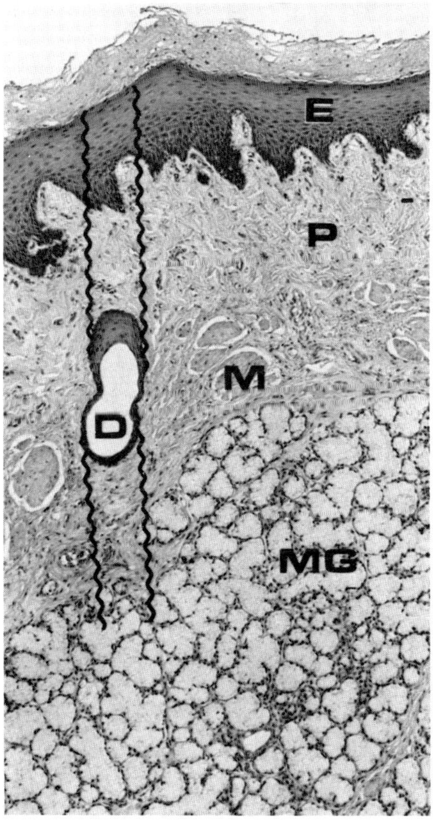

Fig. 10-7. A mucous membrane lined by stratified squamous epithelium (porcine esophagus). The lamina epithelialis (*E*) is covered by a mucoid secretory product and underlaid by the lamina propria (*P*). The lamina muscularis (*M*) is discontinuous. Mucosal glands (*MG*) are responsible for the moistened surface. Their products reach the surface (*wavy lines*) through the excretory duct (*D*) and its continuations. ×16.

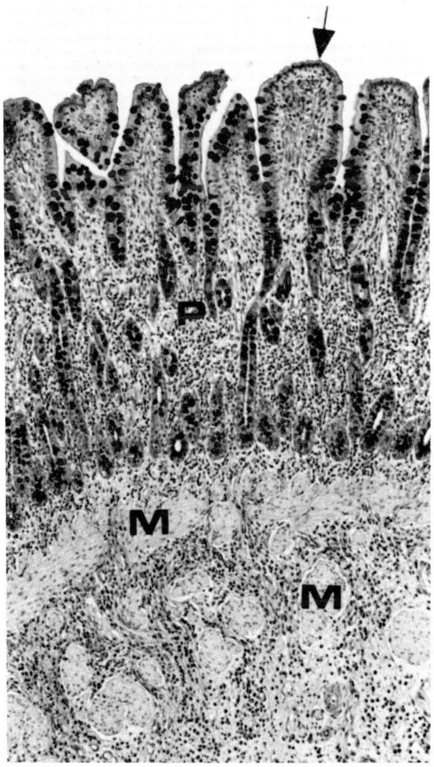

Fig. 10-8. A mucous membrane lined by a simple columnar epithelium (canine jejunum). The epithelium (*solid arrow*) invaginates into the lamina propria (*P*). The lamina muscularis (*M*) consists of longitudinal and circular muscle. The dark cells in the epithelium are mucoid secreting cells. ×16. (Alcian blue and PAS).

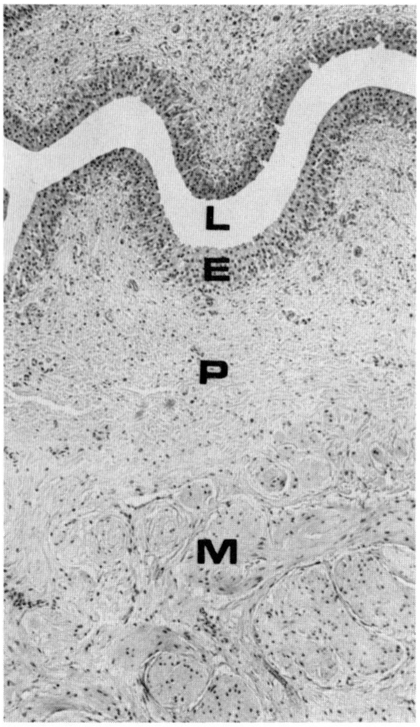

Fig. 10-9. A mucous membrane lined by transitional epithelium. The lumen (*L*) is outlined by transitional epithelium (*E*). The lamina propria (*P*) blends with the tunica submucosa. There is no lamina muscularis mucosae. The tunica muscularis (*M*) is indicated. ×16.

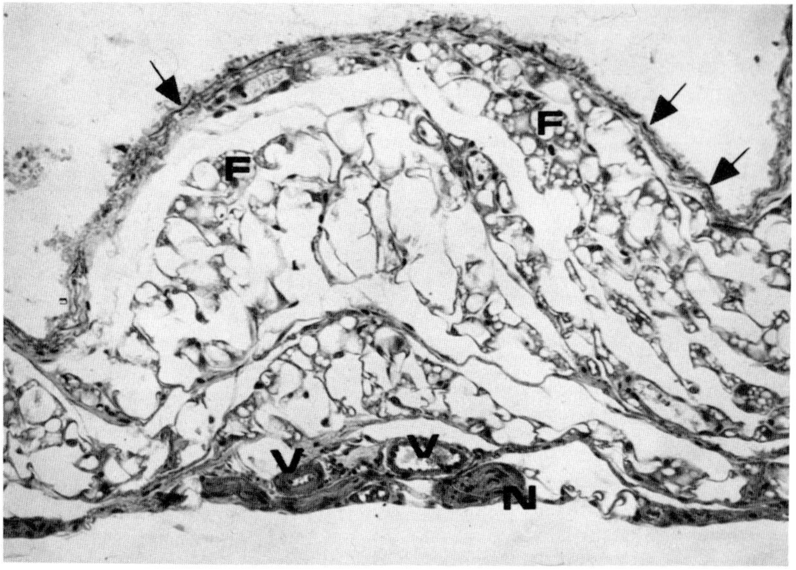

Fig. 10-10. Serous membrane. The mesothelium (*solid arrows*) and its connective tissue is underlaid by a subserosal connective tissue which consists of fat cells (*F*), vessels (*V*) and nerves (*N*). Compare with Fig. 10-5. ×40.

columnar, cuboidal or pseudostratified columnar epithelium occur typically in the digestive, respiratory and reproductive systems (Fig. 10-8). Those lined by transitional epithelium occur in the urinary system (Fig. 10-9).

Serous membranes consist of a layer of mesothelium and associated connective tissue (Fig. 10-10). They line the coelomic spaces and are moistened by the fluids contained within these spaces.

These membranes are simple organs.

11 Musculoskeletal System

General Characteristics

Form and Function. The form of this system is as varied as the form of the muscles and bones of which it is comprised. Some representatives of all of the basic tissues contribute to the formation of this system. The structural component of the system, bone, gives support to the body as well as serving as points of attachment against which the muscles can operate. The contractile portion, skeletal muscle, is the means by which the contractility of the fibers is converted into the work involved in support and locomotion. Dense white fibrous connective tissue in ligaments and tendons constitutes the mechanism for attachment of bone to bone and muscle to bone. Cartilage facilitates growth as well as serving as the substrate for bone to bone contact (articular surfaces). The proper connective tissues bind various parts of the system together and allow for the free passage of blood vessels, lymphatics and nerves.

As an integrated system with numerous component parts, the primary functions are the support and movement of the body.

Bone as an Organ

Growing and Adult Bone. As a tissue, bone consists of those elements discussed previously (Chapter 5). As an organ, however, the interaction of various tissues results in complex relationships which permit a different perspective of form and function. Developing osseous systems are a good example of the complexity of this integrated activity (Chapter 6).

As the long bones of the body grow, they move through space in three dimensions (Fig. 11-1). This growth phenomenon is, of course, the result of integrated cellular and tissue activity. The growth plate is responsible for elongation as well as for the final three-dimensional configuration of the distal and proximal heads. The periosteum is responsible for the thickening or centrifugal growth of the diaphysis, whereas the endosteum is responsible for the thinning of the diaphysis. Of no little significance is the realization that these two envelopes result in *osseous drift*, the three-dimensional movement of the diaphysis through space. Numerous factors, especially mechanical stress, influence the activity at the growth plate and diaphysis. *Modeling* is the response of these activities to varied influencing factors and results in the definitive form of a bone (Fig. 11-2).

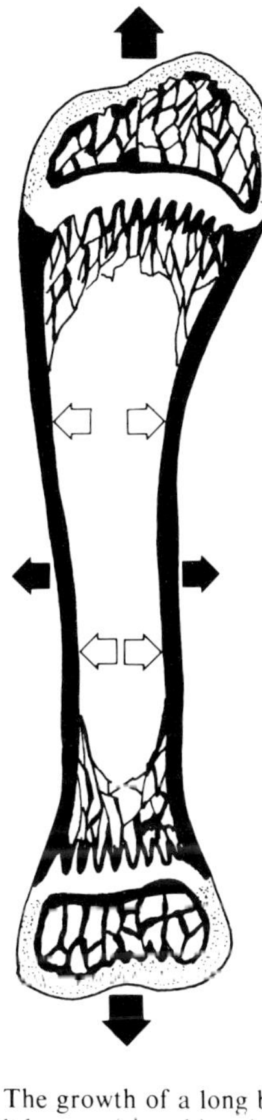

Fig. 11-1. The growth of a long bone. Elongation (*large solid arrows*) is achieved at the growth plate (*white*). The endosteal lining of the diaphysis resorbs bone (*open arrows*), while the periosteum deposits bone (*small solid arrows*). Note the continuity of the growth plate (*white*), articular cartilage (*stipple*) and diaphyseal bone (*black*). All light micrographs are the original magnifications.

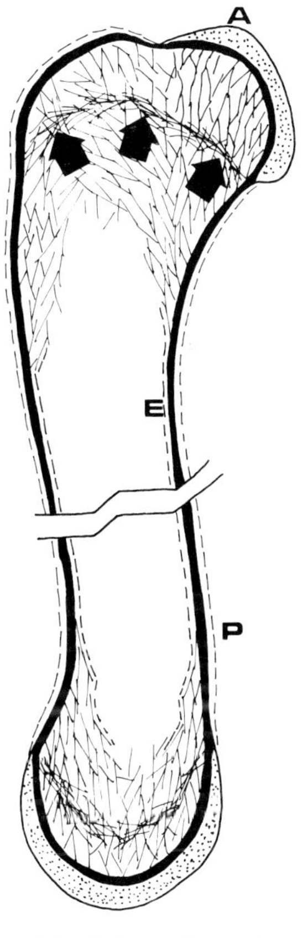

Fig. 11-2. The definitive form of a long bone. The endosteal (*E*) and periosteal (*P*) sleeves are active throughout life. The articular cartilage (*A*) is not covered by the periosteum. Upon closure of the growth plate a synostosis is formed (*arrows*).

In those bones in which proximal and distal secondary ossification centers develop, the peripheral margins of the growth plate are continuous with the cartilage of the articular surfaces (Fig. 11-3). The latter resides on the epiphyseal bone which develops in the secondary ossification center (Fig. 11-4). In those bones in which a secondary ossification center does not develop, a definitive growth plate is not formed. Rather, the growing cartilage is directly continuous with the articular cartilage.

The growth plate is an example of a joint between two bones, those of the epiphysis

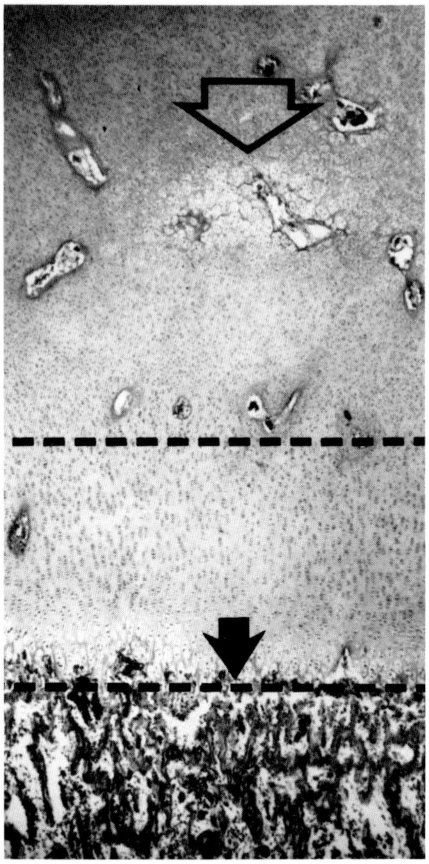

Fig. 11-3. Early stage of secondary ossification center development. The epiphyseal ossification center (*open arrow*) contains hypertrophied chondrocytes. The metaphysis (*solid arrow*) is characterized by osseous replacement of cartilage. *Dashed lines*, approximate limits of the future growth plate. ×10.

and diaphysis. This type of joint is a *synchondrosis* (Fig. 11-4). With age the cartilage of the growth plate is totally replaced by bone. This *synchondrosis* then becomes a *synostosis*. Naturally, this transition represents the completion of bone elongation. Of no little significance, also, is the recognition of what the closure of the growth plate represents. During growth the definitive thickness of the plate was maintained because of the balanced activity of the proliferative cartilage zone and the region of osseous replacement. At closure, the balance of these activities favored the total replacement of the cartilage.

The completion of growth and the achievement of the definitive adult form does not mark the completion of bone changes. *Internal remodeling* still occurs (Chapter 5). It is through this process that bone may respond to various stimuli. During periods of calcium need, for example, mineral may be mobilized by osteoclasia and/or osteolysis. In response to mechanical stress, osteons may form in areas previously devoid of them. Although the definitive form of a bone may not change through such activity, internal alterations occur constantly.

Types of Joints. Bones are held together or connected by a variety of means. Various connective tissues are associated with these articulations. Among them are cartilage, bone and dense white fibrous connective tissue. The functional significance of joints is varied:

1. Stabilize and unite two or more bones.
2. Facilitate movement between two or more bones.
3. Facilitate the growth of bones.

Some of the more commonly encountered joints are *syndesmoses*, *synchondroses*, *synostoses*, *symphyses* and *diarthroses*. Although this list is not complete, it does represent a selection of joints composed of various tissues, as well as demonstrating simple and complex organization.

A *syndesmosis* is the union of bone surfaces by dense white fibrous connective tissue. This is typical, as in the skull, when bones develop from separate ossification centers. The edges of the bones, which grow by appositional growth mechanisms, mark the limits of the *fontanelles*. The fontanelles contain the connective tissue of the joint, as well as the cells responsible for appositional growth. Progressive closure of the fontanelles results in a *suture*. A cranial suture, therefore, is an example of a syndesmosis. However, since all of the cells necessary for the continued deposition of bone are present, syndesmoses of the skull are commonly replaced by synostoses. At this point, the bones cease to grow.

A *synchondrosis* is the union of two bones by hyaline cartilage (Fig. 11-4). The most common example is the growth plate of the long bones. This joint permits a unidirectional growth of diaphyseal bone while it permits fusion of both diaphyseal and epiphyseal bone. Some synchondroses, however (not those of the growth plate), permit a two-dimensional growth of fused bones. The ultimate fate of a synchondrosis is conversion to a synostosis.

A *synostosis* is the fusion of bones by bone. It may occur through syndesmoses or synchondroses. Whereas these two types facilitate growth, a synostosis ensures stability and immobility.

In a *symphysis*, the bones are joined through cartilage, fibrocartilage and/or dense white fibrous connective tissue. The ends of the bones are covered by hyaline cartilage. A dense white fibrous connective tissue or fibrocartilage connects the hyaline cartilage of the adjacent bones. The symphysis pubis and intervertebral joints are different examples of symphyses (Fig. 11-5).

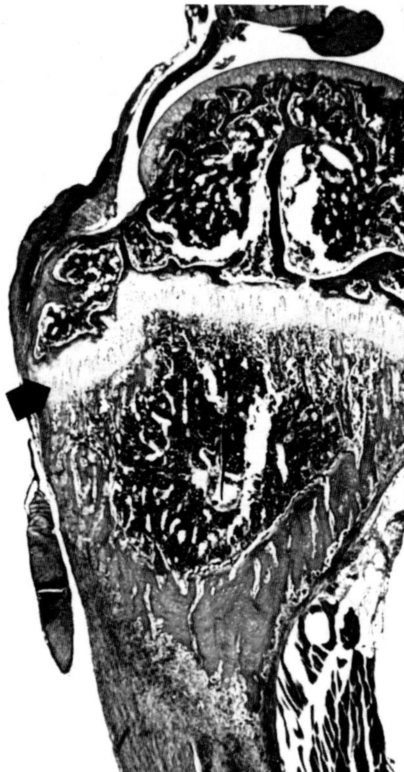

Fig. 11-4. An advanced stage of the development of a secondary ossification center. The epiphyseal growth center is well-developed. The growth plate (*arrow*) is a synchondrosis. ×3.

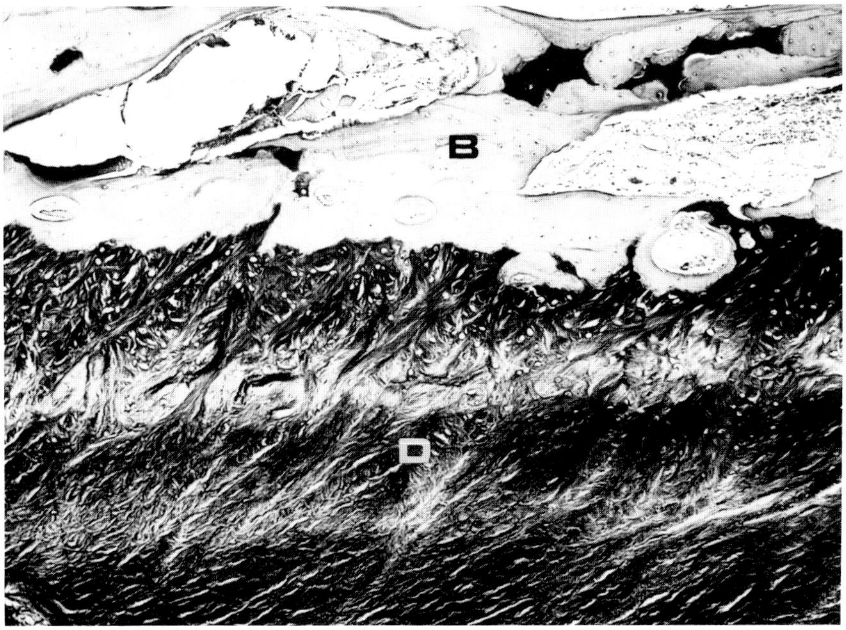

Fig. 11-5. A portion of an intervertebral joint. The bone of a vertebra (*B*) is connected to an adjacent vertebra by an intervertebral disk (*D*) which is composed of fibrocartilage. ×160 (periodic acid-Schiff).

Diarthroses are those articulations that permit the greatest range of movement. They are also the most complex in organization. These types of joints are also referred to as *synovial joints* (Fig. 11-6).

The basic components of a diarthrosis are *articular cartilage* and *articular capsule*.

The articular cartilage is composed generally of hyaline cartilage (Fig. 11-7). In the adult body, the hyaline cartilage of the articular surfaces accounts for the bulk of this tissue. The articular cartilage is divisible into four poorly defined subdivisions. This cartilage is devoid of a perichondrium. The most superficial (surface) layer is composed of small, flattened chondrocytes, the long axes of which are oriented parallel to the articular surface. A transitional (intermediate) zone is characterized by round cells that are slightly hypertrophied. These cells are arranged in columns oriented perpendicular to the surface. A deep zone is characterized by a further delineation of these columns which are composed of large cells. A cartilage mineralization zone is present at the point of union of the articular

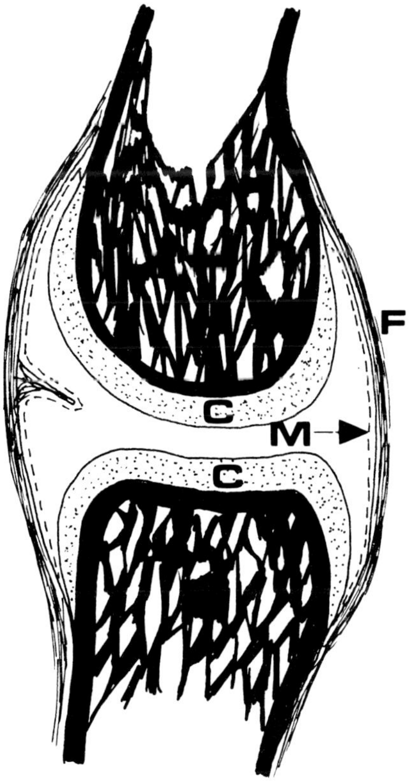

Fig. 11-6. A diagram of a simplified diarthrosis. The articular cartilage (*C*) borders on the joint cavity. The articular capsule consists of a fibrous portion (*F*) and a synovial membrane (*M*).

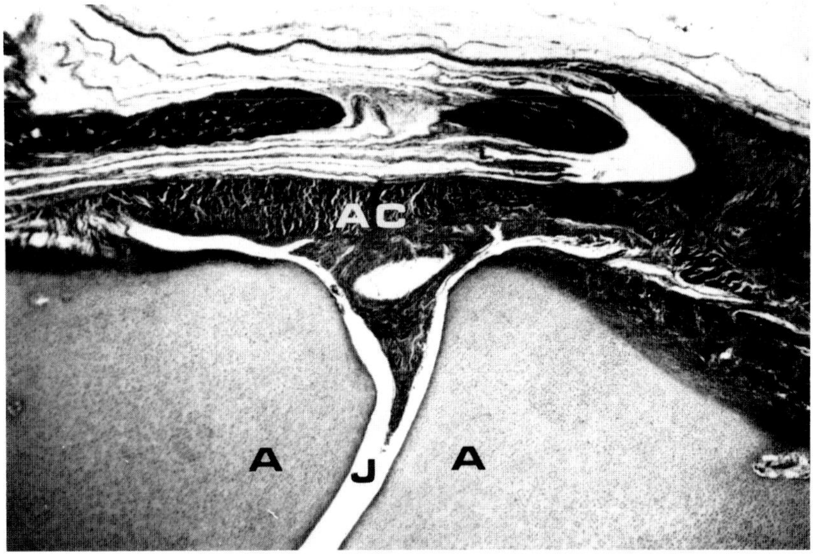

Fig. 11-7. A portion of a synovial joint. The ligaments and muscles traverse the upper part of the micrograph. The articular capsule (*AC*) surrounds the joint and projects into the joint cavity (*J*). The articular cartilages (*A*) of the contributing bones are indicated. ×10.

cartilage with the underlying epiphyseal bone. Cell nests are characteristic of all of the zones except the superficial region. Since a perichondrium is lacking, these isogenous groups are indicative of the significance of interstitial mechanisms in the growth, maintenance and repair of articular cartilage.

The attainment of the adult configuration marks the end of active articular cartilage growth. Since articular cartilage is rather resistant to wear, the replacement and maintenance problems are minimal. Superficial injury to the surface of the joint repairs quite slowly. Extensive injury results in the formation of a *callus*. This situation generally leads to an arthritic condition.

The ***articular capsule*** consists of a ***fibrous layer*** and a ***synovial membrane*** (Fig. 11-7). The fibrous layer is composed of dense white fibrous connective tissue which contains some elastic fibers. The fibrous components of the capsule are continuous with the fibers of tendons and ligaments associated with the joint. The inner surface is incompletely lined by the synovial membrane (Fig. 11-8). This membrane is comprised of flattened cells which are considered fibroblasts. The components of *synovial fluid* are derived from different sources. The mucopolysaccharides (hyaluronic acid) are produced by the synovial cells. Tissue fluids also move across the lining and contribute to the volume of synovial fluid. Macrophages, various leukocytes and synovial cells commonly occur in the synovial fluid, which lubricates the joint. The synovial membrane and accompanying fibrous layer contain numerous folds and projections into the joint space (*synovial villi*), but none of the components of the articular capsule cover the articular surface.

Fibrous, *areolar* and *adipose* synovial membranes are recognized. A fibrous type occurs in conjunction with ligaments and tendons that are subjected to pressure. An areolar type occurs in those joints in which pressure is minimal. Adipose synovial membranes occur over intra-articular deposition of adipose tissue. Thus, they are associated with a cushioning function.

Some ligaments and *menisci* (fibrocartilage) may occur within the joint space.

Bone Marrow. The bone marrow is intimately associated with bone as an organ. It is contained within the medullary cavities as interosseous tissue in all bones of the soma. During postnatal development and growth, all of the marrow is *red bone marrow*. By adulthood, the red bone marrow is confined to a limited number of foci: sternebrae, ribs, vertebrae and cranial bones (Fig. 11-9). The remaining foci will have been replaced with *yellow bone marrow*.

The *red bone marrow* is hematopoietic and is responsible for the production of erythrocytes, granulocytes and platelets

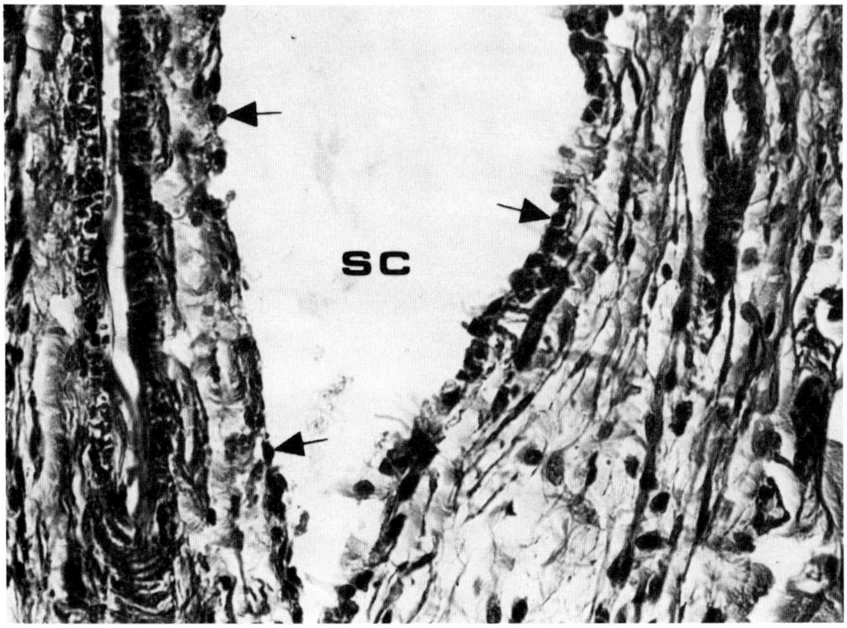

Fig. 11-8. Synovial membrane. The synovial cavity (*SC*) is delimited by a fibrous synovial membrane. The lining cells (*arrows*) are flattened fibroblasts. ×100.

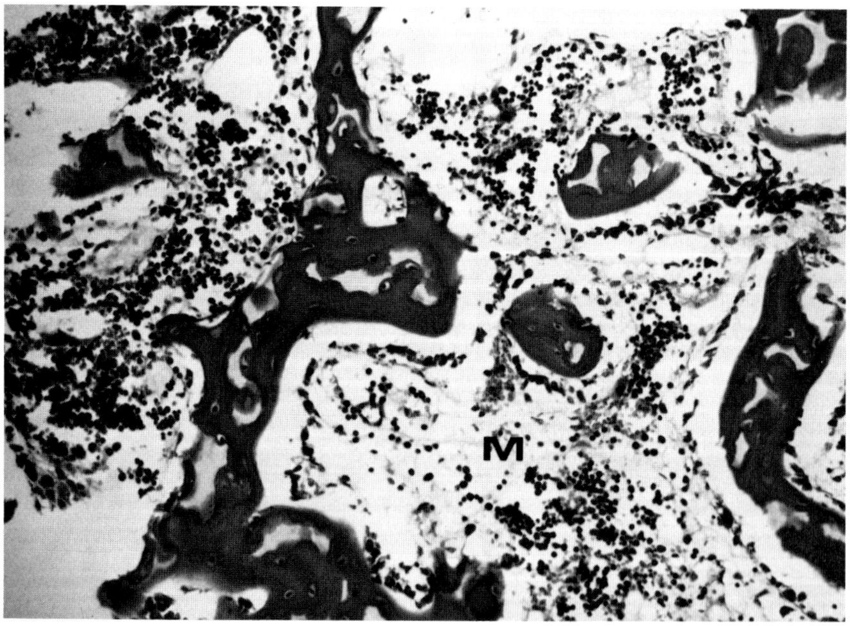

Fig. 11-9. Red bone marrow. The bone marrow (*M*) occupies the interosseous spaces between developing bone and mineralized cartilage of the primary spongiosa. ×40.

(Chapter 15). It consists of phagocytic sinusoids, a reticular fiber framework, free cells and some adipose tissue (Fig. 11-10). The lining cells of the phagocytic sinusoids comprise the *fixed cells* of the organ. The free cells, which include stem cells, intermediate blood cell forms, mature blood cells and fat cells, are intermeshed between the sinusoids. The primary function of this organ is blood cell production. The ultimate functions of the red bone marrow, therefore, are associated with the specific functions of the cells that it produces.

The *yellow bone marrow* develops as adipose tissue replaces the red bone marrow. Under conditions of stress and/or disease, the yellow bone marrow can revert to an active hematopoietic organ.

The specifics of hematopoiesis are discussed in a subsequent section (Chapter 15).

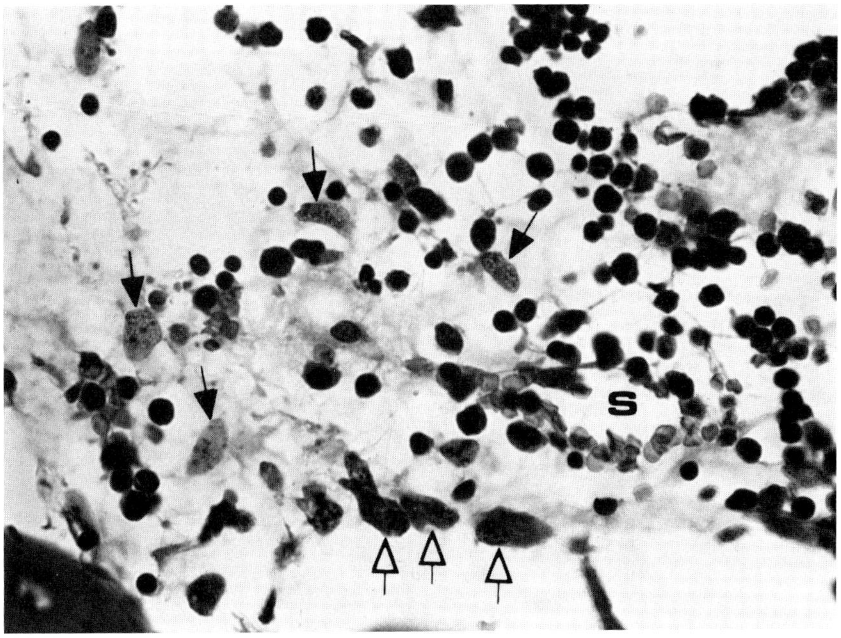

Fig. 11-10. Elements of red bone marrow. The reticular cells (*solid arrows*) are organized as a cellular reticulum. Numerous free blood cells are in various stages of development. A sinusoid (*S*) and displaced osteoblasts (*open arrows*) are also present. ×160.

Muscle as an Organ

Muscle Organization. Although the muscles of the body, at a gross level of examination, assume varied configurations, their microscopic organizational pattern is quite similar. The components of these organs include skeletal muscle, loose and dense connective tissues, vessels and nerves.

Individual muscle fibers are surrounded by a fine network of loose connective tissue which contains reticular fibers, capillaries and nerves (Fig. 11-11). A few connective tissue cells may be encountered. This tissue is referred to as the *endomysium*. Groups of fibers are surrounded by a more coarsely organized loose connective tissue referred to as the *perimysium*. The connective tissue surrounding these bundles or *fascicles*, as well as the contents of this region, is continuous with the endomysium. The perimysial connective tissue is continuous with a dense connective tissue which surrounds the entire mass of muscle. This outermost sheath is referred to as the *epimysium* and may be considered the capsule of the organ. The connective tissue of these three compartments is continuous with the dense white fibrous connective tissue of the tendons.

Bone-Muscle Attachments. The continuation of the proximal and distal connective tissue, as tendons, is terminated in the bones of origin and insertion. (However, some muscles originate and insert in dense white fibrous connective tissue.) At the point of contact with the bones, fibrocartilage is commonly encountered (Fig. 11-12). The actual attachment of the muscle to the bones is achieved by *Sharpey's fibers*. These are coarse collagenous fibers that are anchored deeply in the bone. This relationship is established early in development and results from the appositional growth of bone around the collagenous fibers. This explains the difficulty of reuniting a tendon

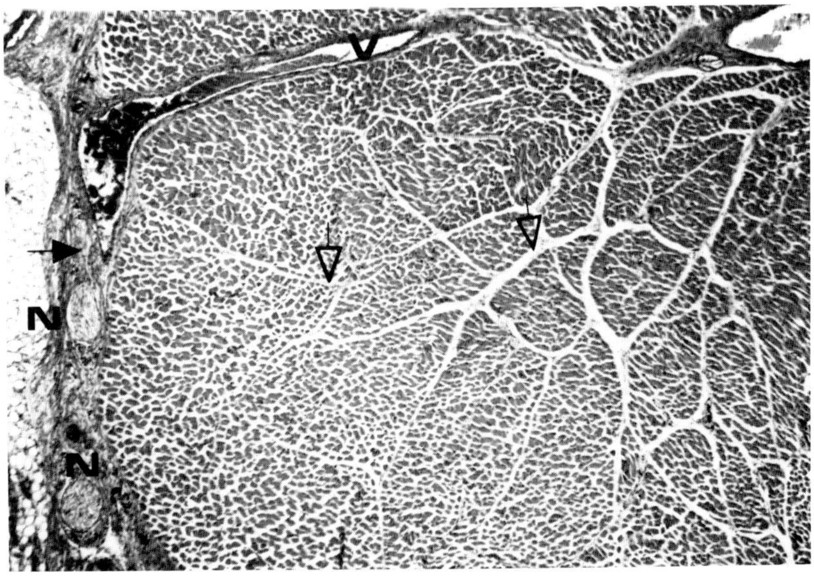

Fig. 11-11. Organization of a muscle. Groups of fibers are surrounded by the perimysium (*open arrows*). This connective tissue is continuous with the epimysial connective tissue (*solid arrow*). Note the occurrence of nerves (*N*) and vessels (*V*). ×10.

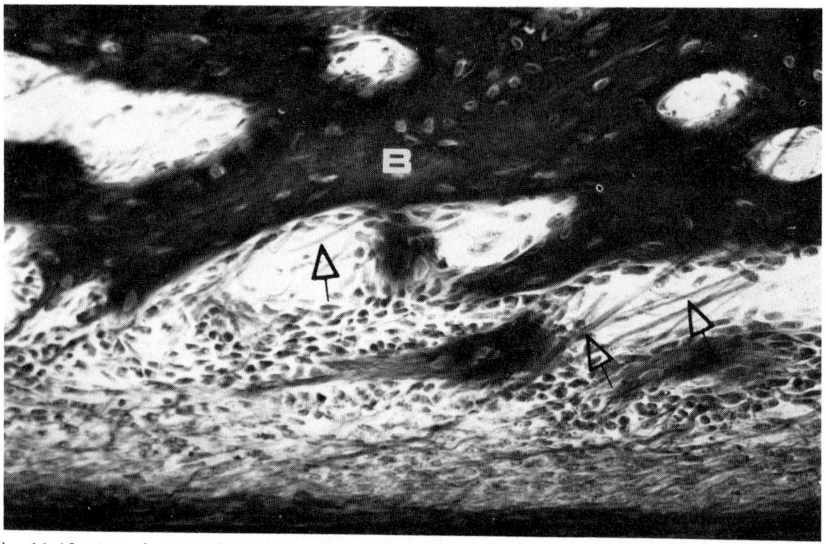

Fig. 11-12. Attachment of muscle to bone. Sharpey's fibers (*arrows*) anchor the dense white fibrous connective tissue to the bone (*B*). ×40.

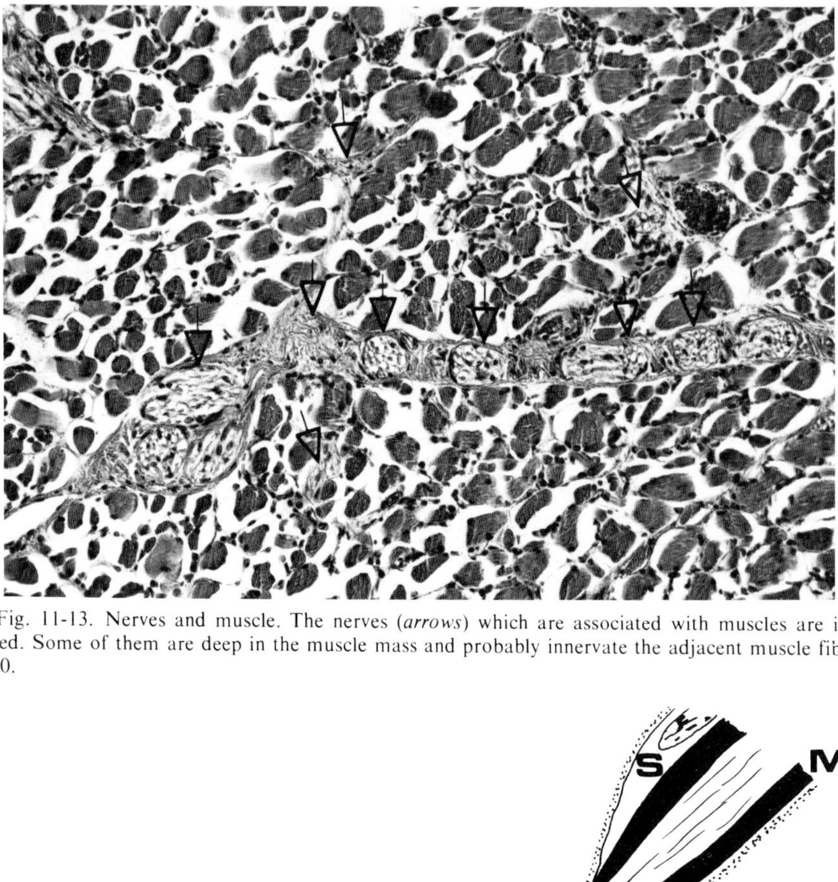

Fig. 11-13. Nerves and muscle. The nerves (*arrows*) which are associated with muscles are indicated. Some of them are deep in the muscle mass and probably innervate the adjacent muscle fibers. ×40.

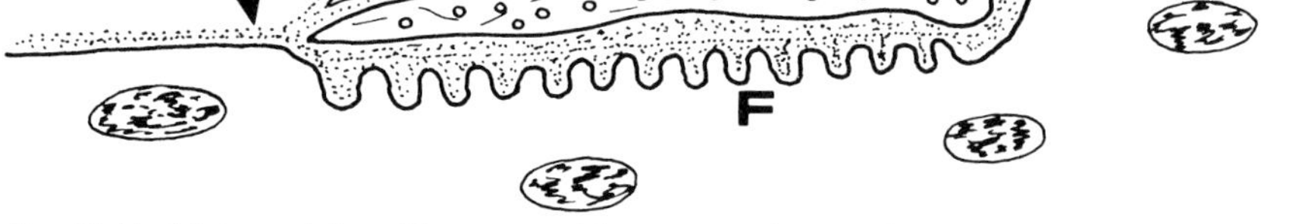

Fig. 11-14. Motor endplate. The nerve, with accompanying myelin sheath (*M*) and Schwann cells (*S*), terminates in a furrow in the skeletal muscle. The muscular portion is highly folded as junctional folds (*F*). Note the disposition of the basal lamina (*arrow*).

(or ligament) to a bone once it has been torn loose from its osseous attachment.

Neuromuscular Relationships. Large nerve fibers enter the epimysial connective tissue, branch throughout the perimysium and send fine terminals into the endomysium (Fig. 11-13). A single nerve may innervate numerous muscle fibers (coarse movers of the body) or each muscle fiber may be innervated by a single nerve (fine movers of the body). The muscle fibers and the nerve that innervates them are called a *motor unit*. The point of junction between the nerve terminal and the muscle fiber is referred to as the *motor endplate* or *myoneural junction* (Fig. 11-14). This relationship is demonstrable with silver and gold impregnation techniques.

As the axon approaches a muscle fiber, the myelin sheath is lost. The sheath of Schwann, however, continues to the point of contact. The enlarged nerve terminal is filled with small synaptic vesicles and mitochondria. The indented muscle fiber at the point of contact has numerous *junctional folds*. The space or cleft between the nerve and muscle is filled with an amorphous substance which probably represents a continuation of the basal lamina through the cleft. The motor endplate is similar to a synapse and represents the means by which a nerve stimulates an effector organ.

More complex neuromuscular relationships exist than those described above. *Neuromuscular spindles* are scattered throughout muscle and are responsible for maintaining the tone of a muscle, as well as minimizing the possibility of damage by excessive stretching of muscles. Spindles mediate their activity through a stretch reflex which involves two neurons at the level of the spinal cord.

Spindles consist of muscle fibers, nerve endings and connective tissue (Fig. 11–15). A loose connective tissue capsule separates the smaller, *intrafusal* fibers of the spindle from the ordinary and larger, *extrafusal* fibers of the muscle mass. Intrafusal fibers vary in length from 2 to 10 mm and are approximately 200 μm in diameter. Two types of intrafusal fibers are present, a *nuclear bag fiber* (Fig. 11–16) and a *nuclear chain fiber* (Fig. 11–17). Of the 20 fibers that may comprise a spindle, the nuclear chain fibers outnumber the nuclear bag fibers by a ratio of 2 or 3 to 1. Both types of fibers are attached to the capsule at their poles.

Both fibers are typically striated. The nuclear bag fiber is enlarged in the center, filled with nuclei and devoid of contractile elements in this area. The smaller and shorter nuclear chain fibers are not expanded in the center, but large nuclei are prominent and contractile elements are missing in this central region. The central regions of both fibers are referred to as the *equatorial regions*.

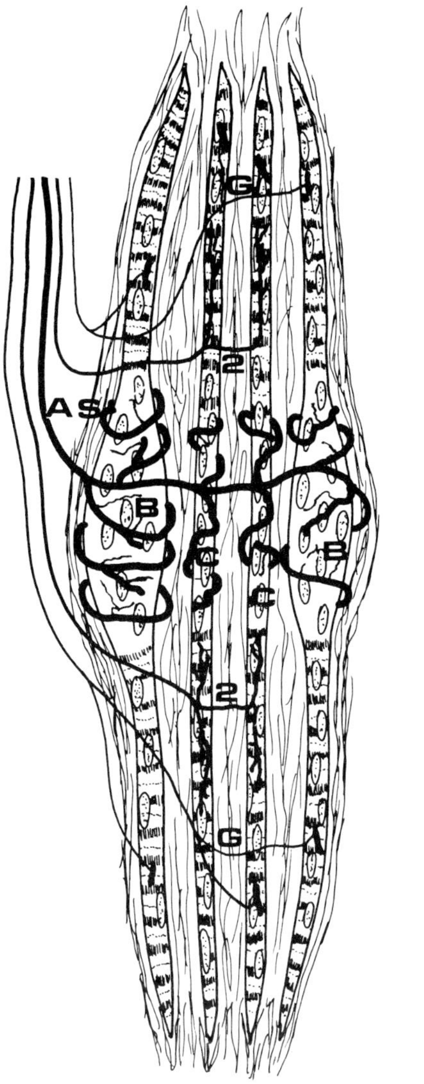

Fig. 11-15. Spindle apparatus. Annulospiral endings (*AS*) encircle the nuclear bag (*B*) and nuclear chain (*C*) fibers. Secondary endings (*2*) originate close to the equatorial region, while gamma efferents (*G*) innervate the intrafusal fibers at their poles. A capsule surrounds the apparatus.

Numerous afferent and efferent nerve endings are associated with these fibers (Fig. 11–15). Afferent endings associated with the equatorial region of both fibers are called *primary* (*annulospiral*) *endings*. When the equatorial region is stretched, these fibers transmit an impulse to the spinal cord which results in a signal to extrafusal fibers of the same muscle mass that causes a contraction. The same input signal from the primaries causes inhibition of other neurons in the spinal cord which results in a relaxation of the antagonistic muscle mass. This accounts for the stretch reflex. This type of activity explains the intuitive thought that when an extensor contracts the corresponding flexor must relax.

The input from the primaries informs the spinal cord and higher brain centers at a subconscious level about the rate of muscle lengthening or stretching and the actual length of the muscle.

Afferent *secondary endings* (*flower spray endings*) originate on either side of the equatorial region (Fig. 11–15). It was thought that their discharge was responsible for inhibition to the antagonistic muscle mass. Currently, they have been shown to evoke a flexor reflex pattern. Their precise function within the spindle is not understood. They do, however, transmit information about muscle length to the central nervous system at a subconscious level.

Small efferent fibers (*gamma efferents*) innervate the intrafusal fibers at their respective poles (Fig. 11–15). Rather than functioning primarily to contract the intrafusal fibers as an end in itself, they are responsible for establishing the degree of stretch on equatorial regions. By accomplishing this, they function to raise or lower the threshold of primary ending discharge and thus make the spindle more or less sensitive to stretching. Once the extrafusal fibers contract, the tension or stretching on the equatorial region would relax and cause a collapse of these areas. By gamma efferent discharge, tension on these regions is maintained throughout the entire range of the contraction. This ensures a constant informational input to the spinal cord and higher brain centers about the degree of stretch or lack thereof in a particular muscle mass.

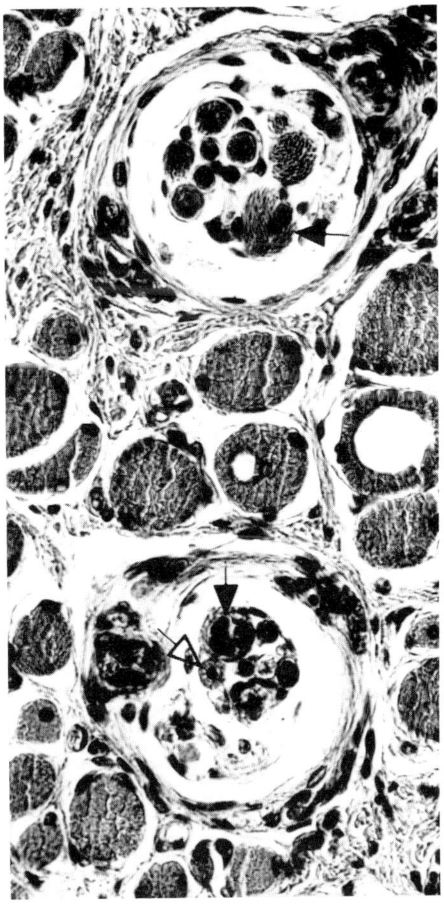

Fig. 11-16. Spindle apparatus from the extraocular musculature of an elk. The spindles are cut in cross-section. Nuclear bag (*solid arrows*) regions and nuclear chain regions (*open arrow*) are indicated. ×100.

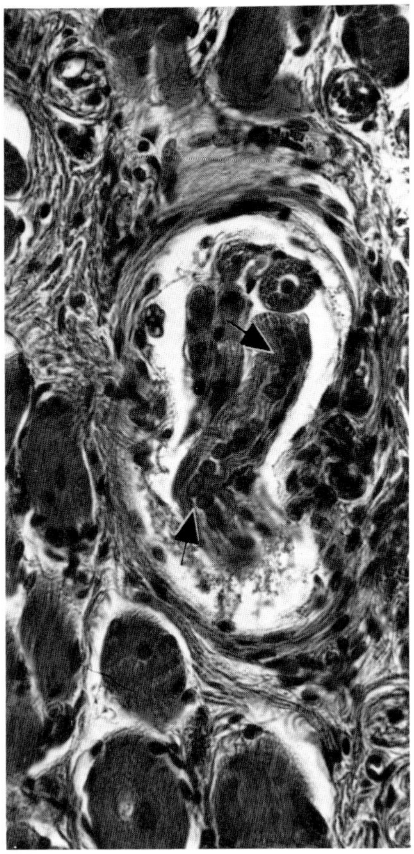

Fig. 11-17. Spindle apparatus from the extraocular musculature of an elk. The spindle is cut obliquely. *Arrows*, equatorial regions of nuclear chain fibers. Note the difference in size between intrafusal and extrafusal fibers. ×100.

Neurotendinous Relationships. *Neurotendinous organs* (*Golgi tendon organs*) are located in the tendons close to their junction with the muscle mass. They consist of collagenous fibers which are contained within a connective tissue capsule. Numerous cells and afferent terminals are also present. They transmit information concerning the amount of stretch or tension on tendons. This type of information, therefore, also indicates the amount of contraction in a mass of muscle. With excessive tension on a tendon, the afferent discharge results in an inhibition to further contraction. Although the informational input is transmitted at a subconscious level throughout the entire range of muscular contraction, ultimately these organs minimize the possibility of tendons being torn from their points of attachment to bone or muscle.

Although the input from spindles and neurotendinous organs is at a subconscious level, conscious input is achieved through other mechanisms. Naked nerve endings (Ruffini-like) are embedded within the connective tissue of joint capsules. Subjected to the compression and tension associated with joint movement, they transmit information which is *kinesthetic*; i.e., information concerning the relative positions of various parts of the body.

References

Bone as an Organ

Arnold, J. S.: Quantitation of mineral of bone as an organ and tissue in osteoporosis. Clin. Orthop. *17:*167, 1960.

Cooper, R. R., Milgram, J. W. and Robinson, R. A.: Morphology of the osteon. An electron microscopic study. J. Bone Joint Surg. *48A:*1239, 1966.

Elliott, H. C.: Studies on articular cartilages. I. Growth mechanisms. Amer. J. Anat. *58:*127, 1936.

Frost, H. M.: New concepts of bone remodelling and of the nature of osteoporoses. J. Med. Surg. *1:*41, 1961.

Frost, H. M.: *Bone Remodelling Dynamics*. Thomas, Springfield, Ill., 1963.

Haines, R. W.: The development of joints. J. Anat. *81:* 33, 1947.

Koch, J. L.: The laws of bone architecture. Amer. J. Anat. *21:*177, 1917.

Roy, S.: Ultrastructure of articular cartilage in experimental hemarthrosis. Arch. Path. *86:*69, 1968.

Silberberg, M., Silberberg, R. and Hasler, M.: Fine structure of articular cartilage in mice receiving cortisone acetate. Arch. Path. *82:*569, 1966.

Muscle as an Organ

Bowman, J. P., Jr.: *The Muscle Spindle and Neuronal Control of the Tongue: Implications for Speech*. Thomas, Springfield, Ill., 1971.

Cohen, L. A.: Contributions of tactile musculo-tendinous and joint mechanisms to position sense in human shoulder. J. Neurophysiol., *21:*563, 1958.

Cooper, S.: Afferent impulses in the hypoglossal nerve on stretching the cat's tongue. J. Physiol. *126:*32P, 1954.

Lentz, T. L.: Development of the neuromuscular junction. J. Cell Biol. *47:*423, 1970.

Matthews, P. B. C.: Muscle spindles and their motor control. Physiol. Rev. *44:*219, 1964.

Nystrom, B.: Muscle-spindle histochemistry. Science *155:*1424, 1967.

Spiro, A. J. and Beilin, R. L.: Histochemical duality of rabbit intrafusal fibers. J. Histochem. Cytochem. *17:*348, 1969.

Yelin, H.: A histochemical study of muscle spindles and their relationship to extrafusal fiber types in the rat. Amer. J. Anat. *125:*31, 1969.

12 Nervous System

General Characteristics

Form and Function. The nervous system is composed of the nervous tissue described previously, as well as connective tissue and vasculature. The anatomical unit of this system is the neuron, while the functional unit is the *reflex arc*.

Anatomically, this system is divisible into two subunits, the *central nervous system* (CNS) and the *peripheral nervous system* (PNS). The CNS consists of the brain, its extensions and the spinal cord. The PNS includes nerve trunks, accumulations of nerve cell bodies (*ganglia*) and nerve terminals. The peripheral nervous system receives stimuli and transmits this information to the CNS, which integrates it, associates it, interprets it and transmits the resulting information via the PNS to various effector organs.

The peripheral nervous system may be subdivided further into a somatic and an autonomic system. The somatic system is responsible for the reception of information from the external environment, its transmission to the CNS and subsequently the carrying of information back to the effector organs.

The autonomic system functions in a similar manner; however, the informational input and subsequent evocation of a response involves the viscera.

The entire nervous system functions in such a manner as to allow the organism to respond to changing internal and external environmental stimuli.

Architecture of the Peripheral Nervous System

Ganglia. Accumulations of nerve cell bodies outside the CNS are referred to as *ganglia*. Corresponding accumulations within the CNS are referred to as *nuclei*. Two main types of ganglia are distinguished, *craniospinal ganglia* (*dorsal root, sensory*) and *autonomic ganglia* (*visceral, motor*).

Ganglia, although variable in size, are usually surrounded by a connective tissue capsule the fine collagenous and reticular fibers of which are scattered throughout the organ as a fine reticulum or stroma (Fig. 12-1). Blood vessels, axons, dendrites, peripheral neuroglia and nerve cell bodies are enmeshed within the supportive framework. Amphicytes are intimately associated with the nerve cell bodies. The amphicytes and the neurons of ganglia are of neural crest ectodermal origin.

The *dorsal root ganglia* are representative of craniospinal ganglia (Fig. 12-1). These globular structures are encapsulated and the connective tissue extensions of the capsule are scattered throughout the ganglia. The predominant neuronal type is pseudounipolar. Their size is quite variable. Each of the neurons is surrounded by amphicytes (Fig. 12-2). These flattened or cuboidal cells are in such intimate contact with the perikaryon that an indentation in the nerve cell body is often apparent. These cells are continuous with the neurolemmal sheath of the nerve fibers. Nerve fibers, usually in distinct fascicles, comprise the remainder of the organ.

The *autonomic ganglia* include those associated with the sympathetic trunk and the parasympathetic ganglia. The latter are located close to or in visceral organs. The *sympathetic ganglia* and the neurons that comprise them are smaller than dorsal root ganglia. Also, the former are comprised primarily of multipolar neurons. The nerve fibers are more diffusely scattered throughout this type of ganglion than in the craniospinal ganglion.

Parasympathetic ganglia, away from the visceral organs, are similar to sympathetic ganglia. Those located within the organs (*intramural ganglia*), however, are not as structured as those described

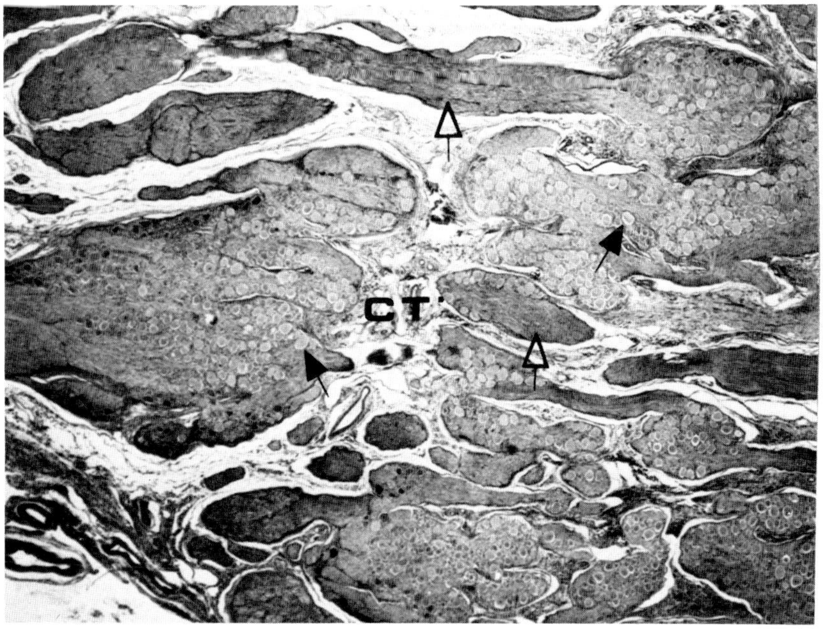

Fig. 12-1. Dorsal root ganglion. The organ consists of nerve cell bodies (*solid arrows*), nerve cell processes (*open arrows*) and connective tissue (*CT*). ×4. All light micrographs are the original magnifications.

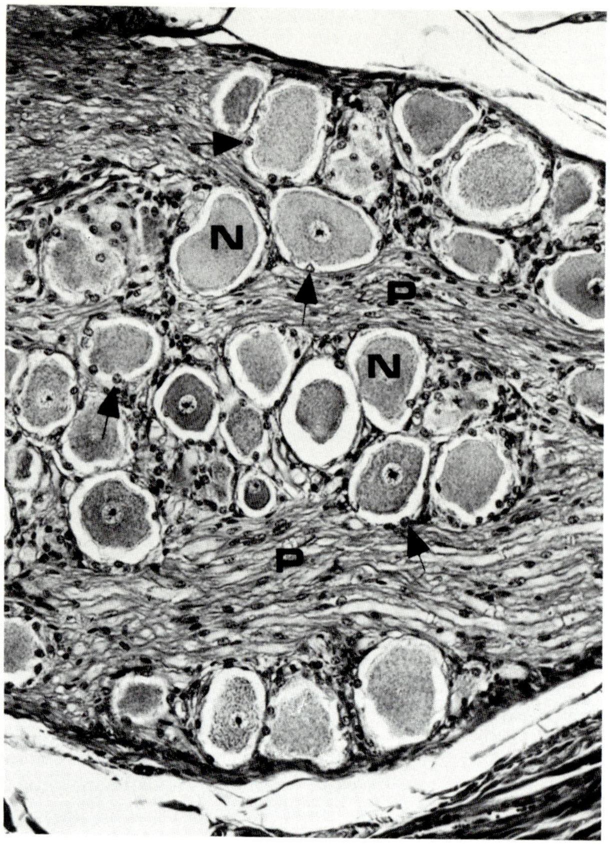

Fig. 12-2. Cells and nerve fibers of a ganglion. The nerve cell bodies (*N*) and the nerve cell processes (*P*) are integral components of a ganglion. Amphicytes (*arrows*) are closely associated with the nerve cell bodies. ×40. (See Fig. 1–17 also.)

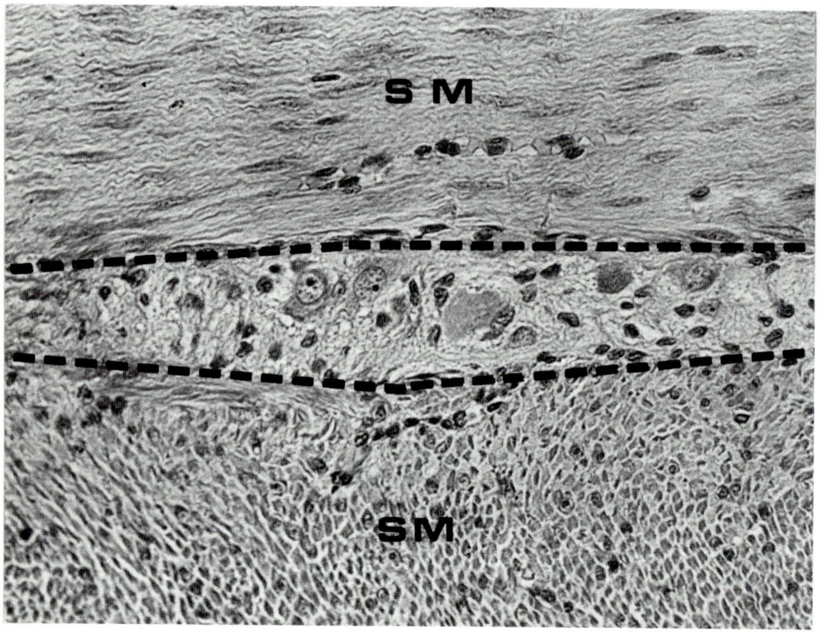

Fig. 12-3. Intramural ganglion from the myenteric plexus. *Dashed lines*, approximate limit of the ganglion, which is interdigitated between two masses of smooth muscle (*SM*). ×100.

previously (Fig. 12-3). They consist of few multipolar nerve cell bodies and fibers. In most instances, these perikarya are devoid of amphicytes. However, small and flattened fibroblasts may replace them.

Nerve Trunks. The organization of peripheral nerve fibers into large trunks follows the basic pattern described for the organization of solid organs (Fig. 12-4). It is almost identical to the pattern of muscle organization.

Individual nerve fibers, myelinated or not, are surrounded by a stroma of fine collagenous fibers with some connective tissue cells and capillaries. This sheath of connective tissue is the *endoneurium* (Fig. 12-5). A number of nerve fibers is grouped as a fascicle (Fig. 12-6). These fascicles are surrounded by one to three layers of cells. Since each of these layers of *perineural cells* is invested with a basal lamina, they are not connective tissue cells. Fine collagenous and reticular fibers as well as fibroblasts may be located between the perineural sleeves. The perineural investments terminate before the end of the nerve. At these points, as well as at points along the nerve where vessels enter, the epineurium is continuous with the endoneurium. This complex sheath is referred to as the *perineurium*. Individual fascicles may be widely separated by this space. The *epineurium* is composed of dense white fibrous connective tissue the contents of which are continuous with the components of the endoneurium.

Afferent Nerve Terminals. The afferent nerve terminals are the means by which an organism perceives various stimuli from its external and internal environment. The reception of varied information once transmitted to the CNS is the basis upon which an integrated response (or lack thereof) is initiated (or not).

These receptors are transducers that convert various types of modalities (pain, touch, warmth, pressure, etc.) into a form usable by the nervous system. Although receptors have been classified in numerous ways, none is totally satisfactory and others overlap to varying degrees. The following is the basis for the different classifications:

1. Source of the stimuli and location of the receptors.
2. Types of modalities transduced by the receptors.
3. Form of the stimuli required to stimulate the receptors.
4. The structure of the receptors.

Although not perfectly satisfactory, the structural basis of classification will be used.

On an anatomical basis, two main subdivisions are used to classify receptors: *free and diffuse*, *encapsulated*.

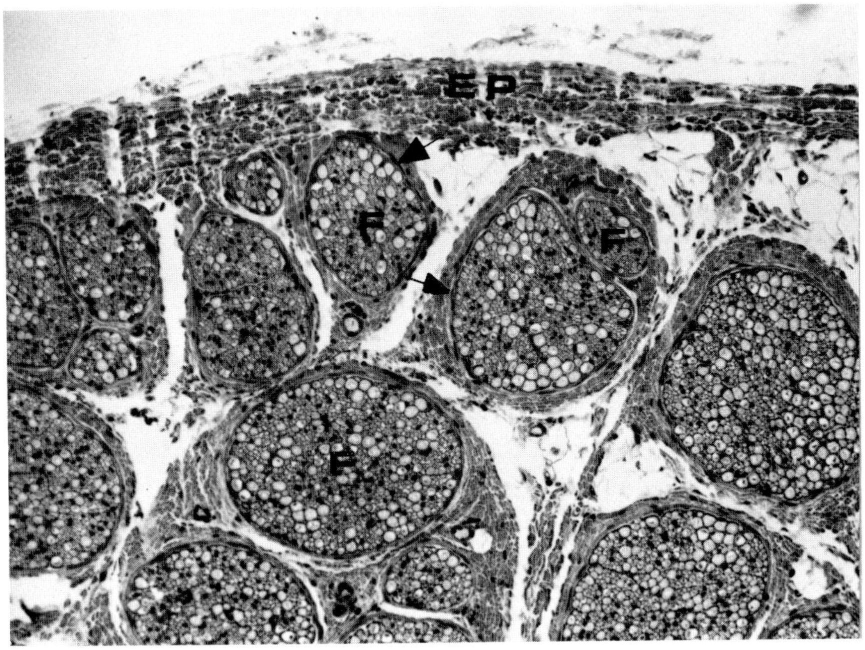

Fig. 12-4. Organization of a nerve trunk. The epineurium (*EP*) surrounds all the fascicles (*F*). Individual fascicles are surrounded by a perineurium (*solid arrows*). The endoneurium surrounds individual nerve cell processes. ×40.

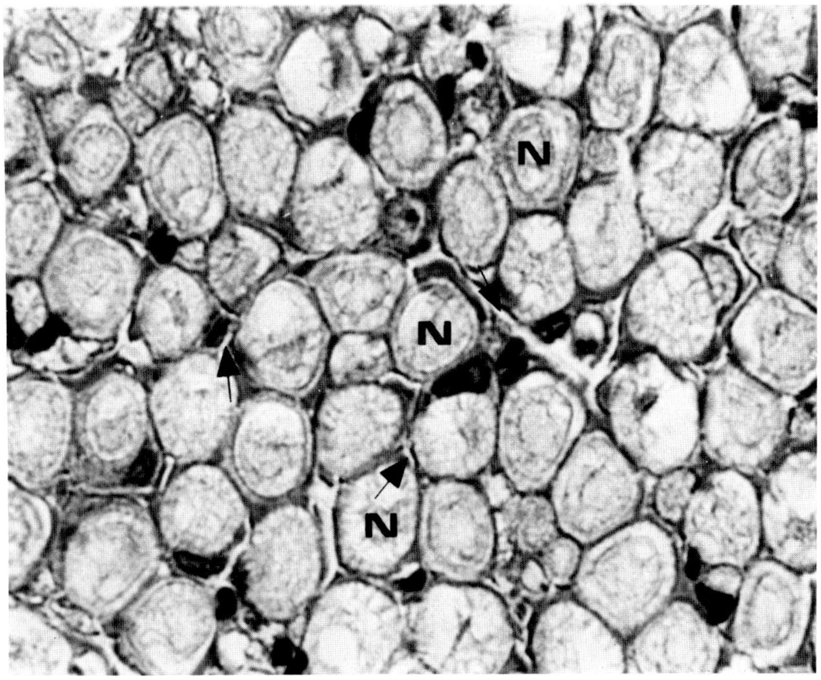

Fig. 12-5. Endoneurium. Individual nerve cell processes (*N*) are surrounded by the connective tissue of the endoneurium (*arrows*). ×320.

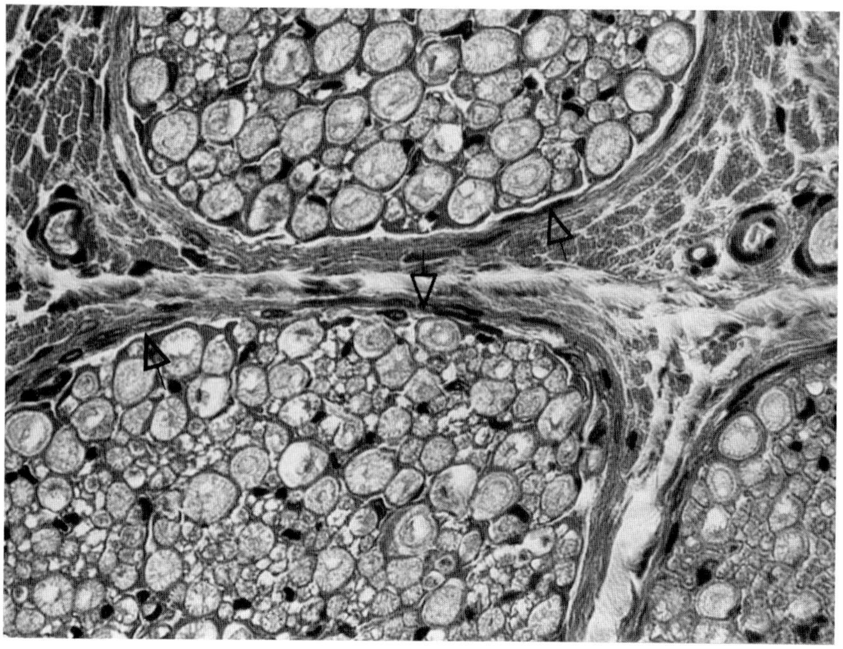

Fig. 12-6. Perineural cells. Layers of perineural cells (*arrows*) surround individual fascicles. ×160.

receptors for tactile discrimination. Merkel's disks may be rudimentary forms of this corpuscle.

Krause's endbulbs are slightly encapsulated, spherical receptors which are located in the skin and associated mucous membranes (especially the conjunctiva). In one type, the nerve terminal enters the granular mass within the capsule and terminates at the opposite pole in a slightly expanded ending. In a second type, the nerve enters the granular mass within the capsule, undergoes arborization and terminates in expanded endings. This type of corpuscle is a cold receptor.

Golgi-Mazzoni corpuscles are similar to Meissner's corpuscles. They are, however, smaller and more thickly encapsulated than Meissner's corpuscles. They are believed to be pressure receptors which occur in the connective tissue of hairless skin and associated mucous membranes. They also occur in the dermis of the glans penis, the digital pads of carnivores and the connective tissue associated with the hoof.

Genital corpuscles are similar to Golgi-

The *free and diffuse nerve endings* are the most ubiquitous of the body. While they are most numerous in the epidermis, they are also found in mucous and serous membranes, muscles, joints and the connective tissue of the viscera. The extensively arborized fibers may be myelinated or unmyelinated and may terminate as flattened or bulblike endings scattered among epithelial or connective tissue cells (Fig. 12-7). They are usually considered touch receptors.

Merkel's disks are modified free nerve endings which are associated with deep epidermal cells. The terminal branches are flattened or disklike and in contact with these modified cells. They generally occur in hairless skin. These receptors are associated with tactile stimulation which is pain associated.

The *encapsulated receptors* vary from slight to heavy encapsulation. These include *Meissner's corpuscles, Krause's endbulbs, Golgi-Mazzoni corpuscles, genital corpuscles, Vater-Pacinian corpuscles, Herbst corpuscles, Ruffini corpuscles, neuromuscular spindles* and *Golgi tendon organs*.

Meissner's corpuscles are one of the most ubiquitous encapsulated receptors of hairless skin (Fig. 12-8). They occur in the dermal papillae of the soles and palms. The corpuscles are about 100 μm long and approximately 25 μm wide. They are slightly encapsulated and contain the terminals of one or more nerves arranged in a helical order around a mass of cells similarly arranged. The overall form is that of an imbricated fir cone. These corpuscles are

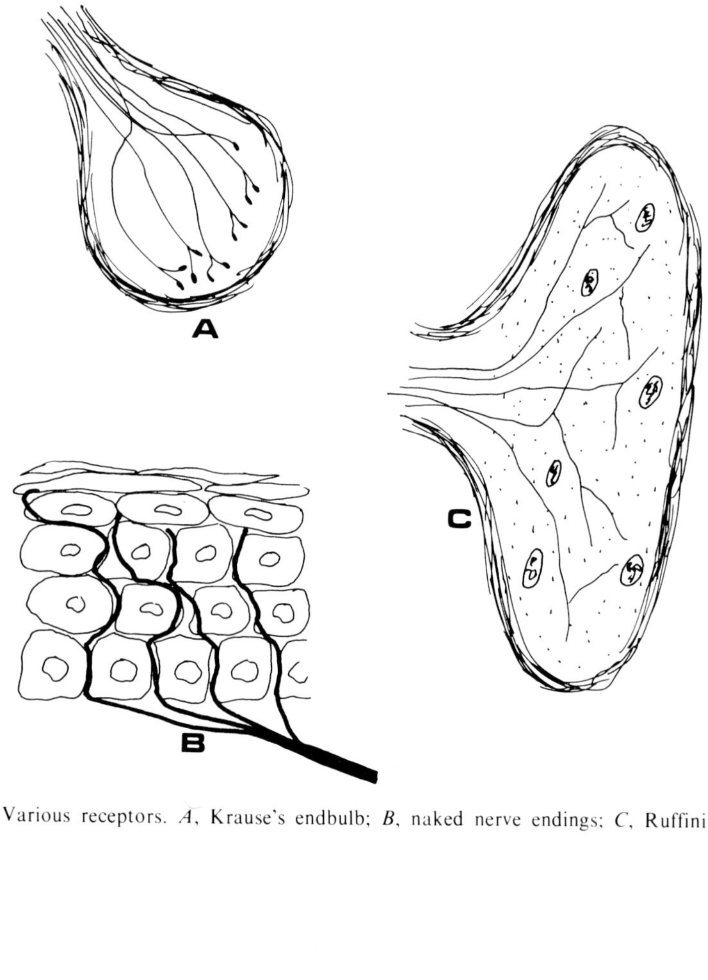

Fig. 12-7. Various receptors. *A*, Krause's endbulb; *B*, naked nerve endings; *C*, Ruffini corpuscle.

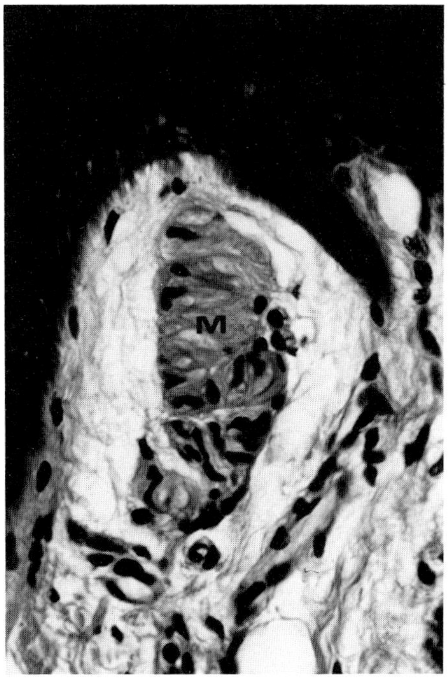

Fig. 12-8. Meissner's corpuscle. The corpuscle (*M*) occupies a dermal papilla. ×115.

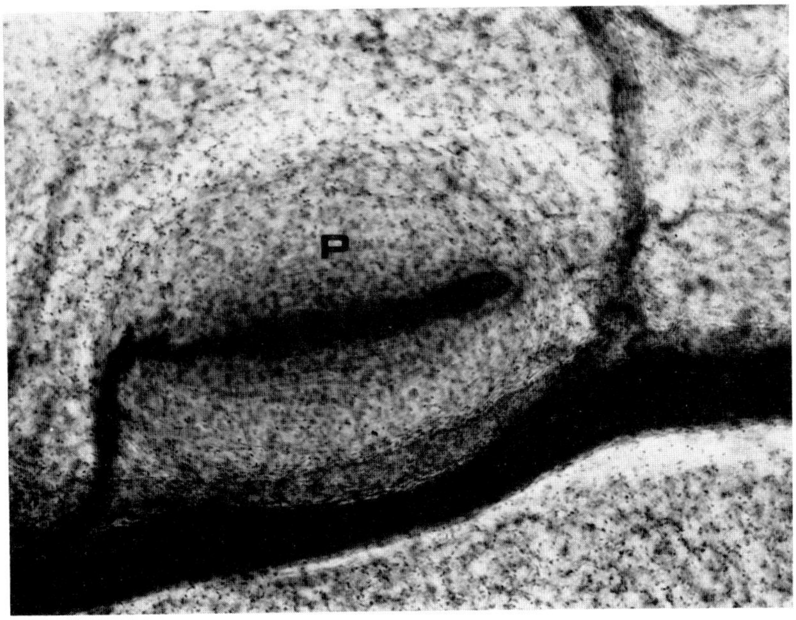

Fig. 12-9. A whole-mount preparation of a Vater-Pacinian corpuscle (*P*) from a mesentery. ×16.

Mazzoni corpuscles. However, the former are larger and more thickly encapsulated than the latter. They may also be lobulated. The number of nerves entering the capsule varies from one to ten. They arborize and form a spiral, interlacing network of naked nerve terminals. These corpuscles occur in the clitoris and glans penis. They are considered to be pressure receptors.

The *Vater-Pacinian corpuscles* are the largest encapsulated nerve endings of the body (Fig. 12-9). They may be 3 to 4 mm long and thus observable with the unaided eye. A single nerve enters the corpuscle and terminates in a bulbous enlargement surrounded by a mass of granular material. Concentric layers of epithelial cells (similar to perineural cells), connective tissue cells and capillaries impart an onion-like appearance (Fig. 12-10). These corpuscles are pressure receptors and are extremely unbiquitous. They occur in the deep connective tissue, mesenteries and serous membranes, as well as the connective tissue of visceral organs, muscle and that associated with tendons and ligaments.

Herbst corpuscles are smaller versions of Pacinian corpuscles. These are pressure receptors and occur in the tongues and beaks of birds.

The *Ruffini corpuscles* are composed of an arborization of nerve fibers interlacing throughout a granular mass which is enclosed by a connective tissue capsule. These corpuscles are believed to be heat receptors, but Ruffini-like receptors are associated with kinesthetic sensations (Chapter 11).

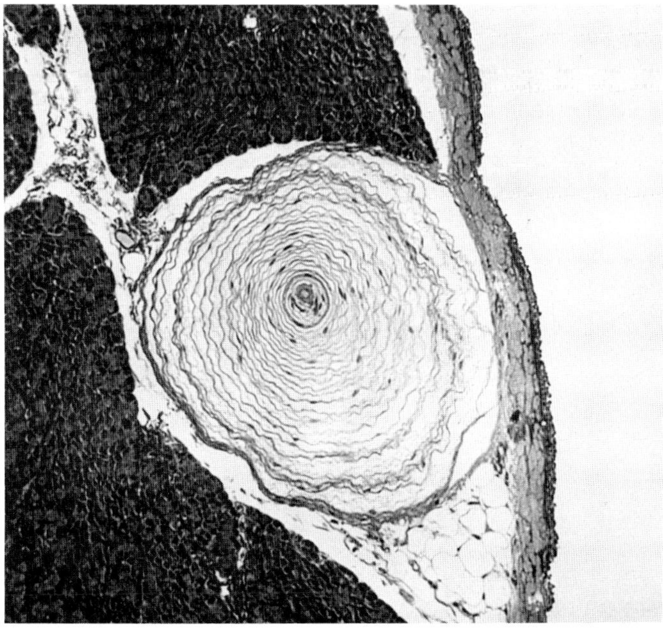

Fig. 12-10. A sectioned Vater-Pacinian corpuscle in the connective tissue of the feline pancreas. The concentric layers of components impart an onion-like appearance. ×25.

Neuromuscular spindles and *Golgi tendon organs* were described with the musculoskeletal system (Chapter 11).

Although numerous receptors and their associated modalities have been described, there is some question relating to the specificity of given afferent terminals for a specific modality. The distinctness of some corpuscles is also questioned. Meissner's corpuscles, Merkel's disks, Golgi-Mazzoni corpuscles, Krause's endbulbs and genital corpuscles are closely related and may be modified forms of one another. Similarly, Pacinian and Herbst corpuscles may be closely related. There is also evidence that receptors continuously break down and reorganize throughout life.

Architecture of the Central Nervous System

Meninges. The central nervous system is well protected by its placement within the bones of the skull and spinal column. Further protection is afforded by the association of dense and loose connective tissue with the CNS (Fig. 12-11). These tissues are disposed as three fibrous membranes totally enclosing the system: *dura mater*, *arachnoidea* and *pia mater*. The dura mater is also referred to as the *pachymeninx;* the arachnoid and pia mater are referred to as the *leptomeninges*. Besides the protection by virtue of the connective tissue, these membranes are intimately associated with *cerebrospinal fluid*. Also, the vascular supply gains access to the CNS via these membranes.

The *dura mater* is a tough dense white fibrous connective tissue covering of the brain and spinal cord which consists of collagen, some elastic fibers and blood vessels (Fig. 12-11). In association with the brain, it consists of two layers. The outer layer is the fibrous periosteum of the inner surface of the cranial bones. This layer contains a number of blood vessels associated with the cranial bones. An inner, poorly vascularized layer blends insensibly with the outer or periosteal layer. These layers become distinct in specific areas of the brain where they separate and form the *dural sinuses*. These sinuses are responsible for the collection of cerebrospinal fluid and its return to the vascular system. The dura is separated from the arachnoid membrane by a *subdural space*.

Since the bones of the skull are not continuous as a unit with the bones of the vertebral column, the periosteum of the inner skull surface is reflected as the periosteum of the outer skull surface at the *foramen magnum*. The dura of the spinal cord, therefore, is a single layer (the inner layer of the cranial dura) and is separated from the periosteum which lines the vertebrae by an extensive space called the *epidural space*. This space is filled with loose connective tissue, adipose tissue and extensive veins and venous sinuses. The epidural space is used for the administration of some anesthetics (*epidural anesthesia*).

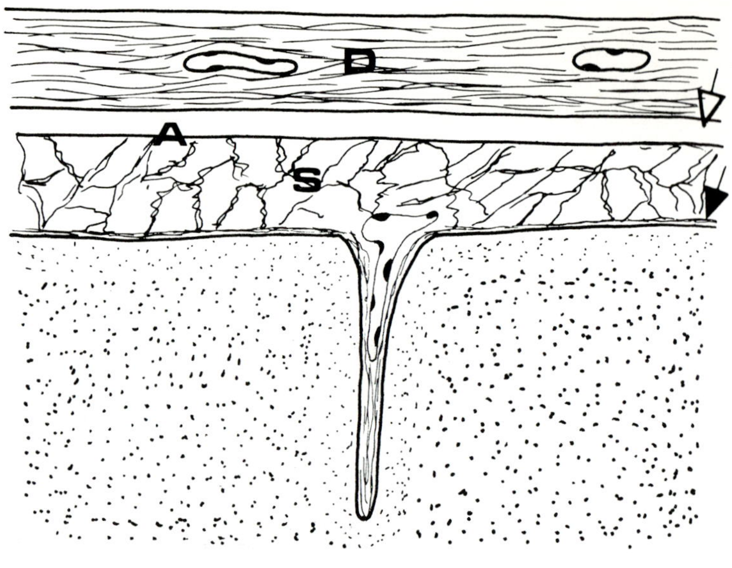

Fig. 12-11. The meninges. The meninges include the dura mater (*D*), arachnoid membrane (*A*) and pia mater (*solid arrow*). Subdural (*open arrow*) and subarachnoid spaces (*S*) are present.

The *arachnoidea* consists of a distinct membrane and numerous fibrous trabeculae on its inner surface (Fig. 12-11). Both are composed of fine collagenous and elastic fibers. The extensive network of trabeculae which extend to the pia mater comprise the supportive framework for the *subarachnoid space*. This space is occupied by cerebrospinal fluid which mechanically protects the central nervous system. Blood vessels, also, are scattered on the floor of this space in the pia mater. Protrusions of connective tissue from the subarachnoid space extend through the inner layer of the dura mater and form *arachnoid villi* (*arachnoid granulations*) which project into the sinuses of the dura. Through this association, cerebrospinal fluid from the subarachnoid space is returned to the blood vascular system.

The *pia mater* is the most intimate protective membrane of the brain and spinal cord (Fig. 12-11). It extends into the numerous depressions and fissures that characterize the CNS. This membrane is composed of very fine collagenous and elastic fibers, as well as small vessels. It is covered by a continuous membrane of flattened cells which are quite similar to the mesothelial lining cells of serous membranes. As blood vessels enter the depths of the nervous tissue they carry with them some of the fine connective tissue components of the pia mater.

Choroid Plexus. The embryonic, tubular nature of the CNS is not lost in the adult, but it is extensively modified. The simple tube of the embryo is converted to large ventricles and a canal in the brain which is continuous with a central canal in the spinal cord. The ependymal lining of this modified tube is also retained in the adult. In specific areas (roof and walls of the ventricles) the ependyma is closely associated with the vascular pia mater, the vessels of which form the *choroid plexuses* (Fig. 12-12). Modified cuboidal ependymal cells with a well-developed brush border are in intimate contact with the highly vascularized underlying pia mater and both are thrown into extensive folds (villi) by the tortuous paths of the vasculature.

Cerebrospinal fluid is a transudate of the vascular bed and is devoid of protein. A few cells, primarily lymphocytes, may occur within this fluid. Produced at the choroid plexuses and from the nervous tissue adjacent to the ventricular system, it is transported across the barrier into the ventricles and canals. The fluid gains access to the subarachnoid space through foramina in the roof of the fourth ventricle. From this point the fluid is returned to the vasculature via the arachnoid villi in the dural sinuses.

Spinal Cord. The spinal cord varies in configuration at the cervical, thoracic, lumbar and sacral levels. The following pattern, however, is similar at all levels of examination prior to the termination of the spinal cord.

The cord is generally round to oval and is surrounded by the pachymeninx (inner layer) and the leptomeninges in a pattern described previously (Fig. 12-13). The bulk of the cord is divided into two distinct areas, *gray matter* and *white matter*. The gray matter is arranged in a pattern often described as an H or butterfly. The *gray matter* consists of nerve cell bodies, unmyelinated fibers, some myelinated fibers, protoplasmic astrocytes, oligodendrogliocytes, microgliocytes, some

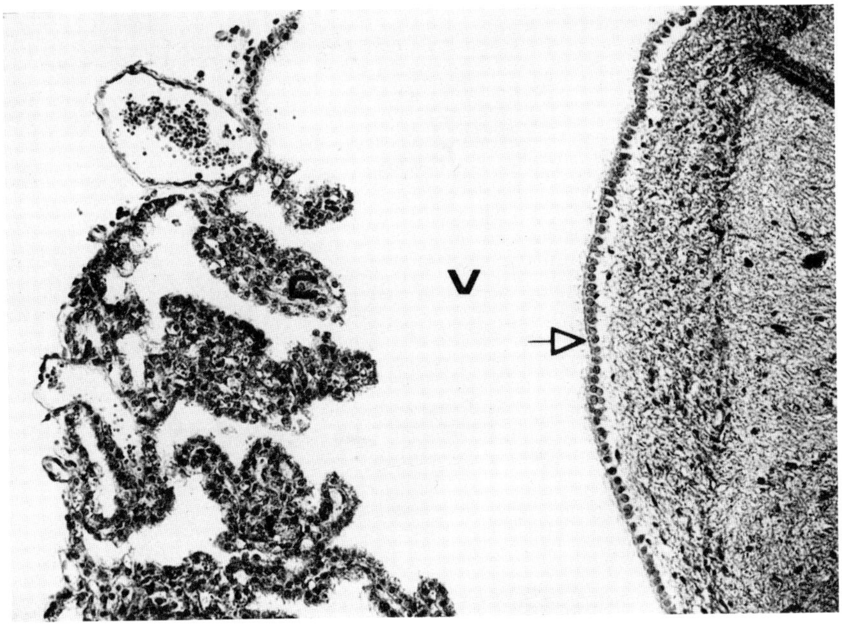

Fig. 12-12. The choroid plexus of the fourth ventricle. The choroid plexus (*C*) is suspended from the roof of the fourth ventricle (*V*) while ependyma (*arrow*) lines the floor of the ventricle. ×40.

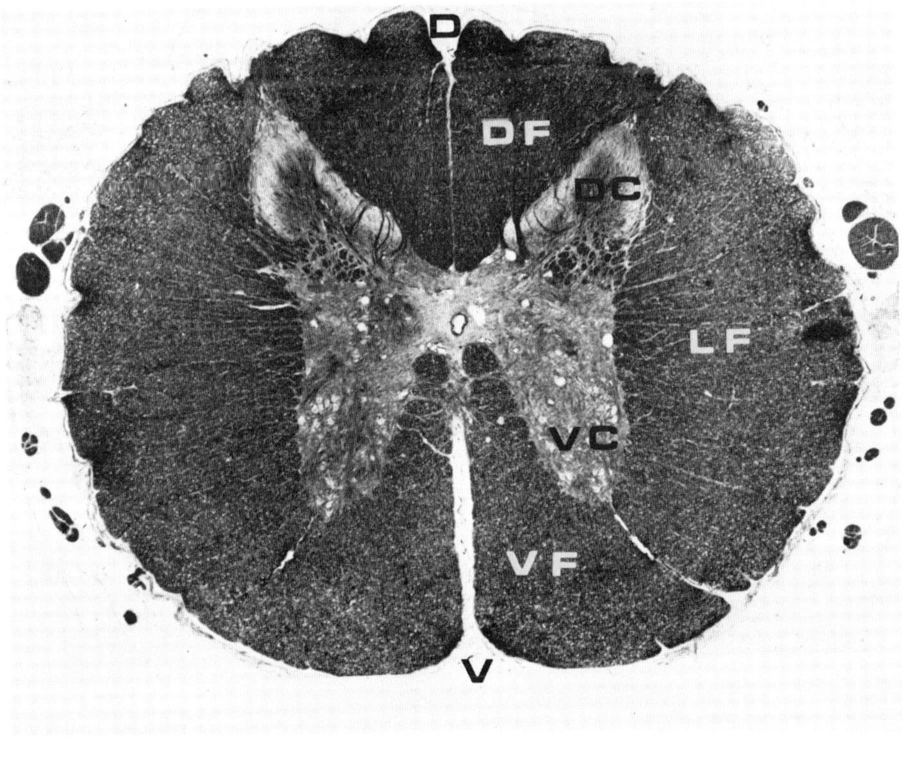

Fig. 12-13. A typical section through the cervical region of the spinal cord. The dorsal (*DC*) and ventral columns (*VC*) are prominent within the white matter. The dorsal (*DF*), lateral (*LF*) and ventral funiculi (*VF*) are indicated. The dorsal (*D*) and ventral (*V*) borders are indicated. ×4 (myelin stain).

blood vessels and associated fine connective tissue fibers. Although neurons are aggregated or scattered throughout the gray matter, they are especially distinct in the *ventral columns*. These large multipolar neurons give rise to axons carrying information to effector organs of the body. Neurons of medium size are located in the *lateral columns* of the thoracolumbar segments. These neurons give rise to axons which connect with autonomic ganglia. Small neurons characterize the *dorsal columns*. Their axons project up and down the spinal cord. The dorsal and ventral columns are especially prominent in the cervical and lumbosacral regions. The spinal canal (lined by ependyma) is contained within the *central intermediate substance* or *gray commissure*.

The *white matter* is composed of myelinated and unmyelinated fibers, scattered neuroglial elements and blood vessels. A *dorsal funiculus* occupies the region between the dorsal columns; a *lateral funiculus* is between two adjacent dorsal and ventral columns; and a *ventral funiculus* is between the two ventral columns.

Brain Stem. The brain stem is a complex structure which is continuous with the spinal cord caudally and higher brain centers rostrally. The organizational constituents are similar to the spinal cord; however, these constituents are distributed differently. Various nuclei and tracts are distributed in a specific manner throughout the brain stem (Fig. 12-14).

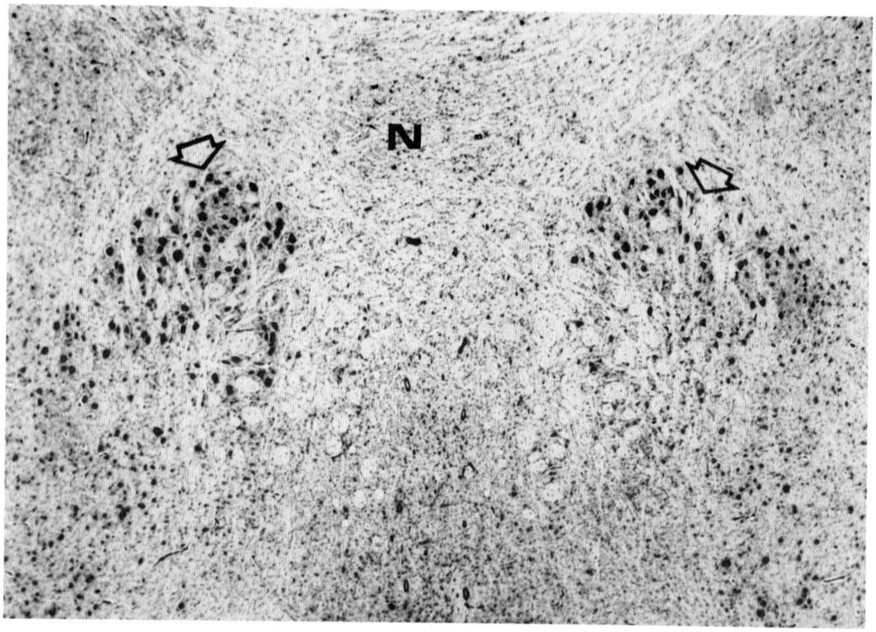

Fig. 12-14. A frontal section through the brain stem of a pig. Nerve cell processes and supportive cells of the neuroglia form the neuropil (*N*). Two prominent nuclei are apparent (*arrows*). ×4.

Cerebellum. The cerebellum is also divided into gray and white matter (Fig. 12-15). The white matter is covered by a thin layer of gray matter. Three distinct zones of gray matter are apparent: an *outer molecular layer*, a *central layer of large cells* (*Purkinje cells*) and a *deep granular layer*. The granular layer is contiguous to the white matter.

The outer molecular layer consists of some small neurons and numerous unmyelinated fibers. The Purkinje cells of the central layer are large, pyramidal cells which are very prominent (Fig. 12-16). *Do not confuse Purkinje cells with Purkinje fibers!* The neurons of the granular layer are small and tightly packed within this region. The details of the connections among these cells, as well as connections with *mossy* and *climbing fibers*, are available in texts of neuroanatomy.

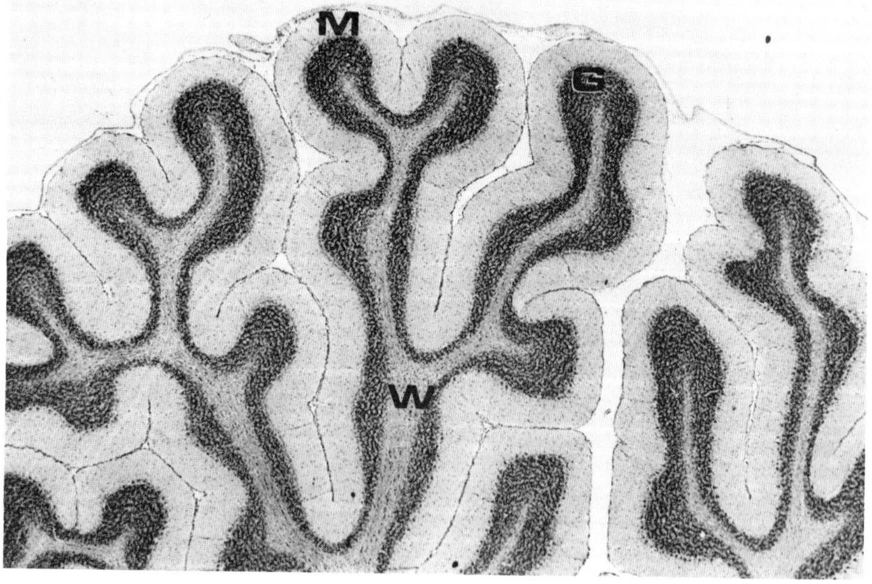

Fig. 12-15. A section through the cerebellum. The molecular layer (*M*) and the granular layer (*G*) are peripheral to the white matter (*W*). ×4.

Cerebrum. Considering the diverse and complex functions of this portion of the brain, it is not unreasonable to assume that its cytoarchitecture reflects this diversity as well as this complexity. Although six layers of cells have been described, the degree of development of each layer varies with the section of cerebral cortex being studied (Fig. 12-17). The gray (outer) area of the cerebral cortex consists generally of the following cellular regions: *molecular*

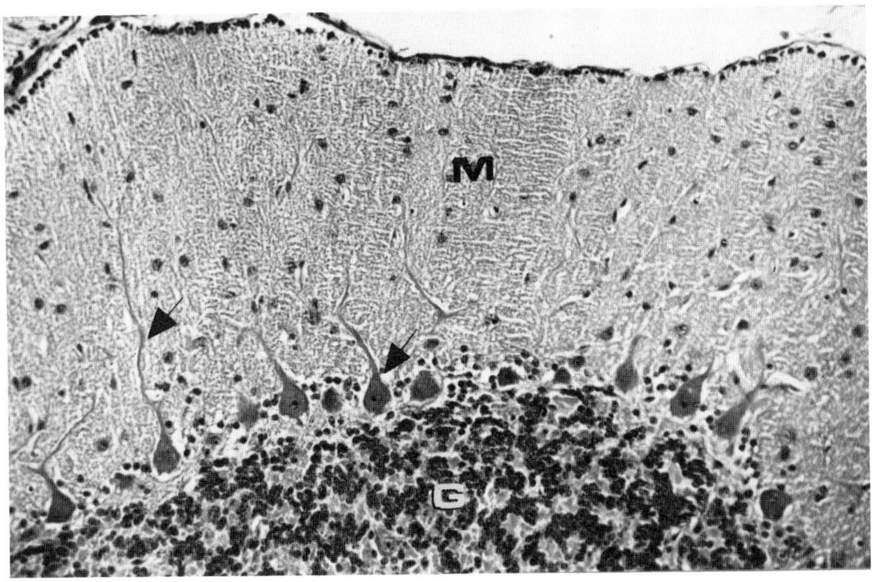

Fig. 12-16. Purkinje cells of the cerebellum. The Purkinje cells (*arrows*) occur at the interface between the molecular (*M*) and granular (*G*) layers. ×40.

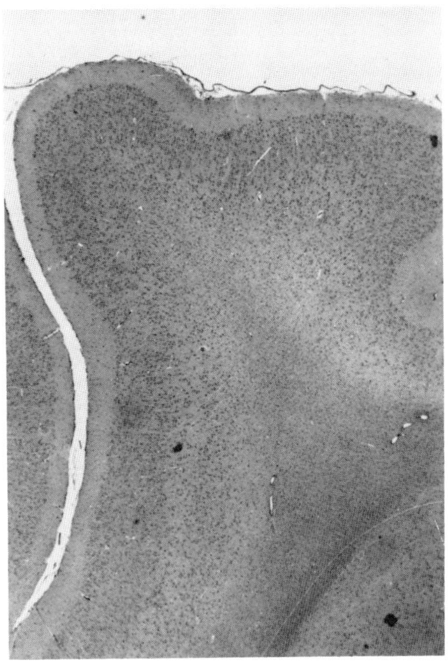

Fig. 12-17. A section through the cerebrum. The occurrence and distribution of the layers of the gray matter differ in various areas of the cerebrum. ×3.

layer, *outer granular layer*, *pyramidal cell layer*, *inner granular layer*, *ganglion* or *inner pyramidal cell layer* and *polymorphic cell layer*. Throughout these areas are neuroglial elements, myelinated and unmyelinated nerve fibers and vessels. The student is referred to a text of neuroanatomy for further discussion of the cerebral cortex.

References

Peripheral Nervous System

Cauna, N.: Structure of digital touch corpuscles. Acta Anat. *32*:1, 1958.

Cauna, N. and Mannan, G.: The structure of human digital Pacinian corpuscles (corpuscula lamellosa) and its functional significance. J. Anat. *92*:1, 1958.

Fernand, V. S. V. and Young, J. Z.: The sizes of the nerve fibers of muscle nerves. Proc. Roy. Soc. (Biol.) *139*:38, 1951.

Gamble, H. J. and Eames, R. A.: An electron microscope study of the connective tissue of human peripheral nerve. J. Anat. *98*:655, 1964.

Grillo, M. A.: Electron microscopy of sympathetic tissues. Pharmacol. Rev. *18*:387, 1966.

Hess, A.: The fine structure of young and old spinal ganglia. Anat. Rec. *123*:399, 1955.

Ortiz-Piçon, J. M.: The neuroglia of the sensory ganglia. Anat. Rec. *121*:513, 1955.

Shanthaveerappa, T. R. and Bourne, G. H.: The "perineural epithelium," a metabolically active, continuous, protoplasmic cell barrier surrounding peripheral nerve fasciculi. J. Anat. *96*:527, 1962.

Central Nervous System

Elliott, H. C.: Studies on the motor cells of the spinal cord. Amer. J. Anat. *70*:95, 1942.

Globus, E. G. and Scheibel, A. B.: Pattern and field in cortical structure. J. Comp. Neurol. *131*:155, 1967.

Herndon, R. M.: The fine structure of the Purkinje cell. J. Cell Biol. *18*:167, 1963.

Maxwell, D. S. and Pease, D. C.: Electron microscopy of the choroid plexus. Anat. Rec. *124*:331, 1956.

Weed, L. H.: Meninges and cerebrospinal fluid. J. Anat. *72*:181, 1938.

13 Cardiovascular System

General Characteristics

Form and Function. The cardiovascular system consists of moieties to pump, transport and distribute required elements to the cells and tissues of the soma. These cardiovascular elements include the heart, arteries, veins and capillaries as well as the lymphatic vessels. The heart is a highly muscularized tube the contractions of which supply the force to move the blood through the system. The arteries carry the blood away from the heart to the capillaries. The capillaries mediate the exchange of materials between the vascular bed and the extravascular tissues. The venous system returns the blood to the heart. Lymphatics arise in the tissue space and return extracellular fluid as lymph to the blood vascular system in the cervical region.

Although a basic scheme of organization is common to all these entities, there are modifications and deviations from the basic pattern to permit a diversity of functional adaptations. Of prime consideration in the construction of the walls of these organs are the following factors:

1. Velocity of the blood moving through the vascular channel.
2. The pressure with which blood is being propelled.
3. The volume of the blood being moved.
4. The requirements for pumping, transportation and distribution.

Some of the morphological factors that must be considered to fulfill the functional aspects mentioned previously are:

1. The size of the lumen of the organ.
2. The thickness of the vessel wall.
3. The resistance and/or elasticity of the vessel wall.
4. The specific function of the organ as reflected in the relationships of mural elements.

The histological aspects of vessel construction cannot be separated from the hemodynamic role they fulfill. The arterial side of the system carries a low volume of blood under high pressure at a high velocity. The capillary system carries a large volume of blood under an appreciably diminished pressure and velocity. The venous system carries high quantities of blood at very low pressures and velocities.

Although various patterns in mural morphology are observed to accommodate the pressure-volume relationships, the basic scheme consists of *tunica intima*, *tunica media* and *tunica adventitia* (Fig. 13-1).

The *tunica intima* is composed of three distinct subdivisions: *endothelium*, *subendothelial coat* and *internal elastic membrane* (Figs. 13-1, 13-2). The endothelium consists of typical squamous cells which line the lumen of the organ. Typically, the nucleus is prominent and may bulge into the lumen, whereas the marginal cytoplasm is difficult to discern with the light microscope. The cells reside upon a basement membrane which separates the endothelium from the peripheral fibroelastic connective tissue and fibroblasts of the *subendothelial coat*. For the most part, these elements are oriented longitudinally (parallel to the long axis of the vessel). Smooth muscle fibers may be present, as well as cells that normally occupy connective tissue spaces. The *internal elastic membrane* is a condensation of elastic fibers that separates the tunica intima from the tunica media.

The *tunica media* consists of a mixture of smooth muscle cells, collagenous fibers, elastic fibers and fibroblasts (Figs. 13-1, 13-3). The smooth muscle cells are arranged in a circular pattern around the lumen. They are in intimate association with collagenous and elastic fibers. *Nervi* and *vasa vasorum*, the nerve and blood supply of the vessels, may be observed in large vessels.

At the junction between the tunica media

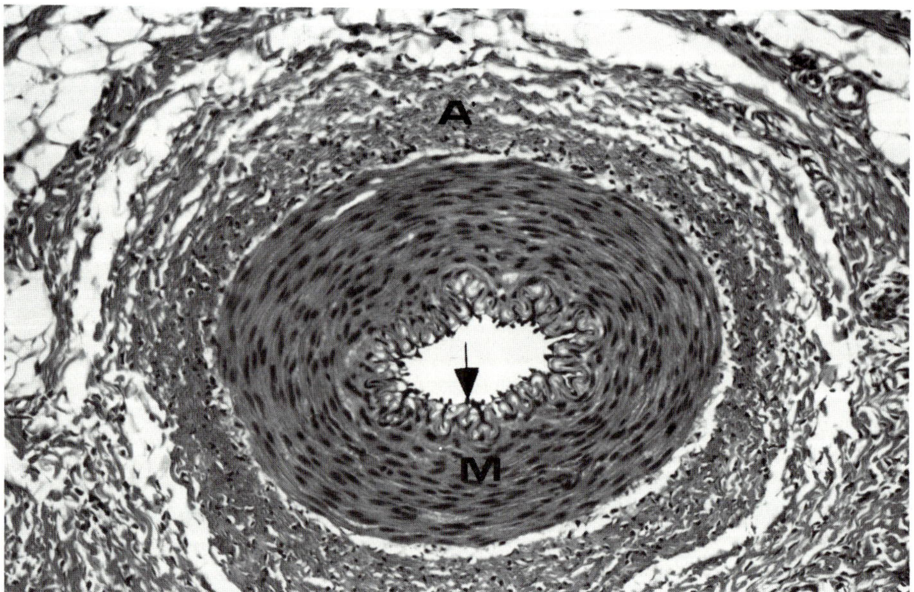

Fig. 13-1. Mural elements of a muscular artery. The three components are tunica intima (*arrow*), tunica media (*M*) and tunica adventitia (*A*). ×40. All light micrographs are the original magnifications. All electron micrographs are the final magnifications.

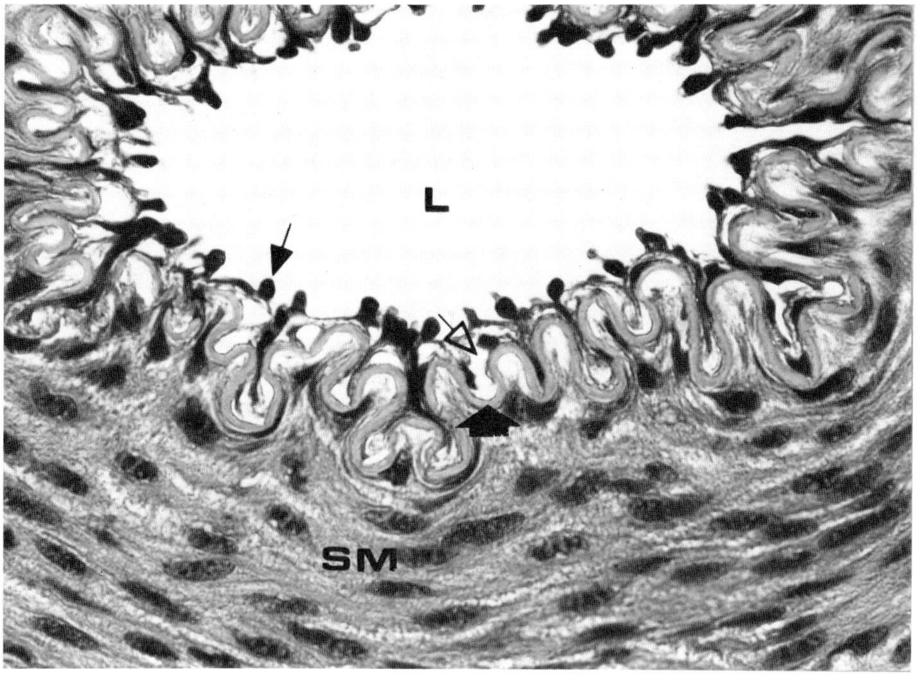

Fig. 13-2. Tunica intima of a muscular artery. The lumen (*L*) of the vessel is lined by endothelial cells (*small solid arrow*) which protrude into it. The subendothelial space (*open arrow*) is accentuated by contraction of the vessel and artifact. The internal elastic membrane (*large solid arrow*) is adjacent to the smooth muscle (*SM*) of the tunica media. ×160.

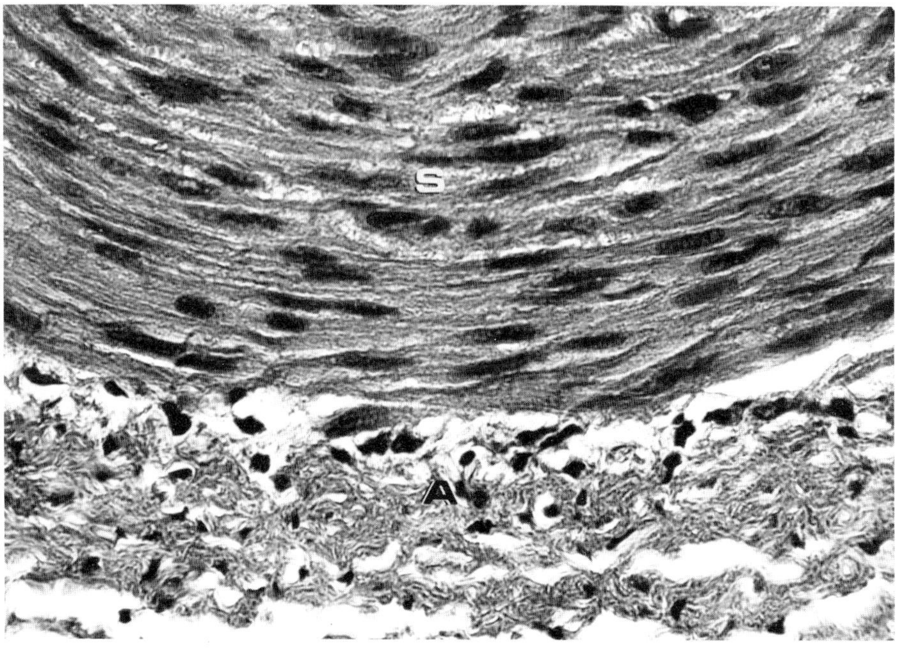

Fig. 13-3. Tunica media and tunica adventitia of a muscular artery. The tunica media contains smooth muscle cells (*S*), while the tunica adventitia (*A*) consists of fibroelastic connective tissue. ×160.

and tunica adventitia, an *external elastic membrane* may be present. It, too, is a condensation of elastic fibers. This membrane demarcates the media from the adventitia. The *tunica adventitia* is formed of this membrane and dense fibroelastic connective tissue (Fig. 13-3). Generally, it is difficult to distinguish the end of the adventitia and the beginning of the surrounding connective tissue. Nervi and vasa vasorum ramify in the tunica adventitia.

It is of utmost importance to realize that the aforementioned entities represent generalizations concerning mural structure. Not all vessels will contain all of the aforementioned moieties; nor, if present, will all of them be represented equally in all vessels. Distinctions between vessels are made on the basis of the variations of mural elements from the generalized scheme.

Exchange System

Capillaries. *Capillaries* are the simplest members of the vascular system, but their function, by virtue of their simplicity, is extremely important. They are the means by which metabolities gain access to and waste products leave the connective tissue space. Capillaries are simple endothelial-lined tubes with a diameter of 7–9 μm. Due to this size limitation, they are able to accommodate a single red blood cell (RBC) at a time. Peripherally, this tube is covered by a basement membrane.

In section with light microscopy a thin rim of acidophilic cytoplasm delimits the extent of the capillary (Fig. 13-4). The dark nucleus of the endothelial cell occurs along the margin of the lumen and may bulge into the lumen. Capillaries are accompanied along their entire length by connective tissue cells, thin collagenous fibers and reticular fibers. Among the many cells closely associated with them, fixed macrophages, mesenchymal cells and Rouget cells are especially prominent.

All capillaries appear somewhat similar with the light microscope. However, there are two basic types. Capillaries may be *continuous*; i.e., there are no interruptions in the continuity of the endothelial cells (Fig. 13-5). This type is found typically in muscle, lungs, nervous system and other organs. The second type is *fenestrated*; i.e., pores are scattered throughout the walls of the endothelium (Fig. 13-6). These pores may be covered by a diaphragm or not. Fenestrated capillaries occur in the endocrine glands, intestines, kidneys and other organs. Whether a capillary is continuous or fenestrated, the associated basal lamina is uninterrupted.

Sinusoids. *Sinusoids* are large areas in the vascular bed which are lined by endothelial or endothelial-like cells (*littoral cells*). They are similar to capillaries but are larger and

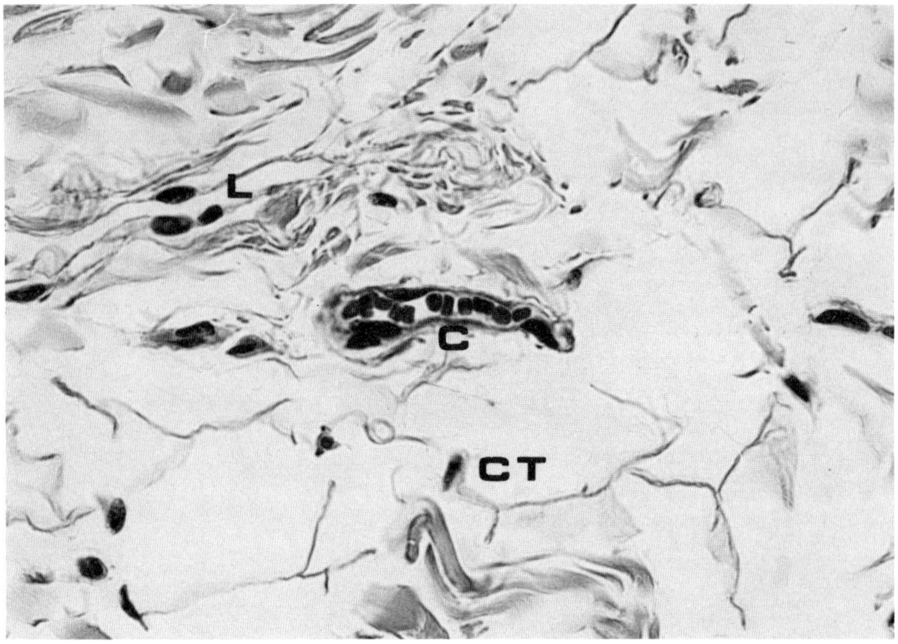

Fig. 13-4. Capillaries in loose connective tissue. The connective tissue (*CT*) contains a blood capillary (*C*) and a lymphatic capillary (*L*). ×160.

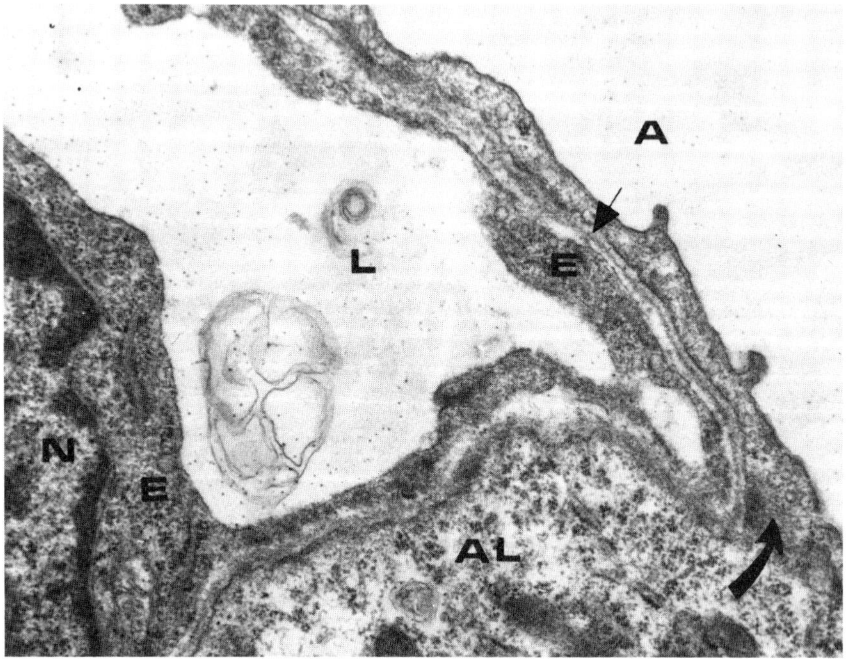

Fig. 13-5. An electron micrograph of a continuous capillary. The alveolus (*A*) of the lung is defined by the perikaryon of the alveolar lining cell (*AL*) and its attenuated process (*curved arrow*). The lumen of the capillary (*L*) is delimited by the endothelial cell (*E*) and its nucleus (*N*). The basal lamina (*small arrow*) is complete and the endothelial lining is continuous. ×20,000.

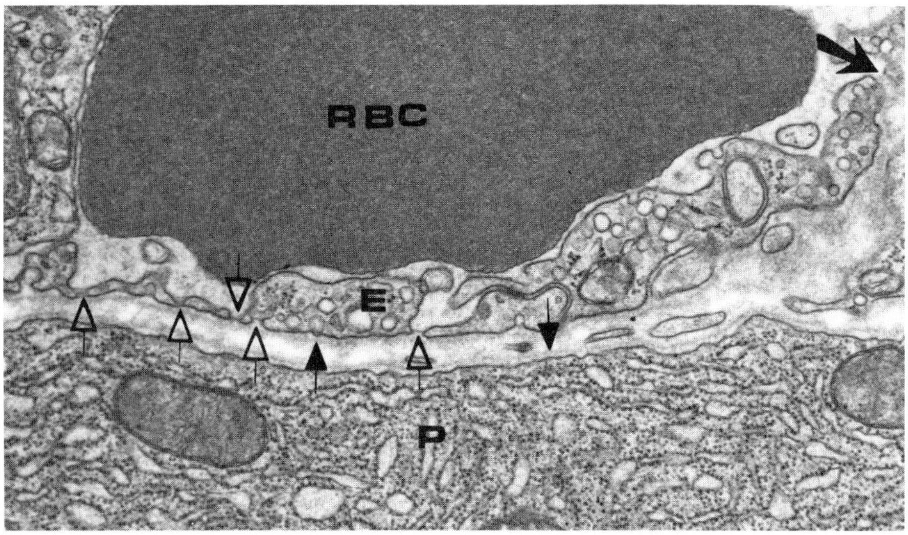

Fig. 13-6. An electron micrograph of a discontinuous capillary. The endothelium (*E*) of a capillary is separated from a pancreatic acinar cell (*P*) by two basal laminae (*small solid arrows*). The capillary contains a RBC. Numerous fenestrations (*open arrows*) are covered by diaphragms, while one fenestration (*large solid arrow*) is not. ×25,000.

irregularly shaped. A basal lamina may be present, incomplete or absent. Some of the lining cells are phagocytic, while others are not. The phagocytic lining cells, members of the reticuloendothelial system, appreciably broaden the function of these vascular channels. If the lining cells of the sinusoids are not phagocytic, then these channels may be considered similar to very large capillaries. Sometimes these nonphagocytic sinusoids are referred to as *sinuses*. Various types of sinusoids may be observed, but their identification requires the electron microscope. Three types of sinusoids have been described: *continuous*, *discontinuous* and *fenestrated*. *Continuous sinusoids* have a complete basal lamina and may be phagocytic or nonphagocytic. *Discontinuous sinusoids* have either an incomplete or no basal lamina and are phagocytic (Fig. 13-7). *Fenestrated sinusoids* are fenestrated, have a continuous basal lamina and are nonphagocytic. Continuous sinusoids occur in the liver of some species, while discontinuous sinusoids are characteristic of the liver, spleen, and bone marrow of most species. Fenestrated sinusoids occur in the pituitary gland and adrenal cortex.

The organization of capillaries and sinusoids is simple compared to the previously described general plan. Actually, these structures represent the two innermost regions of the tunica intima, the *endothelium* and *subendothelial coat*. Increased organization and complexity is achieved by peripheral addition to these elements.

High Pressure System

Arterioles. Gradual transitions from capillaries to arterioles are exemplified by *arterial capillaries*. These structures are 4–5 times larger than capillaries and may contain scattered smooth muscle cells within their walls.

Arterioles have a diameter less than 100 μm (Fig. 13-8). The smallest arterioles consist of a tunica intima devoid of a subendothelial coat. The only recognizable elements are the endothelium and thin internal elastic membrane which appears as a bright scalloped line. The tunica media consists of one to three layers of smooth muscle among which are scattered some fine collagenous fibers and elastic fibers. An external elastic membrane is not present and the loose connective tissue of the tunica adventitia blends insensibly with the surrounding connective tissue.

It is not unusual to observe a scalloped endothelial layer, the individual cells of which appear to protrude into the lumen. This, naturally, is reflected in the internal elastic membrane. It is probably due to excessive contraction of the vessel at the

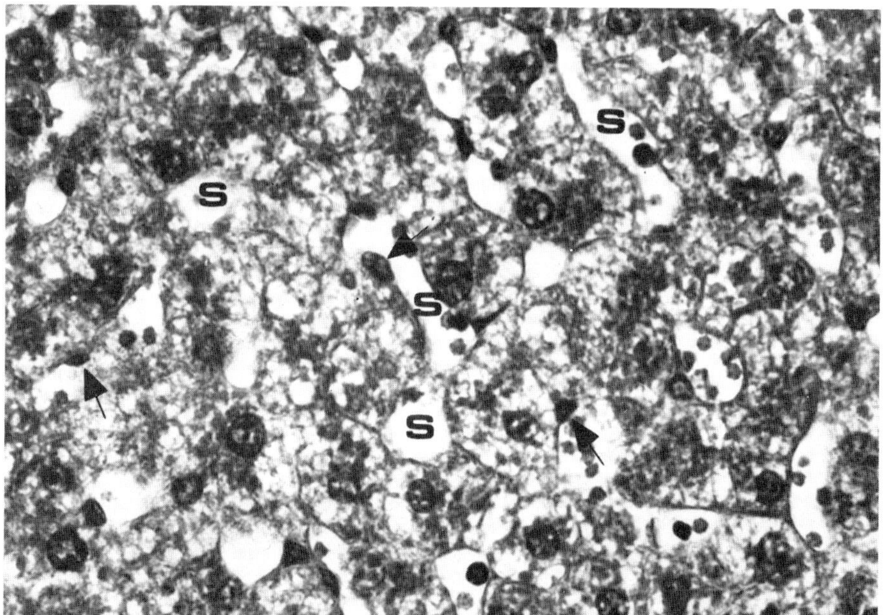

Fig. 13-7. Discontinuous sinusoids from the liver. The sinusoids (*S*) are lined by phagocytic cells (*arrows*). ×160. (See Figs. 17-59, 17-60, 17-62).

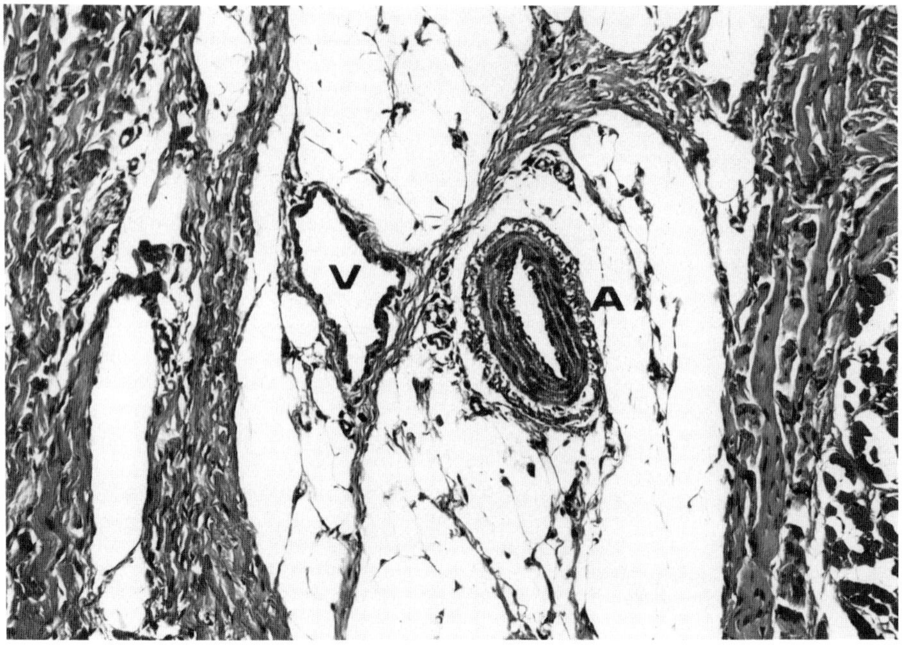

Fig. 13-8. An arteriole and companion venule. The arteriole (*A*) has three layers of smooth muscle in the tunica media. The companion venule (*V*) does not contain smooth muscle. ×40.

time of fixation. This type of change may be observed in larger vessels of the high-pressure system as well.

Small and Medium-sized Arteries. There is no sharp line of distinction between arterioles and small arteries. Rather, there is a continuum of quantitative change from the smaller to larger vessels.

The small and medium-sized arteries are also referred to as *muscular* or *distributing arteries* (Fig. 13-1). The tunica intima of these vessels is typical and consists of three layers. The tunica media consists of circularly oriented smooth muscle cells among which are scattered some collagenous fibers, reticular fibers, elastic fibers and fibroblasts. An external elastic membrane is often well-defined, while the tunica adventitia consists of heavy collagenous fibers, some elastic fibers, and vasa and nervi vasorum.

Elastic Arteries. The *elastic arteries* are the largest arteries in the body (Fig. 13-9). Compared to their luminal volume, they have a rather thin wall.

All the elements of the tunica intima are present. The endothelial layer consists of polygonal cells rather than the expected flattened cells. The subendothelial layer consists of collagenous fibers, elastic fibers, fibroblasts and smooth muscle cells in a loose connective tissue. An internal elastic membrane is present; however, it is not always distinct because the tunica media consists of large quantities of elastic fibers which are oriented in such a manner as to be interpreted as repeating elastic membranes. Between the coarse elastic fibers are fine collagenous fibers, fine elastic fibers, fibroblasts and smooth muscle cells. A distinct external elastic membrane is not present. The connective tissue of the tunica adventitia is thin and blends insensibly with the surrounding connective tissue.

Low Pressure System

Venules. The transition from capillaries to venules is a gradual one. *Venous capillaries* attain large diameters (up to 20 times those of capillaries) and gradually become associated with other mural elements. In distinction to arterial capillaries, venous capillaries usually become associated with connective tissue first and later develop smooth muscle within their walls.

Venules usually consist of a simple endothelial tube surrounded by a loose connective tissue (Fig. 13-8). Smooth muscle cell investment occurs as the venules become small veins. The tunica adventitia of these vessels is quite thick compared to the tunica media.

Small and Medium-sized Veins. These vessels are lined by a thin tunica intima which consists of polygonal endothelial cells

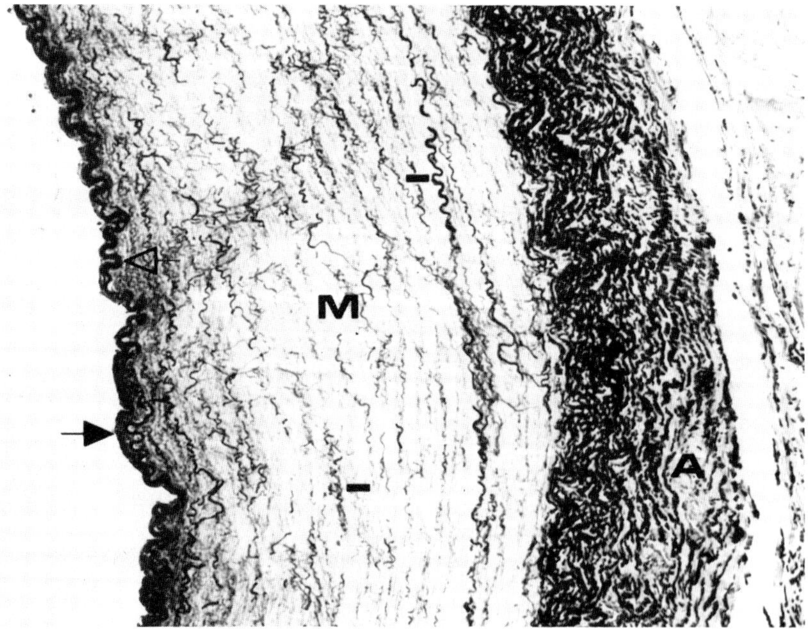

Fig. 13-9. An elastic artery. This section of the aorta is stained for elastic fibers. The tunica intima (*solid arrow*) contains a well-defined internal elastic membrane. The tunica media (*M*) consists of smooth muscle and elastic fibers (*bars*). The tunica adventitia (*A*) has numerous elastic fibers also. ×25 (Van Giesen stain).

and a very small subendothelial connective tissue layer (Fig. 13-10). The tunica media is thin and consists of circularly oriented muscle cells, collagenous fibers and fine elastic fibers. The tunica adventitia is well-developed and comprises the bulk of the wall.

Many of these veins are equipped with *valves* (Fig. 13-11). These are invaginations of the tunica intima into the lumen of the vessel. Valves are lined by flattened endothelial cells and contain a core of subendothelial connective tissue (Fig. 13-12). These intimal modifications are especially prominent in vessels located below the heart.

Large Veins. These vessels represent quantitative changes from the smaller ones. The tunica intima is thicker than observed in smaller veins and an internal elastic membrane may be present. The tunica media consists primarily of collagenous and elastic fibers, while the smooth muscle component is reduced or even absent. The tunica adventitia is well-developed and is the thickest part of the wall. Scattered bundles of smooth muscle may be present within this coat and oriented parallel to the long axis of the vessel. Valves are absent in the venae cavae and the hepatic portal vein.

High and Low Pressure Systems Compared

Like their high-pressure counterparts, the mural organization of veins is quite variable. However, these vessels occur as companion vessels and comparisons are made easily. Generally, the mural elements of a vein of a given size, when compared with the companion artery, are less distinct. The following distinctions will assist in distinguishing these entities from one another in section:

1. Blood is rarely found in sectioned arteries, but it is typically present in veins.
2. The tunica media is well-developed in arteries, while the tunica adventitia is well-developed in veins.
3. Luminal diameters are greater than mural thicknesses in veins, while luminal diameters of arteries are smaller than mural thicknesses.
4. During agonal changes, veins are subject to irregular contractions, while arteries contract more regularly.
5. Internal elastic membranes may be present in arterioles, but these are usually confined to large veins.
6. The tunica adventitia of veins is usually the thickest coat of the wall.

Heart

The heart of endotherms (mammals and birds) consists of four separate chambers: two *atria* and two *ventricles*. The heart is a thick-walled, highly muscularized tube which propels the blood through the body. Two distinct, yet interconnected, circulatory patterns are apparent. Venous blood low in oxygen is returned to the *right atrium*

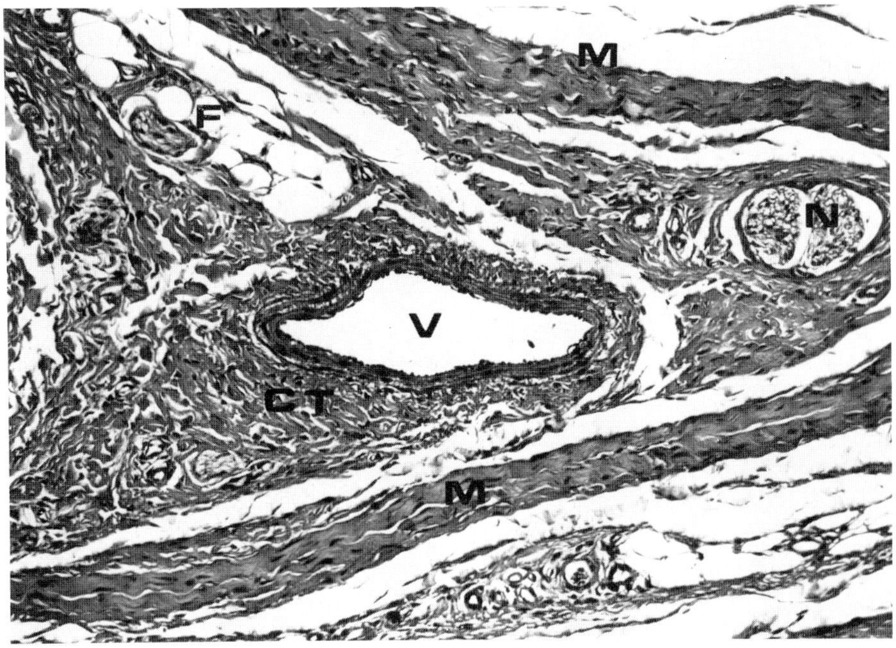

Fig. 13-10. A small vein. The small vein is surrounded by connective tissue (*CT*). Fat cells (*F*), nerves (*N*) and skeletal muscle (*M*) are present also. ×40.

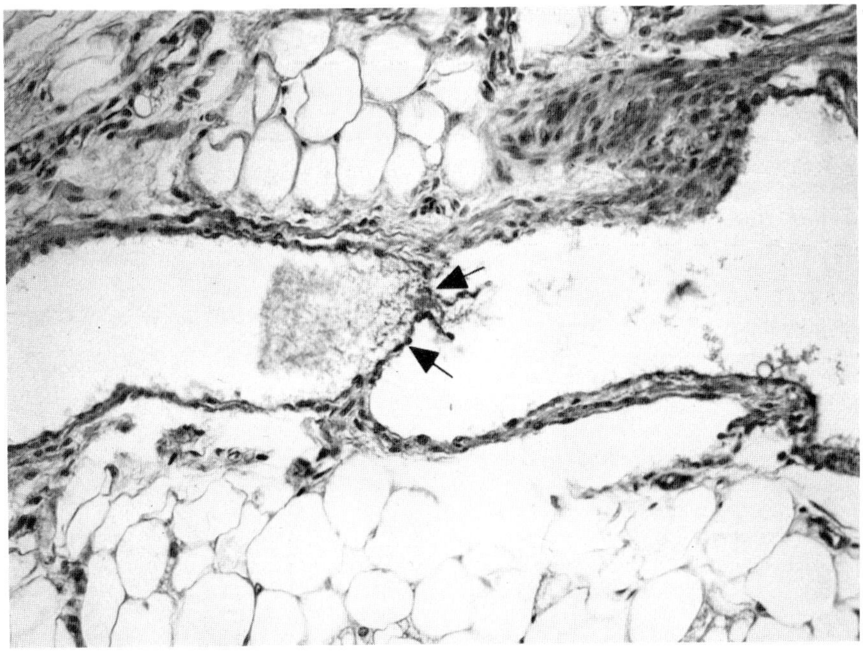

Fig. 13-11. A valve of a vein. The cusps (*arrows*) of the valve prevent a reverse blood flow. ×50.

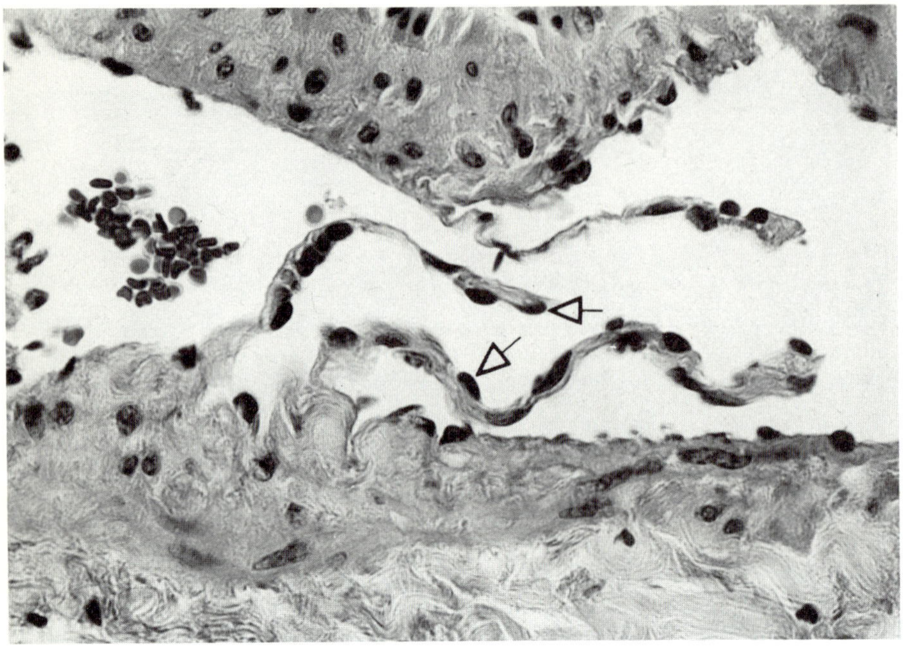

Fig. 13-12. Components of a valve. The cusps are composed of endothelial cells (*arrows*) and subendothelial connective tissue. ×160.

whence it passes through the *right atrioventricular valve* (*tricuspid valve*) into the *right ventricle*. Upon contraction, blood is propelled through the *semilunar valve* of the *pulmonary artery* and carried to the lungs where it is oxygenated. Oxygenated blood returns to the *left atrium* via the *pulmonary vein*. Upon passing through the *left atrioventricular valve* (*bicuspid valve*) into the *left ventricle*, it is propelled through the *semilunar valve* of the *aorta* for distribution throughout the soma.

The mural elements of the heart are organized in a manner similar to the peripheral vessels. The heart consists of three coats: an inner coat, *endocardium*; a middle coat, *myocardium*; an outer coat, *epicardium* (Fig. 13-13).

Endocardium. The endocardium is the cardiac counterpart of the tunica intima. The endocardium consists of: *endothelium* and a *subendothelial coat*. Deep to this there is a *subendocardial coat* (Fig. 13-14). The endothelium consists of polygonal cells that reside on a basement membrane. This lining is continuous with the endothelial lining of the peripheral vessels. The *subendothelial coat* consists of fine collagenous and elastic fibers. This coat is continuous with a deeper or more peripheral *subendocardial coat* of loose connective tissue. It contains collagenous and elastic fibers, adipose cells, smooth muscle fibers, blood vessels, nerves and, in the ventricles, Purkinje fibers. Besides attaching the endocardium to the myocardium, this coat also contains the impulse-conducting system of the heart (Purkinje fibers) in the ventricles.

Myocardium. The *myocardium* is comparable to the tunica media (Fig. 13-15). It

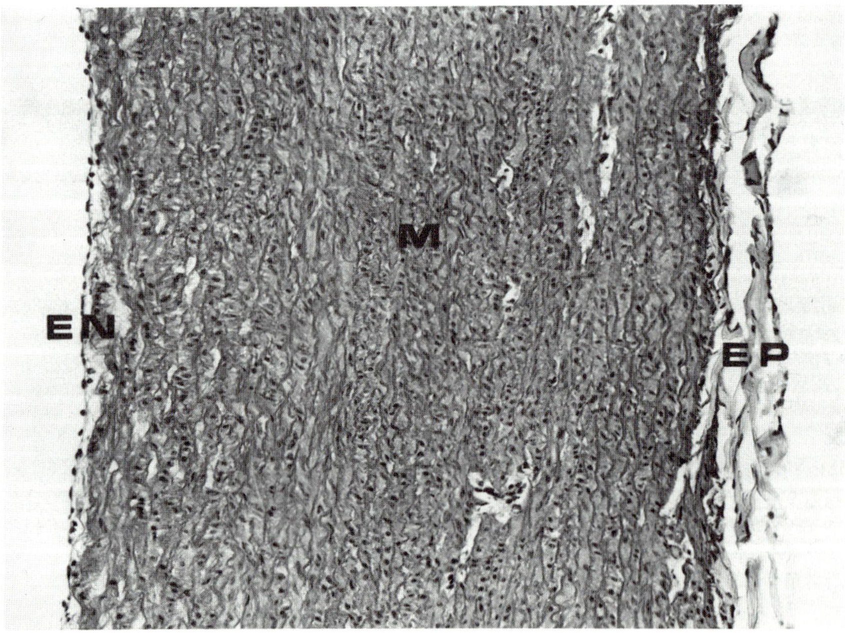

Fig. 13-13. Wall of the atrium. The wall consists of endocardium (*EN*), myocardium (*M*) and epicardium (*EP*). ×40.

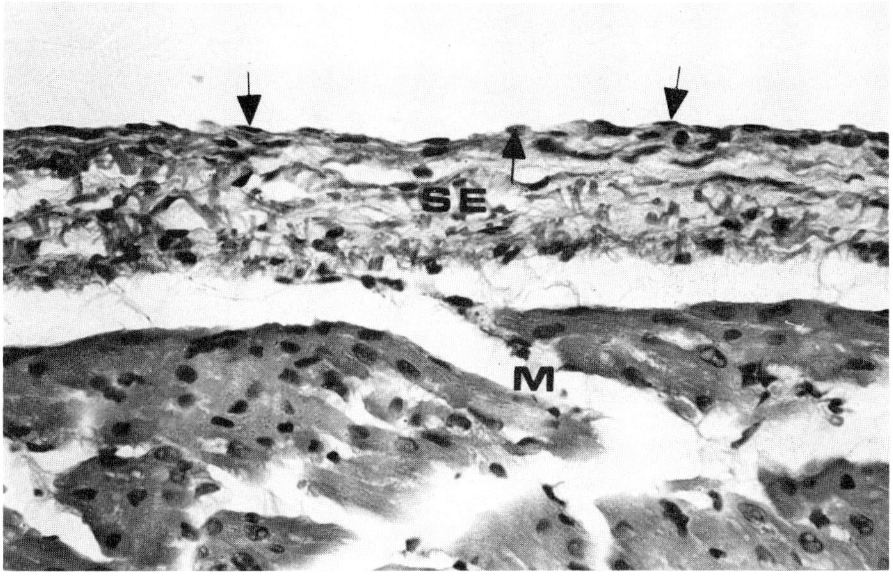

Fig. 13-14. Atrial endocardium. The endothelium (*arrows*) is underlaid by subendothelial connective tissue (*SE*) which is adjacent to the myocardium (*M*). ×100.

consists, primarily, of cardiac muscle. Connective tissue fibers, nerves and blood vessels are also present (Chapter 8).

Epicardium. The *epicardium* is functionally similar to the tunica adventitia (Fig. 13-16). However, the epicardium is actually a serous membrane—the *visceral pericardium* of gross anatomy. The mesothelial lining resides upon a thin layer of loose connective tissue. It is continuous with a loose connective tissue layer which contains variable deposits of adipose tissue, blood vessels and nerves—the *subepicardial coat*.

Cardiac Skeleton. The cardiac muscle and valves are supported by a skeleton of dense white fibrous connective tissue (DWFCT). Some components of this skeleton may also be cartilaginous or osseous. The following elements comprise the cardiac skeleton:

1. Four fibrous rings (*annuli fibrosi*).
2. A fibrous triangle (*trigonum fibrosum*).
3. A fibrous and membranous septum (*septum membranaceum*).

The *annuli fibrosi* are dense white fibrous connective tissue rings which surround the *semilunar valves* of the pulmonary artery and aorta and the two atrioventricular valves. These rings are continuous, directly or indirectly, with the *trigonum fibrosum*. This is a mass of DWFCT between the atrioventricular canals. Similarly, it is continuous with the DWFCT of the interventricular septum—the *septum membranaceum*. These skeletal elements serve as points of attachment for the cardiac muscle mass.

Cartilage and/or bone may occur in the fibrous rings. In the ox, especially, ossification of the fibrous ring associated with the semilunar valve of the aorta is common, resulting in the formation of two *ossa cordis*.

Cardiac Valves. The cardiac valves are invaginations of the endocardium into the lumen of the heart (Fig. 13-17). The connective tissue of the annuli fibrosi is continuous as a supportive core in the valves between the two layers of endocardium. The connective tissue of the atrioventricular valves is continuous with the collagenous fibers of the tendinous cords (*chordae tendineae*) which are attached to the ventricular surfaces of the valves. Naturally, a thin layer of endocardium is reflected over these tendinous cords and is continuous with the endocardium of the papillary muscles. Elastic fibers are more numerous on the side of the valve facing the back pressure.

The semilunar valves are similar to the atrioventricular valves. A dense nodule of collagen or cartilage may be present on the edge of the three cusps. This is referred to as the *nodule of Arantius*.

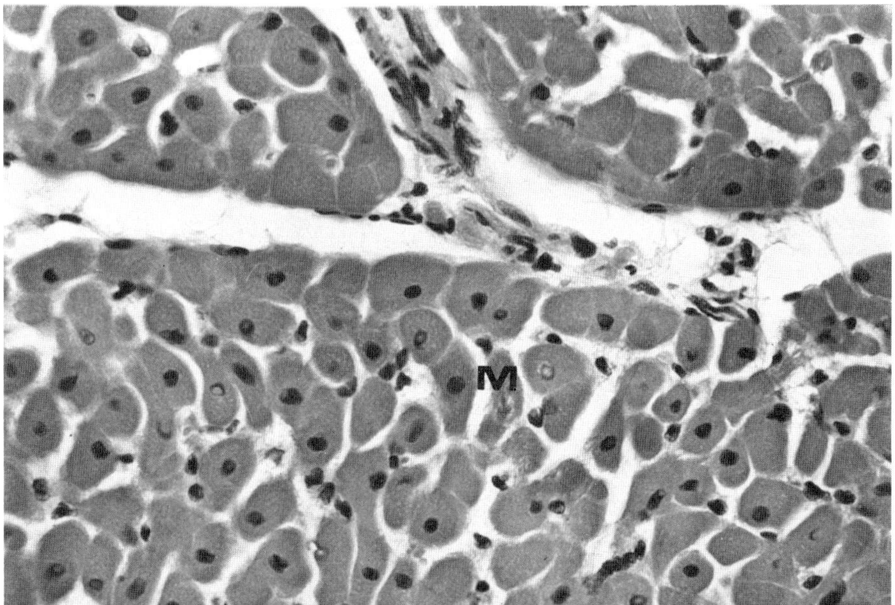

Fig. 13-15. Ventricular myocardium. The myocardium (*M*) consists primarily of cardiac muscle cells. ×100.

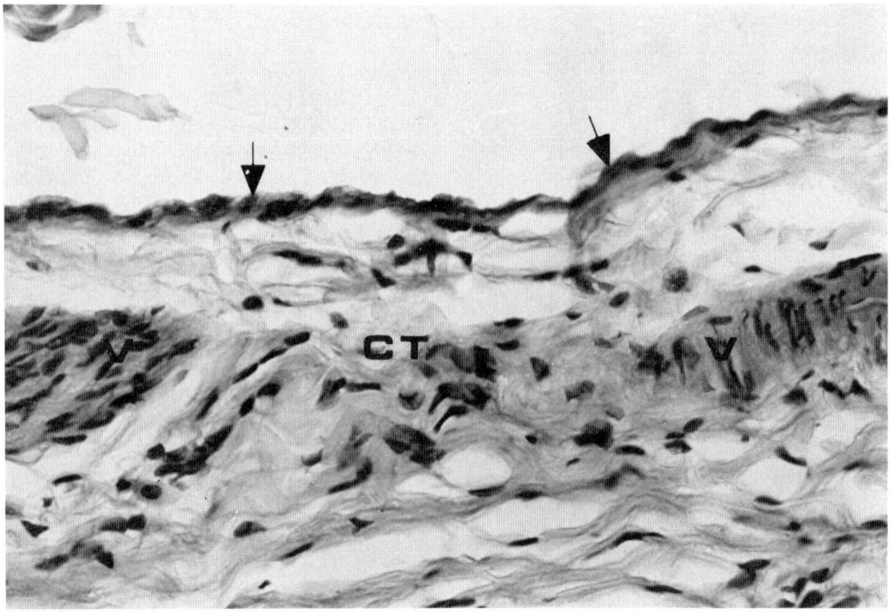

Fig. 13-16. Atrial epicardium. The mesothelial lining (*arrows*) resides upon a layer of connective tissue (*CT*). The smooth muscle is part of vessels (*V*) which have been sectioned obliquely. ×100.

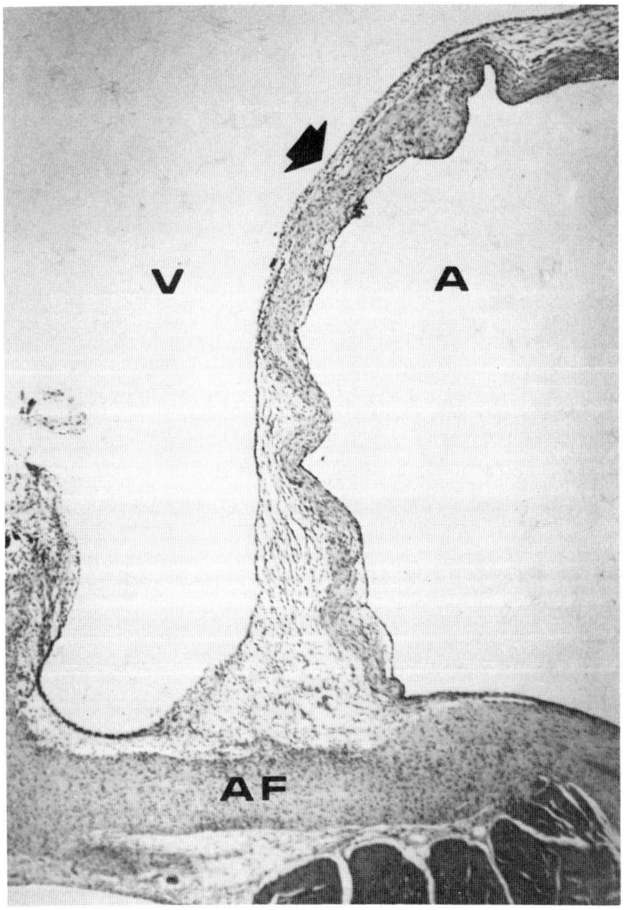

Fig. 13-17. Part of an atrioventricular valve. The valve (*arrow*) separates the ventricle (*V*) from the atrium (*A*). The connective tissue of the fibrous ring (*AF*) is continuous with the core of the valve. ×10.

Lymphatic Vessels

Capillaries and Larger Vessels. Lymph capillaries are very similar to continuous blood capillaries and are most difficult to distinguish from one another in section (Fig. 13-4). Three features generally may be used to make the distinction. Lymph capillaries are partially or completely devoid of a basement membrane. Their abluminal surfaces may have microvilli which anchor the vessel in the connective tissue space. Also, they are generally devoid of formed elements; however, agranulocytes may be encountered.

The larger vessels are not well-organized. Although the three mural regions may be present, they are not well-defined. Generally, the lymphatics have thinner walls than the veins of a corresponding size. Valves occur in lymph vessels of a smaller size than the corresponding appearance of valves in veins.

References

Vasculature

Ahmed, M. M.: The fine structure of endothelium in coronary arterioles. Acta Anat. *69*:327, 1968.

Bennet, H. S., Luft, J. H. and Hampton, J. C.: Morphological classification of vertebrate blood capillaries. Amer. J. Physiol. *196*:381, 1959.

Bruns, R. R. and Palade, G. E.: Studies on blood capillaries. I. General organization of blood capillaries in muscle. J. Cell Biol. *37*:244, 1968.

Fernando, N. V. P. and Movat, H. Z.: The capillaries. Exp. Molec. Pathol. *3*:87, 1964.

Hayes, J. R.: Histological changes in constricted arteries and arterioles. J. Anat. *101*:343, 1967.

Keech, M. K.: Electron microscope study of the normal rat aorta. J. Biophys. Biochem. Cytol. *7*:533, 1960.

Leak, L. V. and Burke, J. F.: Fine structure of the lymphatic capillary and the adjoining connective tissue area. Amer. J. Anat. *118*:785, 1966.

Rhodin, J. A. G.: Fine structure of vascular walls in mammals with special reference to smooth muscle component. Physiol. Rev. *42*:447, 1962.

Wood, J. E.: *The Veins: Normal and Abnormal Function*. Little, Brown, Boston, 1965.

Heart

Eckner, F. A. O., Brown, B. W., Overll, E. and Glagov, S.: Alterations of the gross dimensions of the heart and its structures by formalin fixation: A quantitative study. Virchow Arch. Path. Anat. *346*:318, 1969.

Ghidoni, J. J., Liotta, D. and Thomas, H.: Massive subendocardial damage accompanying prolonged ventricular fibrillation. Amer. J. Pathol. *56*:15, 1969.

James, T. N. and Sherf, L.: Ultrastructure of myocardial cells. Amer. J. Cardiol. *22*:389, 1968.

Merklin, R. J.: Position and orientation of the heart valves. Amer. J. Anat. *125*:375, 1969.

Mitomo, Y., Nakao, K. and Angrist, A: The fine structure of the heart valves in the chicken: I. Mitral valve. Amer. J. Anat. *125*:147, 1969.

Muir, A. R.: Observations on the fine structure of the Purkinje fibers in the ventricles of the sheep's heart. J. Anat. *91*:251, 1957.

Nabors, C. E. and Ball, C. R.: Spontaneous calcification in hearts of DBA mice. Anat. Rec. *164*:153, 1969.

Rhodin, J. A. G., Delmissier, P. and Reid, L. C.: The structure of the specialized conducting system of the steer heart. Circulation *24*:349, 1961.

14 Lymphatic System

General Characteristics

Form and Function. All of the basic tissues of the body are involved, directly or indirectly, in the composition of the lymphatic system. This system, in conjunction with the blood vascular system, comprises an important defensive system for the body, *a secondary defense system*. The primary defense system is in the skin and mucous membranes of the tubular organs of the body. The defensive aspects of this system are achieved by various methods: *production of defensive cells, aggregation of lymphatic tissue scattered throughout the body, transport of lymph via lymphatic vessels, filtration of lymph through lymph nodes* and *phagocytosis of materials during filtration.*

The filtration function is achieved by a variety of mechanisms:

1. Some lymphatic tissues remove foreign substances from the tissue fluid and immediate surroundings (tonsils and other scattered lymph nodules).
2. Some are designed to remove foreign substances from the lymphatic fluid (lymph nodes, hemolymph nodes).
3. Others remove substances from the blood (spleen, hemal nodes).

The phagocytic function is achieved through the activity of phagocytic cells that line sinusoids. These cells are integral parts of the *reticuloendothelial system.*

The tissues and organs of the lymphatic system may be grouped into morphologically distinct subdivisions accordingly:

1. Diffuse, unencapsulated lymphatic tissues (subepithelial lymphatic tissue associated with somatic orifices in the respiratory, digestive and urogenital tracts).
2. Dense, unencapsulated lymphatic tissue (subepithelial accumulations of lymphatic tissue associated with the respiratory, digestive and urogenital tracts).
3. Dense, encapsulated tissues scattered throughout the body (lymph nodes, spleen, hemal nodes, hemolymph nodes, thymus, bursa of Fabricius).

Organs of the Lymphatic System

Lymph Nodes. These organs are dense, encapsulated components of the system that are scattered throughout the body. Although their precise location is variable, they occur constantly in specific regions of the body. Lymph nodes are usually bean-shaped and vary in size from about 1 mm to several centimeters. The nodes, sometimes called glands, consist of a *capsule, stroma, cortex, medulla, nodules and hilus* (Fig. 14-1).

The capsule consists of dense white fibrous connective tissue (DWFCT) which is continuous with trabeculae of the same tissue. The latter subdivide the organ into smaller compartments. Smooth muscle and elastic fibers are rarely present as stromal components. The fine stromal elements of the organ are reticular fibers (Fig. 14-2).

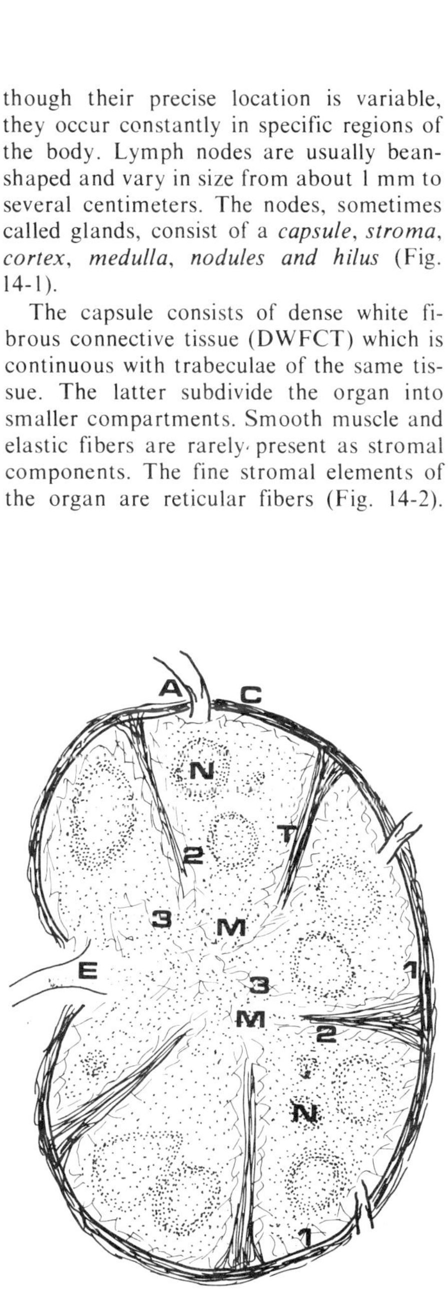

Fig. 14-1. Organization of a lymph node. *A*, afferent lymphatics; *C*, capsule; *T*, trabeculae; *N*, nodules; *M*, medullary cords; *E*, efferent lymphatics; *1*, subcapsular sinus; *2*, trabecular sinus; *3*, medullary sinus. All light micrographs are the original magnifications.

Two distinct regions of the organ are apparent, an outer *cortex* and an inner *medulla*. The cortex consists of nodules, trabeculae, fine stromal elements and lymph sinuses (Fig. 14-3). The *medulla* contains the same elements, but they are arranged differently. This lymphatic tissue is arranged as aggregates of cells in cords (*medullary cords*) which are separated by connective tissue and lymph sinuses (Fig. 14-4). The hilus is a connective tissue space which contains efferent or afferent lymphatic vessels. The connective tissue of the capsule is continuous with that of the hilus through the trabeculae.

An immunologically competent and active nodule (*secondary nodule*) consists of a *germinal center* and outer *corona* (Fig. 14-5). The *germinal center* contains lymphopoietic cells, plasma cells and their progenitors and lymphocytes. These centers are paler than the peripheral corona due to the presence of fewer cells as well as to their pale-staining characteristics. As lymphocytes are produced, they migrate peripherally to form the corona or *cortex of the nodule*. Following a period of activity, the germinal centers regress and the nodule returns to its original configuration as a *primary nodule* devoid of a germinal center. Immunologically incompetent animals do not possess germinal centers. Following antigenic insult, however, germinal centers appear.

The *medullary cords* contain accumulations of plasma cells and their progenitors, some lymphocytes and macrophages. In ideal preparations, these regions are clearly delimited by large medullary sinusoids.

Although the lymph nodes may be likened to a sponge, large spaces are present which clearly delineate the flow of lymph through the organ. *Afferent vessels* enter at the capsule and empty into a prominent *subcapsular* or *marginal sinusoid* which separates the capsule from the underlying cortical parenchyma. Percolation of lymph continues through the *cortical sinuses* and nodules into the *medullary sinusoids*. The latter are confluent with *efferent lymphatic vessels* at the hilus of the organ. Flow through a lymph node is unidirectional—capsule to hilus.

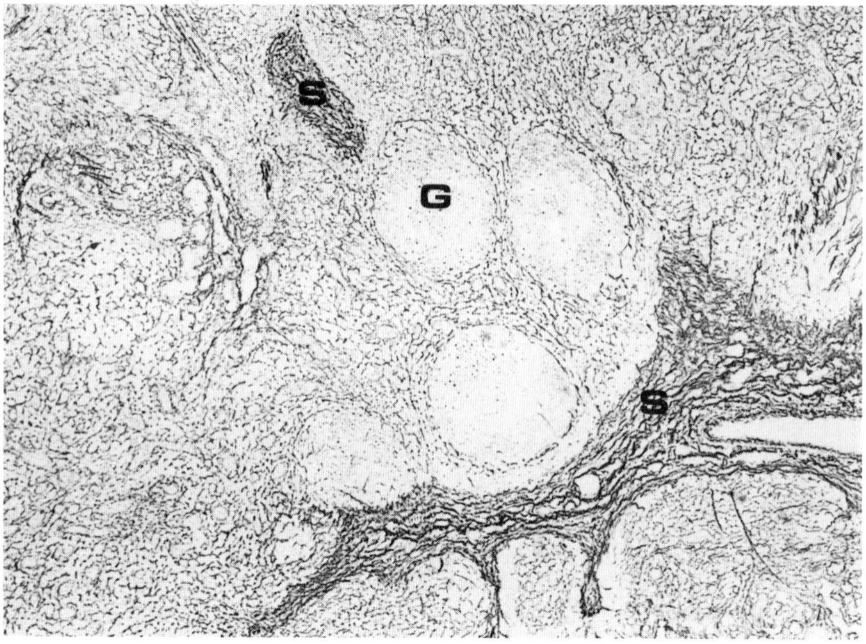

Fig. 14-2. Stromal elements of a lymph node. The stroma of the trabeculae (*S*) is composed of reticular and collagenous fibers, while other interstitial regions of the lymph node are composed of reticular fibers. The germinal center of the nodules (*G*) contains a minimal amount of these fibers. ×16 (reticular stain).

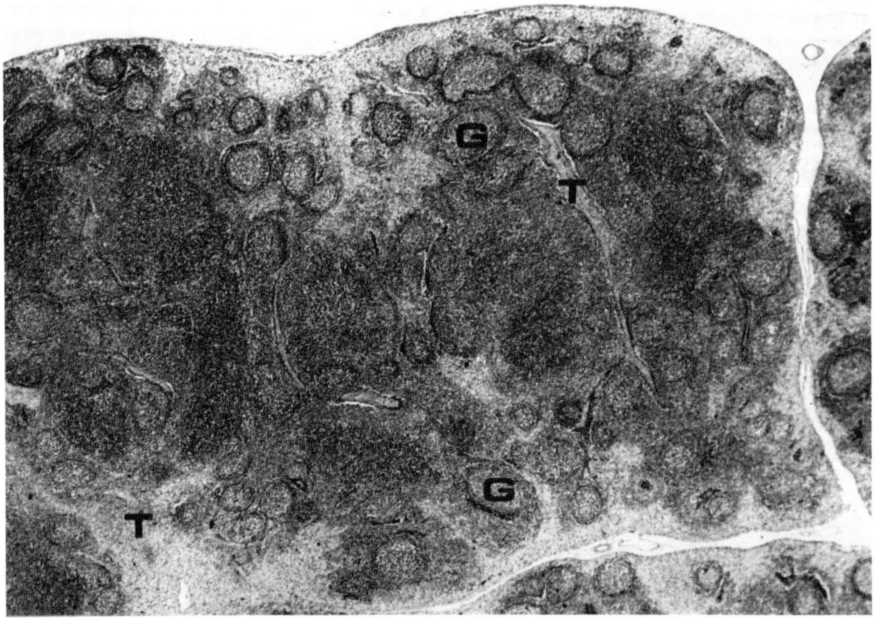

Fig. 14-3. An equine lymph node. The cortex consists of nodules with germinal centers (*G*), trabeculae (*T*) and lymphatic sinuses. ×4.

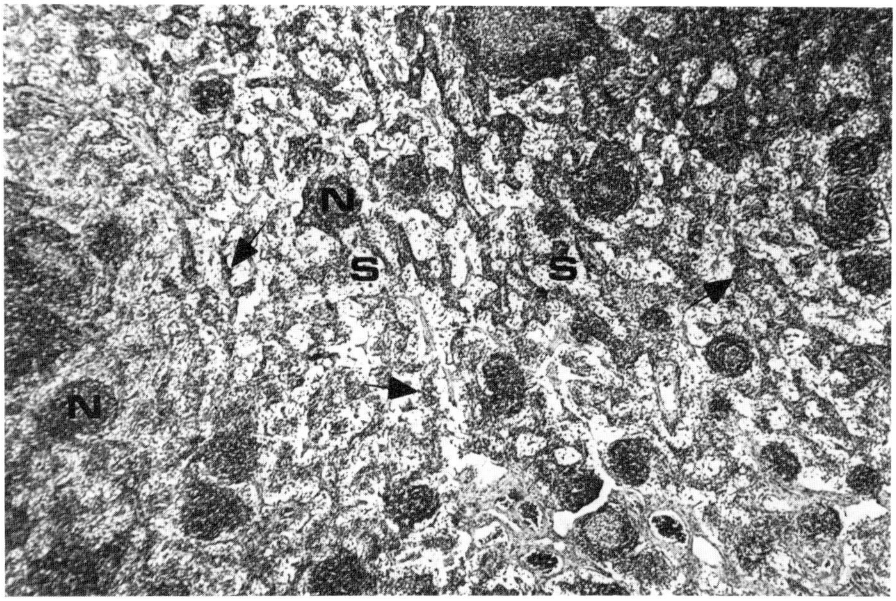

Fig. 14-4. The medulla of a canine lymph node. Nodules (*N*) are scattered throughout this region. The primary constituents, however, are lymphatic sinuses (*S*) and medullary cords (*arrows*). ×10.

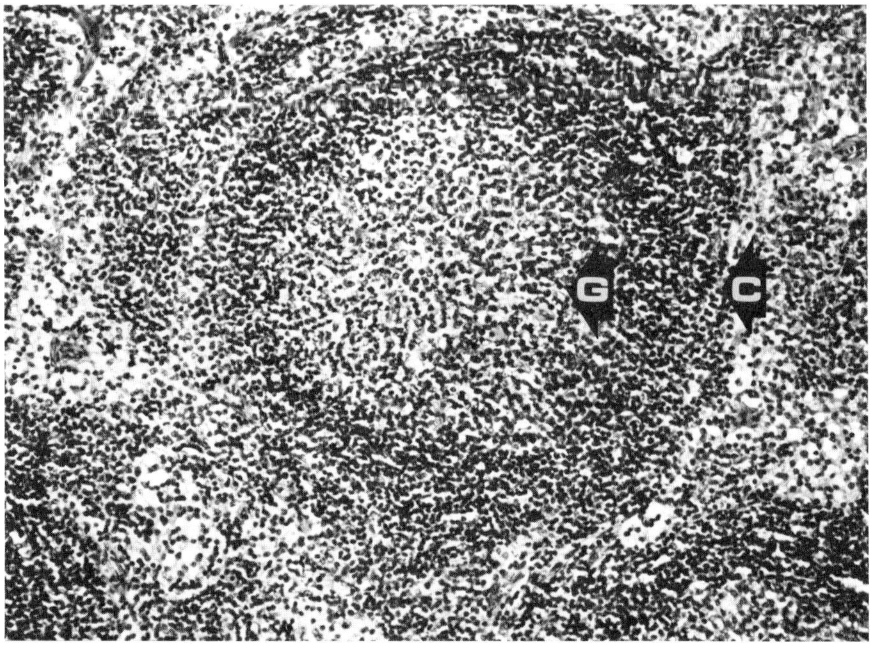

Fig. 14-5. A lymphatic nodule. The nodule consists of a central germinal center (*G*) and an outer corona (*C*). ×40.

Nutritive vascular supply and nerves enter and depart at the hilus.

The primary functions of lymph nodes are to *produce lymphocytes*, to *filter and phagocytose foreign materials* and to *produce antibodies*.

The porcine lymph node has the reverse pattern of that observed in other species (Fig. 14-6). Lymphatic nodules are located in the central or medullary regions of the organ, while the medullary cords and related aggregates of cells are located at the peripheral or cortical region. Flow of lymph, similarly, is the reverse of other domestic species; i.e., it enters at the hilus and emerges at the capsular area. Because of this particular arrangement, it is both tempting and probably most nearly correct to refer to the primary constituents as medullary nodules and cortical cords. Since most histologists are aware of this structural difference, as long as the species is specified it is unnecessary to reverse the terminology.

Important variations in lymph nodes occur in many species. In the horse, a fusion of cortical nodules is common. The ox possesses very large germinal centers. In swine, the nodules are inverted and extremely numerous. The age and physiological state of the organism appreciably alter the lymph node morphology in all species.

Hemal Nodes and Hemolymph Nodes. The sinusoids of *hemal nodes* are filled with blood rather than lymph (Fig. 14-7). Also, lymph vessels are not demonstrable. The capsule and trabeculae contain smooth muscle fibers. Otherwise, the organ looks much like a typical lymph node. These organs, however, have been described as miniature spleens.

Hemal nodes occur in ruminants in retroperitoneal positions along the vertebral column and in association with some of the visceral organs. They also occur in the jugular furrow.

Hemolymph nodes, as believed by some, are simply hemorrhagic lymph nodes. However, there is evidence that these are separate and distinct entities. These organs receive blood and lymph supplies that intermix in the sinusoids. Thus, they represent an intermediate form of lymphatic organ between the two aforementioned extremes.

These occur in the perirenal region of the sheep and goat and have been observed in the lumbar area of the ox.

Because of the significance of lymph nodes in diagnostic histopathology, it is important to be aware of the aforementioned variations. These, otherwise, may be mistaken for hemorrhagic lymph nodes.

Solitary Lymph Nodules. These accumulations of lymphatic tissue are scattered throughout the body. These solitary nodules, with prominent germinal centers, are associated with the digestive, respiratory and uro-

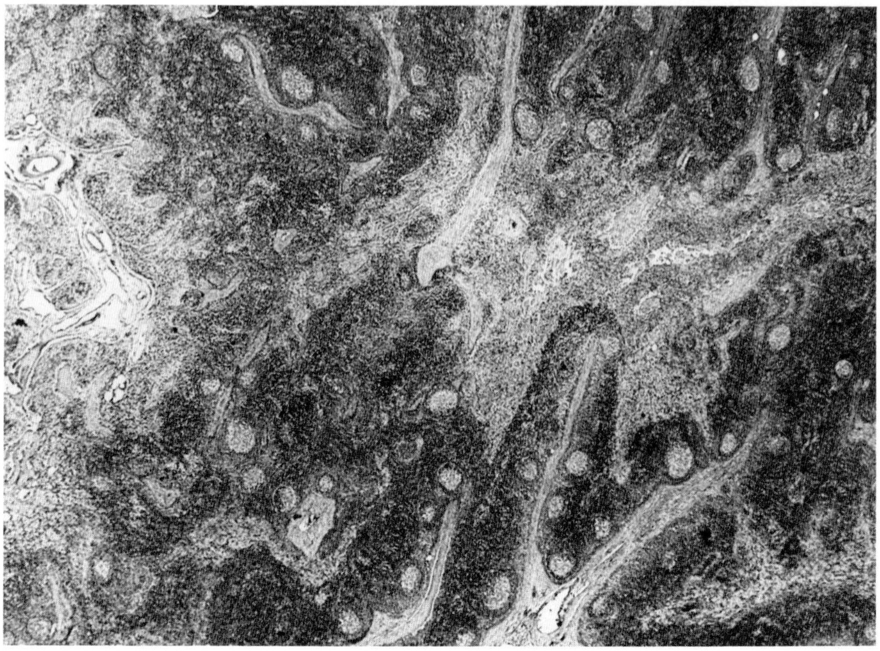

Fig. 14-6. A porcine lymph node. The organization of the lymph node is the reverse of that which occurs in other animals. ×10.

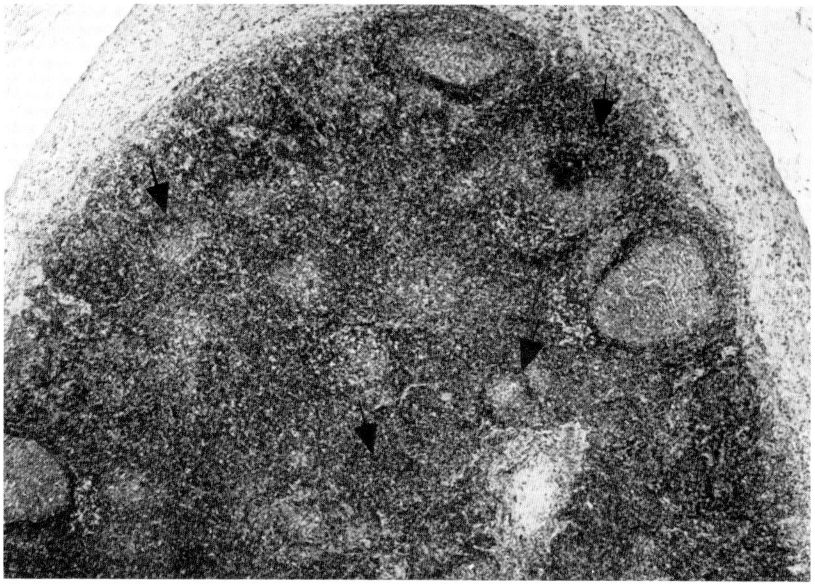

Fig. 14-7. A bovine hemal node. The organ is similar to a lymph node. Sinusoids (*arrows*), however, are engorged with blood. ×10.

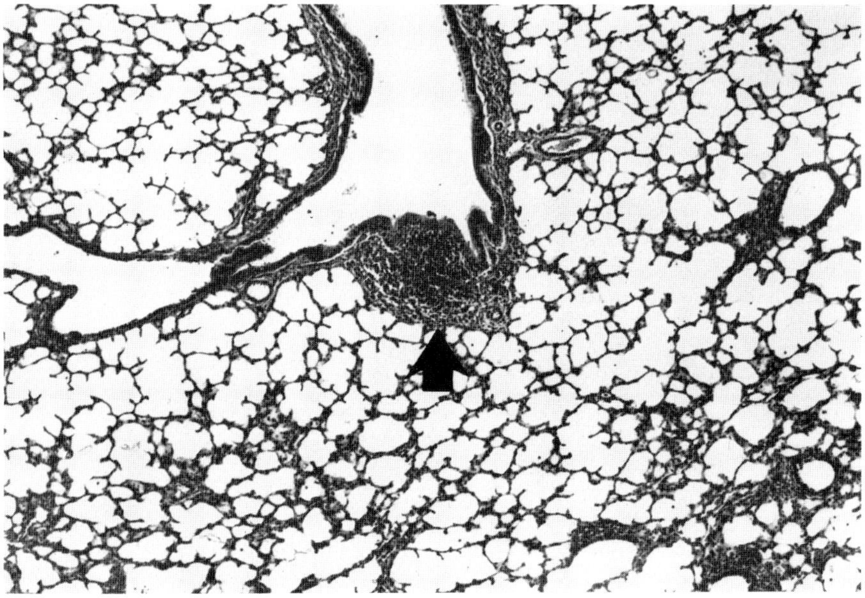

Fig. 14-8. Lymph nodule in the lung. The lymph nodule (*arrow*) is closely associated with a bronchiole. ×16.

genital tracts (Fig. 14-8). The lymphocytes from the corona migrate into the surrounding lamina propria mucosae. These solitary nodules are not intercalated into the lymphatic drainage by specific efferent vessels but are surrounded by vessels that function similarly. Some of these nodules may be encapsulated. They occur in the lamina propria mucosae, tunica submucosa and occasionally in the tunica adventitia.

Aggregated Lymph Nodules. Accumulations of lymph nodules are encountered in scattered foci throughout the soma (Fig. 14-9). In some instances the nodules are quite large and may even become confluent. The Peyer's patches of the intestinal wall are a good example of these. Often, aggregated lymph nodules are referred to as tonsils, in which case Peyer's patches may be considered "intestinal tonsils."

Tonsils. Tonsils are formed of solitary or aggregated nodules and diffuse lymphatic tissue (Fig. 14-10). They form a "pharyngeal ring" along the tract from the mouth to the pharynx in the lamina propria mucosae in close association with the epithelial lining. They are basically accumulations of dense, encapsulated lymphatic tissue similar to the nodules of lymph nodes. The germinal centers are large, the cortices are dense and there is extensive infiltration of lymphocytes into the surrounding connective tissue and associated epithelium.

Although all tonsils are similar, there are two distinguishable groups that are defined on the basis of tonsillar tissue relationships

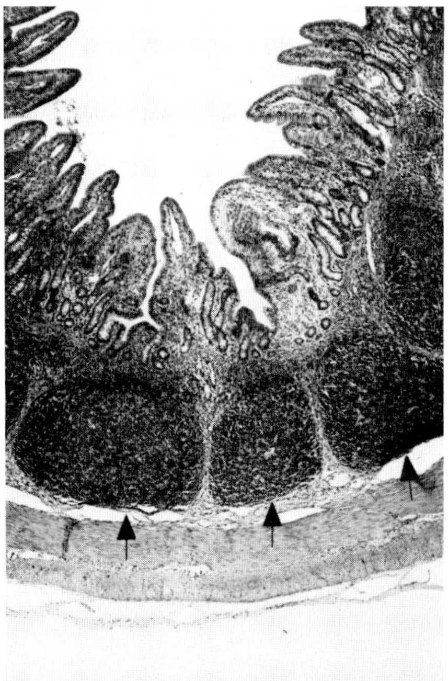

Fig. 14-9. Peyer's patches in the wall of the ileum. The Peyer's patches (*arrows*) are examples of aggregated lymph nodules. ×8.

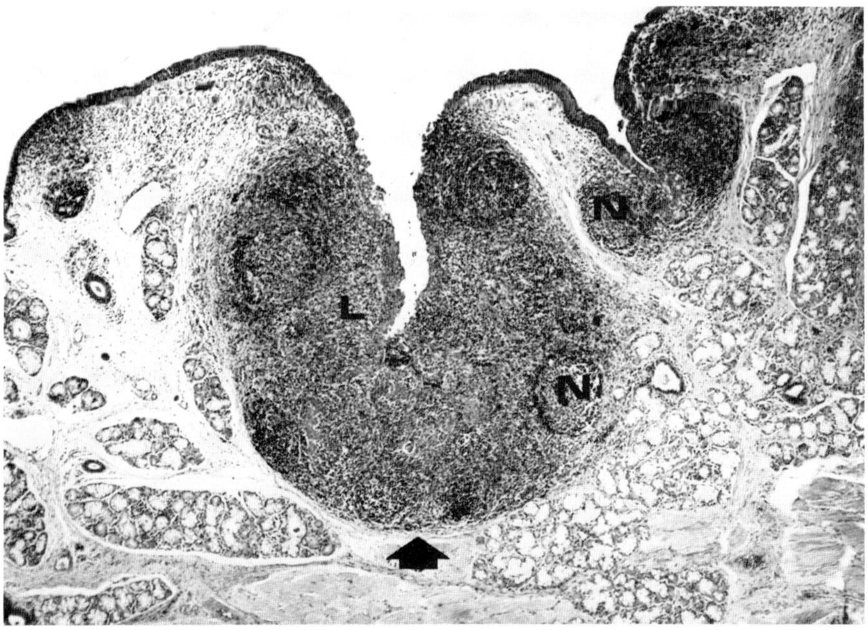

Fig. 14-10. A tonsil without crypts. The tonsil (*arrow*) is composed of nodular (*N*) and loose lymphatic (*L*) tissue. The tunica mucosa is slightly folded. Extensive lymphocytic infiltration into the lamina propria and lamina epithelialis is apparent. ×10.

with the surface epithelium with which they are associated. These are *tonsils with crypts* and *tonsils without crypts*. The *crypt* is a blind and sometimes branched invagination of the surface epithelium. A crypt and the associated lymphatic tissue is referred to as a *tonsillar follicle* (Fig. 14-11). A group of follicles constitutes a tonsil of this type. A *tonsil without crypts* is formed by a single lamina of lymphatic tissue which may be secondarily bulged outward or slightly folded to increase surface area (Fig. 14-10).

The invaginations of the tunica mucosa are significant because they serve as foci of infection and corresponding inflammatory processes.

The morphological features and specific sites of tonsillar tissue vary among domestic species.

1. Tonsils with crypts (follicular tonsils): palatine tonsils in man, horse, ruminant, swine; lingual tonsils in man, horse, ruminant, swine; tubal tonsils in swine; paraepiglottic tonsils in sheep, goat, swine.
2. Tonsils without crypts: palatine tonsils in carnivores; pharyngeal tonsils in all domestic animals except carnivores; tubal tonsils in ruminants.

Tonsils do not possess afferent lymphatic channels. Rather, material is either filtered into the organ or carried to it by cells from the surrounding connective tissue space. Efferent lymphatic channels exist.

Avian Lymphatic Tissue. Most avian species do not possess lymph nodes, with the exception of swamp, sea and shore birds. Solitary accumulations of lymphatic tissue as nodules characterize the walls of the digestive tract, serous membranes and skin (Fig. 14-12).

Spleen. The spleen is related to other blood-forming organs and is the largest mass of lymphatic tissue in the body (Fig. 14-13). Despite its size and multiplicity of function, it is not essential for life. Among its numerous functions are *blood cell formation, hemoglobin and iron metabolism, red blood cell destruction, blood filtration, blood storage* and *phagocytosis*.

The capsule of the organ is covered by a thin layer of mesothelium. The associated connective tissue of this serous membrane blends with the DWFCT of the capsule. In a manner similar to that of lymph nodes, trabeculae of DWFCT extend into the parenchyma and effectively subdivide it into smaller compartments (Fig. 14-14). Smooth muscle fibers and elastic fibers are important structural components of the capsule and trabeculae of this organ (Fig. 14-15). These are continuous with the primary stromal elements, the reticular fibers. The arrangement of the capsular and trabecular smooth muscle is species variable. These components allow for large volume changes, whereas the smooth muscle fibers empty the organ of its blood.

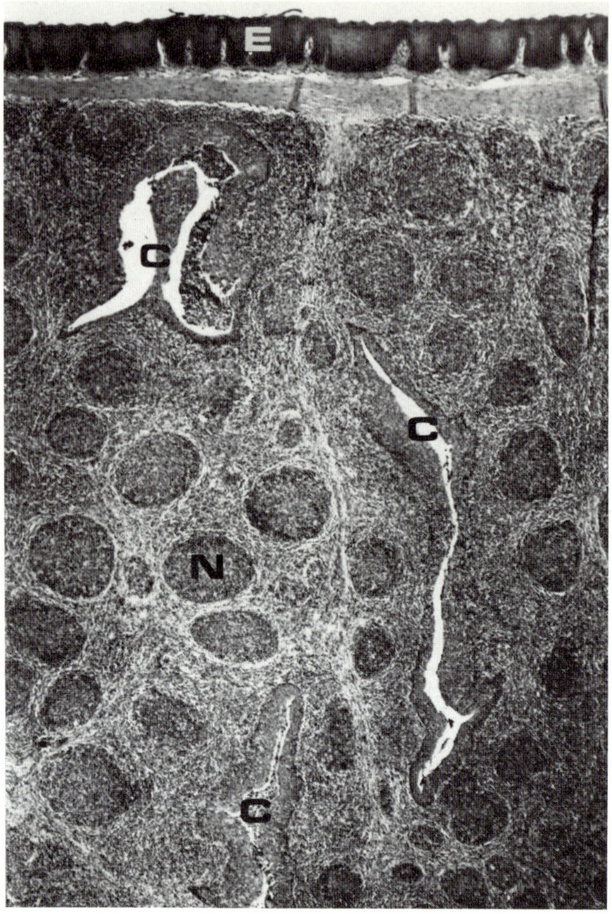

Fig. 14-11. A tonsil with crypts. Nodular (*N*) and loose lymphatic tissue are the primary components. The lamina epithelialis mucosae (*E*) is highly folded and forms extensive crypts (*C*). ×10.

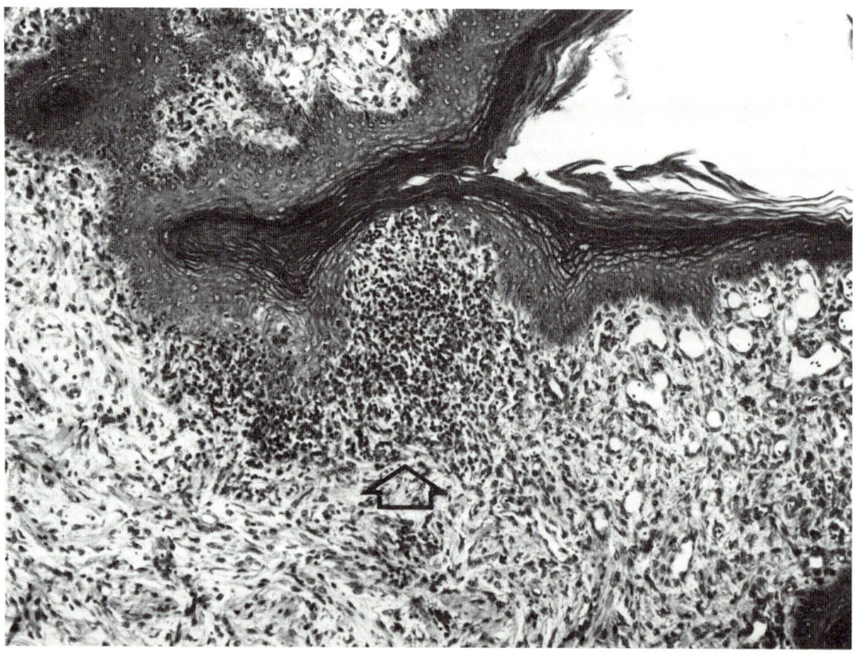

Fig. 14-12. The comb of a bird. The dermis contains a lymphatic nodule (*arrow*) and loose lymphatic tissue. ×40.

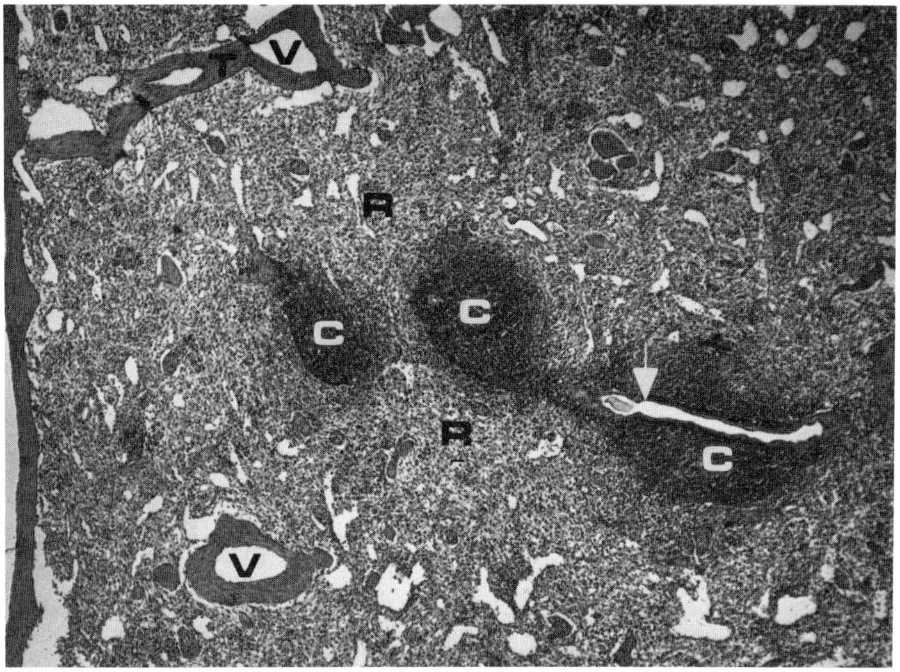

Fig. 14-13. General organization of the spleen. Trabeculae (*T*) invaginate into the parenchyma from the capsule. They contain arteries and veins (*V*). The parenchyma consists of splenic corpuscles (*C*) which contain nodular arterioles (*arrow*). The corpuscles are surrounded by red pulp (*R*). ×10.

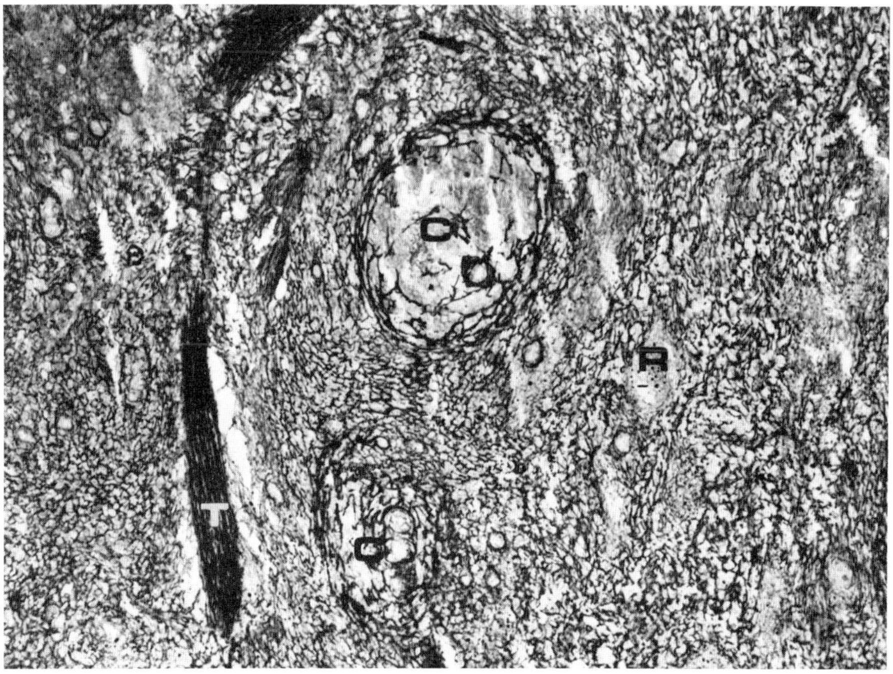

Fig. 14-14. Stromal elements of the spleen. The trabeculae (*T*) consist of DWFCT while the remaining stroma is reticular fibers. Splenic corpuscles (*C*) are delineated by the red pulp (*R*). ×40 (reticular stain).

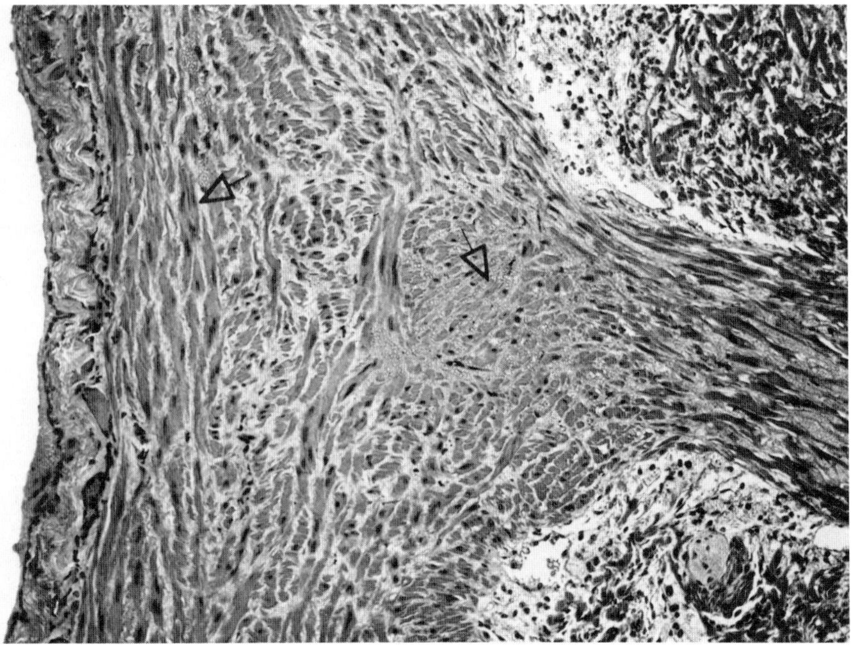

Fig. 14-15. Smooth muscle of the capsule and trabeculae of the spleen of a deer. The smooth muscle (*arrows*) is a prominent feature of this spleen. ×40.

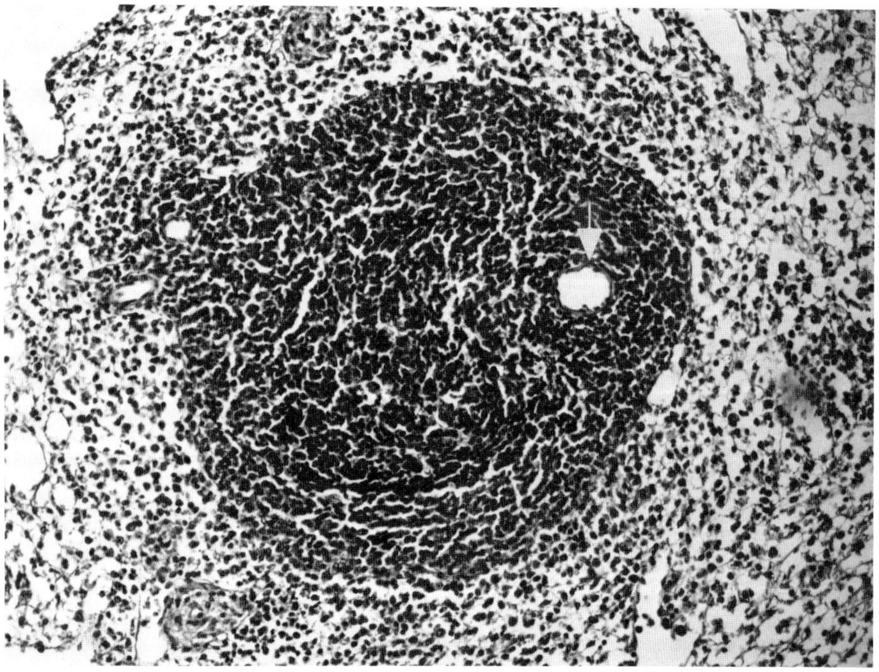

Fig. 14-16. A splenic corpuscle. This nodule contains a nodular arteriole (*arrow*) in a paracentral position. ×40.

Blood vessels enter the spleen proper by following trabecular pathways. Because of the nature of the mural elements and the trabeculae, it is very difficult to define clearly the typical mural divisions as outlined previously. A prominent hilar region of DWFCT extends along the length of the organ. Nerves and vessels enter and leave in this region. Efferent lymphatic vessels occur in the capsule, hilus and trabeculae.

Like other lymphatic organs the spleen is a mixture of phagocytic sinusoids, reticular fiber stroma and a very cellular parenchyma. There is, however, no distinct cortex or medulla. The parenchyma consists of two distinct regions which are arranged in a random pattern. These regions are termed the *white pulp* and *red pulp*. Lymph nodules (*splenic corpuscles*) comprise the white pulp (Figs. 14-13, 14-14). However, careful examination will reveal the presence of an arteriole, mistakenly called the *central artery*, which occupies a central or paracentral position. It is sometimes referred to as the *nodular arteriole* (Fig. 14-16). It is not observed in all sections because the plane of section may parallel its course. The presence of nodules is dependent upon the same factors that influence germinal center development or regression in lymph nodes. The cellular constituents of these nodules are the same as those of lymph nodes.

The areas between the splenic corpuscles and trabeculae are the areas of the red pulp, so named because of the extensive vascularity. The red pulp consists of splenic sinusoids and splenic cords (Fig. 14-17). The splenic sinusoids are discontinuous and are lined by phagocytic reticular cells. These sinusoids open into the splenic cords. The cords are composed of granulocytes, granulocyte progenitors, primitive reticular cells and phagocytic reticular cells. In some species smooth muscle fibers also occur (Figs. 14-18, 14-19). The sinusoids and cords are an integral filtration and phagocytic unit with many fixed and wandering macrophages. These phagocytic cells, of course, are responsible for the removal of cellular detritus and foreign substances from the blood. A yellow-brown pigment, *hemosiderin* (a breakdown product of hemoglobin), is usually present in the phagocytic cells of the sinusoids and cords (Fig. 14-20).

An understanding of the circulatory pattern through the spleen is essential for a general comprehension of its function (Fig. 14-21). *Splenic arteries* enter at the hilus and divide into *trabecular arteries*. These arteries leave the trabeculae and enter the splenic parenchyma. Upon entering the parenchyma lymphocytes accumulate in the adventitia of the vessels. This sheath of lymphocytes progressively increases to the magnitude of a splenic corpuscle. The ves-

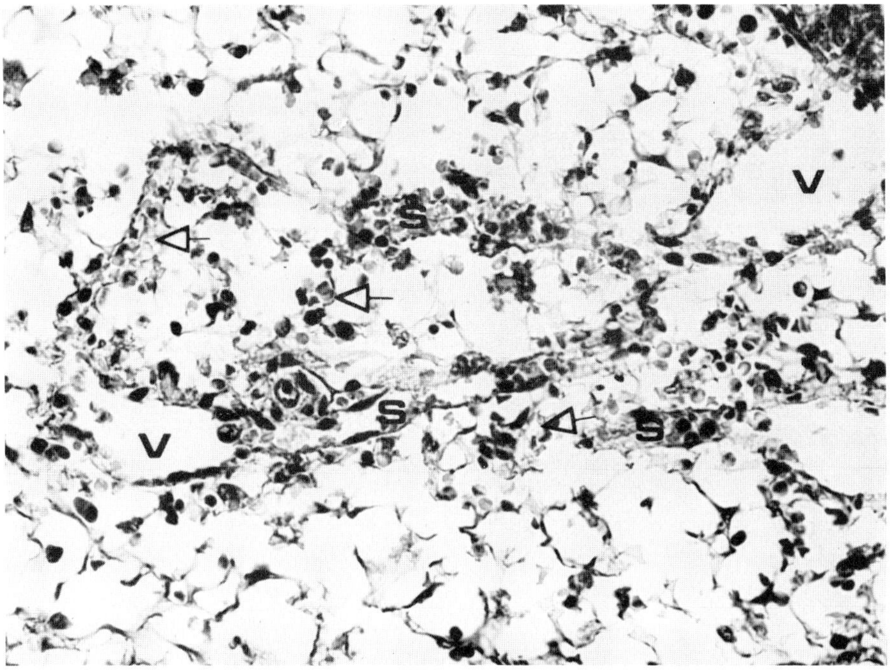

Fig. 14-17. Red pulp of the spleen. The red pulp consists of splenic sinusoids (*S*), splenic cords (*arrows*) and venous sinuses (*V*). ×100.

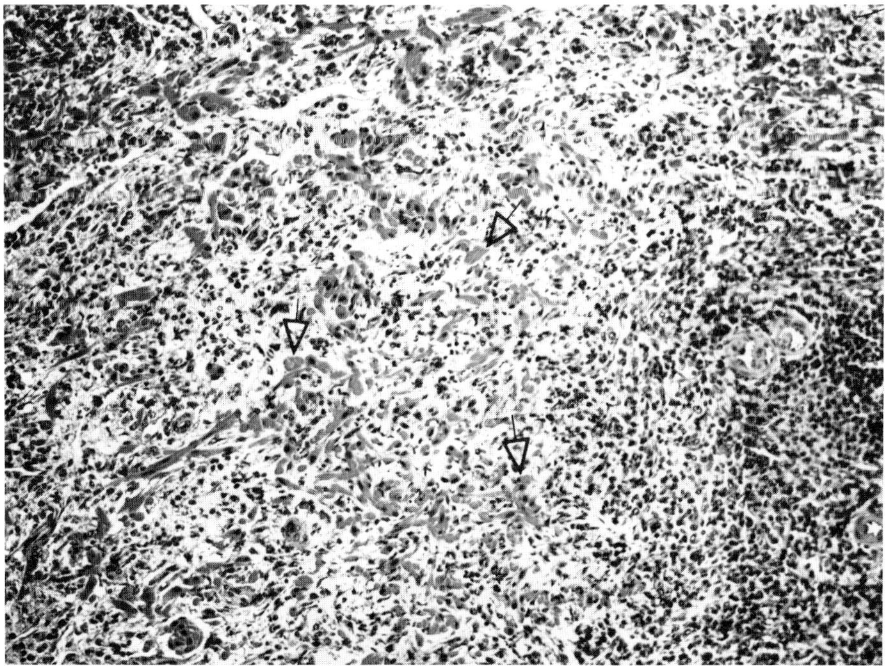

Fig. 14-18. Red pulp of a deer spleen. The smooth muscle fibers (*arrows*) are prominent features of this organ. ×40.

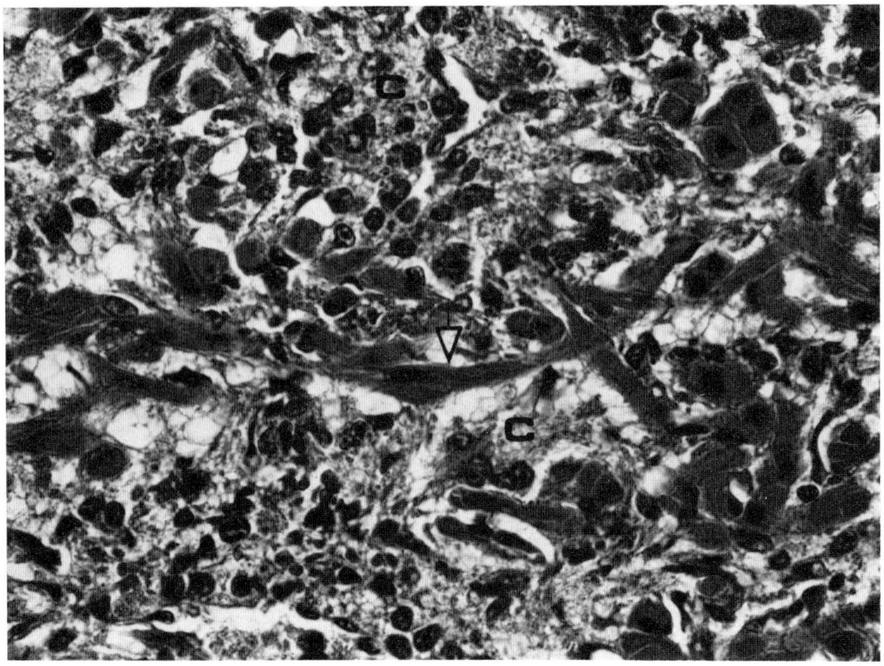

Fig. 14-19. Red pulp of a deer spleen. The smooth muscle fibers (*arrows*) and splenic cords (*C*) are well-defined. ×100.

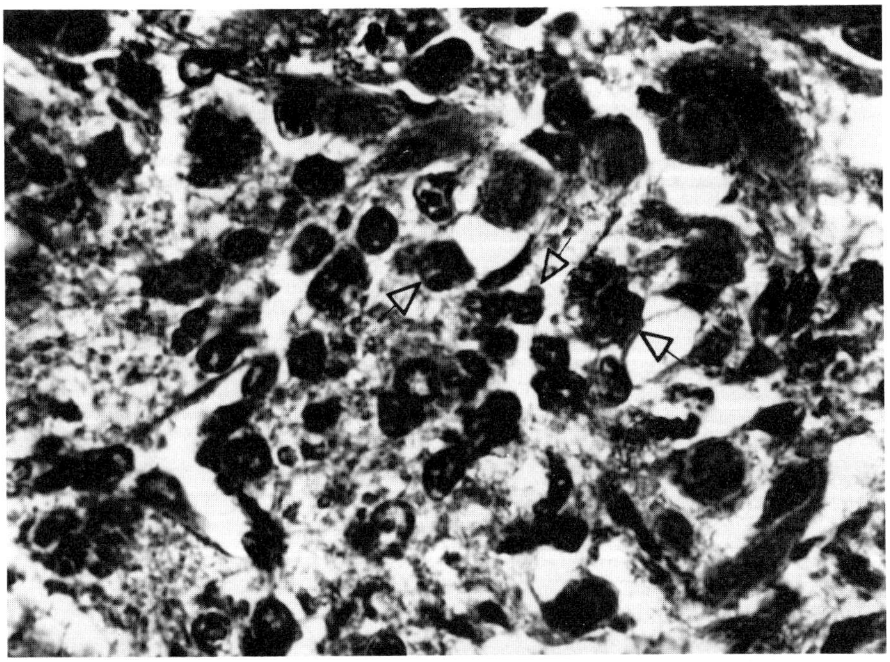

Fig. 14-20. Phagocytic cells of the splenic sinusoids and splenic cords. The phagocytes (*arrows*) contain large quantities of hemosiderin. ×320.

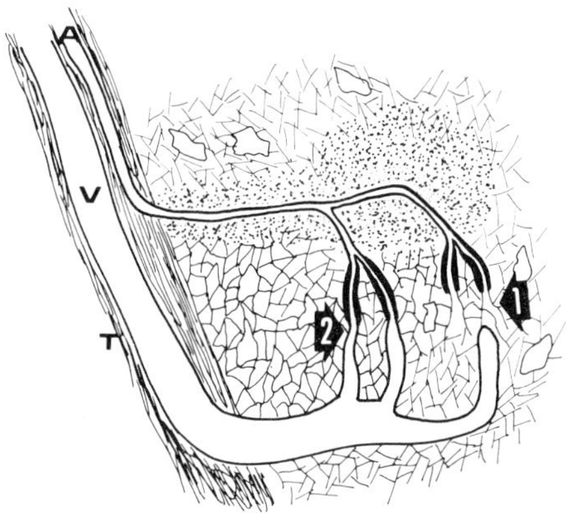

Fig. 14-21. Splenic circulation. The blood may pass from the terminal arterial capillaries into the red pulp and then into the venous sinuses (*1*) or it may pass directly from the arterial capillaries into the venous sinuses (*2*). An artery (*A*) and a vein (*V*) are indicated within a trabeculum (*T*). (Redrawn and modified from Ham, A. W.: *Histology*, Lippincott, Philadelphia, 1969.)

sel is then referred to as the *nodular arteriole*. Branches from this vessel supply capillaries in the white pulp and marginal region of the white pulp. They empty into the *red pulp sinuses* or into *pulp veins*. The nodular arteriole emerges from the white pulp and divides into several smaller branches, the *penicillar arterioles*. The penicillar arterioles are divisible into three regions: *red pulp arterioles*, *sheathed arterioles* and *terminal arterial capillaries*. The sheathed arterioles are branches of the red pulp arterioles and have thickened walls (*sheath of Schweigger-Seidel*), composed of concentric laminae of reticular cells and reticular fibers (Fig. 14-22). The termination of the arterial capillaries is a subject of much controversy. In the *closed theory*, the blood from the terminal arterial capillaries opens directly into the venous sinuses. This presumably occurs in man, rat and dog. In the *open theory*, the arterial capillaries terminate in the open reticulum of the red pulp and filter into the venous sinuses. This is supposedly characteristic of the mouse, cat, horse, ox and swine. Some authors claim that both methods are utilized, while others claim that the circulation may change between both extremes. The question is academic: both methods achieve blood filtration.

Two basic types of spleens have been described, *defensive* and *storage* types. The first type has few trabeculae and muscle fibers but abundant lymphatic tissue (lagomorphs, man). The storage type has many trabeculae and smooth muscle fibers. It is relatively large and has less white pulp than the other form (horse, dog, cat). Intermediate forms are typical of ruminants and swine. Although red blood corpuscular destruction is typical of all spleens, it is especially well demonstrated in horses and swine.

Thymus. Because of embryological origin, the thymus may be more closely related to the endocrine system than the lymphatic system. There is evidence that the thymus elaborates a humoral factor which is involved in immunological competency. The thymus is responsible for lymphocytopoiesis during early postnatal life and lymphocytes of thymic origin populate other lymphatic organs (*peripheralization*). The thymus is active until the age of puberty at which time involution begins and continues through old age. The bulk of evidence in support of the immunological role of this organ justifies its being included with the lymphatic system.

Both lobes of the organ are covered by a capsule of DWFCT from which septa of similar tissue arise and subdivide the organ into lobules (Fig. 14-23). These septa extend to the corticomedullary junction. The incomplete septation results in the lobules being continuous with each other. In some sections, however, some lobules will appear to be completely encased by the capsular

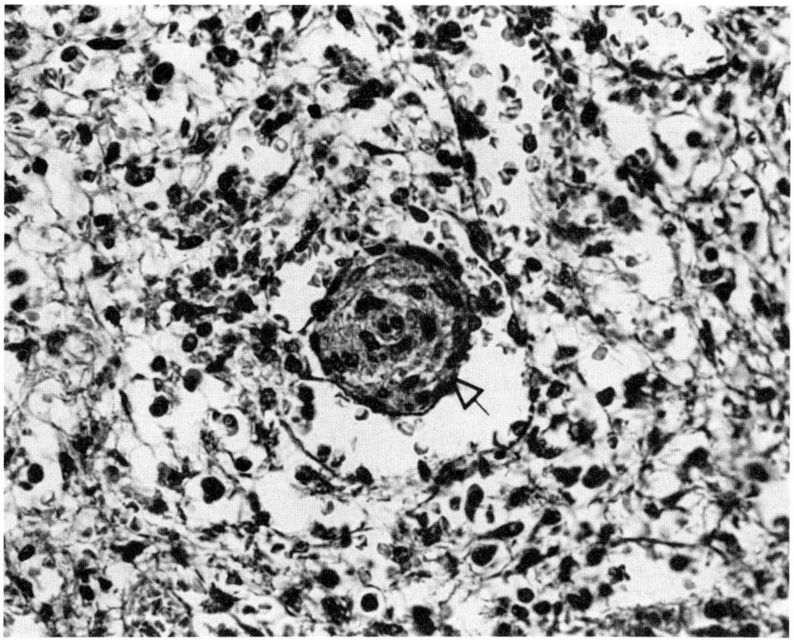

Fig. 14-22. A sheathed arteriole from the splenic red pulp. The sheathed arteriole (*arrow*) is surrounded by concentric whorls of reticular cells and fibers. ×100.

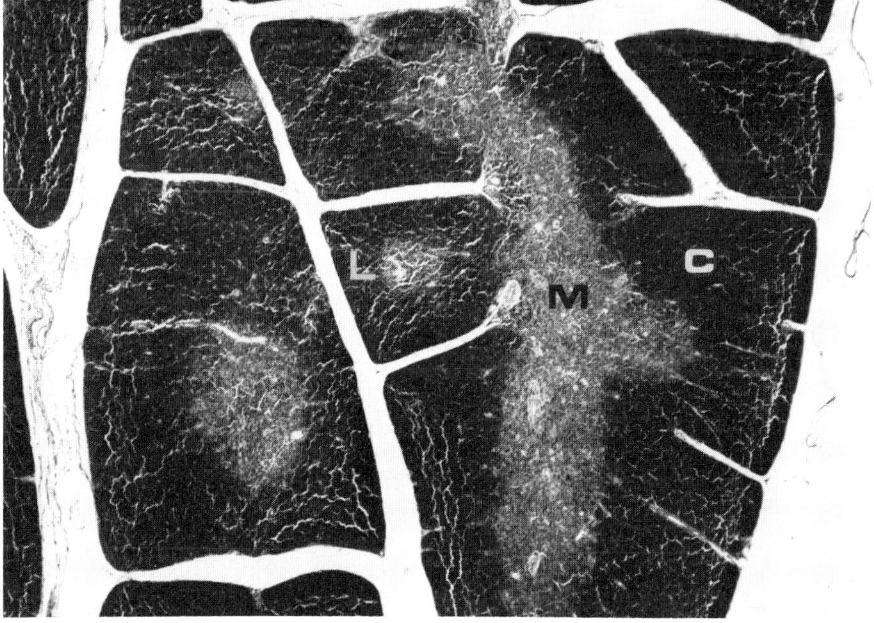

Fig. 14-23. The thymus gland. The connective tissue capsule subdivides the organ into lobules (*L*). The cortex (*C*) and medulla (*M*) are clearly defined. There are no lymph nodules. The organ may be considered to be one large nodule. ×10.

and septal tissue. Reticular connective tissue comprises the bulk of the stroma.

The organ is composed of a distinct *cortex* and *medulla* (Fig. 14-23). Lymph nodules do not occur. The *cortex* consists of dense accumulations of small lymphocytes (*thymocytes*) which obliterate the reticular cells and reticular fiber stroma. Endodermally derived reticular cells are intercalated between the blood capillaries and the cortical parenchyma. These *epithelial-reticular cells* contribute to the blood-thymus barrier.

The *medulla* of the organ consists of a similar cellular and fibrous stroma as the cortex (Fig. 14-24). The thymocytes of this region are not as dense; thus, the reticular cells are readily observed. The definitive feature of the organ, however, is the presence of *thymic corpuscles* (*Hassall's corpuscles*) which occur in the medulla (Fig. 14-25). These acidophilic bodies vary in diameter from 20 μm to more than 100 μm. They are concentric whorls of cells (probably reticular cells) in various stages of degenerative change. The hyaline-appearing cells can undergo keratinization and even mineralization. Pyknosis and karyolysis are common. They are often observed in advanced stages of involution. The peripherally located reticular cells of the bodies are continuous with the cellular stroma. Despite their being rich in gamma globulins, their exact role in immunity is unknown.

Involution of the thymus is characterized by a reduction and eventual loss of the cortex. Eventually, the cortex and medulla are indistinguishable from each other. This is accompanied by a vascular and connective tissue invasion. Much adipose tissue is also apparent. The entire organ is eventually replaced by connective tissue.

Bursa of Fabricius. This structure is characteristic of birds (Fig. 14-26). It is a blind sac which opens on the dorsal wall of the proctodeum. It is often referred to as the "*cloacal tonsil*" or "*cloacal thymus*." The wall of the organ is extensively folded and covered by a simple columnar or pseudostratified columnar epithelium. Lymphatic nodules are located between the folds of the epithelium and seem to produce follicle-like structures. Germinal centers are present. These are referred to as medullary structures, while the darker coronal regions are referred to as cortical areas. This organ resembles tonsils and the thymus, but it seems to function in a manner similar to that of the thymus.

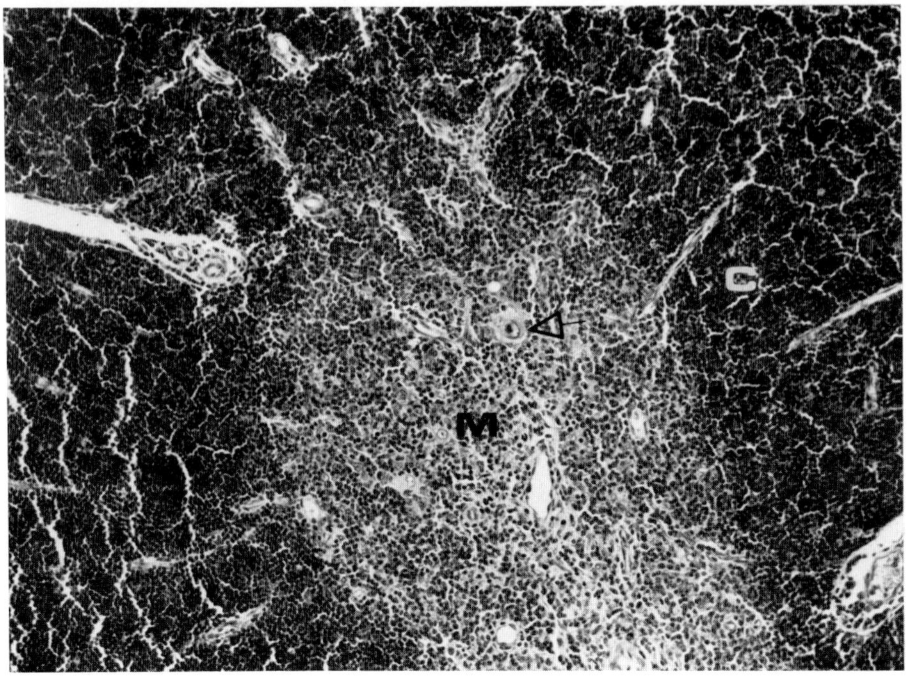

Fig. 14-24. The cortex and medulla of the thymus gland. The cortex (*C*) contains more dense aggregations of thymocytes than does the medulla (*M*). A characteristic thymic corpuscle (*arrow*) is present. ×40.

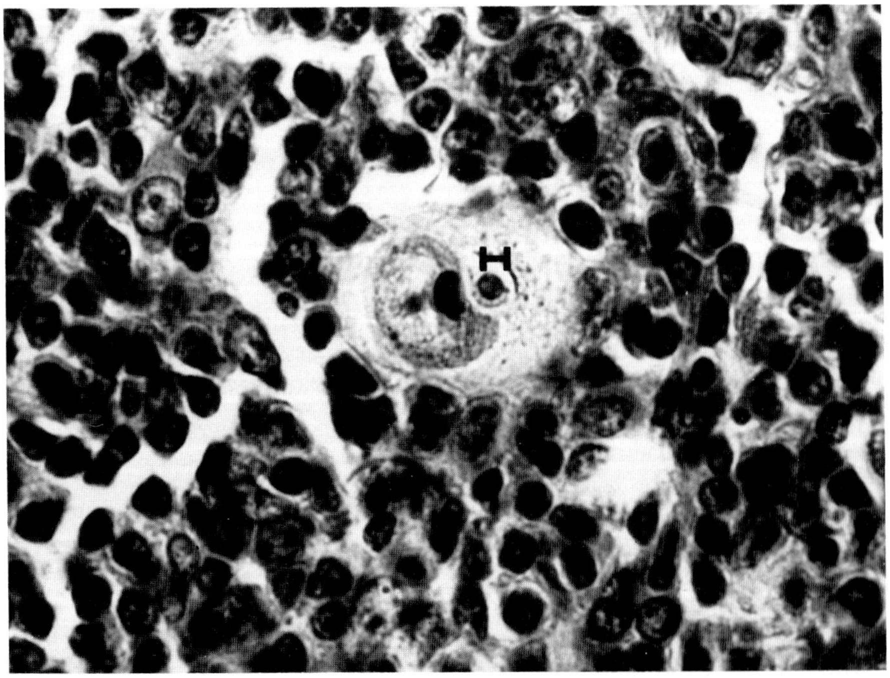

Fig. 14-25. A thymic corpuscle. The thymic or Hassall's corpuscle (*H*) is a morphological feature of the medullary portion of this organ. ×320.

References

Clark, S. L., Jr.: The reticulum of lymph nodes in mice studied with the electron microscope. Amer. J. Anat. *110*:217, 1962.

Edwards, V. D. and Simon, G. T.: Ultrastructural aspects of red cell destruction in the normal rat spleen. J. Ultrastruct. Res. *33*:187, 1970.

Fujisaki, S.: The fine structure of Hassall's corpuscles and reticular cells in the mouse thymus. Acta Med. Biol. *14*:107, 1966.

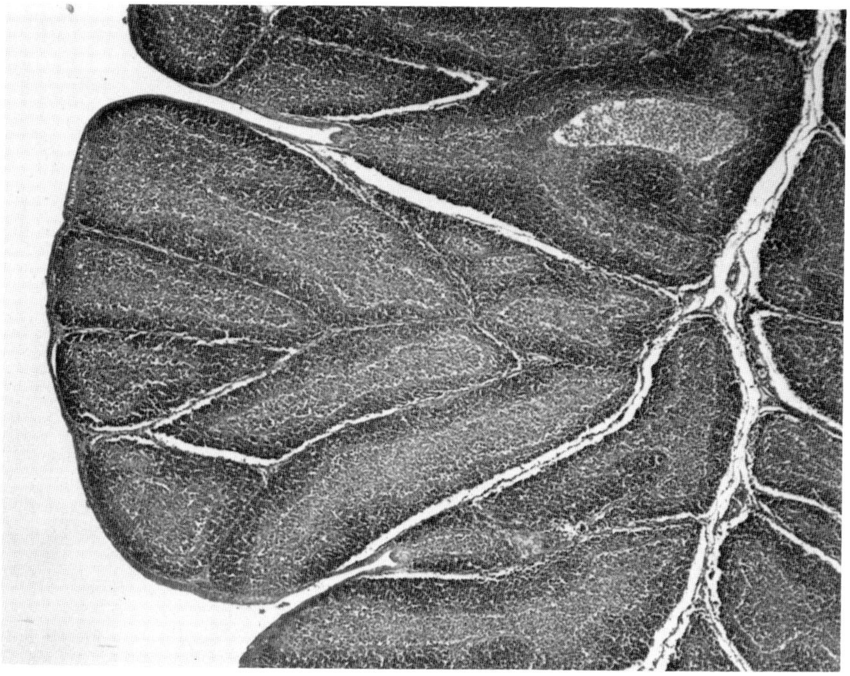

Fig. 14-26. The avian bursa of Fabricius. Lymphatic nodules are aggregated in such a way as to impart the appearance of the thymus gland. ×10.

Hoshino, T., Takeda, M., Abe, K. and Ito, T.: Early development of thymic lymphocytes in mice, studied by light and electron microscopy. Anat. Rec. *164:* 47, 1969.

Jaroslow, B. N.: Genesis of Hassall's corpuscles. Nature *215:*408, 1967.

Levin, P. M.: The development of the tonsil of the domestic pig. Anat. Rec. *45:*189, 1930.

Meyer, A.: Hemal nodes in bovines and goats. Amer. J. Anat. *21:*359, 1917.

Moe, R. E.: Electron microscopic appearance of the parenchyma of lymph nodes. Amer. J. Anat. *114:* 341, 1964.

Movat, H. Z. and Fernando, N. V. P.: The fine structure of the lymphoid tissue during antibody formation. Exp. Molec. Pathol. *4:*155, 1965.

Murray, R. G., Murray, A. and Pizzo, A.: The fine structure of the thymocytes of young rats. Anat. Rec. *151:*17, 1965.

Payne, F. and Breneman, W. R.: Lymphoid areas in endocrine glands in the fowl. Poult. Sci. *31:*155, 1952.

Peck, H. M. and Hoerr, N. L.: The intermediary circulation in the red pulp of the mouse spleen. Anat. Rec. *109:*447, 1951.

Roberts, D. K. and Latta, J. S.: Electron microscopic studies on the red pulp of the mouse spleen. Anat. Rec. *148:*81, 1964.

Tehver, J. and Grahame, I.: Capsule and trabeculae of spleens of domestic mammals. J. Anat. *65:*473, 1931.

Yamori, T. and Mori, Y.: Electron microscopic observation of reticuloendothelial system. Tohoku J. Exp. Med. *81:*330, 1964.

15 Hematopoiesis

General Characteristics

Form and Function. The replacement of all cells, as has been presented previously (Chapter 1), is predicated upon the occurrence of stem cells associated with the various tissues. Blood cell replacement is achieved through the activities of stem cells that are confined to specific areas. These areas of *hematopoiesis* differ in the prenatal, postnatal and adult animal. During early prenatal development, hematopoiesis begins in the blood islands associated with the yolk sac endoderm. It becomes widespread in the fetus and includes mesenchyme and blood vessels, liver, spleen, thymus, lymph nodes and bone marrow. Postnatal formation of erythrocytes, granulocytes and platelets is confined primarily to the red bone marrow. The spleen also is involved to a lesser degree in erythropoiesis. A progressive reduction in red bone marrow occurs throughout adolescence and hematopoietic activity is confined to the marrow cavities of the sternebrae, ribs, vertebrae and cranial bones. This reduction in hematopoiesis results from a conversion of *red bone marrow* to *yellow bone marrow* (Chapter 11).

During early development, the thymus is the primary organ of lymphocytopoiesis. The spleen and remaining lymphoid tissues then become responsible for the production of agranulocytes throughout the life of the organism.

Hematopoiesis is one of the most controversial areas of histology. Although the progress of differentiation of specific cell types is easily described, the nature of the stem cell or cells has not been clarified satisfactorily. As a result there are three theories on the nature and fate of the stem cell or stem cells. The *monophyletic* theory supports the premise that *all* blood cells arise from a single stem cell, the *hemocytoblast*. The *diphyletic* theory supports the premise that there is a separate stem cell (*lymphoblast*) for the agranulocytes and a separate stem cell (*myeloblast*) for the granulocytes and erythrocytes. The *polyphyletic* theory supports the idea that separate stem cells give rise to the erythrocytes and granulocytes, lymphocytes and monocytes.

Since the monophyletic theory has the most wide acceptance, the subsequent description of blood cell differentiation is predicated upon that premise. Moreover, the description of the cells is based upon their reactivity with a Romanowsky-type (polychromed methylene blue and eosin) stain.

Myeloid Elements

General Characteristics. The bone marrow of the body consists of hematopoietic and nonhematopoietic types. The red bone marrow (hematopoietic) is of concern here. The interstitial regions between sinusoids contain free cells that are involved in blood cell production. Red bone marrow, therefore, is a secretory organ.

Three formative sequences occur in the *myeloid tissue: erythropoiesis, granulocytopoiesis* and *thrombocytopoiesis*. Various terminology has been applied to the free cells involved in these sequences. Those in Scheme 15-1 and associated terminology are the most widely accepted.

The myeloblasts give rise to all of the granulocytes. Each of the intermediates in this series is described as neutrophilic, eosinophilic or basophilic.

Trends in Development. The differentiation of mature red blood corpuscles and granulocytes is characterized by sequential changes which typify the developmental process.

The early cells in the sequence are large and become smaller with maturation. The nucleus, as well, is large and decreases with maturation. In the erythrocytic series, the nucleus is extruded from the cell.

The nucleus of early cells is light-staining and acidophilic. With maturation it becomes darker and basophilic. Similarly, the cytoplasm of early cells is basophilic and becomes progressively acidophilic with the maturation process.

The nuclei of stem cells are round and light-staining. The chromatin is disposed in a fine reticulated distribution. With maturation the nuclei become indented, lobed or segmented and the chromatin stains more darkly and is clumped.

Early cells are devoid of granules. In the granulocytic series, early granules are nonspecific and are replaced by the specific granulocytic inclusion granules.

Early cells have one or more nuclei which are not apparent as development progresses toward the definitive cell type.

Also, mitotic activity is high in more primitive cells in normal development.

Similar trends are characteristic of the agranulocytic series also.

Erythropoiesis. The following cells comprise the erythrocytic series: *hemocytoblast, rubriblast, prorubricyte, rubricyte, metarubricyte, reticulocyte, mature red blood corpuscle*.

Primitive reticular cell
|
Hemocytoblast

(myeloblast)	(megakaryoblast)	(rubriblast)
promyelocyte	promegakaryocyte	prorubricyte
myelocyte	megakaryocyte	rubricyte
metamyelocyte	metamegakaryocyte	metarubricyte
band cell	platelet	reticulocyte
mature granulocyte		RBC

Scheme 15-1

The *hemocytoblast* is approximately 15 μm in diameter and has a deeply basophilic cytoplasm and a large, round, pale-staining, vesicular nucleus. It can undergo mitosis or differentiate from primitive reticular cells.

The *rubriblast* (*proerythroblast, pronormoblast*) is an intermediate between the hemocytoblast and the prorubricyte which is described by some authors. The nucleus of this cell is primitive and somewhat smaller than that of the hemocytoblast. Also, the cytoplasm is more basophilic than that of the hemocytoblast. This cell is the first cell in the erythrocytic series.

The *prorubricyte* (*basophilic erythroblast, basophilic normoblast*) is smaller than the two previous forms and has a coarsely distributed chromatin in the nucleus and an intensely basophilic cytoplasm. The nucleoli are either poorly defined or absent. Mitotic activity is high.

The *rubricyte* (*polychromatophilic erythroblast, normoblast*) is a small cell with a small, round and dense nucleus. Nucleoli are not apparent. The cytoplasm has a mottled basophilic and acidophilic appearance due to the presence of hemoglobin and ribonucleic protein.

The *metarubicyte* (*orthochromatic erythroblast, normoblast*) is characterized by an acidophilic cytoplasm which is very similar to the mature red blood corpuscle. Following extensive mitotic activity, the nucleus becomes very condensed and eventually pyknotic. The nucleus is lost either by simple extrusion from the cell or by *karyolysis*.

The resulting enucleated cell is the *reticulocyte* (*polychromatophilic erythrocyte, diffusely basophilic erythrocyte*). The cytoplasm is diffusely basophilic, and with special staining techniques (supravital dyes such as cresyl blue or neutral red) a fine cytoplasmic reticulum is demonstrable. Although this reticulum is normally lost within the myeloid tissue during the transition to mature red blood corpuscles, some reticulocytes occur normally in the peripheral blood.

The increased cytoplasmic basophilia represents the accumulation of ribonucleoproteins for cellular synthesis. Hemoglobin, first synthesized by the rubricyte, results in a mottled cytoplasmic appearance. Increased synthesis of hemoglobin and a reduction of the appropriate cellular organelles characterizes the metarubricytic stage. A continuation of this process results in the mature RBC. Importantly, the circulating RBC's of the embryo are nucleated and probably represent metarubricytes.

Granulocytopoiesis. The following cells comprise the granulocytic series: *hemocytoblast, myeloblast, promyelocyte, myelocyte, metamyelocyte, band cell, mature granulocyte.*

The *hemocytoblast* was described with the erythrocytic series.

The *myeloblast* has a diameter of 15 to 20 μm. The basophilic cytoplasm is unevenly stained and is darker at the periphery than in the perinuclear region. The nucleus is large, finely reticular and red-staining. Two or more nucleoli may be observed.

The *promyelocyte* (*progranulocyte*) is a large cell which may even be larger than the hemocytoblast. The nucleus is round with coarsely distributed chromatin. Nucleoli are not readily observed. The cytoplasm, although basophilic, contains acidophilic regions. Granules are present and vary from acidophilic to basophilic. There is a gradual decrease in *nonspecific granules* and a gradual increase in *specific granules*. A promyelocyte becomes a myelocyte when the specific granulocyte can be identified on the basis of the staining affinity, size and shape of the specific granules. Promyelocytic mitotic activity is high.

The *myelocyte* (*basophilic myelocyte, eosinophilic myelocyte, neutrophilic myelocyte*) is the first recognizable stage of the specific granulocytes. The nucleus is smaller and the chromatin is more coarse than the previous stages. Also, the nucleus is more oval than round and a slight indentation may be apparent. The decreased cytoplasmic basophilia is complemented by an increase in the number of specific granules. Mitotic activity of these cells is especially high.

The *metamyelocyte* (*basophilic metamyelocyte, eosinophilic metamyelocyte, neutrophilic metamyelocyte*) is characterized by a bean-shaped or horseshoe-shaped appearance. The cytoplasm is slightly acidophilic and filled with specific granules. Progressive indentation results in the lobed nuclear appearance of the mature granulocytes.

Neutrophilic granulocytes are the most predominate granulocytes of the myeloid tissue and peripheral blood. Immature forms of neutrophils are commonly encountered in the peripheral blood. A *neutrophilic metamyelocyte* is also referred to as a *juvenile*. The progressive indentation of the nucleus results in a neutrophil referred to as a *neutrophilic band cell* (*neutrophilic stab cell, neutrophilic nonsegmented*). The nucleus of this cell is characteristically horseshoe-shaped. The subsequent lobulation of the nucleus results in a mature cell referred to as a *neutrophilic segmenter* (*PMN, polymorphonuclear neutrophilic granulocyte, neutrophilic filamented, neutrophilic polymorphonuclear* or, simply, *neutrophil*).

Platelet Formation. The cells that comprise the platelet formation series are: *hemocytoblast, megakaryoblast, promegakaryocyte, megakaryocyte, metamegakaryocyte* and *platelets*.

The *hemocytoblast* was described with the erythrocytic series.

The *megakaryoblast* has a lightly basophilic cytoplasm and a nucleus that stains red and is finely granular. The peripheral cytoplasm has pseudopods and a foamy appearance.

The *promegakaryocyte* is larger than the previous cell type and two nuclei may be present. The cytoplasm is slightly basophilic and contains numerous basophilic granules. Cytoplasmic blebs with a foamy appearance may be apparent at the periphery of the cell.

The *megakaryocyte* is larger than the previous cell type. Karyokinesis occurs and as many as 16 nuclei may form. These, however, subsequently fuse to form the characteristic bulged and lobed nucleus of this cell. The cytoplasmic volume is large and acidophilic. Vacuoles and pale-staining areas are scattered among the evenly distributed, lightly basophilic granules.

The *metamegakaryocyte* is the largest cell in the series. Except for the aggregation of cytoplasmic granules and the appearance of platelets at the cellular periphery, it is similar to the megakaryocyte.

This series of cellular changes is characterized by an increase in size and number of nuclei per cell—the reverse in the general trend in the aforementioned series. Mitoses occur in which nuclear separation (*karyokinesis*) is not accompanied by a cytoplasmic separation (*cytokinesis*). Platelets form from metamegakaryocytes by an exocytotic process in which they pinch off from the cell surface.

Lymphoid Elements

General Characteristics. The development of agranulocytes (lymphocytes, plasma cells, monocytes and macrophages) occurs in the lymphoid organs previously discussed (Chapter 14). The developmental sequences leading to the mature cell forms are not as clearly defined in these series as they are in the previously described ones. Scheme 15-2 represents some of the known and conjectured relationships among the agranulocytes.

Agranulocytopoiesis. The germinal tissue of lymph nodes and other lymphatic organs contains all or most of the aforementioned intermediate and mature cell types. The previous diagram is not to be construed as a definitive scheme for the origin and relationships of the agranulocytes. Rather, it does represent a workable model which is consistent with the current literature. The terminology used is a simplification and a compromise between the various names that are used to describe similar cells in these series.

Primitive reticular cells have been described previously (Chapter 3). These cells are the stem cells of all hematopoietic tissues as well as those cells referred to as reticuloendothelial cells. These cells are the

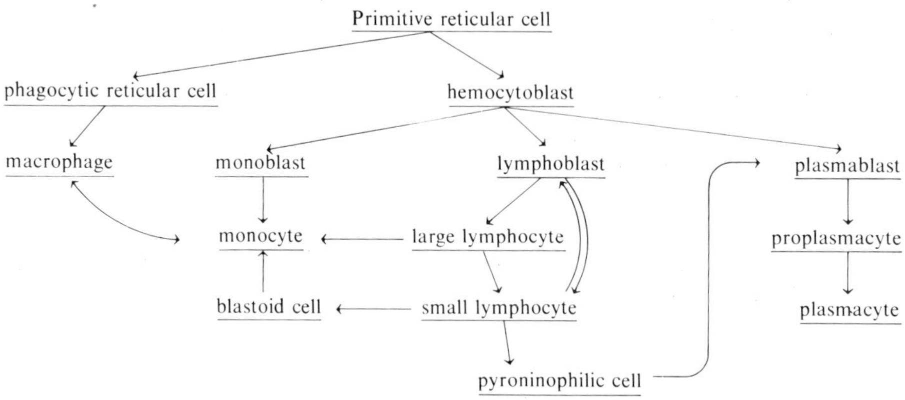

Scheme 15-2

ones that are associated with reticular fibers, form a lining of certain blood vessels and lymphatic vessels and are phagocytic. Some reticular cells are phagocytic. These cells, *phagocytic reticular cells*, are similar to the more primitive cell type. There is some evidence that phagocytic reticular cells are capable of becoming macrophages. The reticuloendothelial cells and all macrophages comprise the *reticuloendothelial system*.

The *hemocytoblast* was described with the section on erythropoiesis. In the agranulocytic series, the hemocytoblasts are capable of differentiating into lymphocytes, plasmacytes and monocytes.

The *lymphoblasts* are the largest cells of this series. They have large, round, vesicular nuclei with one or two prominent nucleoli. Their cellular limits are well-defined. These round cells have an extensive basophic cytoplasm. (They are often referred to as *large lymphocytes*.) With subsequent differentiation these cells become smaller, and their nuclear contents are more coarsely arranged. At this time they are referred to as *large lymphocytes*. (Some authors, however, refer to these cells as *prolymphocytes* or *medium-sized lymphocytes*.) The subsequent division of this intermediate results in *small lymphocytes*. Small lymphocytes are not fixed postmitotic cells. Under proper antigenic stimulation they are capable of dedifferentiating into lymphoblasts which then give rise to more small lymphocytes.

The small lymphocyte has also been implicated in the plasmacytic series. The small lymphocyte is converted into a pyroninophilic cell under antigenic stimulation. This large cell has a basophilic cytoplasm and a large quantity of ribonucleoprotein which accounts for its specific staining affinity. This pyroninophilic cell or *immunoblast* gives rise to plasma cells.

The *plasmablasts*, *proplasmacytes*, *monoblasts* and *promonocytes* are not recognizable as distinct entities in normal blood cell production. In certain types of hematopoietic disorders, however, they are easily recognized.

References

Ackerman, G. A.: Ultrastructure and cytochemistry of the developing neutrophil. Lab. Invest. *19:*290, 1968.

Behnke, O.: An electron microscope study of the megakaryocyte of the rat bone marrow. I. The development of the demarcation membrane system and the platelet surface coat. J. Ultrastruct. Res. *24:*412, 1968.

Calhoun, L. M.: Bone marrow of horses and cattle. Science *104:*423, 1946.

Calhoun, L. M.: A cytological study of costal marrow. I. The adult horse. Amer. J. Vet. Res. *15:*181, 1954; II. The adult cow. Amer. J. Vet. Res. *15:*395, 1954.

Campbell, F. R.: Nuclear elimination from the normoblast of fetal guinea pig liver as studied with electron microscopy and serial sectioning techniques. Anat. Rec. *160:*539, 1968.

Fedorko, M.: Formation of cytoplasmic granules in human eosinophilic myelocytes: An electron microscopic autoradiographic study. Blood *31:*188, 1968.

Johnson, F. R. and Roberts, D. B.: The growth and division of human small lymphocytes in tissue culture: An electron microscopic study. J. Anat. *98:*303, 1964.

Kaihotsu, N.: Electron microscopic studies on the maturation process of neutrophilic leucocytes. Kobe J. Med. Sci. *13:*47, 1967.

Kato, K.: Monophyletic scheme of blood cell formation for clinical and laboratory reference. J. Lab. Clin. Med. *20:*1243, 1935.

Loutit, J. F.: Transplantation of haemopoietic tissue. Brit. Med. Bull. *21:*118, 1965.

Pease, D. C.: An electron microscopic study of red bone marrow. J. Hemat. *11:*501, 1956.

Scott, R. E. and Horn, R. G.: Fine structural features of eosinophil granulocyte development in human bone marrow. J. Ultrastruct. Res. *33:*16, 1970.

Wetzel, B. K., Horn, R. G. and Spicer, S. S.: Fine structural studies on the development of heterophil, eosinophil and basophil granulocytes in rabbits. Lab. Invest. *16:*349, 1967.

Wu, A. M., Till, J. E., Siminovitch, L. and McCulloch, E. A.: A cytological study of the capacity for differentiation of normal hemopoietic colony-forming cells. J. Cell Physiol. *69:*177, 1967.

Yamada, E.: The fine structure of the megakaryocyte in the mouse spleen. Acta Anat. *29:*267, 1957.

16 Integumentary System

General Characteristics

Form and Function. The integumentary system is comprised of all of the tissues previously discussed as well as structures derived from the external body covering. The latter includes the epithelial covering and its associated connective tissue. The *epidermis* is stratified squamous epithelium, while the *dermis* varies from loose connective tissue to dense white fibrous connective tissue (DWFCT). Of the many derivatives and associated structures, the following are representative: hair, nails, claws, feathers, horns, antlers, sweat glands, mammary glands, hooves and others. Because of the vast number of diversified structures in this system, it can be expected that the integumentary system fulfills numerous and varied functions.

The outer keratinized layer of the skin is an effective *barrier* against invasion by foreign organisms. This layer also is an effective *barrier against desiccation* of the more fluid organs located beneath it. Through numerous glands associated with the skin, the integument is an effective organ of *excretion*. These glands, by virtue of their fluid secretory products, are also effective means of *temperature regulation*. The integument is also significant in *calcium homeostasis* by virtue of its synthesis of vitamin D. The pigmentation of the skin also *protects the body against damaging ultraviolet radiation*. Highly cornified regions of the skin are aids to *locomotion*. *General behavioral patterns*, *sexual behavioral displays* and *mechanical protection* are also afforded the organism by this system. The integumentary system is also a very extensive *sensory organ*.

Integument

Epidermis and Dermis. The *epidermis* is composed of distinct layers that comprise the outer layer of the body (Figs. 16-1, 2-7). However, the relative amounts of these layers will vary from region to region. The most basal layer is termed the *stratum germinativum* (Fig. 2-8). It varies from one to a dozen or more cell layers thick. This zone is further divisible into two distinct strata. That which abuts on the basement membrane is termed the *stratum basale* or *stratum cylindricum*. The cells of this zone vary from cuboidal to columnar. A *stratum spinosum* or *parabasal layer* is located peripheral to the basal layer (Fig. 2-9). It varies in thickness and is characterized by *apparent* intercellular bridges. The cells gradually change from a polyhedral to a squamous configuration. Pigment, when present, extends into this zone as far as the transition into the next region of the epidermis. The stratum germinativum is of variable thickness. It is usually thick in hairless regions of the body and rather thin in heavily haired regions.

The *stratum granulosum* contains flattened rhomboidal or squamous cells which possess keratohyalin granules (Fig. 2-10). The granules are also of variable occurrence

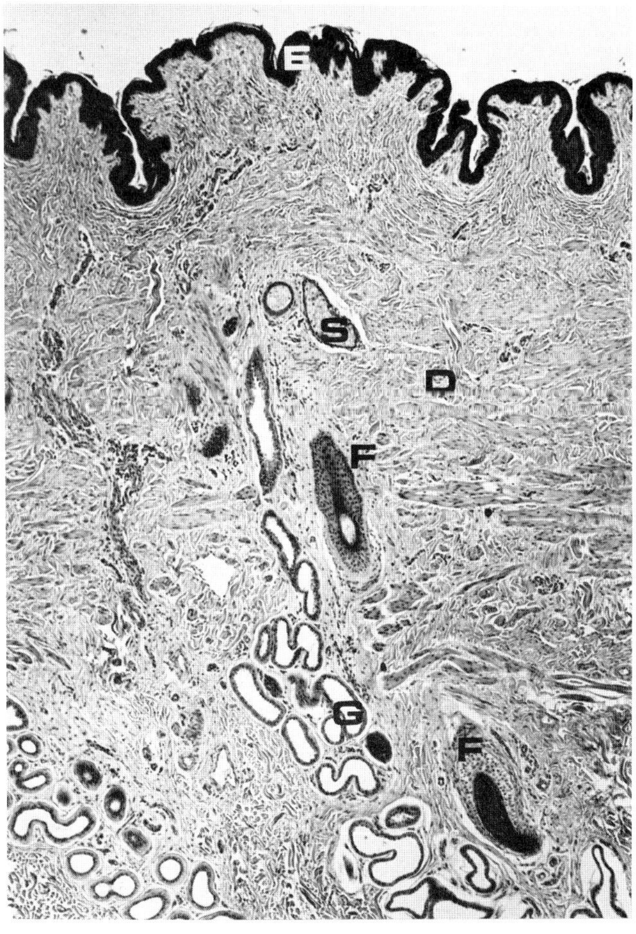

Fig. 16-1. Ovine haired skin. The epidermis (*E*) is underlaid by an extensive dermis (*D*) which contains hair follicles (*F*), sebaceous glands (*S*) and tubular glands (*G*). ×10. All light micrographs are the original magnifications.

and may be absent in regions where hair is abundant. The term *intermediate layer* is applicable to this zone.

The *stratum lucidum* consists of several layers of homogeneous, translucent, squamous cells that are only slightly stainable (Fig. 2-10). Keratohyalin granules are no longer visible, but a substance called eleiden is present. This zone is especially prominent in very thick epidermal regions of the body, such as the footpads of carnivores.

The superficial *stratum corneum* consists of several to many layers of anucleated, squamous, cornified (keratinized) cells (Fig. 2-11). A fibrous protein, keratin, is abundant. In noncornified areas, the term *superficial layer* is used. Dead cells are sloughed from the peripheral portion of this zone.

The *dermis* or *corium* is separated from the epidermis by a typical basement membrane. Two zones are described in the dermis, a *papillary* and a *reticular area* (Fig. 16-2). They are, however, quite similar and blend insensibly with each other. The connective tissue of the papillary region is areolar and varies to DWFCT in the reticular zone. The term reticular does not refer to the presence of reticular fibers; rather, it refers to the reticular arrangement of the collagenous fibers of the region. Elastic fibers, which usually stain a bright pink with routine hematoxylin and eosin (H and E) are prominent in both zones.

Dermal papillae extend into the epidermis (Fig. 16-2). Corresponding *epidermal pegs* are also evident in such zones. This is the means by which the epidermis and dermis become highly interdigitated. The dermal papillae probably serve to increase surface contact with the epidermis and contain numerous blood vessels and various special receptor terminals of nerves.

Lymphatic tissue, glands and smooth muscle also occur in the dermis. The cell population of the dermis may include all cells listed with loose connective tissue.

The skin (epidermis and dermis) resides upon a *hypodermis* or subcutaneous layer of connective tissue. It is a loose connective tissue which may contain extensive quantities of adipose tissue. This zone then blends insensibly with the underlying DWFCT of the fascia.

Hair. These modifed epidermal structures are of variable occurrence in the system and serve various functions: *insulation*, *protection* and *sensory reception*. Hairs develop as localized thickenings of the epidermis which subsequently invaginate into the underlying connective tissue and may extend into the hypodermis.

A connective tissue sheath from the dermis is oriented circumferentially around the *hair follicle* (Fig. 16-3). A basement membrane (*glassy membrane*) separates the connective tissue from the epithelium of the follicle. The *external root sheath* is essentially a continuation of the *stratum basale*, *stratum spinosum* and *stratum granulosum* of the epidermis (Fig. 16-4). An internal root sheath, an apparent continuation of the *stratum corneum*, may be subdivided into three regions: a peripheral *Henle's layer*, an intermediate *Huxley's layer*, and an inner *cuticle of the root sheath* (Fig. 16-4). *Henle's layer* consists of a single layer of flattened cells. *Huxley's layer* consists of several layers of cells which contain *trichohyalin* granules, a substance similar to keratohyalin. The *cuticle of the root sheath* is a single layer of cornified cells which abuts the cuticle of the hair. These cells interdigitate with the cornified cells of the cuticle of the hair.

The hair consists of three regions: an outer *cuticle*, an inner *cortex* and a central *medulla* (Fig. 16-4). The *cuticle* is a single layer of enucleated, cornified cells which interdigitate with the cuticle of the root sheath. The *cortex* comprises the bulk of the hair shaft. It consists of several layers of flattened, cornified cells which contain "hard keratin." Pigment may be present and numerous air spaces characterize the intercellular spaces. The *medulla* may be absent in some hairs. When present, it consists of cornified, cuboidal cells which are separated by air spaces. The cuticular, cortical and medullary characteristics are so specific that identification to species is possible with careful examination.

The hair follicle terminates in a cone-shaped epidermal peg (*hair bulb*) which defines the limits of the *dermal papilla* (Fig. 16-5). The dermal papilla ensures the close association of the vascular bed to the rapidly growing epidermis in this region. Hair growth is achieved in a simple fashion. The epidermal cells at the apex of the papilla give rise to medullary cells. The epidermal cells lateral to the apex give rise to cortical cells and cuticular cells. The cells at the depths of the epidermal pegs give rise to the inner root sheath, while more laterally located cells give rise to the outer root sheath. The growth of a hair, therefore, is achieved by the simple apposition of new cells from the depths of the follicle. It is similar to typical skin growth.

A sheath of smooth muscle, the *arrector pili muscle*, attaches to the connective tissue

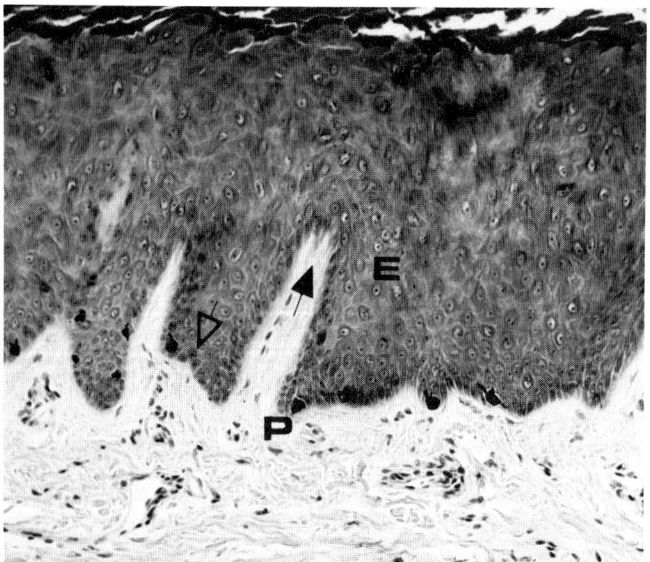

Fig. 16-2. Papillary and reticular zones of the dermis. The papillary zone (*P*) is immediately adjacent to the epidermis (*E*) and is continuous with the reticular zone (*R*). Dermal papillae (*solid arrow*) and epidermal pegs (*open arrow*) are well-developed. ×40.

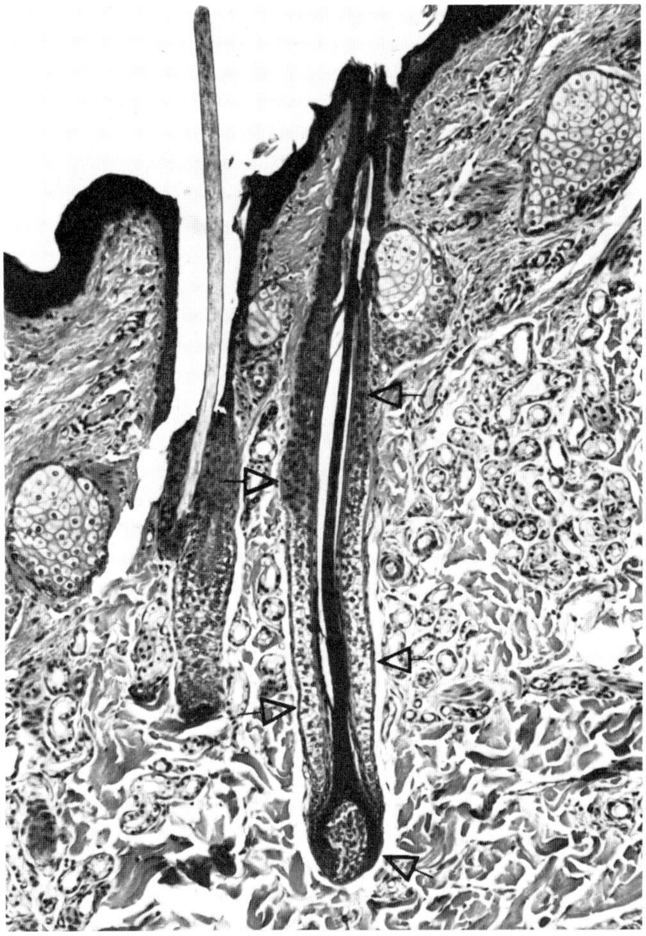

Fig. 16-3. Hair follicle. The margins of the follicle (*arrows*) have been partially separated from the surrounding connective tissue. ×25.

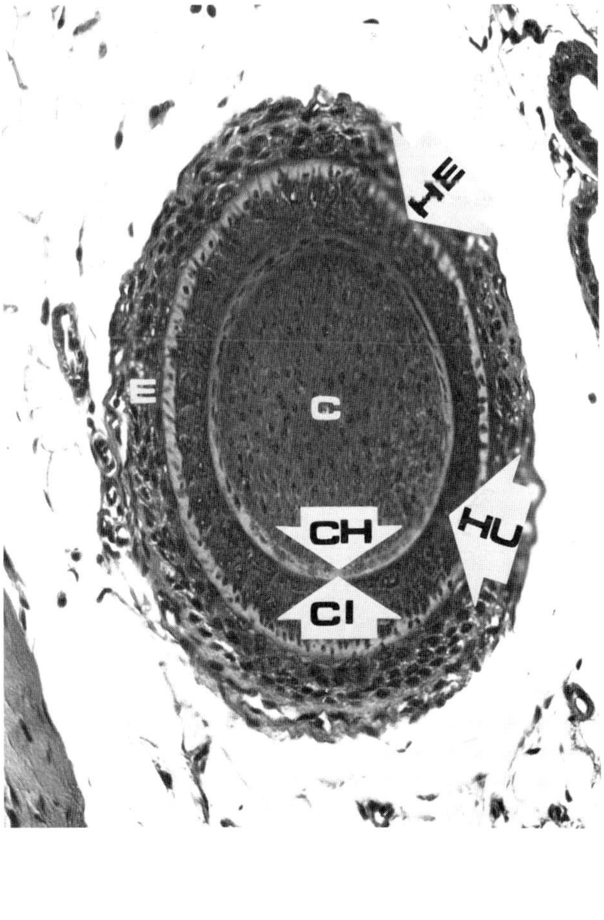

Fig. 16-4. A cross-section of a hair follicle. The external root sheath (*E*) surrounds the hair and is separated from the connective tissue by a glassy membrane (not apparent). The internal root sheath consists of Henle's layer (*HE*), Huxley's layer (*HU*) and an inner cuticular layer (*CI*). The hair consists of cuticular layer (*CH*) and cortex (*C*). A medulla is not present. ×63.

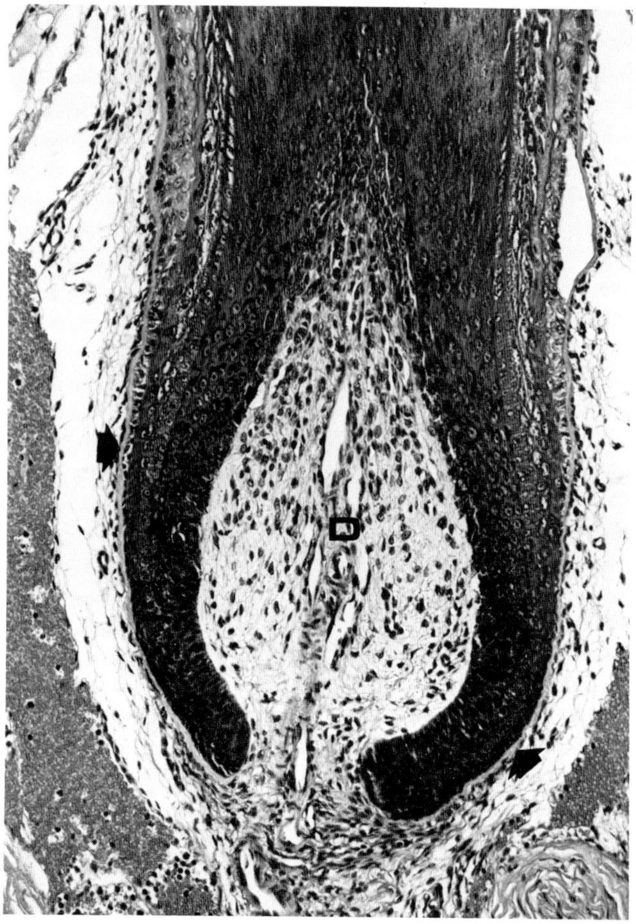

Fig. 16-5. Hair bulb and dermal papilla. The cone-shaped hair bulb surrounds the dermal papilla (*D*). The glassy membrane (*arrows*) is apparent. ×40.

associated with the hair follicle and the connective tissue of the papillary region associated with the skin proper (Fig. 16-6). Its contraction not only erects the hair but probably expresses the sebaceous glands which are located between the mass of muscle and the hair follicle.

In the horse and large ruminants, the hairs are evenly distributed on the body. In other domestic species (pig, cat, dog), the hairs are arranged in groups (*hair beds*). In the dog, a hair bed contains two to four clusters of hair follicles. Each cluster of hair follicles consists of usually one *principal* or *guard hair* and three to nine *auxiliary* or *wool hairs*. A guard hair is approximately 150 μm in diameter and has a cuticle, cortex and medulla. The wool hairs are approximately 70 μm in diameter and are devoid of a medulla. Although a cluster usually has one surface opening, separate openings may be present. In the latter case they open in close association with each other. Clustering of hairs may be as exaggerated as in the chinchilla in which as many as 75 hairs may comprise a cluster with a single surface opening. The single guard hair is approximately 15 μm in diameter while the numerous wool hairs are maximally 11 μm in diameter.

Sensory Hair. These structures are also referred to as *tactile hairs* or *sinus hairs* (Fig. 16-7). Although the distribution of this type of hair is rather specific, the structure of the hair and follicle is similar to nonsensory or normal hairs. The connective tissue sheath adjacent to the glassy membrane is thickened and separated by connective tissue trabeculae from a peripherally located connective tissue sheath. The intertrabecular spaces are filled with venous blood contained within the venous sinuses. Free nerve endings and Merkel's disks are associated with the epidermal cells and connective tissue fibers.

Avian Integument

Epidermis and Dermis. The epidermis of avian skin is quite thin, loose and dry (Fig. 16-8). Although much thinner than the mammalian counterpart, three strata are defined: *stratum basale*, *stratum spinosum* and *stratum corneum*. The connective tissue adjacent to the epidermis is composed of fine collagenous fibers; however, a papillary region is not defined. The connective tissue becomes more dense in the depths of the corium and abuts on a very extensive subcutis. Lymphoid tissue is extensive in the corium and subcutis. The corium and epidermis are devoid of glands.

Feathers extend from the epidermis into the corium and assume a configuration similar to hairs. Although they are both epidermal structures, they probably have a different phylogenetic origin.

Feathers. Feathers are of epidermal origin and, like their mammalian counterparts, develop within a follicle. The base of the follicle, however, is not continuous over the dermal papilla. Thus, the core of the feather contains remnants of vascular connective tissue (feather *pulp*).

The principal parts of the feather are the *quill* (*calamus*) and the *vane* (*vexillum*) (Fig. 16-9). The quill is contained within the follicle and contains two foramina (*proximal umbilicus* and *distal umbilicus*). As the quill grows, the dermal papilla retracts leaving behind the desiccated central *pulp*. The *vane* is the continuation of the quill above the skin surface. It consists of a *rachis*, which is actually the continuation of the quill, and *barbs*. The barbs project laterally from the rachis in an oblique and parallel manner. The barbs possess *proximal* and *distal barbules* which are oriented at right angles to the barbs and parallel to the rachis. The distal barbules have hooklets which engage the indentations of the proximal barbules. This relationship establishes a relatively nonporous and flexible sheet that sheds water and facilitates flight.

Down feathers have a small and thin rachis. The barbs are devoid of barbules. Thus, these feathers are loose and fluffy; they serve as good insulation.

Filoplumes are feathers with a hair-like structure. They are scattered over the body but are especially predominant structures on the head and neck.

Specialized Structures. There are numerous other epidermal modifications in birds: scales, toe pads, claws, beaks, wattles, spurs and combs. Claws, spurs and beaks are similar to the mammalian claw, while toe pads may be compared to the pads of carnivores. Scales are comparable to those of reptiles and occur on the legs of all birds as well as on the wings of penguins. Wattles and combs are diverticuli of the skin which contain extensive vasculature, mucous connective tissue and fat. In some birds (turkey), erectile tissue may be present.

Glands of the Skin

The glands of the skin are generally those that are associated with hairs. These are the *sebaceous glands* and the *tubular skin glands*. The former deposit their excretory product into the follicle, or they may empty independently on the skin surface. The tubu-

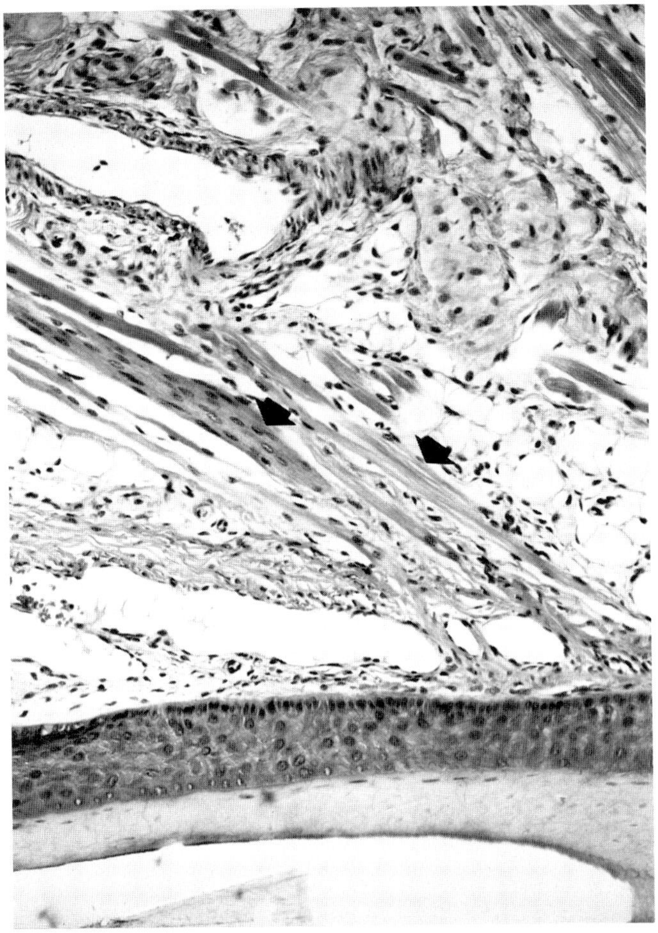

Fig. 16-6. Arrector pili muscle. This muscle (*arrows*) attaches to the hair follicle and papillary region of the dermis. ×40.

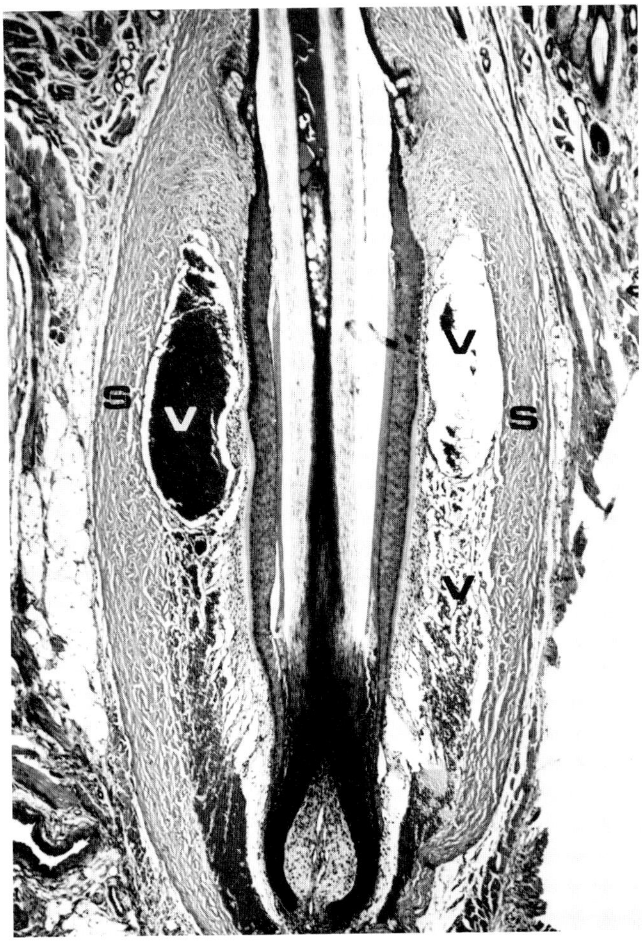

Fig. 16-7. Sinus hair surrounded by a well-developed connective tissue sheath (*S*) which contains venus sinuses (*V*). ×10.

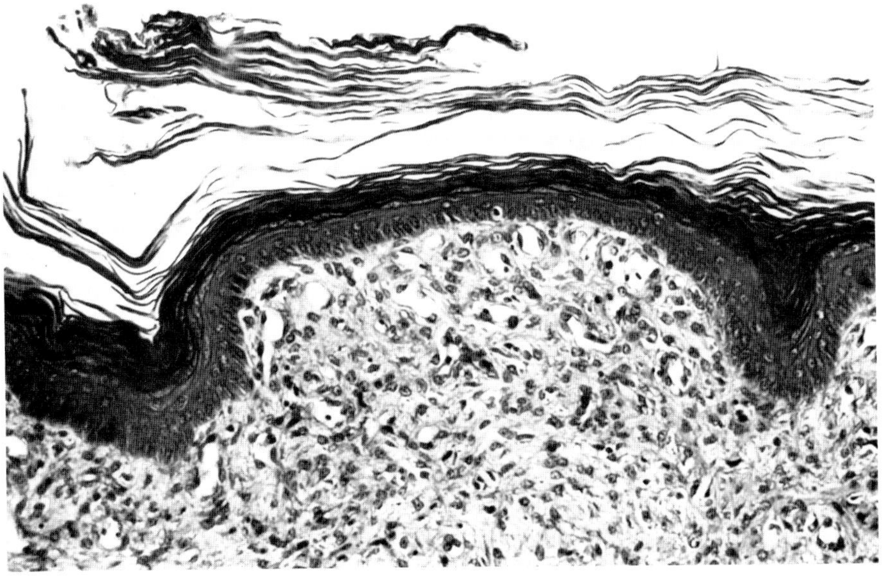

Fig. 16-8. Avian skin. The layers of the epidermis are reduced. ×63.

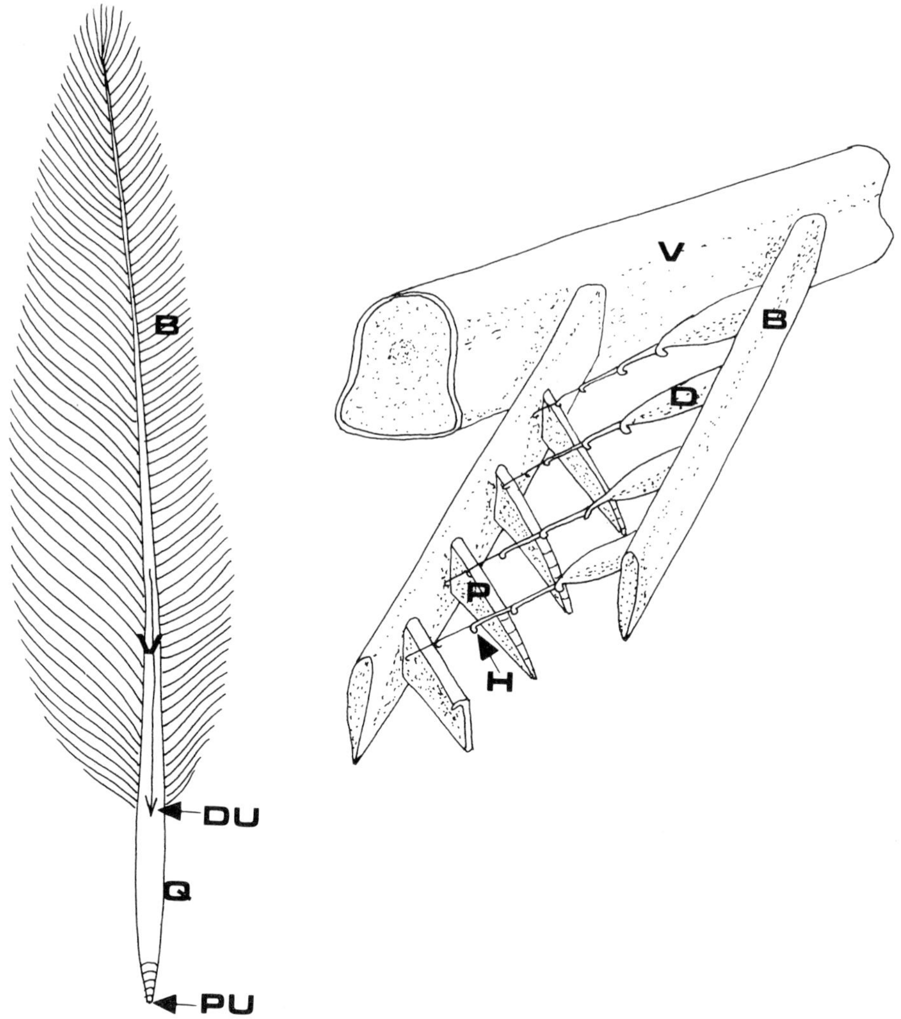

Fig. 16-9. The main parts of a feather. *Q*, quill; *PU*, proximal umbilicus; *DU*, distal umbilicus; *V*, vane; *B*, barbs; *D*, distal barbule; *P*, proximal barbule; *H*, hooklets.

lar skin glands are in close association with the follicles but generally open independently on the skin surface.

Sebaceous Glands. Sebaceous glands in association with hairs are evaginations of the epithelial lining of the root canal in the form of simple, branched alveolar glands (Fig. 16-10). They vary in size from 0.2–2.0 mm. The *peripheral cell layer* (*basal cell layer*) is either squamous or cuboidal epithelium which resides on a basement membrane (Fig. 16-11). These are the stem cells of the gland and function in a manner similar to the stratum basale of the skin. Because of the holocrine nature of sebaceous glands, this layer assures a copious supply of cells. The lumen of the alveolus is almost completely filled with polyhedral cells. As they are derived peripherally they are forced to the center of the gland during which time they accumulate lipids and undergo degeneration. Numerous examples of pyknosis and karyolysis are usually present. The accumulated lipids (fatty acids, cholesterol) and the entire cell constitute the secretory product, *sebum*.

The basal cells of the alveolus are connected to the root canal by a short and wide excretory duct which is lined by a stratified squamous epithelium. Although the mechanism for the regulation of secretory activity is not understood, it is believed that the contraction of the arrector pili muscle expresses the gland. The secretory product, therefore, enters the follicle and then spreads over the surface of the skin.

The functions of sebaceous glands are varied: sebum diminishes the possible entry of microorganisms into the skin; the secretory product diminishes water loss; it contains precursors to vitamin D; sebum keeps the hairs and outer skin surface soft and pliable.

Some areas are devoid of sebaceous glands: foot pads, hooves, claws, horns and others.

Sebaceous glands that are not hair associated are discussed with special skin glands.

Tubular Skin Glands. The tubular glands of the skin are simple, coiled, tubular structures. They are extensively developed in the horse and man and are absent in the bird. There are two general types: *merocrine* and *apocrine*.

The adenomere consists of a low cuboidal epithelium in the merocrine glands, while the epithelial lining of the adenomere of apocrine glands is a low columnar type. Blebs on the luminal surface are indicative of the apocrine secretory mechanism. The adenomeres of both types of glands are arranged as a *glomus* (a tuft or ball). The glomus is connected to the surface or most usually to the neck of the root canal above the opening of the sebaceous gland by a loosely coiled or straight excretory duct which consists of a single or double layer of cuboidal cells. Myoepithelial cells are associated with the adenomeres.

While the merocrine tubular glands are the primary sweat glands of man, they are usually restricted to the footpads of other animals (Fig. 16-12). The apocrine tubular gland is the predominant sweat gland in domestic animals (Figs. 16-13, 16-1). In man, these glands are usually confined to the mammary, axillary, pubic and perineal regions. In the cat, these glands are not as extensive as in other animals. They are confined to the anal and oral regions, the lower jaw and footpads. The canine has extensive tubular glands over the entire body, but apparently they are minimally functional as sweat glands.

Sweat glands serve as a cooling mechanism for the body, as well as an excretory organ. The secretory product is mostly water (serous) and slightly alkaline. In the horse, however, it is strongly alkaline and contains albuminoids, serum globulins and some urea.

Special Skin Glands

Glands of the Anal Region. These glands may be divided into three types according to their association with the rectum and anus: *anal glands*, *glands of the anal sac* and the *circumanal* or *perianal glands*.

The *anal glands* are present in the dog and pig. They are tubuloacinar glands which are located within the lamina propria of the rectum but open into the anus (Fig. 16-14). They secrete either a mucoid (dog) or fatty (pig) substance (Fig. 16-15). Nodular and diffuse lymphatic tissue may be associated with the lamina propria of this region. Also, venous erectile tissue may be present.

The *anal sacs* or *perianal sinuses* are paired, lateral cutaneous diverticula of the anus which are lined by a stratified squamous epithelium which is keratinized. Each

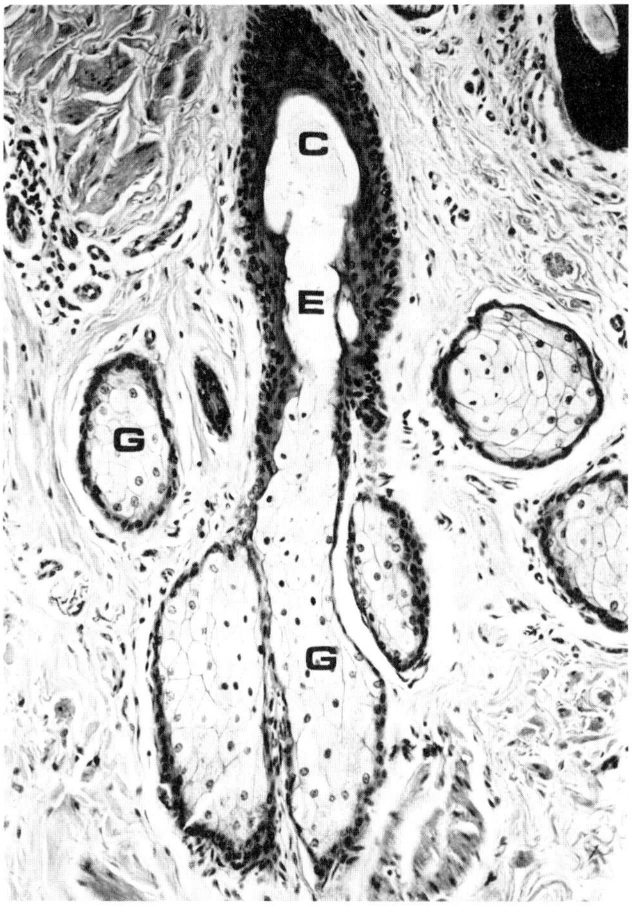

Fig. 16-10. Sebaceous glands and hairs. The sebaceous glands (*G*) are connected to the root canal (*C*) by an excretory duct (*E*). ×40.

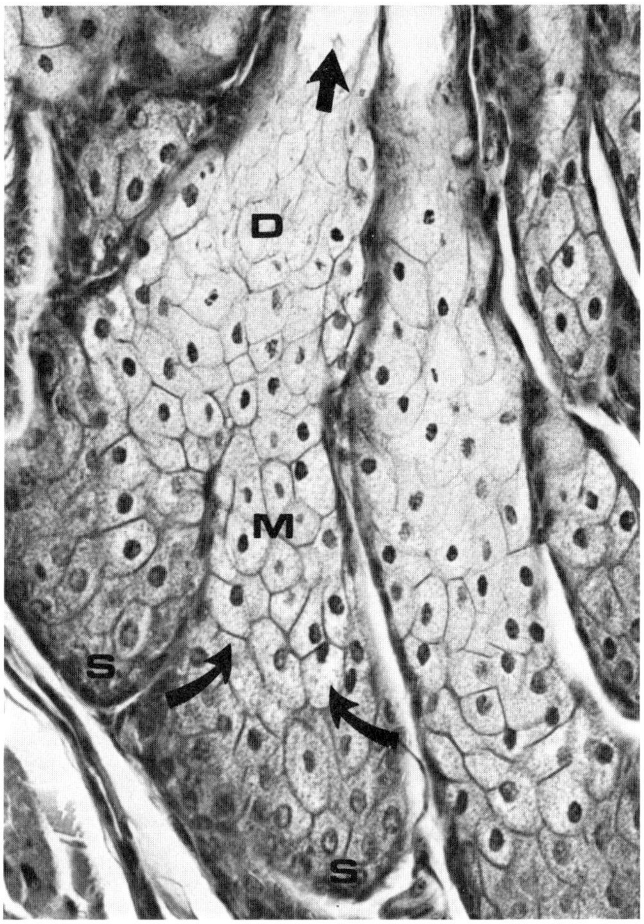

Fig. 16-11. Secretory sequence in a sebaceous gland. The stem cells (*S*) migrate from the periphery (*curved arrows*), mature (*M*), disintegrate (*D*) and are propelled to the excretory duct (*straight arrow*). ×100.

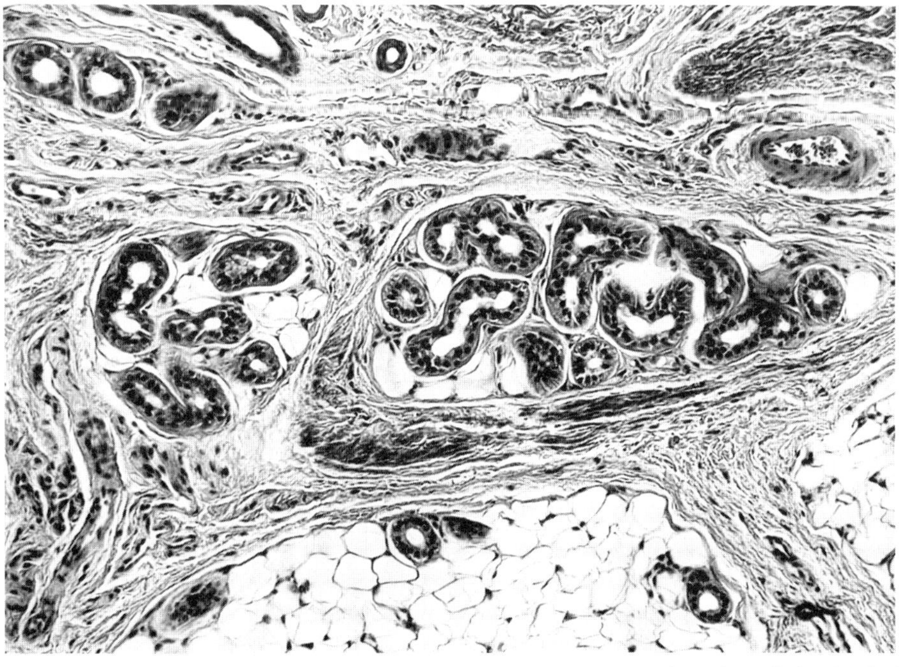

Fig. 16-12. Merocrine tubular glands of the feline footpad. These are not the typical tubular glands of domestic animals. ×40.

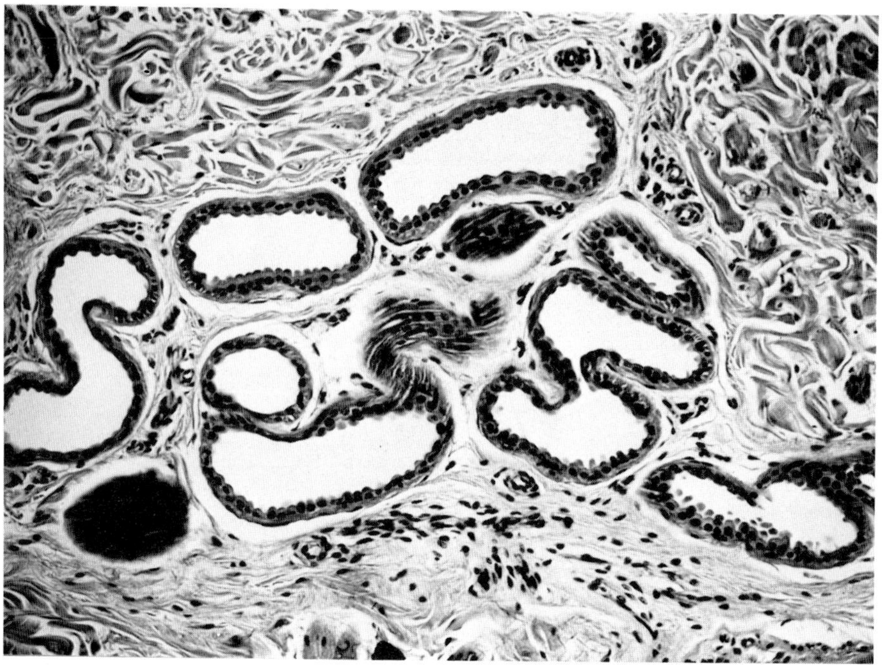

Fig. 16-13. Apocrine tubular glands of the ovine skin. These are the typical sweat glands of domestic animals. ×40.

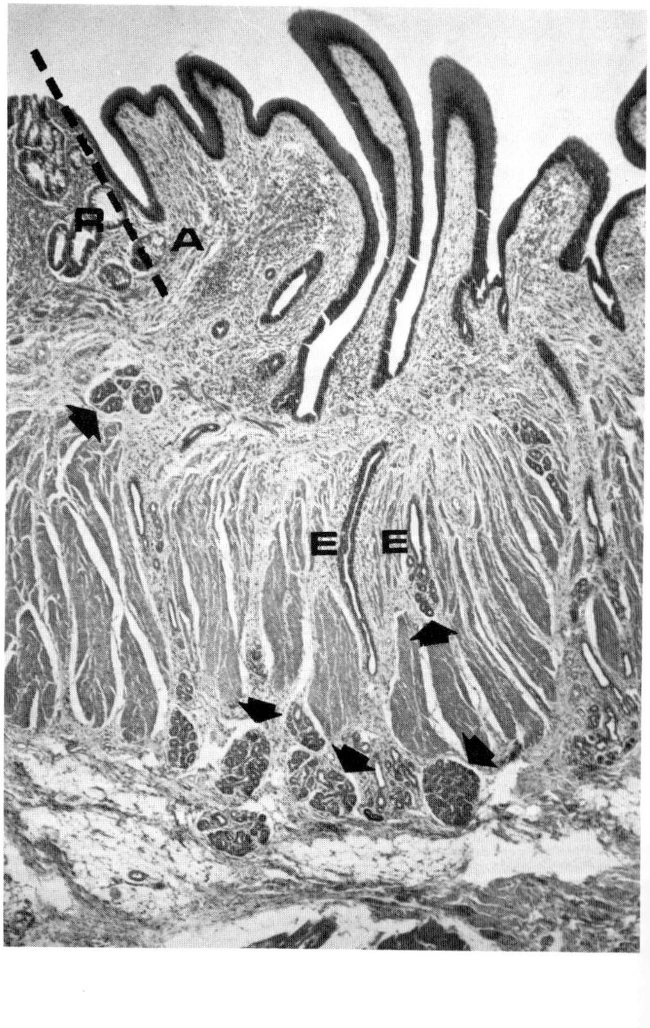

Fig. 16-14. Porcine anal glands. The anal glands (*arrows*) are located at the junction (*dashed line*) between the rectum (*R*) and the anus (*A*). The excretory ducts (*E*) of these glands open to the anus. ×10.

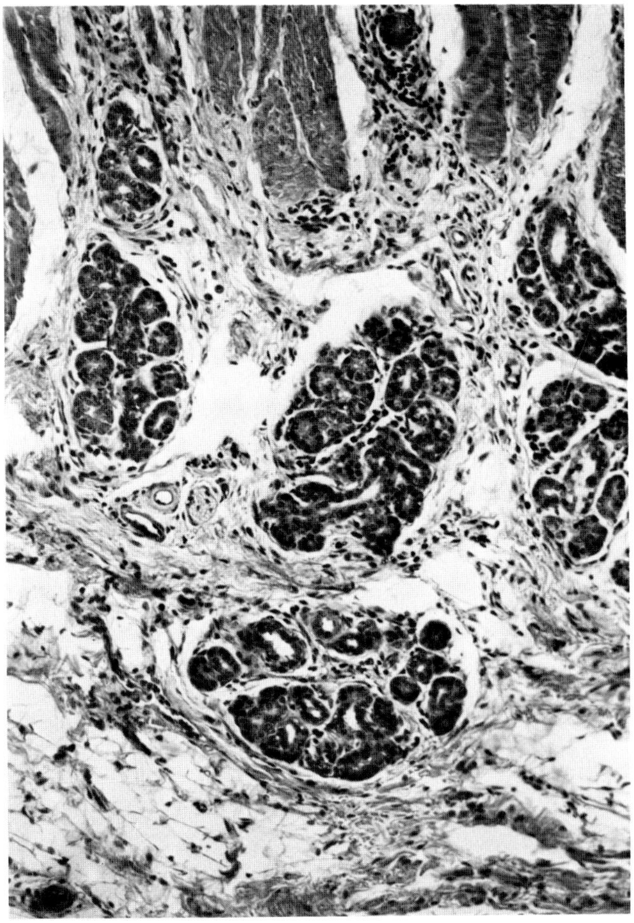

Fig. 16-15. Adenomeres of porcine anal glands. These tubuloalveolar glands secrete a lipid material. ×40.

sac, itself, is not glandular but has numerous glands opening into it (Fig. 16-16). The sac is located between the internal and external anal sphincters. It is supported by a loose connective tissue (lamina propria and submucosa) which is typical of the region and underlaid by a dense fibroelastic connective tissue. Because of the association with the sphincters, much smooth and skeletal muscle is present in the connective tissue.

The anal sac is present in carnivores and many rodents. In the dog, the glands of the anal sac are apocrine tubular; in the cat, apocrine tubular glands and sebaceous glands are present. In both species, both types of glands open into the excretory duct or neck of the anal sac.

The excretory products of the glands of the anal sac, sloughed cells and excrement may occlude the opening of the sacs to the anus. In dogs they may have to be expressed periodically.

The *glands of the circumanal region* comprise two main types: *sebaceous glands* and *circumanal glands* (Fig. 16-17). The former are typical and may or may not be associated with hairs.

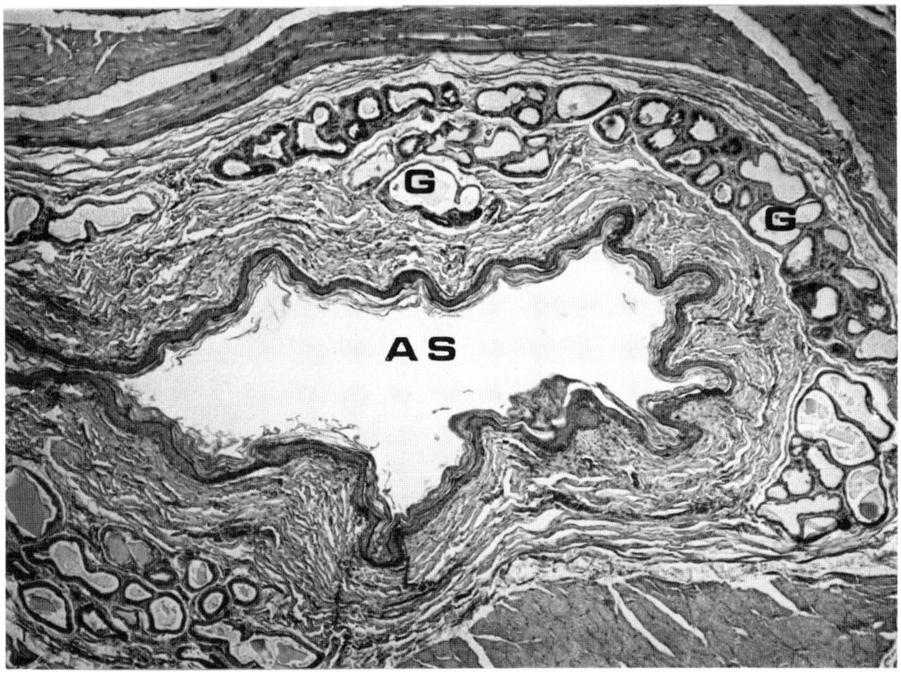

Fig. 16-16. Canine perianal sinuses. The anal sacs (*AS*) are paired diverticula of the anus into which numerous apocrine tubular glands (*G*) deposit their secretory products. ×10.

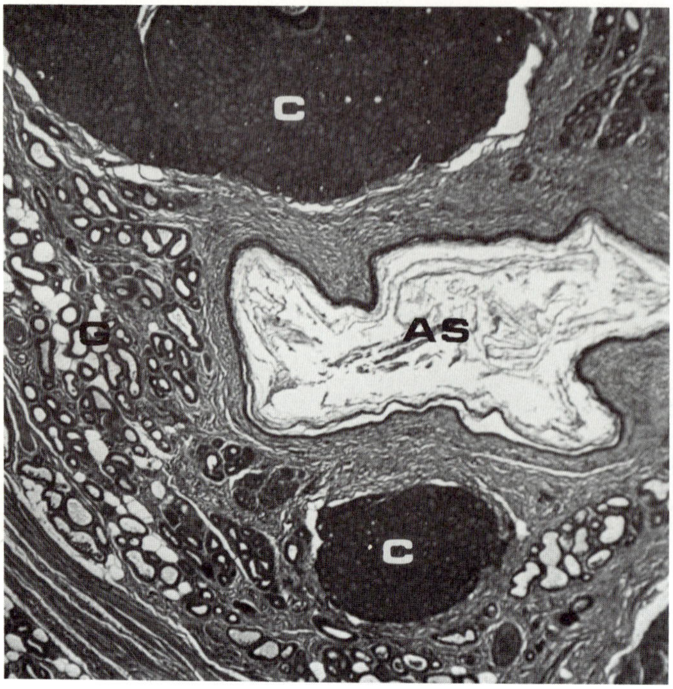

Fig. 16-17. Canine circumanal glands. The circumanal glands (*C*) are solid masses of cells which may be in close association with the anal sacs (*AS*). *G*, apocrine tubular glands. ×10.

The circumanal glands of the dog are nonpatent masses of parenchymal cells which have often been described as *hepatocyte-like* (Fig. 16-18). These cells have a finely granular, acidophilic cytoplasm and pale nuclei. Numerous proteinaceous granules are present. The cells are usually polygonal, but some of them at the periphery of the organ assume a tall columnar configuration.

Nonpatent ducts from the circumanal glands have been reported to connect with the sebaceous glands of the region. It is concluded, therefore, that these glands are nonsecretory, abortive sebaceous glands. Because of the association of these solid masses of cells with sebaceous adenomeres, it is common to refer to the sebaceous and nonsecretory solid masses as circumanal glands. Many of the latter, however, are located some distance from sebaceous endpieces.

These solid masses are predisposed to neoplasia.

Mammary Gland. The following description generally applies to all species but is especially applicable to the cow.

The organ is a compound, tubuloalveolar gland which is believed to be a modified sweat gland (Fig. 16-19). Although it is normally described as being an apocrine gland, this method of secretion refers to the elaboration of lipids, while the protein and carbohydrate components of milk are elaborated by the merocrine method.

The mammary gland consists of the *teats* and *udder*. The udder consists of a capsule,

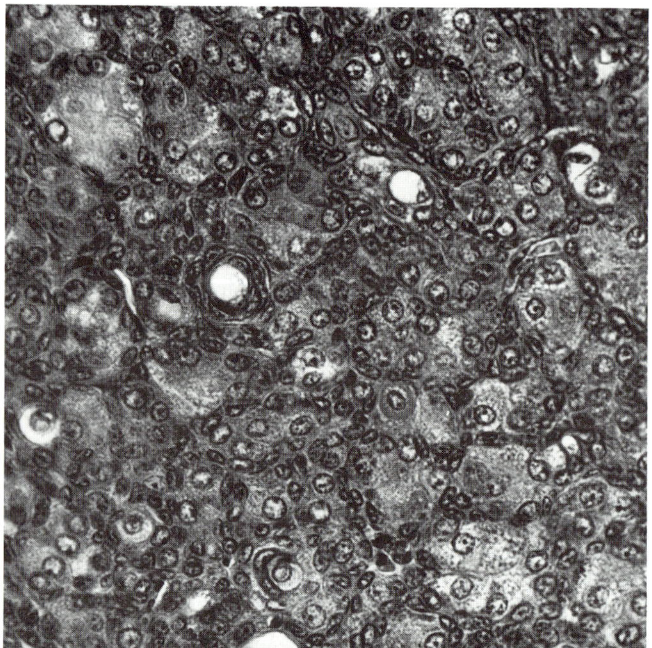

Fig. 16-18. Parenchyma of the circumanal glands. The parenchyma consists of a solid mass of polygonal cells which are acidophilic. Although ducts are present, they become nonpatent as they leave the gland. ×100.

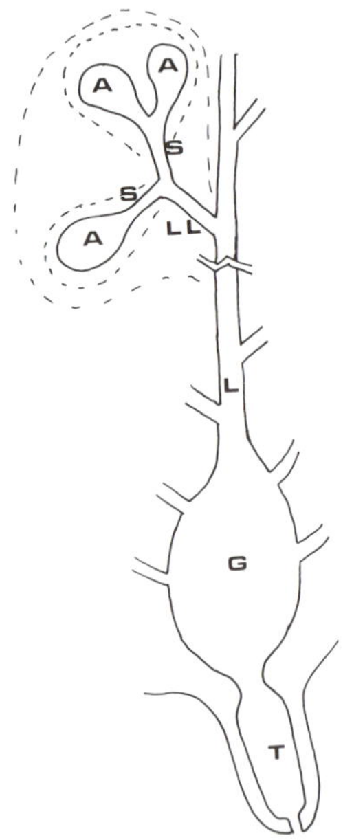

Fig. 16-19. Diagram of the bovine mammary gland. *A*, alveoli; *S*, secretory tubule (intralobular duct); *LL*, lobular duct; *L*, lobar duct; *G*, gland sinus; *T*, teat sinus. Groups of alveoli are organized as lobules. Numerous lobules form lobes.

interstitial connective tissue, secretory epithelium and a system of excretory ducts. The distribution of connective tissue and parenchyma is a function of the secretory activity of the gland. Actively lactating glands have much parenchyma and little connective tissue, while the reverse is true of nonlactating glands.

For a cow to produce 40 lb of milk per day, approximately 8 tons of blood must pass through the udder. This same amount of milk is produced, secreted, suspended and subsequently removed from the udder in a short milking period from a sac of tissue that weighs approximately 50 lb. These relationships necessitate extensive secretory tissue, blood supply and supportive connective tissues.

The following description is applicable to the lactating mammary gland (Fig. 16-20). The secretory portions of the organ include the epithelial lining of the *alveoli* and the initial portion of the *intralobular ducts* (*secretory tubules*). During lactation, the cells assume a columnar configuration with their apical borders protruding into the lumina (Fig. 16-21). Typical apical blebs are indicative of the apocrine secretory method. The accumulation of fat droplets is manifested by the foamy appearance of the cells. These small droplets may become confluent and form a single large droplet. The lateral cell borders usually are indistinct. The nucleus may be basally displaced or may be positioned apically during the secretory process. It may even be discharged into the lumen and become part of the secretory product.

Many cells may occur in the lumina of the gland (Fig. 16-22). These may include sloughed secretory cells, macrophages and leukocytes, all of which then comprise part of the secretory product. These cells may occur in the secretory product throughout lactation. However, macrophages and leukocytes are especially prominent during early lactation when they comprise part of the *colostrum*. Colostrum functions as a laxative, but most importantly in some species it imparts a passive immunity to the nursing offspring until immunological competency is gained.

Following the formation and secretion of milk, the cells become much lower. This can be the result of a diminished or terminated secretory phase or the result of mechanical distortion due to the accumulation of the secretory product in the lumen. Not all the cells of a given secretory unit or all the secretory tubules and alveoli will be in the same state of activity at any given moment. Rather, a broad range of activity may be observed even in a highly active gland.

One or two *alveoli* drain into a single *secretory tubule* (Fig. 16-19). This tubule or *intralobular duct* is lined by cuboidal epithelium, except in the initial secretory por-

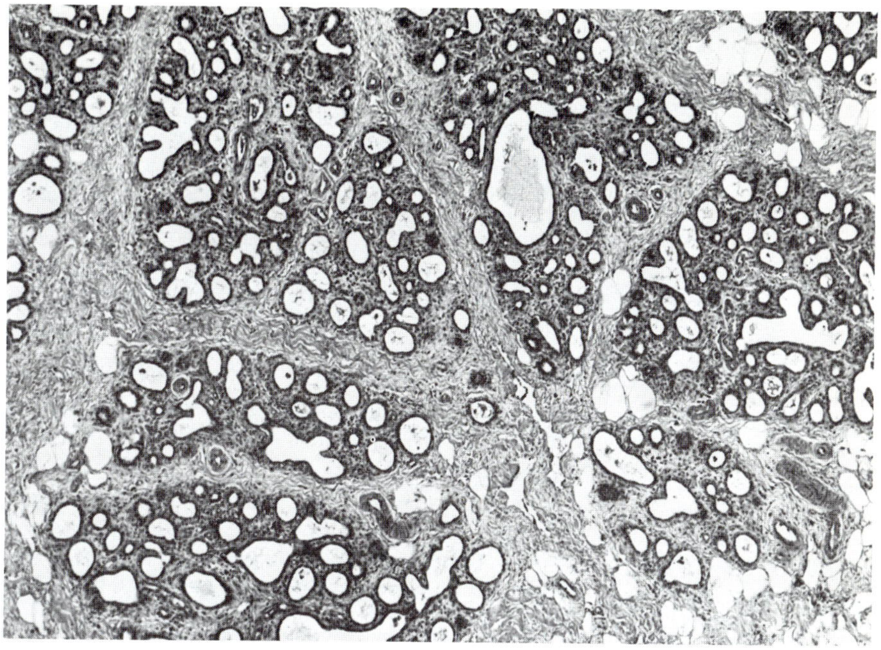

Fig. 16-20. Lactating bovine mammary gland. The parenchyma of the organ is predominant. Compare with Fig. 16-24. ×16.

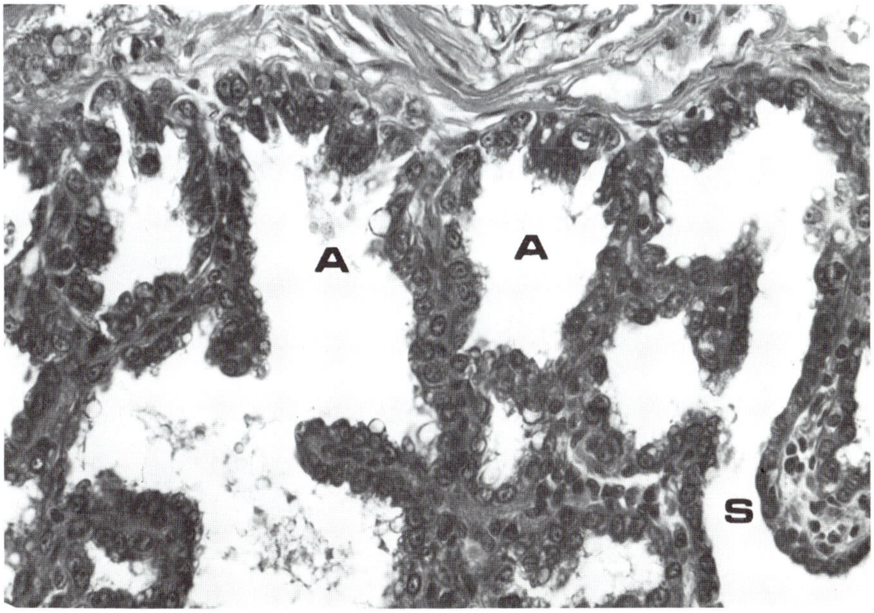

Fig. 16-21. Adenomeres of a lactating bovine mammary gland. The alveoli (*A*) are lined by a columnar epithelium with apical blebs. The secretory tubules (*S*) are lined by a cuboidal epithelium. ×100.

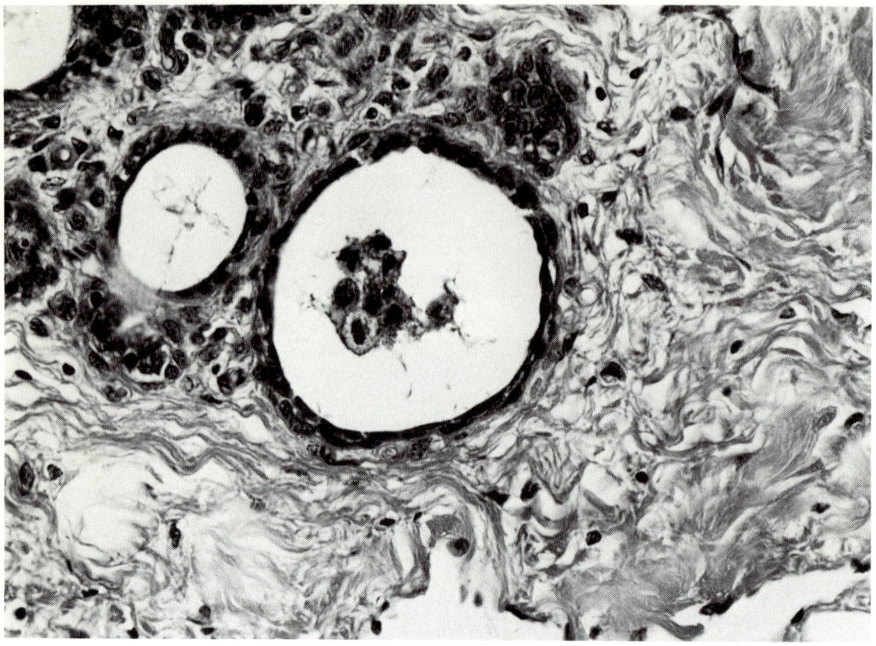

Fig. 16-22. Cells within an alveolus. The cells may be sloughed epithelial cells or migratory cells from the connective tissue. ×100.

tion which is lined by a columnar epithelium. The intralobular ducts drain into a *lobular duct* which is lined by a cuboidal or columnar epithelium which is nonsecretory. The lobular duct is the primary excretory duct for a lobule and numerous lobular ducts drain into a *lobar duct*. The lobar duct is the primary excretory duct for a lobe and is lined by a bistratified columnar epithelium. Besides serving as excretory pathways for milk, the ducts may undergo expansion and serve as storage areas for milk. Numerous lobar ducts drain into the *gland sinus* (*gland cistern*, *lactiferous sinus*) which is lined by the same type epithelium. This is a common chamber at the base of each quarter of the udder. The volume of this cistern is quite variable. A slight constriction or *annulus* separates the *gland sinus* from the *teat sinus* (*teat cistern*); the latter is lined by a bistratified columnar epithelium. The annulus that separates the teat sinus from the gland sinus is not always apparent and is justification for referring to both sinuses collectively as the *lactiferous sinus*. The teat sinus is continuous with the outside via the *streak canal* (*papillary duct*, *teat canal*). The internal orifice of this canal is marked by an abrupt change to stratified squamous epithelium (keratinized). The tunica mucosa of this area is organized into longitudinal folds referred to as the *rosette of Furstenburg*. The epithelium of the teat canal continues through the external orifice and is continuous with the epidermal covering of the teat.

The connective tissue of the gland varies with its position within the organ. The sparse amount of intralobular connective tissue is areolar and contains an extensive capillary network. Numerous myoepithelial cells are intimately associated with the alveoli and secretory tubules. Interlobular (intralobar) and interlobar connective tissue is areolar. Numerous elastic and collagenous fibers, as well as blood vessels, lymphatics and nerves are present. Bundles of smooth muscle fibers are present and associated with large ducts. Helically arranged elastic fibers are also associated with large ducts.

The capsule of the organ is a fibroelastic connective tissue which is especially rich in elastic fibers. This capsule divides the organ into four quarters. The external lamina of the capsule is DWFCT and comprises the *lateral suspensory ligament*. The *medial suspensory ligament* is especially rich in elastic fibers. The disposition of the capsule and connective tissue stroma is typical of solid organs.

The tunica mucosa and associated connective tissue (lamina propria and submucosa) of the teat sinus and teat canal are in close association and are actually continuous with the dermis (corium) and epidermal covering of the teat. The lamina epithelialis is bistratified columnar epithelium underlaid with a lamina propria of areolar connective tissue which is rich in elastic fibers. There is no distinct submucosa. A tunica muscularis consists of strands of smooth muscular fibers. In the area of the internal orifice of the streak canal they are disposed as a sphincter. At the junction between the teat sinus and gland sinus this muscle also forms a sphincter. Extensive longitudinal blood vessels, thick-walled veins and lymphatic vessels are associated with the smooth muscle layers, especially in the areas of the sphincters (Fig. 16-23). The connective tissue peripheral to the smooth muscular fibers is the corium. It is typical, except that it is especially rich in elastic fibers. The epidermal covering of the teat in the cow is hairless and nonglandular.

In the nonlactating mammary gland, the parenchyma is greatly reduced and replaced by areolar connective tissue (Fig. 16-24). Extensive lymphocytic infiltration into the connective tissue and parenchyma is typical. Extensive adipose tissue may be present. The predominant loss of parenchyma is associated with the alveoli and secretory tubules. The remaining parenchyma is primarily the duct system. During mammary gland development, the alveoli are believed to be derived from the residual duct system.

During advanced stages of milk production, there is a gradual involution of the udder which eventually leads to a morphology associated with inactivity. Throughout lactation, but especially apparent in advanced stages, *corpora amylacea* are common (Fig. 16-25). These are concretions of casein (milk protein) and cellular detritus.

There are numerous gross and subgross anatomical differences among the mammary glands of domestic species. Although there are some histological differences, they are academic. The number of teats, gland cisterns and teat canals per teat vary. The number of teat canals per teat in various species are: ruminants, 1; sow, 2 to 3; mare, 2 to 4; queen, 4 to 7; bitch, 8 to 20; woman, 15 to 24.

Uropygial Gland. The uropygial gland is also referred to as the *oil* or *preen gland* (Fig. 16-26). It is the only cutaneous gland that occurs in birds, and it is especially well developed in aquatic species. It consists of numerous sebaceous adenomeres which empty into a common duct or sinus and empty on the surface on a common papilla. The papilla contains smooth muscle fibers which extend around the excretory duct. The heavily encapsulated, bilobed duct is situated above the last sacral vertebra. Because of its unique structure and size, this gland is considered a specialized sebaceous skin gland.

Miscellaneous Glands. Besides the previously described glands, numerous others are considered as specialized skin glands. Even the remaining specialized glands are not unique histologically but have a unique and/or interesting gross relationship to other structures. However, these specialized glands are usually not associated with hairs. They will not be considered independently. They include, among others, the following: sebaceous glands of the porcine carpus; sebaceous and tubular glands of the preputial pouch of the boar; sebaceous preputial glands of the stallion; sebaceous glands of

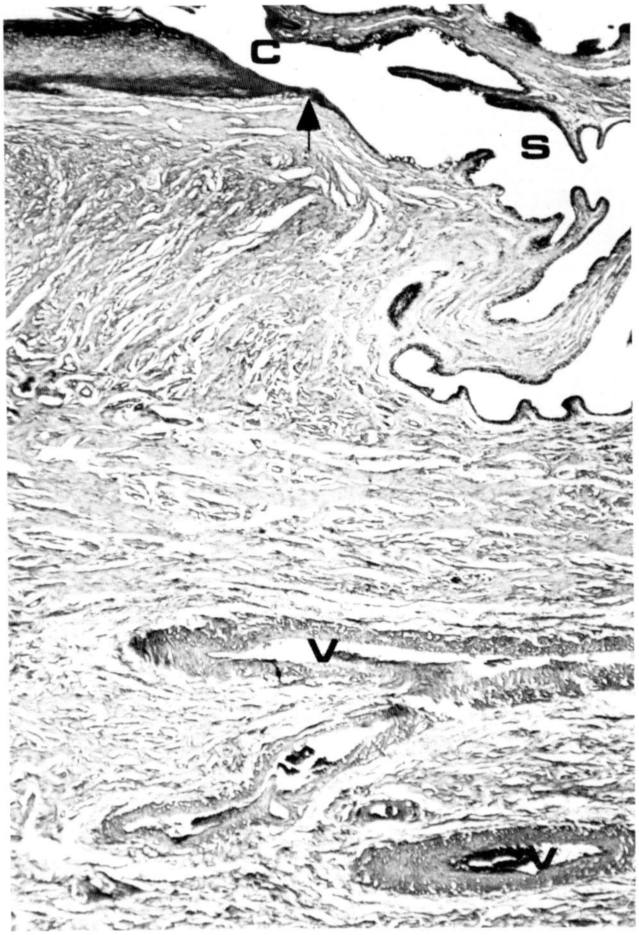

Fig. 16-23. Junction between the teat sinus and the streak canal. The junction (*arrow*) between the teat sinus (*S*) and the internal orifice of the streak canal (*C*) is marked by a transition from bistratified columnar to stratified squamous epithelium. Vessels (*V*) are oriented longitudinally in this region. ×10.

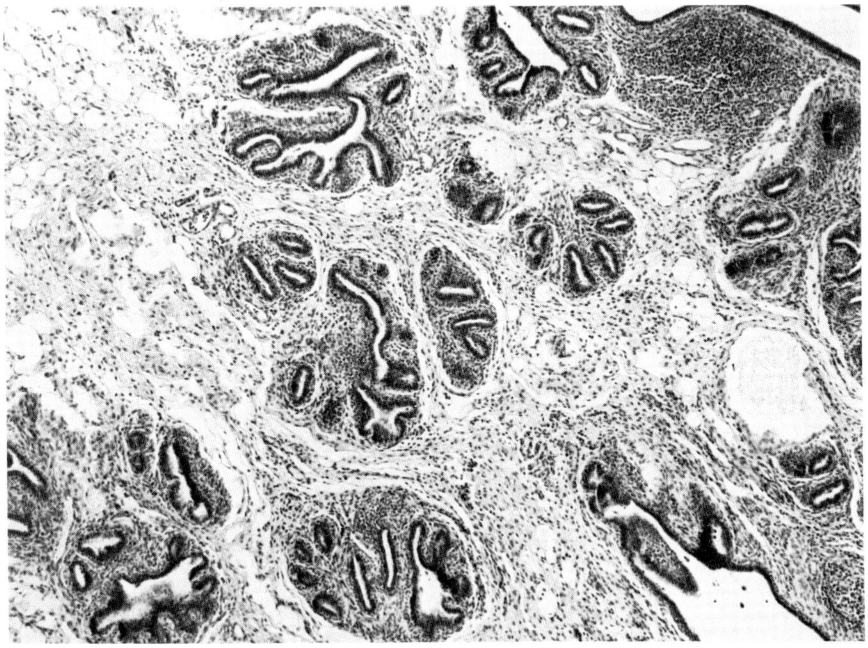

Fig. 16-24. A nonlactating bovine mammary gland. The parenchyma is reduced while the amount of connective tissue is increased. Compare with Fig. 16-20. ×16.

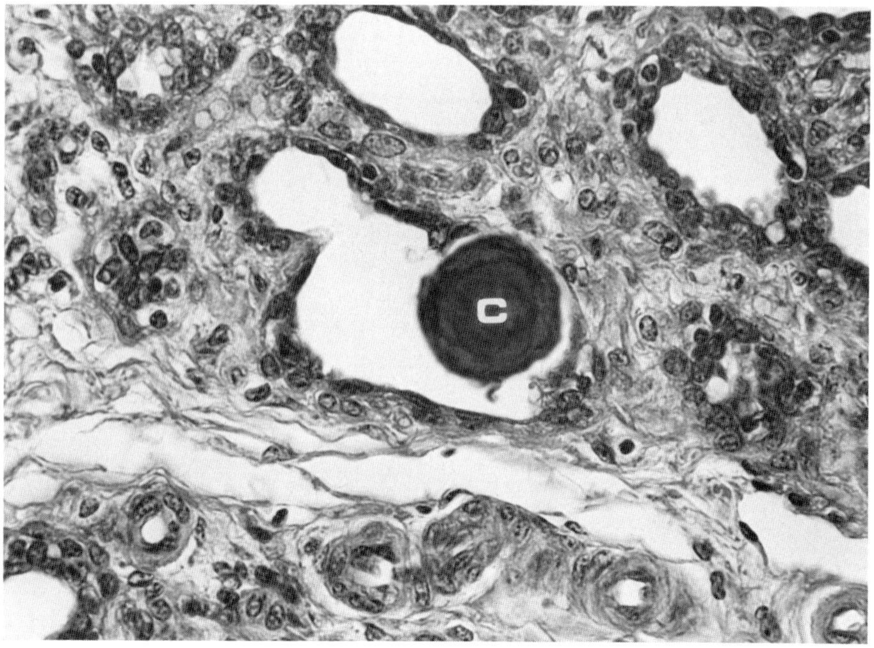

Fig. 16-25. Amylaceous corpuscle in an alveolus of the bovine mammary gland. The corpuscle (*C*) is a concretion of milk protein and cellular debris. ×100.

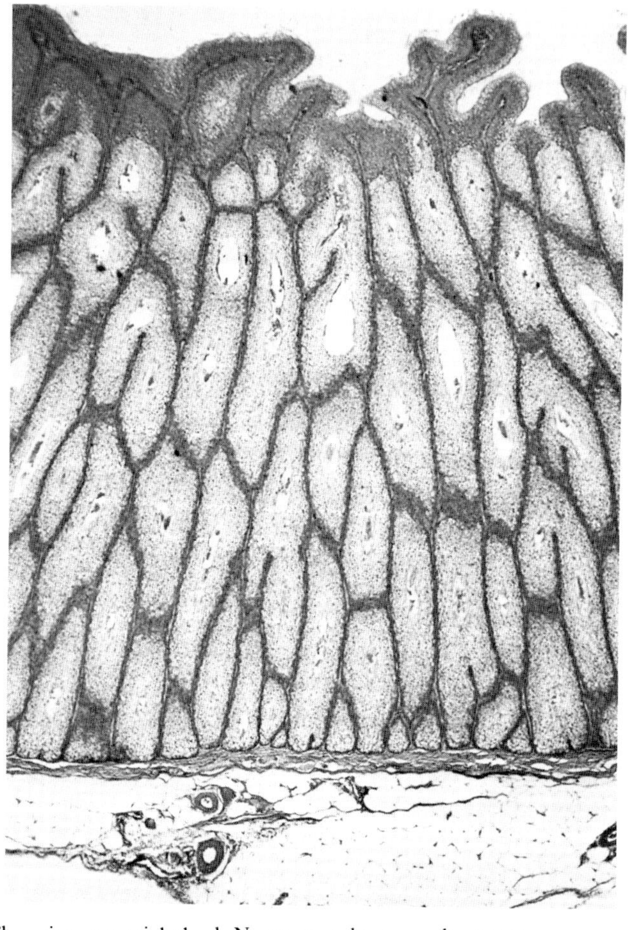

Fig. 16-26. The avian uropygial gland. Numerous sebaceous adenomeres are grouped to form this gland. ×10.

the labia, vulva and external auditory meatus; tubular serous glands of the planum nasolabiale of the ox.

Hooves and Claws

Equine Foot. The hoof is the insensitive cornified layer of the epidermis. The foot, however, includes the hoof, dermis and all the structures contained therein (Fig. 16-27). The hoof is much like any other epidermally derived structure. The unique morphology of the hoof is achieved by the different relationships between the epidermis and related dermis or corium. This is manifested in two distinct ways. In some regions, the dermis is papillated; i.e., typical but pronounced dermal papillae and corresponding epidermal pegs are present. In other regions the papillae and epidermal pegs are confluent. As a result, the adjacent epidermal and dermal regions are *laminar*.

Most parts of the hoof are formed of cornified material which is arranged in a tubular manner. Some regions, however, are nontubular. One region is laminar. The hoof, therefore, is composed of *tubular*, *intertubular* and *laminar horn* (keratin).

The hoof may be divided into the following distinct regions histologically: *periople*,

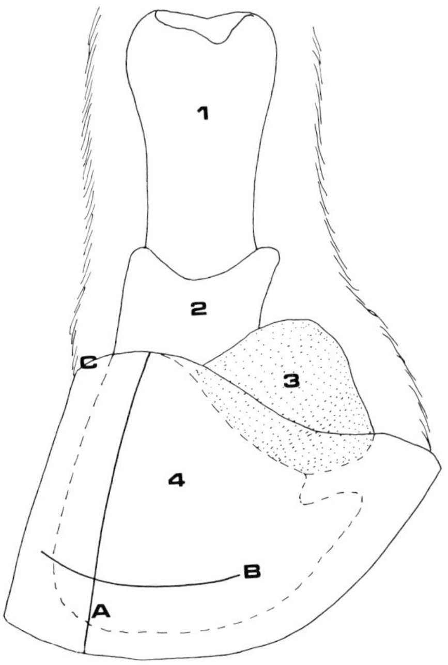

Fig. 16-27. Simplified diagram of the equine foot. *1*, first phalanx; *2*, second phalanx; *3*, cartilage; *4*, third phalanx. The cornified wall of the hoof is demarcated from the typical integument at the coronet (*C*). The *line* at *A* (perpendicular to the ground surface) represents the plane of section for Figs. 16-28, 16-30, 16-31, 16-33 and 16-34. The line at *B* (parallel to the ground surface) represents the plane of section for Figs. 16-29, 16-32 and 16-35.

coronet, *laminae*, *bars*, *sole* and *frog* (Fig. 16-28). Corresponding to these epidermal regions are areas of the corium that bear the same name. Thus, there is a *perioplic epidermis* and a *perioplic corium*, etc.

The perioplic, coronary and laminar epidermises comprise the *wall* of the hoof (Fig. 16-29). In older horses, the coronary and laminar epidermises are the primary constituents of the wall.

The *perioplic epidermis* is referred to as the *stratum externum* or *stratum tectorium* (Fig. 16-30). It is composed of soft, thin, white, shiny and cornified material which extends over the wall and *bulbs*. The perioplic epidermis is the means by which the hoof is directly attached to the epidermis of the skin. It may be absent in older animals. It is probably the means by which water loss from the hoof is diminished. The associated *perioplic corium* is papillated. These papillae are highly vascularized and oriented perpendicular to the ground surface. This orientation results in a downward growth of the perioplic epidermis.

The *coronary epidermis* is also referred to as the *stratum medium* (Fig. 16-31). Normally, it is devoid of a stratum granulosum and a stratum lucidum. This is typical of most parts of the hoof. It is composed of very prominent tubular and intertubular horn which comprises the bulk of the hoof wall (Fig. 16-32). The tubular horn is elaborated in a manner that may be compared to the growth of hairs (Fig. 16-33). The spaces between the tubular horn are filled with intertubular horn. The tubules of horn arise from the germinal epithelium which covers the lateral and distal portions of the dermal papillae. The intertubular horn is elaborated from the germinal epithelium in the depths of the epidermal pegs. The papillae of this region are elongated and are oriented perpendicular to the ground surface. This orientation results in the cornified cells being elaborated in a similar relationship to the ground surface; i.e., the tubular horn is perpendicular to the ground also.

The *epidermis of the laminar region* (*stratum lamellatum*) is composed of nontubular horn (Fig. 16-34). This horn is elaborated at a very slow pace in a plane which is perpendicular to the stratum medium of coronary origin. It fuses with the stratum medium and

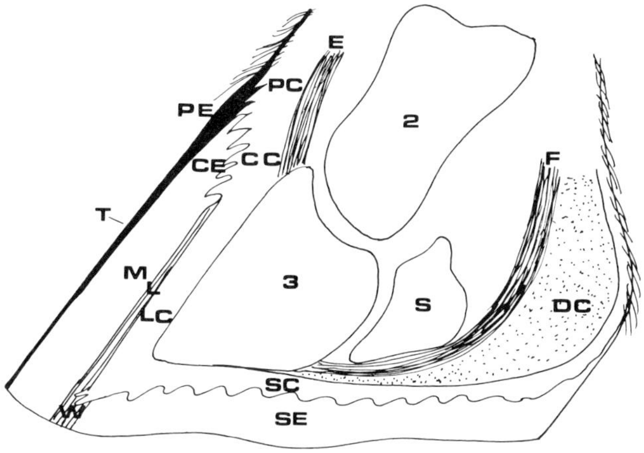

Fig. 16-28. Longitudinal section of the equine foot. *2*, second phalanx; *3*, third phalanx; *S*, sesamoid bone; *F*, flexor tendon; *E*, extensor tendon; *DC*, digital cushion; *PC*, perioplic corium; *PE*, perioplic epidermis; *T*, stratum tectorium; *CC*, coronary corium; *CE*, coronary epidermis; *M*, stratum medium; *LC*, laminar corium; *L*, stratum lamellatum; *SC*, sole corium; *SE*, sole epidermis; *W*, white line.

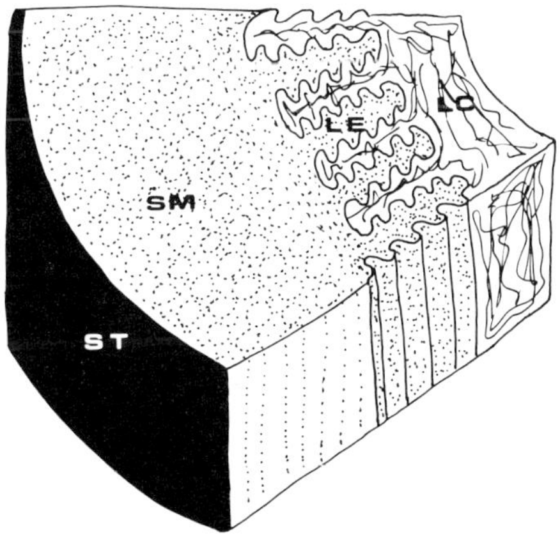

Fig. 16-29. Cross-section through the wall of the equine hoof. The stratum tectorium (*ST*) covers the stratum medium (*SM*). The latter is continuous with the stratum lamellatum (*LE*). The laminar corium (*LC*) has primary and secondary papillae.

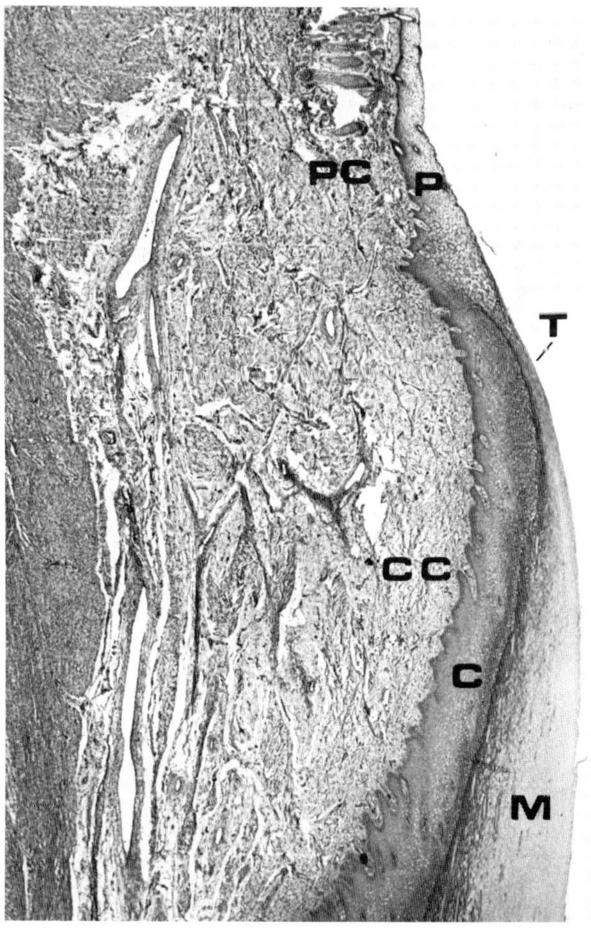

Fig. 16-30. Longitudinal section through the perioplic and coronary region of the equine foot. The perioplic corium (*PC*) is papillated and underlies the perioplic epidermis (*P*). The latter is continued as the stratum tectorium (*T*). *CC*, coronary corium; *C*, coronary epidermis; *M*, stratum medium. ×4.

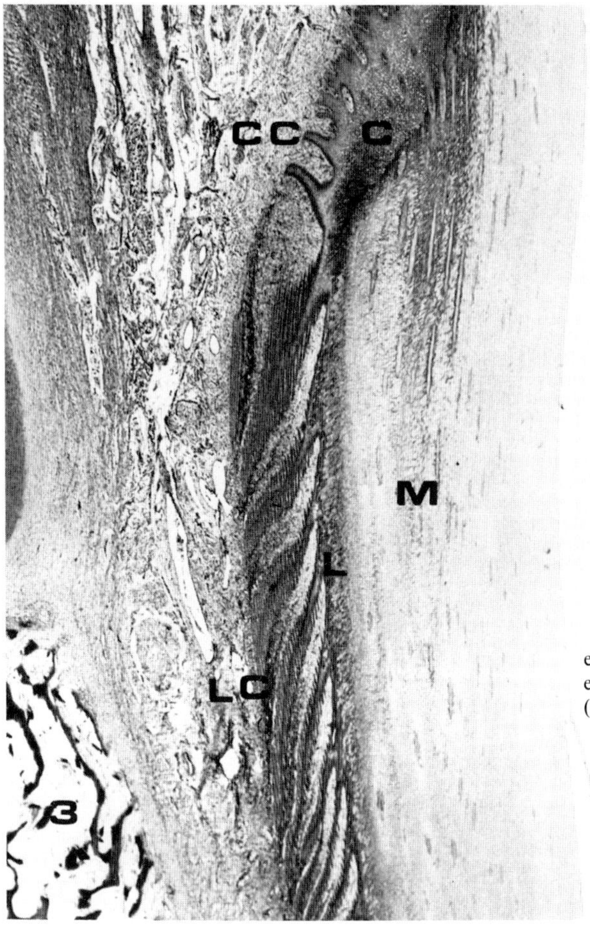

Fig. 16-31. Longitudinal section through the coronary and laminar region of the equine foot. The coronary corium (*CC*) is papillated and associated with the coronary epidermis (*C*) or stratum medium (*M*). The laminar corium (*LC*) and laminar epidermis (*L*) are distal to the coronary region. A portion of the third phalanx (*3*) is visible. ×40.

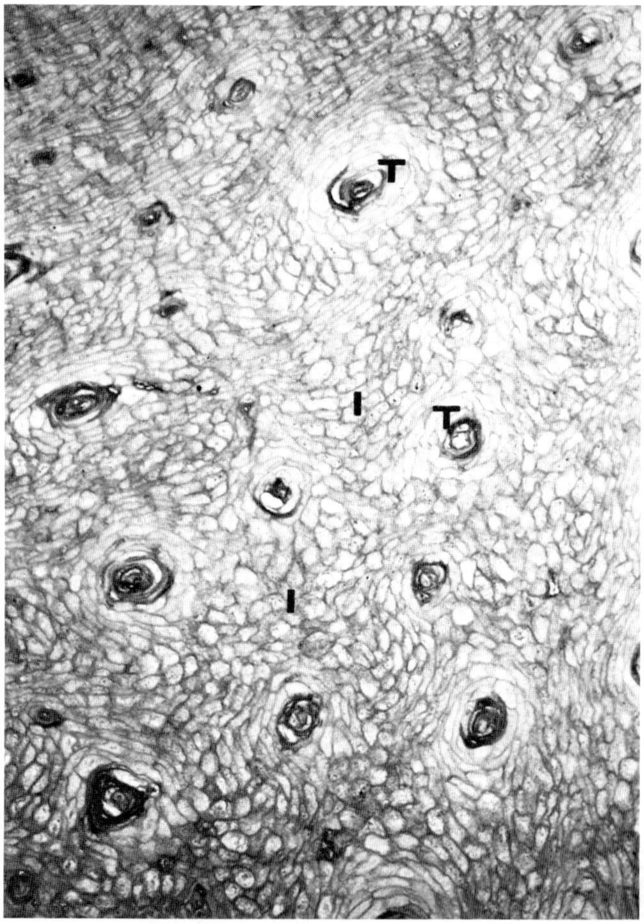

Fig. 16-32. Organization of the stratum medium of the equine hoof. The stratum medium is composed of tubular (*T*) and intertubular (*I*) horn. ×40.

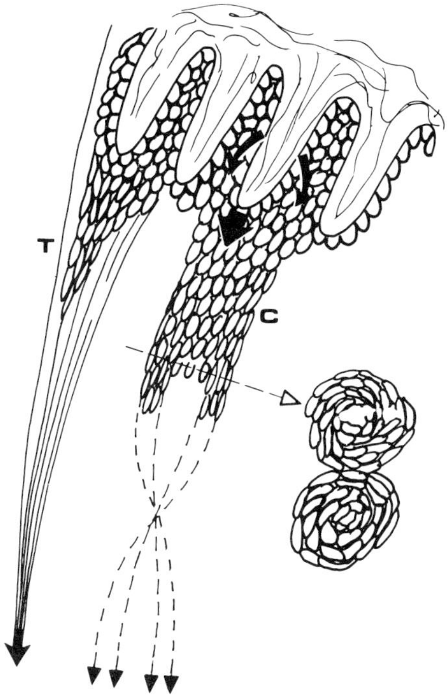

Fig. 16-33. Scheme for the elaboration of tubular and intertubular horn. The perioplic epidermis elaborates cornified cells which elongate and become the stratum tectorium (*T*). The coronary epidermis (*C*) elaborates cells from the depths of the epidermal pegs (*curved arrows*) which become intertubular horn. The epithelium on the lateral and distal portions of the dermal papillae elaborate cornified cells which become tubular horn. The central cells of the tubular horn disintegrate. In cross-section the tubular horn is composed of concentric whorls of cornified cells with hollow centers.

assists in holding the wall proper to the foot. The orientation and configuration of the dermal papillae are altered in this region. The dermal papillae and corresponding epidermal pegs are converted to elongated ridges which are oriented perpendicular to the ground surface. By analogy, the fingers of the hand would represent dermal papillae and the intervening spaces would represent the epidermal pegs. Successive stacking of one hand upon the other converts the confluent papillae and pegs to ridges or laminae. There are *primary* and *secondary laminae* in this region (Fig. 16-35). The secondaries are oriented at an acute angle to the primaries. The primary epidermal laminae are composed of stratum spinosum and horn. Collectively, these areas are referred to as the *insensitive laminae*. The remaining secondary laminae, with the germinal epithelium and associated dermal structures, are referred to as the *sensitive laminae*. The insensitive laminae continue to the ground surface as the laminae of the wall. The junction between the laminae of the wall and *epidermis of the sole* is called the *white line*.

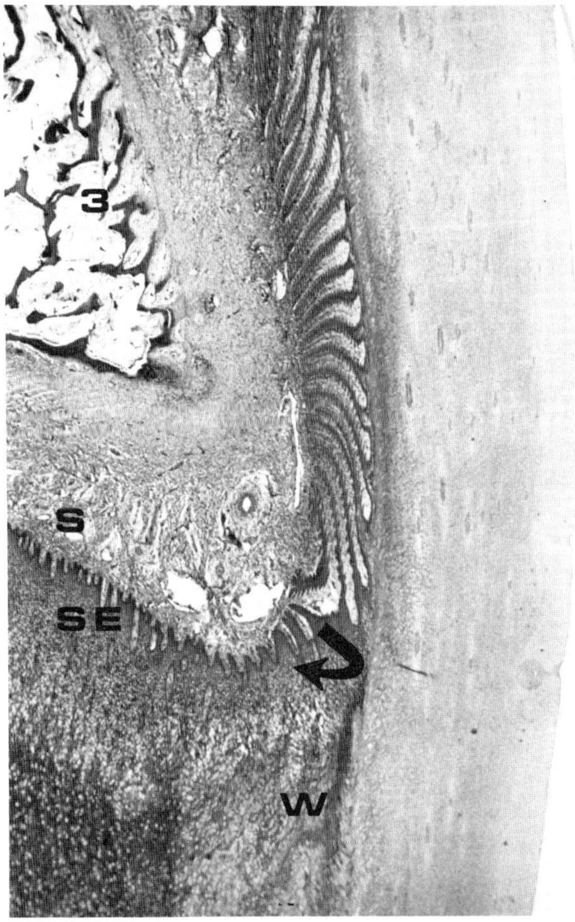

Fig. 16-34. Longitudinal section through the laminar and sole region of the equine foot. The corium and epidermis of the laminar region is continuous (*curved arrow*) with the sole corium (*S*) and sole epidermis (*SE*). The point of transition or reflection of the epidermis is continued to the ground surface as the white line (*W*). *3*, third phalanx. ×4.

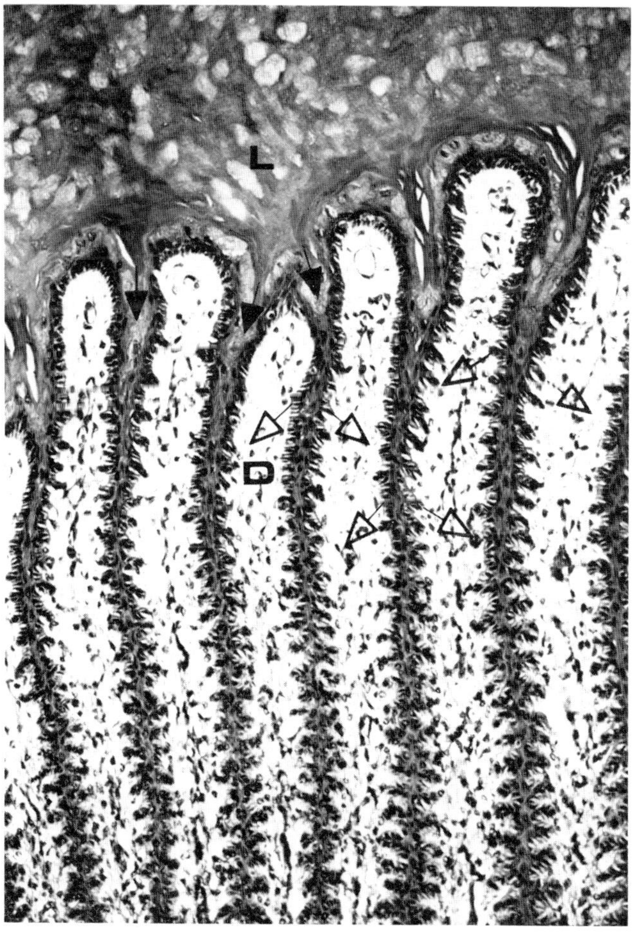

Fig. 16-35. Sensitive and insensitive laminae of the equine foot. The stratum lamellatum (*L*) and the primary epidermal pegs (*solid arrows*) comprise the insensitive laminae. The secondary pegs, as indicated by the orientation of the *open arrows*, constitute the sensitive laminae in conjunction with dermal components (*D*). ×100.

The epidermis and corium of the laminar region are oriented perpendicular to the ground surface. At the white line these structures are reflected around the corner of the wall and become parallel to the ground surface. This point of reflection results in the fusion of horn material which is oriented differently. Thus, the white line is formed. The white line is an important landmark for shoeing horses. A properly oriented nail driven peripherally to the white line will not touch any sensitive structures of the foot.

The *epidermis of the bars, sole* and *frog* is similar to the papillated regions described previously. However, the papillae are not as elongated as those described previously and the horn material is softer than that which composes the wall.

The corium of the foot is a continuation of the loose connective tissue which comprises the corium of the skin. The corium of the foot, however, does contain numerous elastic fibers. In the region of the coronary corium, an extensive venous plexus is present. In most instances, the corium of the foot is intimately associated with the fibrous periosteum of the enclosed osseous structures. These relationships aid not only in shock absorption but also in attaching the hoof to the deeper structures of the foot. The laminar corium attaches the laminar region to the third phalanx and assists in the suspension of the foot within the hoof. The corium of the frog contains modified sweat glands which invaginate from the horn of the frog.

A *digital cushion* occupies the space between the bones and tendons of the foot and the ground surface of the hoof. This fibroelastic connective tissue, which is rich in adipose tissue, is an effective shock absorber.

Ruminant and Porcine Claws. An understanding of the complexity of the equine hoof and related structures facilitates the understanding of similar structures in other species, because the latter are more simple histologically.

Although there are many gross differences between these and the equine hoof, there are only a few significant histological differences (Fig. 16-36). The claws of these species consist of: *wall*, *sole* and well-developed *bulbs*. The laminar epidermis consists of primary laminae only (Fig. 16-37). These occur with a greater frequency than in the horse. The orientation of the papillae of the sole is more craniad than in the horse. Usually, there are more zones of the epidermis apparent.

Claws of Carnivores. The claws of carnivores consist of a wall and sole. The coronary epidermis and associated corium comprise the majority of the wall and consist of long dermal papillae and corresponding epidermal pegs. Laminar epidermis and associated corium are restricted to the dor-

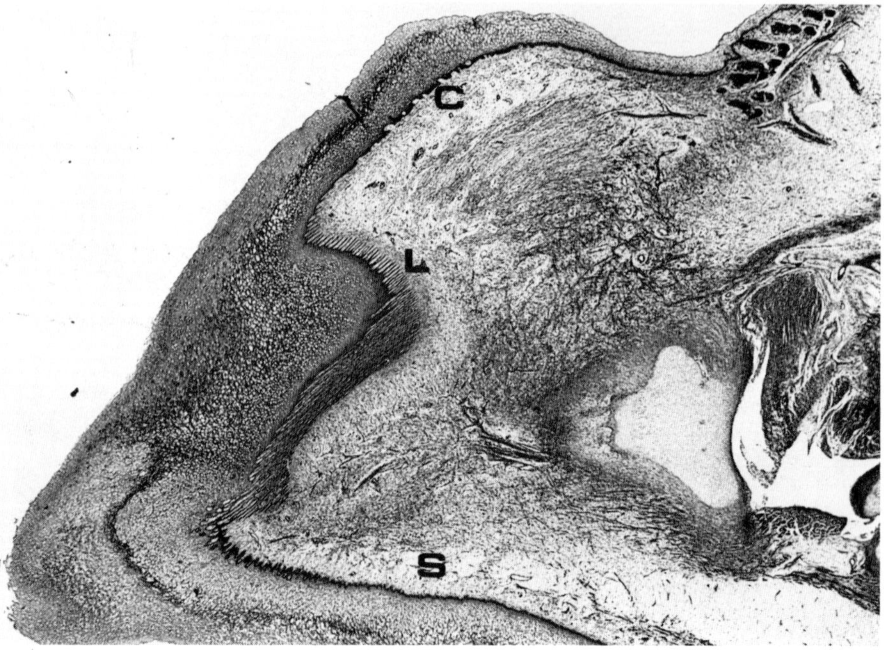

Fig. 16-36. Longitudinal section through the ovine fetal claw. The coronary (*C*), laminar (*L*) and sole (*S*) epidermis and corium are indicated. ×4.

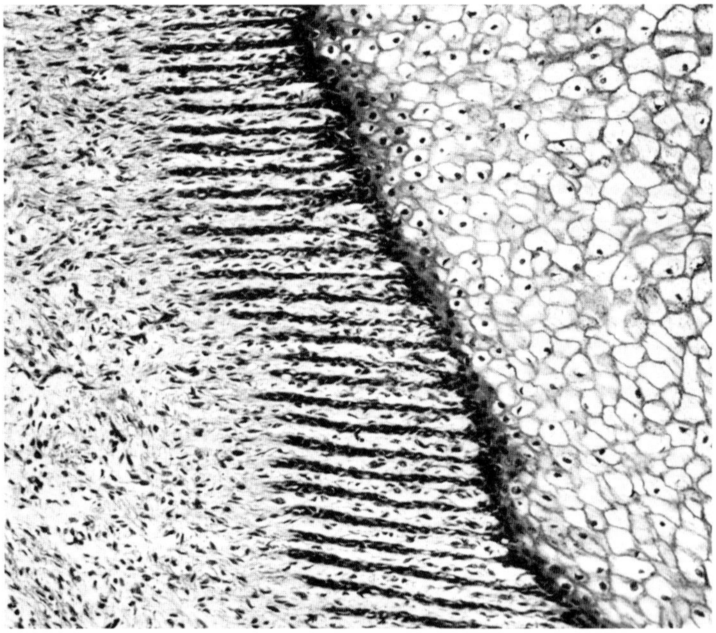

Fig. 16-37. Laminae of the fetal bovine claw. Only primary laminae are present. ×40.

solateral aspects of the wall. The sole corium consists of thick papillae.

Integumentary Appendages

Horns of the Ox. The horn of the ox consists of three basic components: *os cornua*, *corium* and *epidermis*. The *os cornua* or *frontal process* is an outgrowth of the frontal bone. The medullary cavity of the os cornua is continuous with the diploe of the frontal bone. It is covered by typical integumentary corium which is papillated. The associated epidermis gives rise to tubular horn and some intertubular horn. At the base of the horn the epidermis gives rise to soft horn, the *epikeras*, which is similar to the perioplic epidermis of the hoof.

Cellular proliferation of the basal cells of the epidermis is slow and the horn continues to elongate at a very slow pace.

Antlers of Cervids. The antlers of deer and associated species consist of bone and velvet. These structures undergo cyclic growth, maturation and shedding which is intimately associated with the seasonal breeding habits of these species. The bone develops by a modified type of endochondral ossification. During growth, the cartilage-like material is located at the end of each *tine*. It mineralizes and osseous replacement occurs. Eventually, as in the growth plate, the osseous replacement occurs at a faster rate than cartilage differentiation and "closure" occurs. At that point the core of the antler is bone which is continuous with the *pedicle* of the frontal bone. Throughout development, the developing bone is covered by the integument, *velvet*. Upon maturation, the velvet becomes necrotic and is removed by rubbing. The bony protuberance remains as the mature antler. An abscission zone develops at the base of the antler (similar to that which occurs in leaves) and it is dropped. At this point, the entire process begins again.

Besides being a biological curiosity, much information about chondrogenic and osteogenic processes may be had by the study of antler growth. Some species grow as much as 25 lb of bone during the 3-month active growing period at a rate of up to 1 cm per day at the antler tip. No mammalian growth process compares with it. Although antlers are usually confined to males, the female caribou and reindeer are antlered.

Miscellaneous Appendages. The horn of the pronghorn is very similar to the horn of the ox. However, the cornified material is shed annually.

The frontal process of the giraffe is similar to the antler. However, it is not shed.

The horn of the rhinoceros consists of matted hair.

Dewclaws, Chestnut and Ergot. *Dewclaws* of ruminants, swine and dogs represent vestigial digits covered by horn material and associated dermis similar to the horn material characteristic of the species. A bony core may or may not be present (limb and species variable).

Chestnuts and *ergots* are areas of the equine epidermis which are highly keratinized and consist of tubular and nontubular horn (Fig. 16-38). They are devoid of hairs and glands. Some authorities consider these to be vestiges of some of the digits.

References

Chase, H. B.: Growth of the hair. Physiol. Rev. *34*:113, 1954.

David, L. T.: Histology of the skin of the Mexican hairless swine (*Sus scrofa*). Amer. J. Anat. *50*:283, 1932.

Findlay, J. D. and Yang, S. H.: The sweat glands of Ayrshire cattle. J. Agric. Sci. *40*:126, 1950.

Godall, A. M. and Yang, S. H.: Myoepithelial cells in bovine sweat glands. J. Agric. Sci. *42*:159, 1952.

Hausman, L. A.: Structural characteristics of the hair of mammals. Amer. Natur. *44*:496, 1930.

Hibbs, R. G.: The fine structure of human exocrine sweat glands. Amer. J. Anat. *103*:201, 1958.

Moffat, G. H.: The growth of hair follicles and its relation to the adjacent dermal structures. J. Anat. *102*:527, 1968.

Montagna, W.: *The Structure and Function of the Skin*. 9th ed. Academic Press, New York, 1962.

Munger, B. L.: The cytology of apocrine sweat glands. I. Cat and monkey. Z. Zellforsch. *67*:373, 1965.

Stump, J. E.: Anatomy of the normal equine foot, including microscopic features of the laminar region. J. Amer. Vet. Med. Ass. *151*:1588, 1967.

Toker, C.: Observations on the ultrastructure of a mammary ductule. J. Ultrastruct. Res. *21*:9, 1967.

Webber, A. F., Kitchell, R. L. and Sautter, J. H.: Mammary gland studies. I. The identity and characterization of the smallest lobule unit in the udder of the dairy cow. Amer. J. Vet. Res. *16*:255, 1955.

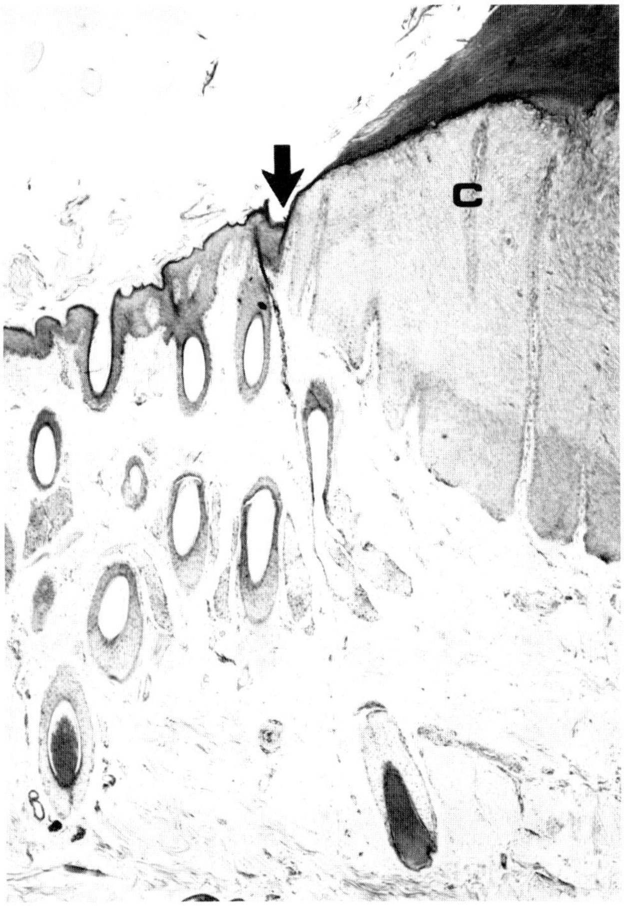

Fig. 16-38. Equine chestnut. The point of transition (*arrow*) from typical epidermis to chestnut (*C*) is marked by an increase in epidermal thickness and keratinization. ×10.

17 Digestive System

General Characteristics

Form and Function. The alimentary canal is a modified tube which generally conforms to a basic pattern (Chapter 10). This pattern of mural organization does vary from organ to organ but is usually modified in such a way that it is readily recognized as conforming, to a lesser or greater degree, to the basic pattern.

The diverse functions of this system are reflected in the numerous histological modifications that are apparent from mouth to anus. These vary from the heavily mineralized teeth to the numerous glands that are associated with this tubular system. Among the more obvious functions of this system are *prehension and mastication of food*, *conversion of foodstuffs* to a form acceptable to the soma and the *elimination of waste materials*. Some of the less obvious but important functions are *production of enzymes and digestive juices*, *vitamin production*, *detoxification of harmful materials* and *elaboration of essential body metabolites*. There are numerous other specific functions, but these will be discussed with the individual organs.

This system, because of its histological diversity, represents an excellent opportunity to study the types of variations that are manifested in the living animal.

Oral Structures

General Characteristics of the Buccal Cavity. This portion of the digestive system represents the greatest variation from the typical mural morphology. Numerous organs of diverse function occupy this region and tend to alter the tubular morphology. Generally, this portion of the system may be described as an extension of the skin which has been modified as a mucous membrane; i.e., it is lined by stratified squamous epithelium and kept moist by the secretions of numerous mucous and serous glands.

The lamina epithelialis is stratified squamous epithelium with varying degrees of cornification. Large epithelial papillae with cores of connective tissue project from the surface epithelium in some species. These assist in the prehension and mastication of food (ruminants).

The lamina propria blends insensibly with the tunica submucosa. Usually, the lamina propria is described as being devoid of glands; it possesses only the excretory ducts of the submucosal glands which are generally referred to as buccal glands. These are either mucous, serous or mixed glands.

The submucosal tunic blends with and rests upon the fascia associated with the underlying skeletal muscle. If absent, the lamina propria then assumes this relationship. In some instances, the skeletal muscle is replaced by bone. Then, the lamina propria or tunica submucosa will rest upon the periosteum of the associated bony structures.

Because the general histological appearance of the buccal cavity is quite uniform, only a few of the unique or different structures will be described.

Lip. This is the mucocutaneous junction, the point of transition from the epidermis to the mucous membrane of the buccal cavity (Fig. 17-1). The external surface is covered by a thin layer of keratinized stratified squamous epithelium. Hairs, sebaceous glands and tubular sweat glands are encountered more frequently on typical skin than on the lips. In large ruminants, the middle region of the dorsal lip is modified as the *muzzle* (*planum nasolabiale*). This region has a thick layer of keratinized epithelium which has numerous furrows on the surface. In small ruminants and the pig (*planum rostrale*), similar modifications are apparent; however, hairs are present. In carnivores, the planum is devoid of hairs and glands.

At the point of actual transition, the thin epidermis becomes the thickened cutaneous mucous membrane of the buccal cavity. It is keratinized in species whose diets contain much roughage (ruminants, horse). It is nonkeratinized in the pig and carnivores. The degree or absence of keratinization is diet-dependent.

The core of the lip is composed of fibroelastic connective tissue and skeletal muscle

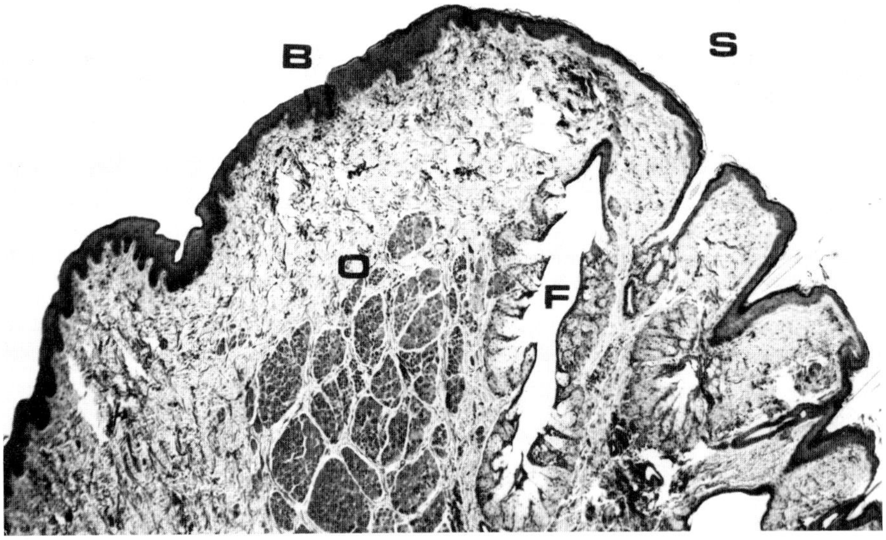

Fig. 17-1. A section through the feline lip. The buccal surface (B) is a mucous membrane. The skin (*S*) is typical and contains hair follicles (*F*) and associated sebaceous glands. The orbicularis oris muscle (*O*) is in the center of the structure. ×10. All light micrographs are the original magnifications. All electron micrographs are the final magnifications.

(*orbicularis oris*). On the integumentary side of the lip the dermis and hypodermis are typical. On the labial side the lamina propria and tunica submucosa are typical although not distinct from one another. Submucosal glands (*labial glands*) are present. They are mucous in small ruminants and carnivores and mixed in other species. These glands are branched tubuloalveolar types. They are serous glands in the bovine nasal planum. The tunica muscularis is skeletal muscle (orbicularis oris).

Cheek. The lamina epithelialis, lamina propria and tunica submucosa of the cheek are similar to the structure of the lip (Fig. 17-2). Serous or mucous *buccal glands* occupy the submucosal connective tissue space.

Hard Palate. The *hard palate* is composed of a keratinized stratifed squamous epithelium which is especially thick and highly keratinized in the *dental pad* of ruminants (Fig. 17-3). The lamina propria-submucosa is typical and is continuous with the fibrous periosteum of the bony roof of the buccal cavity. Adipose tissue and an extensive vascular bed are present. The posterior region of the hard palate of most species has numerous branched tubuloalveolar glands which may be mucous or mixed.

Soft Palate. The soft palate is a fibrous and muscular posterior extension of the hard palate. On its dorsal aspect (nasopharynx) it is covered by a pseudostratified ciliated columnar epithelium (*respiratory epithelium*), while its ventral side is covered by a typical cutaneous mucous membrane. The connective tissue core may contain glands similar to those in the hard palate. Lymphatic nodules are frequently encountered. The palatine tonsil of the pig is entirely within the soft palate.

Tongue. The tongue is a cranial projection from the ventral floor of the buccal cavity which is covered by stratified squamous epithelium and contains a core of connective tissue and skeletal muscle. Structures of significance which are part of the lingual composition are *lingual papillae*, *taste buds* and *lyssa*.

The lamina epithelialis consists of epithelium which is variously keratinized. Numerous epidermal pegs and dermal papillae comprise the epithelial and connective tissue junction (*papillary body*). Extensive invaginations of the dermal papillae into the epithelium result in evaginations of the mucous membrane as *lingual papillae*. In horses and ruminants the posterodorsal aspect of the tongue has a thickened mucous membrane which gives rigidity to this structure. The lamina propria and tunica submucosa are typical and blend with the connective tissue (epimysium) of the core of intrinsic and extrinsic lingual musculature.

The *lyssa* is characteristic of carnivores. It attaches the ventral portion of the tongue to the floor of the buccal cavity. It consists of

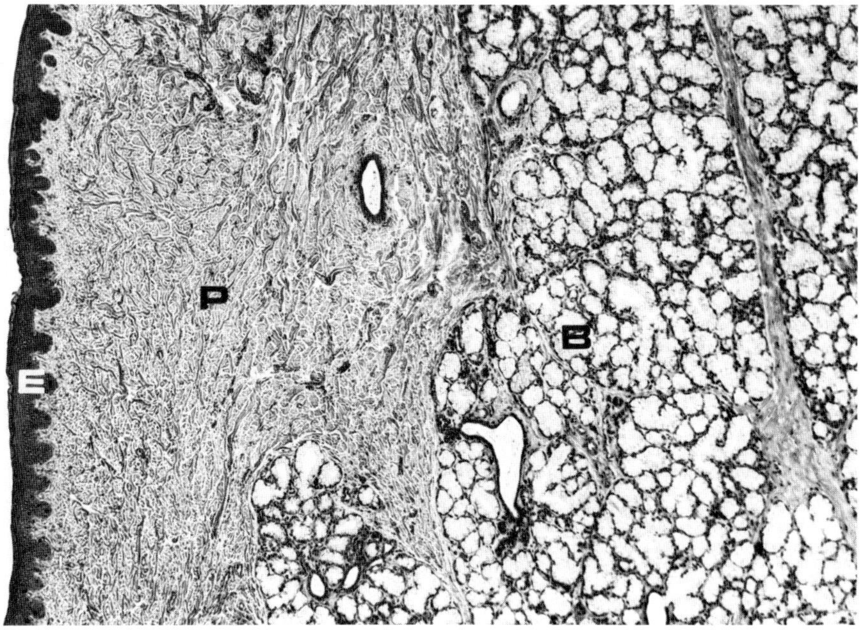

Fig. 17-2. A section of the feline cheek. The lamina epithelialis mucosae (*E*) is underlaid by a typical lamina propria (*P*). Numerous mucous buccal glands (*B*) are present. ×16.

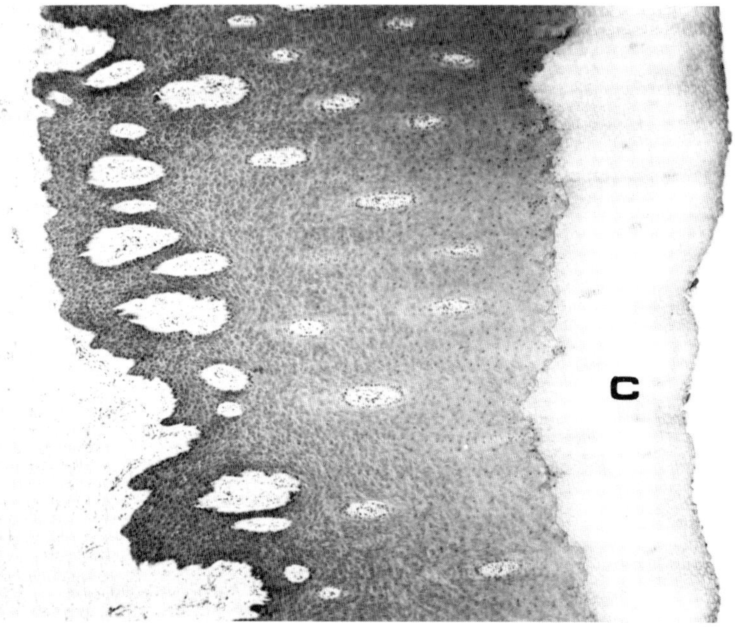

Fig. 17-3. The bovine dental pad. This structure replaces the upper incisors of ruminants. It is a thick lamina epithelialis which is highly cornified (*C*). ×10.

dense white fibrous connective tissue (DWFCT), some adipose tissue, skeletal muscle and occasionally some cartilage. In the pig it consists primarily of adipose connective tissue. It is not well-developed in horses and ruminants.

Lingual papillae are generally confined to the dorsal aspect of the tongue. These differ in size, form, number, distribution and function. Also, they are species-variable. The lingual papillae include the following; *filiform, lenticular, foliate, fungiform* and *circumvallate*.

Filiform papillae are the most numerous and are especially well-developed in the cat and ruminants wherein they serve mechanical functions (Fig. 17-4). These include prehension of foodstuffs and rasping activities. The keratinized papillae are shaped like rose thorns with their curvature directed caudad. The core of connective tissue is typical lamina propria.

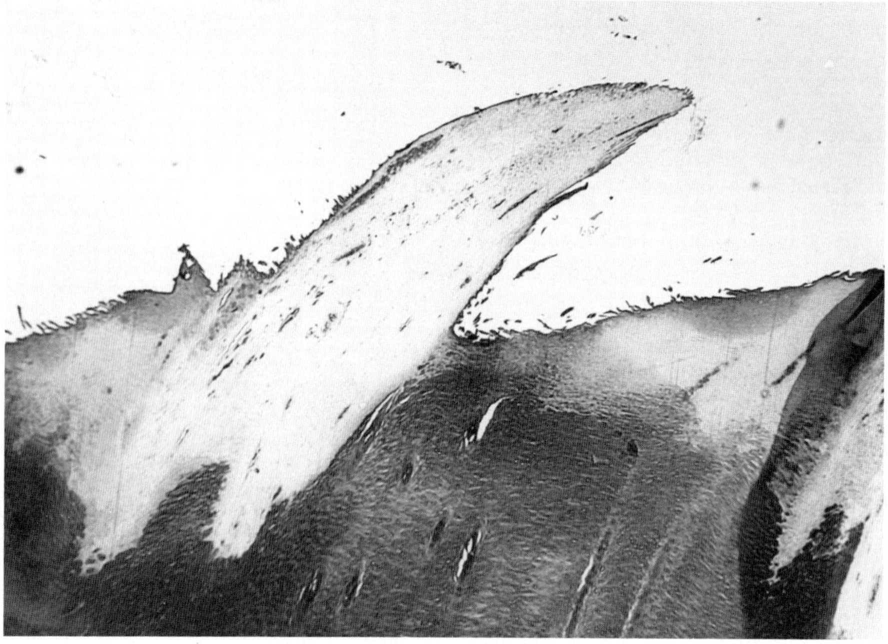

Fig. 17-4. A typical filiform papilla. ×10.

Lenticular papillae also serve mechanical functions (Fig. 17-5). The papillae are shaped like a double convex lens. They are especially prominent on the dorsum linguae of ruminants.

Fungiform papillae are mushroom-shaped papillae which serve a mechanical and gustatory function (Fig. 17-6). Taste buds may be present. These papillae are not as keratinized as the previous types. The primary papillation of the lamina propria is prominent and secondary papillations may be present. The connective tissue core, which may contain diffuse lymphatic tissue, is typical.

Foliate papillae are leaf-shaped and are separated from each other or the associated mucous membrane by an invagination of the mucous membrane (Fig. 17-7). These papillae are gustatory. The epithelium of these papillae is nonkeratinized. Finger-like projections from the lamina propria are present. Branched, tubuloalveolar serous glands of the lamina propria-submucosa open into the base of the *epithelial furrow*. These glands are *von Ebner's glands*. Taste buds occupy the lateral walls of the epithelial lining.

Circumvallate papillae are the largest papillae and those least encountered (Fig. 17-8). These papillae are not elevated above the lamina epithelialis and are surrounded by a deep furrow. Numerous taste buds are located in the lateral walls of the lamina epithelialis. The prominent connective tissue core is typical lamina propria. Branched, tubuloalveolar serous glands (von Ebner's glands) open into the base of the furrow and cleanse this region of foodstuffs.

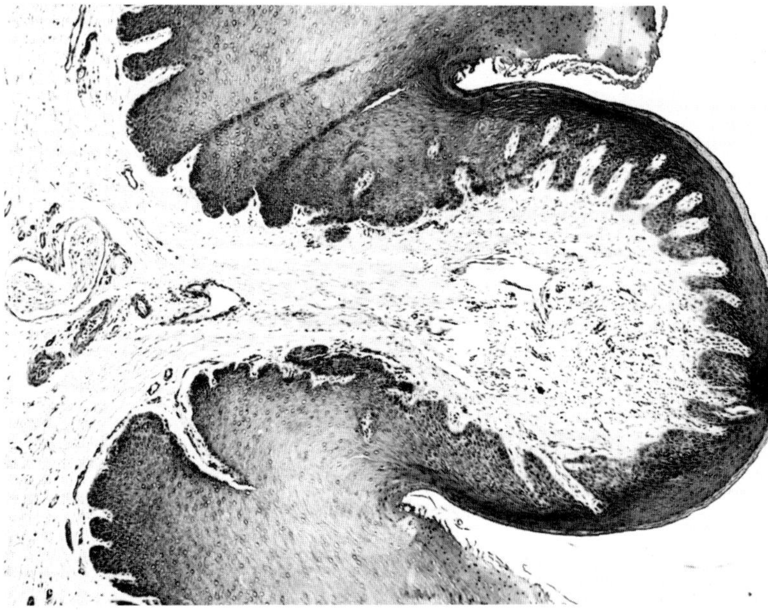

Fig. 17-5. A typical lentiform papilla. ×16.

The *taste buds* are the receptors for gustatory sensations which occur in the lateral walls of foliate, fungiform and circumvallate papillae (Fig. 17-9). Although their shape is variable, they usually assume an onion-like configuration. They extend

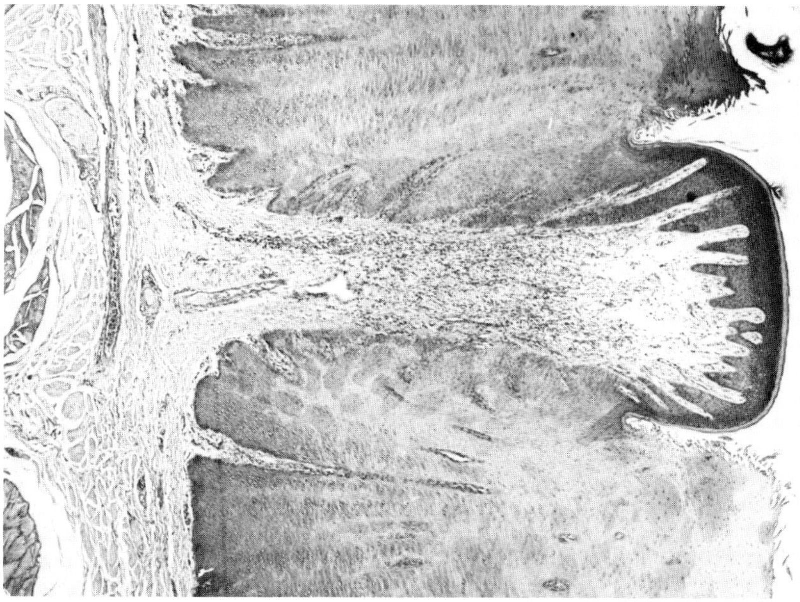

Fig. 17-6. A typical fungiform papilla. This structure may be gustatory. ×10.

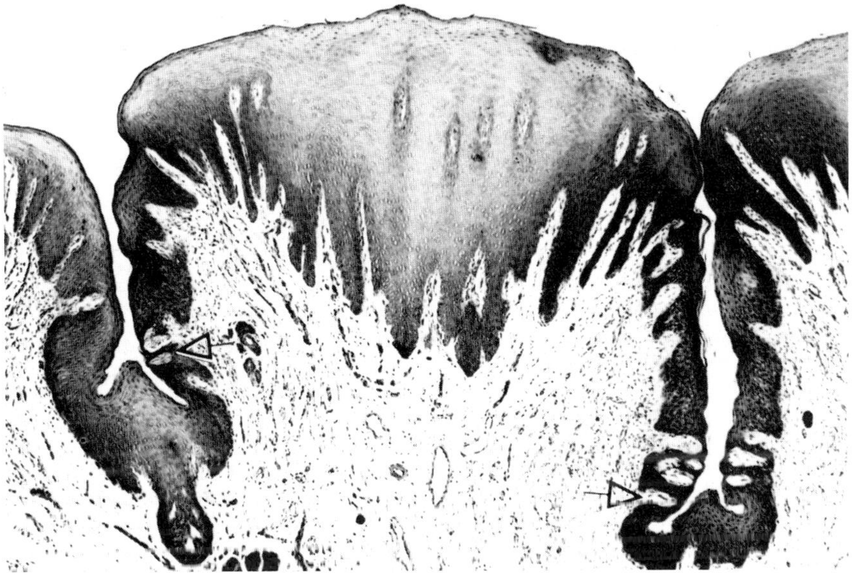

Fig. 17-7. A typical foliate papilla. These papillae are gustatory. *Arrows*, taste buds. ×16.

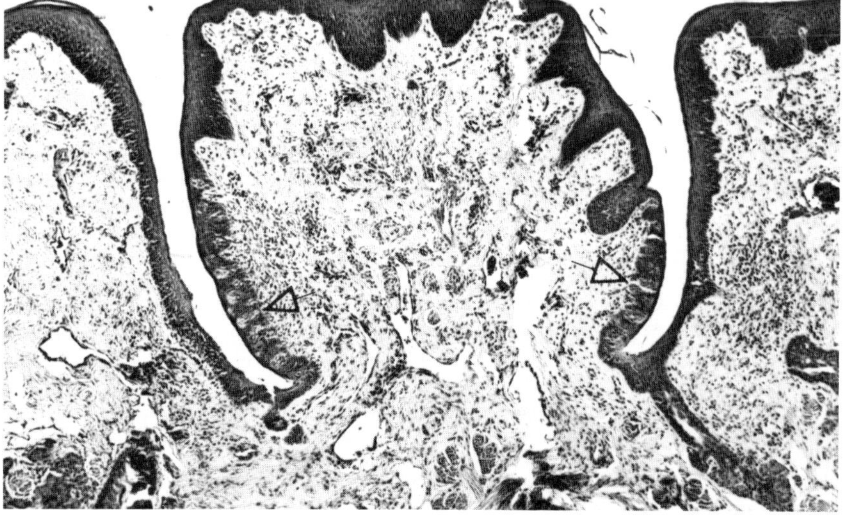

Fig. 17-8. A typical circumvallate papilla. Taste buds (*arrows*) are present. ×16.

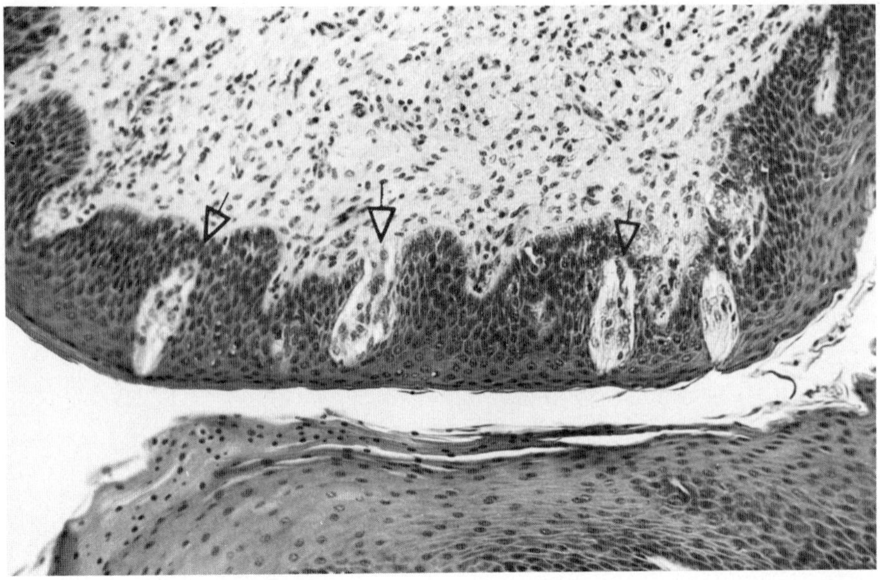

Fig. 17-9. Taste buds associated with circumvallate papillae. The taste buds (*arrows*) are intraepithelial structures. ×40.

from the superficial layer of the lamina epithelialis to the base of this lamina. An opening, the *taste pore*, is present at the surface. "Taste hairs," as extensions of the sensory cells, are closely associated with the pore.

Two types of cells comprise the taste bud (Fig. 17-10): *supporting cells* (*sustentacular*) and *gustatory cells* (*neuroepithelial*). Both cells are elongated or spindle-shaped. The *gustatory cell* (sensory cell) has a dense, acidophilic cytoplasm and a vesicular, elongated nucleus. The sustentacular cell has a vacuolated, acidophilic cytoplasm and a dense, elongated nucleus. Nuclear morphology is usually the distinguishing diagnostic feature. Numerous nonmyelinated fibers terminate on the sensory cells as *intragemmal fibers* or around the taste bud as *perigemmal fibers*.

Tonsils. Since the buccal cavity and associated structures are subjected to varied insults from foreign materials and microorganisms, numerous diffuse and aggregated accumulations of lymphatic tissue are present in the lamina propria-submucosa of this region. Invasion of lymphocytes into the lamina epithelialis from the associated connective tissue is a common occurrence in this region.

The tonsils are important, auxiliary protective organs of the posterior portion of the buccal cavity (Chapter 14).

Salivary Glands

General Remarks. These glands develop as evaginations of the gut lining. Although they are located at various distances from the buccal cavity, they are attached to it by their excretory ducts. They are best described as compound tubuloalveolar glands which elaborate mucous, serous or mixed secretory products. The mucoid product aids in bolus formation and also as a lubricant. The serous product moistens foodstuffs, aids in the adjustment of pH of the upper digestive tract, aids in the dissolution and tasting of foodstuffs and initiates a limited amount of carbohydrate hydrolysis. However, among the domestic species the pig seems to be the only animal that has a sufficient amount of salivary amylase to be of any consequence. Also, the salt content of the secretory products may assist in general somatic electrolyte regulation.

These glands conform to the pattern that typifies the compound, tubuloalveolar glands of the body. The following pathway from secretion to excretion is apparent: *alveolus—intercalated duct—secretory tubule* (*intralobular duct*)*—interlobular duct* (*intralobar duct*)*—lobar duct—excretory duct*. Specific differences in these glands, as compared to other compound tubuloalveolar glands, are related to the alveoli, intercalated ducts and secretory tubules (*striated ducts*). Striated ducts do not occur in purely mucous glands.

The adenomeres may be serous, mucous or mixed and may have serous demilunes (Fig. 17-11). The cells responsible for these secretions and their relationships were discussed in a previous section (Chapter 2). The *intercalated ducts* are small tubules that are lined by a low cuboidal epithelium (Fig. 17-12). They connect the alveoli to the striated ducts and are nonsecretory. The *striated ducts* are lined by a columnar epithelium which is characterized by infranuclear striations that result from dense accumulations of mitochondria and numerous infoldings of the basal plasmalemma (Fig. 17-13). These cells produce a serous-type product which consists of salts and water. At the point of transition from secretory tubule to smaller excretory duct, a bistratified columnar epithelium may be apparent. The entire excretory duct system is lined by a pseudostratified columnar epithelium at the opening into the buccal cavity.

Myoepithelial cells surround the alveoli and assist in the movement of the secretory products from the adenomeres.

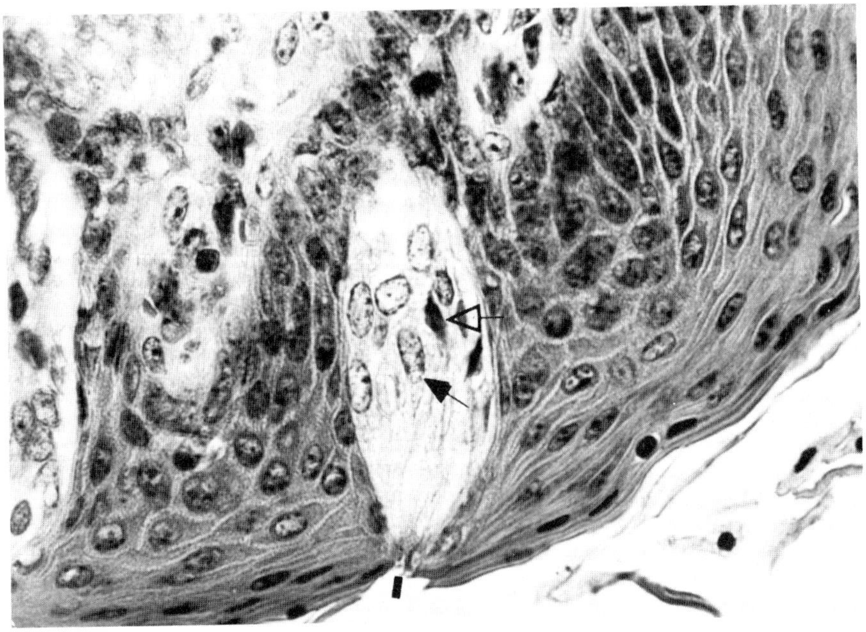

Fig. 17-10. The cells of taste buds. The sustentacular cells (*open arrow*) and gustatory cells (*solid arrow*) are spindle-shaped cells. The taste pore (*bar*) opens on the epithelial surface. ×160.

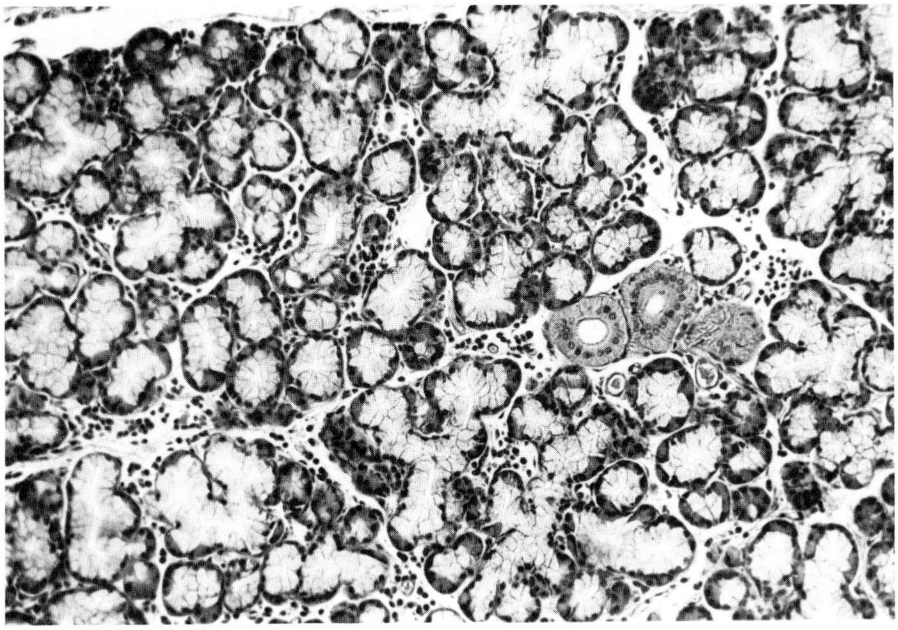

Fig. 17-11. An equine sublingual salivary gland. This is a mixed gland. ×40.

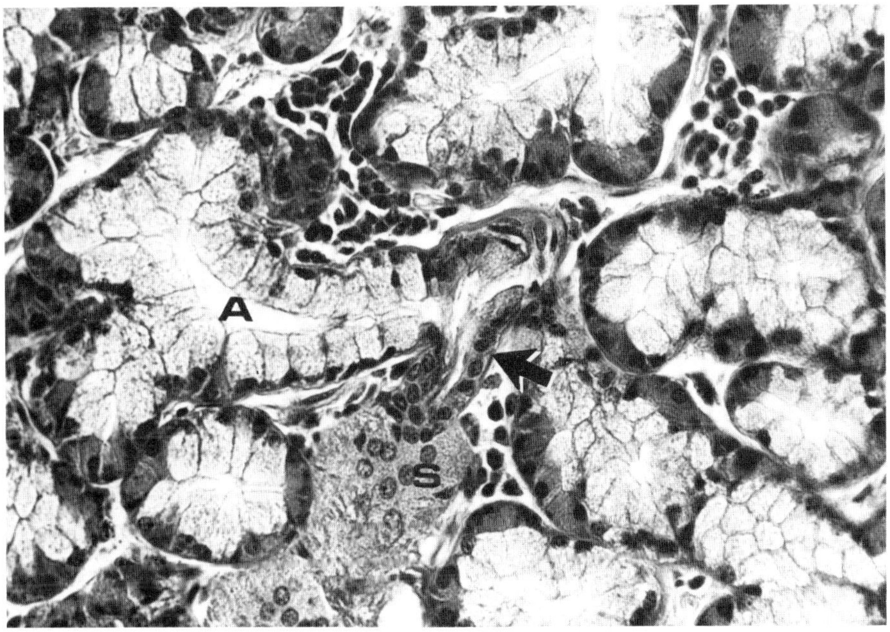

Fig. 17-12. Alveolus, intercalated duct and striated duct of a mixed salivary gland. The alveolus (*A*) is lined by mucous cells and serous demilunes. The intercalated duct (*arrow*) connects alveoli to striated ducts (*S*). ×100.

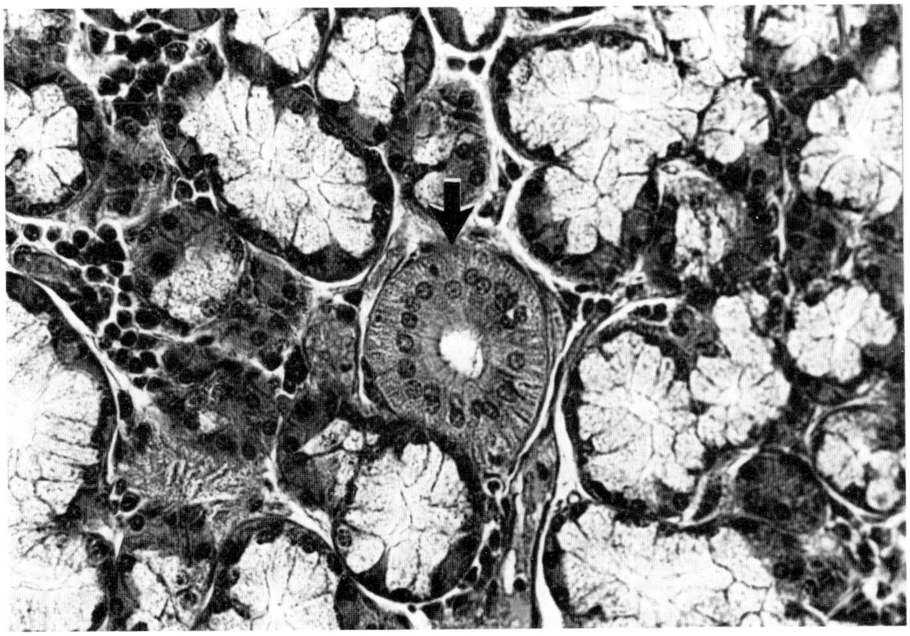

Fig. 17-13. Striated duct of a mixed salivary gland. The striated duct (*arrow*) is lined by columnar epithelium with basal striations. ×100.

The intralobular connective tissue consists of reticular or areolar connective tissue. It is more coarse in association with the larger excretory ducts. The lobar connective tissue is coarse and continuous with the coarse connective tissue of the capsule.

Parotid Gland. The parotid gland generally conforms to the previous description for salivary glands. This gland is a serous gland in all domestic animals, man and rodents (Fig. 17-14). It may be a mixed gland in young puppies and lambs.

Mandibular Gland. This gland also conforms to the previous description for salivary glands. It is a mucous gland in the dog (Fig. 17-15); serous in rodents; mixed in the horse, man and ruminants.

Sublingual Gland. Its morphology also conforms to the previous description. It is a mucous gland in rodents and the dog; mixed in ruminants, man and the horse (Fig. 17-16).

Miscellaneous Glands. Although the lingual, buccal and labial glands are not as large or as definitive as the previously described glands, they are, nevertheless, salivary glands. The nature of these glands is variable according to species and location. The *labial glands* are mucous in sheep and carnivores; serous in large ruminants, pig and horse; and mixed in man. The *dorsal buccal glands* are mucous in large ruminants, carnivores and horses; whereas the *ventral buccal glands* of these species are serous. The buccal glands of man and pig are mixed. Von Ebner's glands are serous, whereas the lingual glands of carnivores and sheep are mucous.

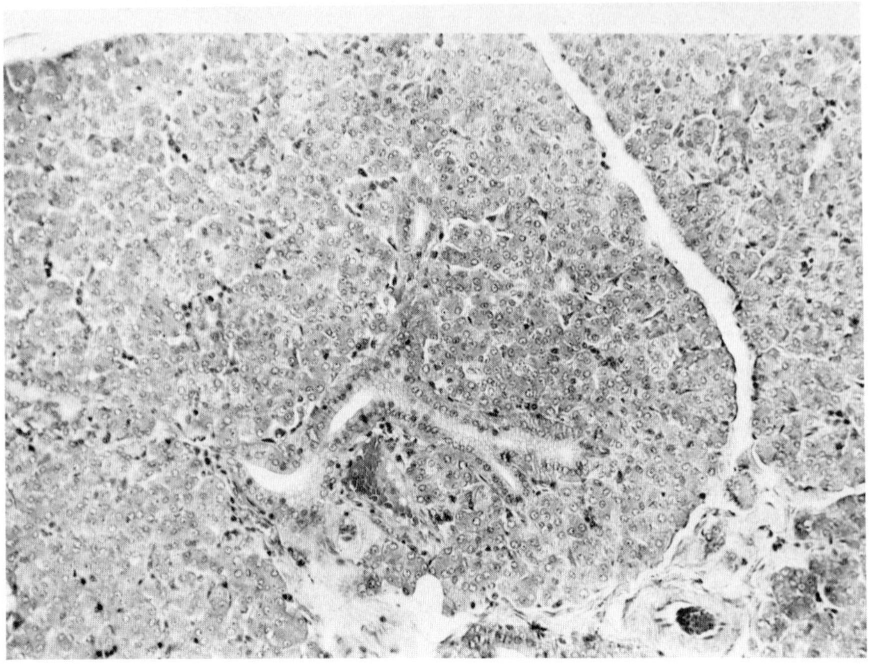

Fig. 17-14. Canine parotid salivary gland. This is a serous gland. ×40.

Teeth

General Characteristics. Although mammalian teeth differ in gross and subgross appearance, they consist of the same components: *enamel*, *dentine*, *cementum* and *pulp*. Teeth are either simple or complex. *Brachydont* (*simple*) teeth do not continue to grow at the completion of eruption (Fig. 17-17). Further, these teeth are divisible into a definitive *crown*, *neck* and *root*. The *hypsodont* (*complex*) teeth of ruminants, rodents and the horse are constantly erupting structures (Fig. 17-18). These teeth do not possess a definitive crown, neck and root. Rather, they are considered to be composed of root only. The hypsodont teeth include the cheek teeth of ruminants, all of the teeth of the horse, the incisorform teeth of rodents and the canine teeth of the pig.

Different teeth are modified for various functions: tearing, shearing or crushing of foodstuffs. Also they are excellent protective devices.

Development of Simple Teeth. The development of teeth requires contributions from the epithelium and the underlying connective tissue (Fig. 17-19). An epithelial ridge,

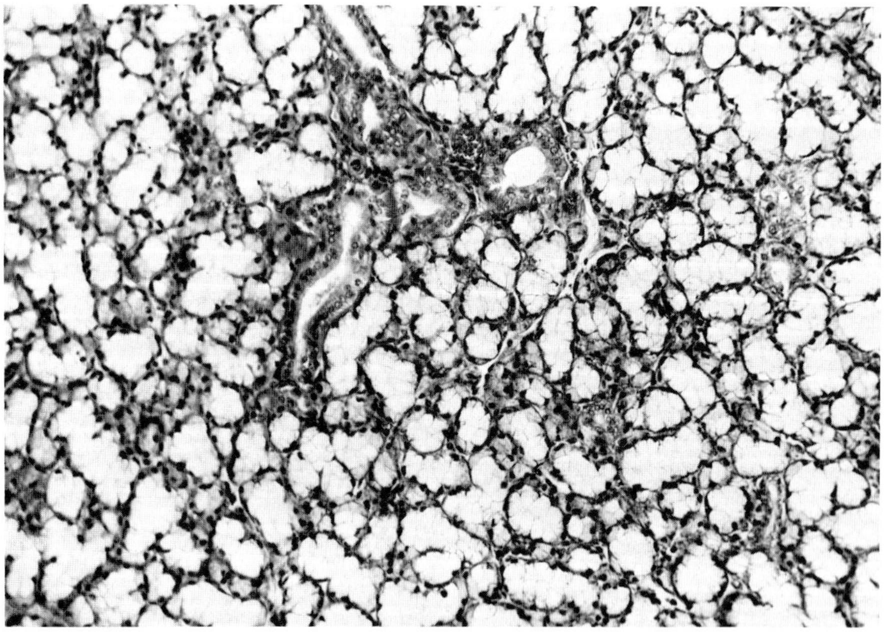

Fig. 17-15. Canine mandibular salivary gland. This is a mucous gland. ×40.

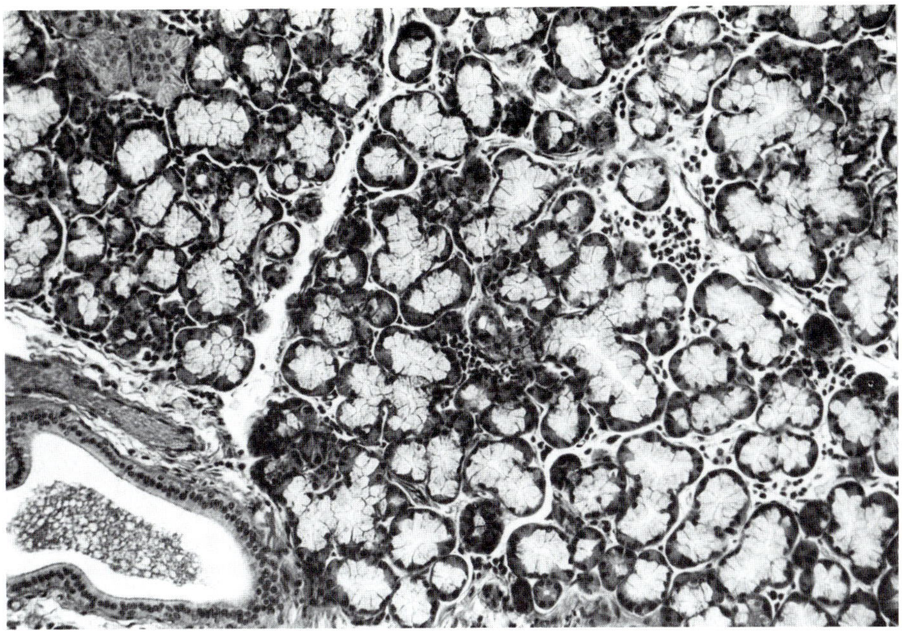

Fig. 17-16. Equine sublingual salivary gland. This is a mixed gland. ×40.

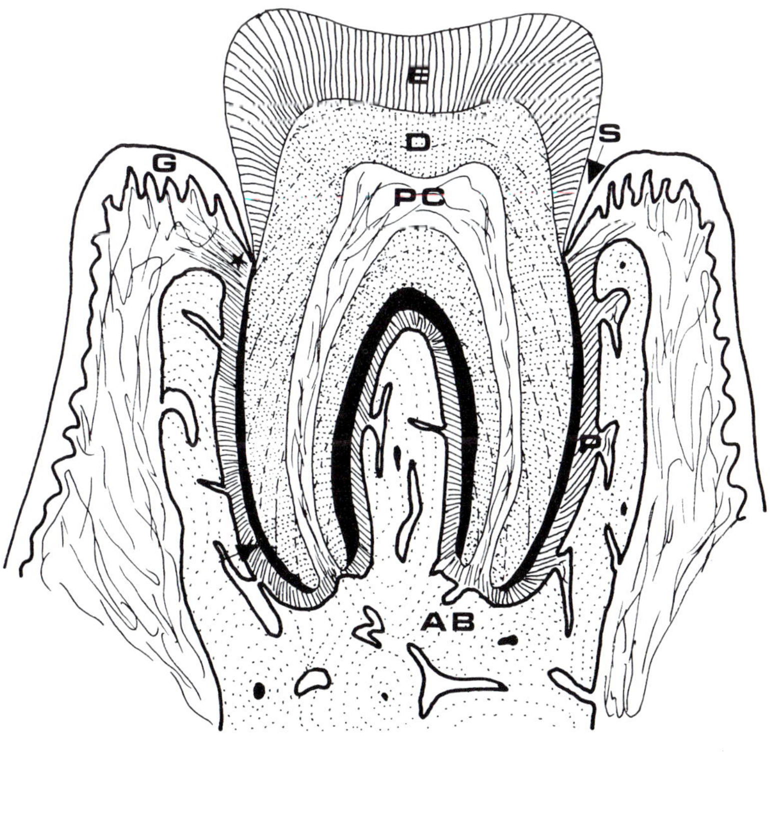

Fig. 17-17. A brachydont molariform tooth. The enamel (*E*) and dentine (*D*) above the epithelial attachment (*star*) constitute the crown of the tooth. The dentine and cementum (*arrow*) below the epithelial attachment are the roots of the tooth. The gingiva (*G*) forms a gingival sulcus (*S-arrow*) along the margin of the crown above the gingival attachment at the neck. The periodontal ligament (*P*) attaches the cementum to the alveolar bone (*AB*) and suspends the tooth in the alveolus. The pulp cavity (*PC*) is continuous throughout the tooth.

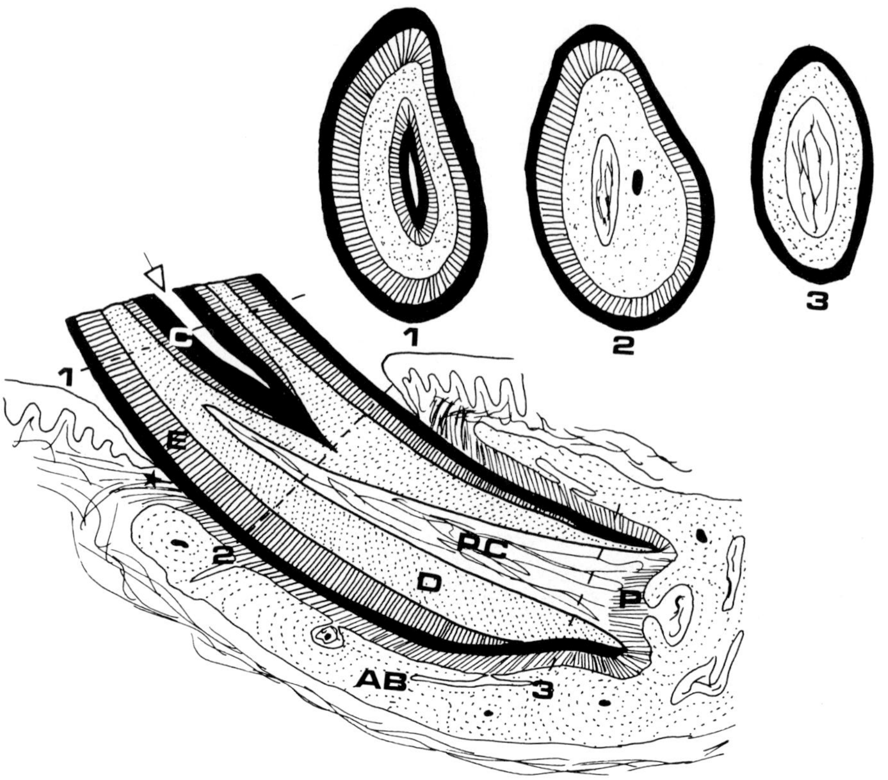

Fig. 17-18. A hypsodont incisorform tooth. The entire tooth is covered by cementum (*C*). This material also fills and lines the infundibulum (*arrow*). The gingiva is reflected and attaches to the tooth (*star*), and the periodontal ligament (*P*) attaches the cementum to the alveolar bone (*AB*). The enamel (*E*) is adjacent to the dentine (*D*). The pulp cavity (*PC*) contains loose connective tissue, vessels and nerves. The levels of the cross-sections (*1*, *2*, *3*) are indicated on the *in situ* tooth.

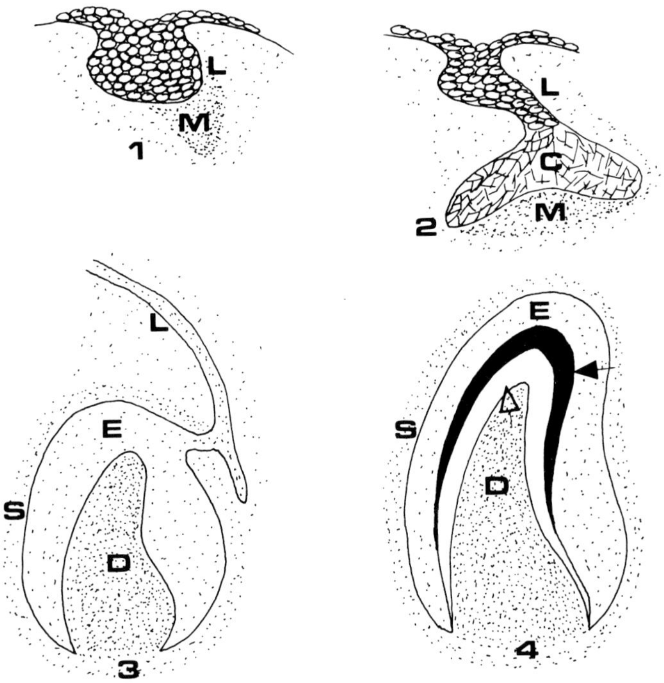

Fig. 17-19. Early development of a tooth. *L*, dental lamina; *M*, condensed mesenchyme; *C*, cap stage; *E*, enamel organ; *S*, dental sac; *D*, dental papilla; *solid arrow*, enamel; *open arrow*, dentine. The gingival epithelium proliferates as the dental lamina and is associated with condensed mesenchyme (*1*). Progressive growth of the dental lamina results in the cap stage (*2*). The enamel organ is formed during the bell stage (*3*). The dental sac and dental papilla are well-defined. Enamel and dentine form subsequently (*4*). The relationship of tooth development to the alveolar bone is not indicated.

dental lamina, develops in the *dental arch* of each jaw and grows into the underlying mesenchymal region. Proliferation of the epithelium along the lateral border of the lamina further extends this structure into the mesenchyme. From this lateral extension, the *enamel organs* of the *deciduous teeth* (*milk teeth*) arise. At a later period, medial or lingual outgrowths of the dental lamina give rise to enamel organs of the *permanent teeth*. Proliferation of the invading epithelium as a solid mass of cells continues to the *cap stage* accompanied by a mesenchymal condensation at the base of the cap (Fig. 17-20).

By complementary growth of the epithelium and associated mesenchymal tissue of the *dental papilla*, the *bell stage* is achieved (Fig. 17-21). The epithelium is now the *enamel organ* and is divisible into distinct regions: *inner enamel epithelium*, *stellate reticulum* and *outer enamel epithelium* (Fig. 17-22). The *inner enamel epithelium* consists of columnar cells, *ameloblasts*, which are separated from the dental papilla by a basement membrane. This epithelium is continuous with the *outer enamel epithelium* at the lower edges (rim) of the bell. This outer epithelium is composed of small, flattened cells. The center of the enamel organ is composed of the *stellate reticulum*. The central cells, previously tightly packed, are separated by extensive intercellular spaces. These cells are stellate in appearance. The region of contact between the stellate reticulum and the inner enamel epithelium is occupied by cuboidal cells, the *stratum intermedium* (Fig. 17-22). As development of the tooth progresses, the stellate reticulum (*enamel pulp*) atrophies and the outer enamel epithelium collapses upon the inner enamel epithelim.

The dental papilla is entrapped within the confines of the enamel organ. A thin layer of columnar cells differentiate from the mesenchyme along the inner surface of the basement membrane, the odontoblasts. The remainder of the papilla becomes the pulp of the tooth. It consists of blood vessels, nerves and loose connective tissue.

An indistinct mass of connective tissue circumscribes the enamel organ and dental papilla. The connective tissue of this *dental sac* is continuous with the connective tissue of the dental papilla. The dental sac is of importance because it gives rise to the following:

1. It gives rise to the *alveolar bone* and periosteum surrounding the root.
2. It forms a layer of *cementum* peripheral to the dentine of the root.
3. It forms a network of anchoring collagenous fibers which connect the cementum of the root to the alveolar bone, the *periodontal membrane*.

The sequence of tooth development includes the differentiation of enamel, dentine and cementum. The deposition of enamel is

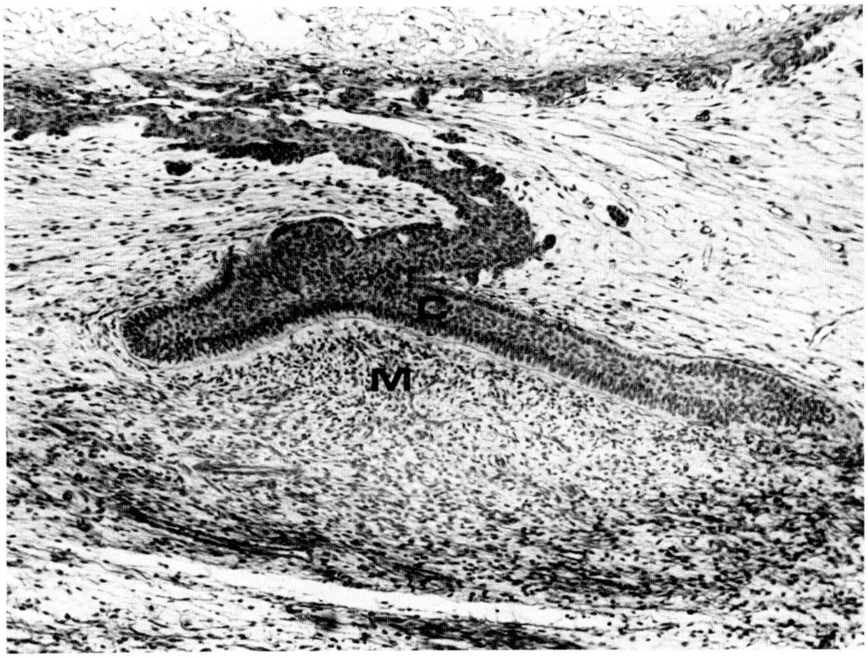

Fig. 17-20. Cap stage of a secondary tooth bud. The enamel organ is still a condensed mass of epithelial cells (*C*) associated with a condensation of mesenchyme (*M*). ×25.

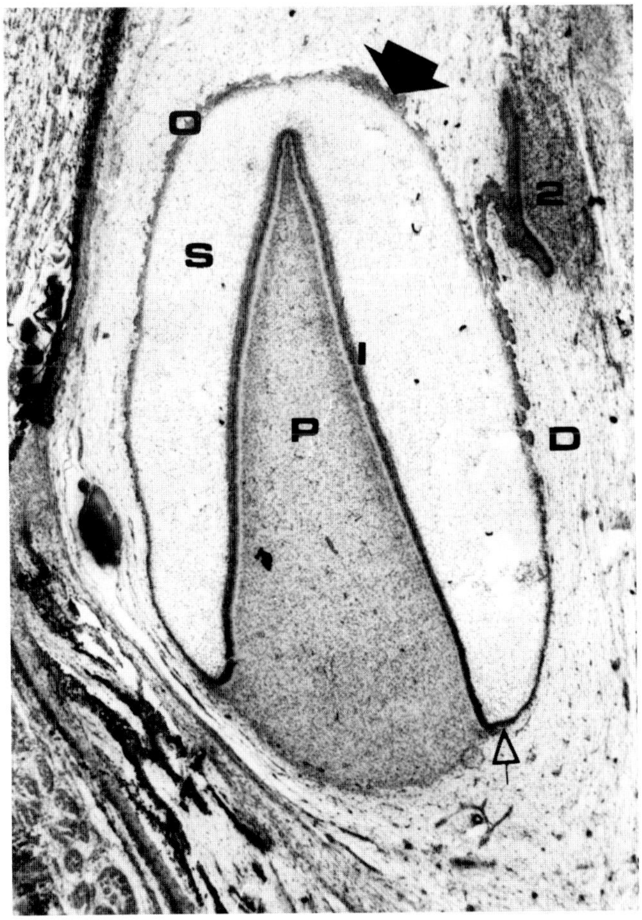

Fig. 17-21. Enamel organ in an early bell stage. The enamel organ (*solid arrow*) has a permanent tooth bud attached to it (*2*). The enamel organ consists of an outer enamel epithelium (*O*) which is continuous with inner enamel epithelium (*I*) at the rim of the organ (*open arrow*). The stellate reticulum (*S*) is between the inner and outer epithelia. The organ surrounds a mesenchymal condensation, the dental papilla (*P*). *D*, dental sac. ×6.

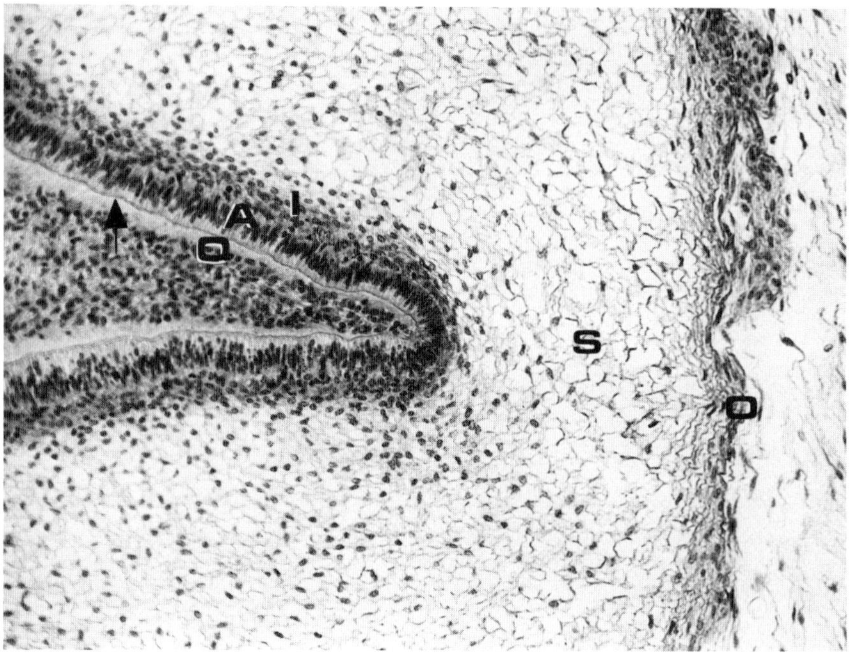

Fig. 17-22. Components of the enamel organ. The outer enamel epithelium (*O-right*) is adjacent to the stellate reticulum (*S*). A layer of cuboidal cells, stratum intermedium (*I*), underlies the inner enamel epithelium which is composed of ameloblasts (*A*). The ameloblasts are separated from the odontoblasts (*O-left*) of the dental papilla by a basement membrane (*arrow*). ×40.

achieved by the secretory activity of the ameloblasts. This appositional process proceeds from the apex of the papilla toward the gingiva and rim of the bell. This process is initiated following the deposition of secretory products from the odontoblasts. The odontoblasts secrete their products in such a way that predentine and dentine are deposited at the apex of the papilla, laterally toward the rim and in a direction opposite to enamel deposition. This process, also, is appositional. The activities of the ameloblasts and the odontoblasts result in the formation of the *crown* of the tooth.

At the point of continuity between the inner and outer enamel epithelium (the future *neck* region of the tooth) a fold of epithelium develops and grows downward as the *epithelial root sheath* (*sheath of Hertwig*). Dentine continues to develop in this region. Instead of enamel, however, the mesenchyme interdigitates itself between the odontoblasts and the root sheath and cementum develops. The root, therefore, consists of cementum and dentine. And, the transition from crown to root is the *neck* of the tooth.

As the aforementioned processes are occurring, the dental sac gives rise to the alveolar bone and other structures. The downward growth of the root exerts pressure against the stationary alveolar bone which results in a translation of upward movement or *eruption*.

During eruption, the crown of the tooth breaks through the enamel organ and gingiva. The ameloblast activity ceases at eruption. The continued deposition of the root during eruption, however, results in the definitive position of the tooth being achieved.

The subsequent development of the enamel organ of the permanent teeth follows the same steps outlined. As the permanent tooth bud develops, its growth exerts pressure against the root and associated structures of the deciduous tooth which results in resorption. The loss of the deciduous tooth is followed closely by its permanent tooth replacement.

Cellular and Matrix Components of Teeth. The cellular components of teeth include *ameloblasts*, *odontoblasts*, *cementoblasts* and various connective tissue cells. The matrix components include *enamel*, *predentine*, *dentine*, *cementum* and *periodontal membrane*.

The ***ameloblasts*** are columnar cells which in cross-section appear hexagonal (Fig. 17-23). These polarized cells have an elongated, basally positioned nucleus. The basal part of the cell is rich in mitochondria. The apical portion of the cell is rich in granular endoplasmic reticulum and Golgi apparatus. At the apex of the cell, *Tome's processes*

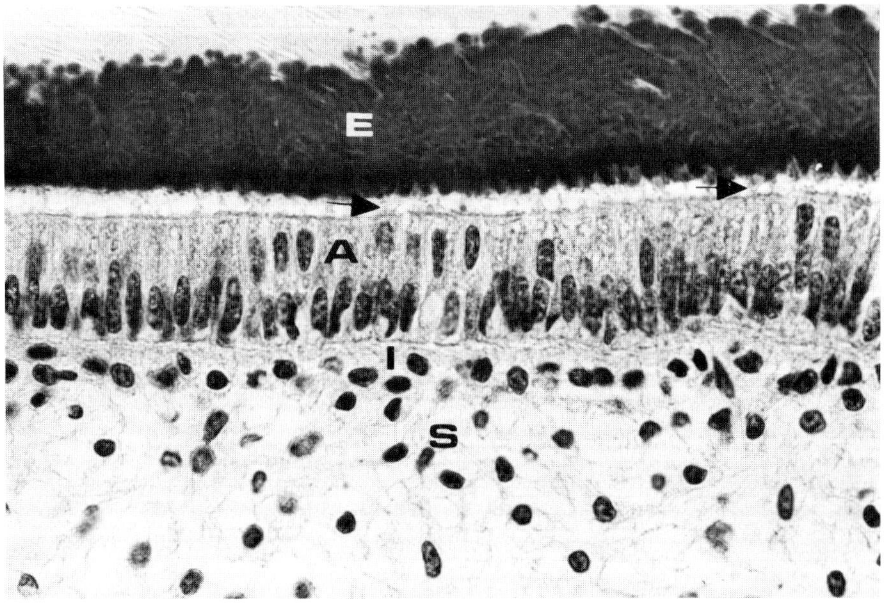

Fig. 17-23. Layer of ameloblasts. The ameloblasts (*A*) are intimately associated with the stratum intermedium (*I*) which is continuous with the stellate reticulum (*S*). Enamel (*E*) has been deposited and Tome's processes (*arrows*) are apparent. ×160.

(prismatic extensions of the ameloblast apical cytoplasm) are apparent. Material for enamel formation is secreted through these processes in the form of rods as a slightly mineralized substance. During the secretory processes, the ameloblasts retreat before their advancing front of secretory products. The result is an acellular enamel composed of rods and inter-rod material. Enamel consists of approximately 95–97% of inorganic material in the form of apatite crystal. It is the hardest substance in the body. Upon completion of enamel formation, the ameloblasts disintegrate. Enamel, therefore, is incapable of repair.

Odontoblasts are not as tightly packed together as the ameloblasts (Fig. 17-24). These columnar cells are also polarized. The predominant organelles are the apically disposed granular endoplasmic reticulum and a large supranuclear Golgi apparatus. The initial secretory product of the odontoblasts is predentine. It is deposited initially at the dentinal-enamel junction. It is not a uninterrupted layer. Rather, it contains *odontoblastic processes* (*Tome's fibers, dentinal fibers*). As predentine is secreted the odontoblasts retreat before the advancing front, but their processes remain and are contained within *dentinal tubules*. Subsequent mineralization of predentine results in *dentine*. This method of secretion is similar to the relationship between osteoid seam and mineralizing bone. Dentine, however, contains about 69% inorganic substances.

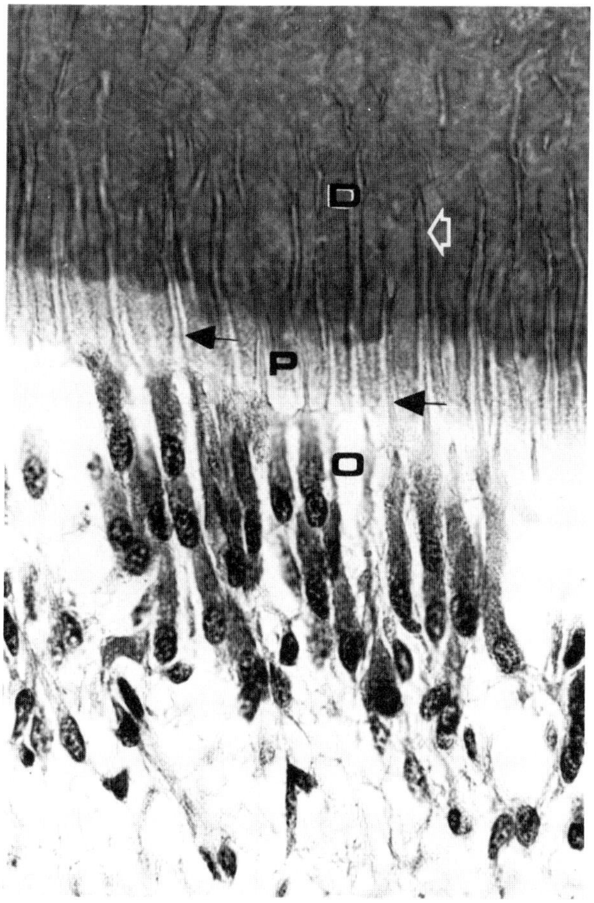

Fig. 17-24. Layer of odontoblasts. The odontoblasts (*O*) have apical processes, dentinal fibers (*solid arrows*), which extended into dentinal tubules (*open arrow*). Predentine (*P*) is deposited and then mineralized as dentine (*D*). ×160.

Unlike ameloblasts, odontoblasts do not disintegrate upon the completion of their secretory activity. Rather, they are viable and potentially functional cells throughout the life of a tooth.

Cementoblasts are differentiated from the dental sac and give rise to *acellular cementum* and *cellular cementum*. This material with its contained *cementocytes* is very similar to woven or immature bone. Sharpey's fibers become embedded in this material by an appositional growth of cementum around the collagenous fibers. This process is similar to the means by which the collagen of tendons is incorporated in and attached to bone.

The *periodontal membrane* consists of coarsely bundled collagenous fibers and fibroblasts. These fibers are embedded in the cementum and associated alveolar bone as Sharpey's fibers. These fibers anchor the tooth in the *alveolus* (*socket*) and are the fibers ruptured during tooth extraction.

Brachydont Dentition. The *crown* of the tooth is covered by enamel and is that portion of the tooth visible above the *gingiva* (Fig. 17-17). The crown is composed of enamel and dentine. The dentine is visible on the surface in worn teeth from which the enamel has been removed by constant abrasion. The *neck* of the tooth is the point of transition between the crown and the root. It is, importantly, the point of *epithelial attachment* to the cementum. The *gingival crevice* or *gingival sulcus* is the depression between the tooth and gingiva above the point of epithelial attachment. The point of the gingiva adjacent to the crown is termed the *gingival crest*. The gingival sulcus and epithelial attachment are especially significant in periodontal disease. *Tartar* or *calculus* commonly accumulates on the tooth in the gingival sulcus.

The root is composed of dentine and cementum in apposition to one another. The periodontal membrane serves as the suspension mechanism between the alveolar bone and cementum of the root.

The dental pulp is a loose connective tissue rich in vascular supply and nerves. It is bounded by the dentine of the crown and root (or roots).

Hypsodont Dentition. The constantly erupting teeth are morphologically somewhat different from the brachydont teeth (Fig. 17-18). This difference is based upon some alterations in the developmental sequence. In brachydont teeth the enamel organ is intact until the time of eruption. In hypsodont teeth, the enamel organ is ruptured prior to eruption. This brings the connective tissue of the dental sac in close association to the newly formed enamel. As a result, cementum is deposited on the enamel. Also, the resulting morphology of the mature hypsodont tooth, especially the *infundibular recess*, requires that the enamel organ is more complex in surface morphology than that of simple teeth.

In brachydont teeth, the eruption of the crown is accompanied by the disintegration of the ameloblasts. In hypsodont teeth, ameloblasts do not disintegrate. They continue their activity for an extended period beyond eruption.

Although hypsodont teeth are described as root teeth without a definitive crown, neck and root, this is not entirely true. A typical root (cementum and dentine) is confined to the lower portion of the tooth.

Pharynx and Esophagus

Pharynx. The *oropharynx* is an extension of the buccal cavity and connects it with the esophagus. The lamina epithelialis is stratified squamous epithelium. Varying degrees of keratinization are species-variable. The lamina propria is typical and contains tonsils, individual lymph nodules and scattered leucocytes. Numerous papillae are obvious and resemble dermal papillae of the skin. Although a typical lamina muscularis is not present, a layer of elastic fibers delimits this space from the tunica submucosa. The latter is typical and contains branched tubuloalveolar mucous glands. The tunica muscularis is composed of striated muscle which is not oriented in any particular manner. The tunica adventitia is typical and blends with the accompanying deep fascia.

Esophagus. This structure is a muscular tube that is modified for the voluntary and involuntary movement of foodstuffs to the caudal portions of the alimentary canal.

The lamina epithelialis is stratified squamous epithelium. Varying degrees of cornification may be apparent. It is especially apparent in those species which ingest hard, dry foodstuffs.

The lamina propria is typical and in some species may contain numerous lymph nodules and scattered lymphatic tissue (man and pig). These are especially prominent at the esophageal-gastric junction. Small blood vessels, lymph vessels and nerves are present.

The lamina muscularis mucosae is typical but of variable occurrence (Fig. 17-25). This muscular layer is continuous with the elastic fiber layer of the pharynx. In man it is a thick and complete layer. In the horse, ruminants and the cat, it consists of scattered muscle bundles which may eventually fuse in the aboral portion of the esophagus. In the dog and pig, it is absent in the cervical portion; it may become complete near the stomach (Fig. 17-26).

The tunica submucosa is typical and contains numerous branched tubuloalveolar mucous glands. These glands are present the entire length of the canine esophagus; in the pig they are present in the cervical portion but sparse in the thoracic portion; in ruminants, the horse and cat they are present in the cervical portion.

The tunica mucosa and tunica submucosa have longitudinal folds that permit expansion of the esophagus.

The tunica muscularis consists of striated muscle, smooth muscle or a mixture of both. The inner and outer lamina may be distinct in the aboral portions. Striated muscle, smooth muscle or a mixture of both vary according to species: in ruminants and the dog it is entirely striated (Fig. 17-27); in the pig the cervical portion consists of striated muscle, the thoracic portion is mixed and the caudal portion consists of smooth muscle; in the horse and cat it consists of striated muscle to the middle portion and then consists of smooth muscle.

The tunica adventitia is typical in the cranial portion. It is replaced by a tunica

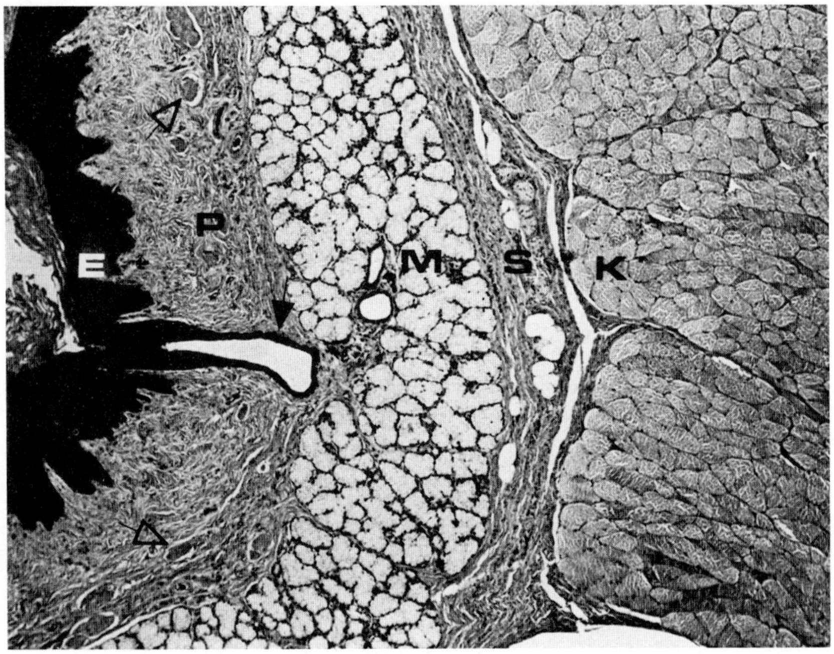

Fig. 17-25. Porcine esophagus (lower cervical region). The lamina epithelialis (*E*) is supported by a lamina propria (*P*). The lamina muscularis consists of scattered bundles of smooth muscle (*open arrows*). Mucous glands (*M*) are continuous with the epithelial lining via excretory ducts (*solid arrow*). A tunica submucosa (*S*) is adjacent to the skeletal muscle (*K*) of the tunica muscularis. ×12.

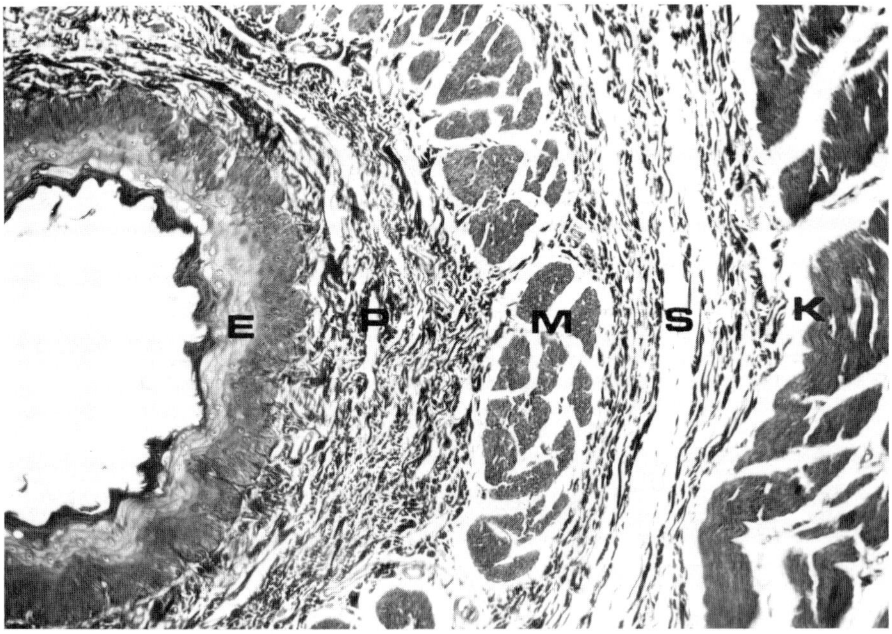

Fig. 17-26. Canine esophagus (thoracic region). The lamina epithelialis (*E*) and lamina propria (*P*) are typical. The lamina muscularis (*M*) is extensive. The tunica submucosa (*S*) is adjacent to the skeletal muscle of the tunica muscularis (*K*). ×40.

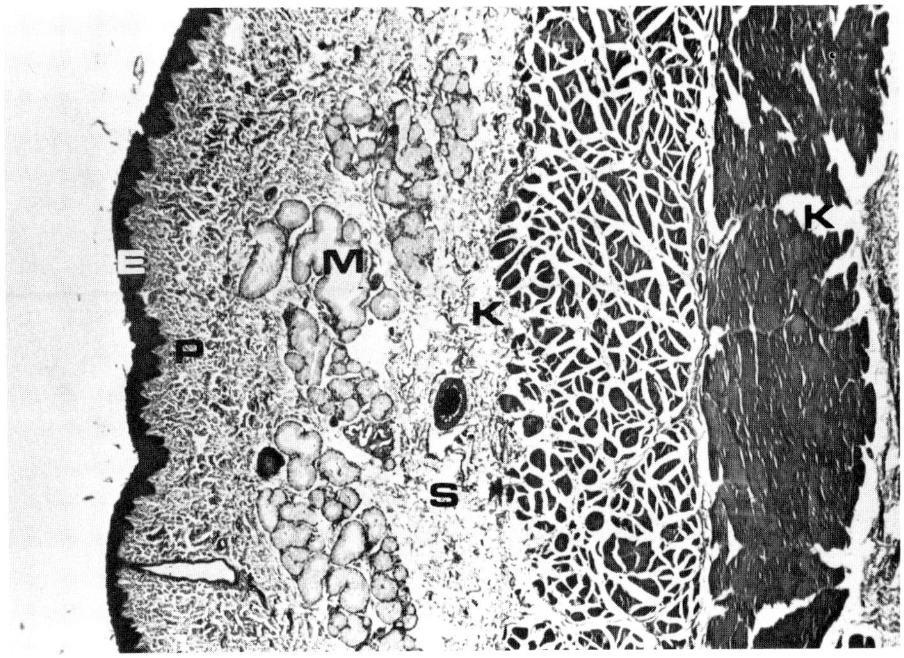

Fig. 17-27. Canine esophagus (cervical region). The lamina epithelialis (*E*), lamina propria (*P*), mucous glands (*M*) and tunica submucosa (*S*) are typical. The lamina muscularis is not present, while the tunica muscularis consists of skeletal muscle (*K*). ×10.

serosa in the caudal portion. The tunica serosa is also typical.

Glandular Stomach

General Characteristics. This organ is a continuation of the muscularized tube of the alimentary canal. It is modified as a saclike structure. Foodstuffs, which are delayed in this structure, are subjected to the enzymatic action of gastric juice and acid hydrolysis. The muscular contractions of the organ also induce mechanical mixing and breakdown of these substances.

The mural elements of the glandular stomach are typical. It conforms to the general pattern described for tubular organs. Regional differences in the tunica mucosa, however, exist. As such, four regions of the stomach are described: an *esophageal region* and *cardiac*, *fundic* and *pyloric gland regions* (Fig. 17-28).

Esophageal Region. This region of the stomach is lined by a nonsecretory, stratified squamous epithelium which may be keratinized. In carnivores, man and the pig, this region is very limited. In ruminants, it is extensive and subdivided into the *rumen*, *reticulum* and *omasum*. These chambers will be described with the compound stomach.

Cardiac Gland Region. This region is not equally developed in all species (Fig. 17-29). The beginning of this region is marked by a transition from stratified squamous to columnar epithelium. This point of transition is called the *margo plicatus* in the horse. The tunica mucosa is highly folded and the

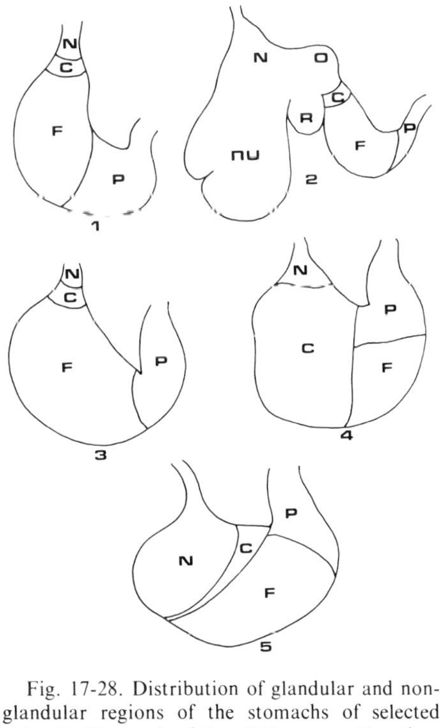

Fig. 17-28. Distribution of glandular and nonglandular regions of the stomachs of selected animals. *N*, nonglandular; *RU*, rumen; *R*, reticulum; *O*, omasum; *C*, cardiac region; *F*, fundic region; *P*, pyloric region; *1*, man; *2*, ruminant; *3*, dog; *4*, pig; *5*, horse.

surface has numerous invaginations called *gastric pits* (*foveolae gastricae*). These pits are present throughout all regions of the stomach.

The lamina epithelialis is lined by a single cell type—a mucus-secreting columnar cell, which is polarized. The apical portions of the cells are filled with granules that are precursors of mucin. The nucleus is flattened against the basal border. These cells are more cuboidal in the gastric pits close to the opening of the cardiac glands.

The *cardiac glands* are branched tubular, coiled glands which may be divided into a neck and body region (Fig. 17-30). The neck, at the opening to the gastric pit, as well as the upper portion of the gland, is lined by cuboidal cells. These are mucus-secreting cells which migrate from the pit to the surface replacing sloughed cells. As they migrate, they become columnar. The remaining cells of the body of the gland are columnar, mucus-secreting cells. In the dog, some *parietal cells* may be present. In the pig, some *chief cells* are present. *Argentaffin cells* are also present.

The cardiac glands are nonspecific glands that secrete mucus.

The lamina propria is typical. Although the actual amount of connective tissue is not extensive because of the presence of cardiac glands, the region is thick. The connective tissue is interdigitated between the cardiac glands.

A lamina muscularis mucosae is present, but its arrangement is variable. It may consist of two to four layers. Strands of the muscular tissue extend into the interglandular areas of the lamina propria in a manner similar to the connective tissue.

The tunica submucosa is present and typical. Adipose tissue is present, as well as blood vessels and nerves. The nerves form a *submucosal plexus* (*Meissner's plexus*).

The tunica muscularis is present and typical. A *myenteric plexus* (*Auerbach's plexus*) is interdigitated between the inner and outer laminae of muscle.

The tunica serosa is present and typical.

Fundic Gland Region. This region of the stomach is essentially similar to the configuration described for the cardiac region. The primary differences are in the configuration of the glands and the types of cells contained within the glands (Fig. 17-31).

The glands of this region, *fundic glands*, are branched tubular glands which are longer but less frequently branched than the cardiac glands (Fig. 17-32). Three areas of the glands are demonstrable: *base*, *neck* and *isthmus* (the region that opens into the gastric pit). Four cell types are distinguishable in the fundic glands: *chief cells* (*zymogen cells*), *argentaffin cells* (*enterochromaffin cells*), *parietal cells*, *mucous neck cells*. Occasionally, a fifth type of cell, a *transitional cell*, is described in the isthmus.

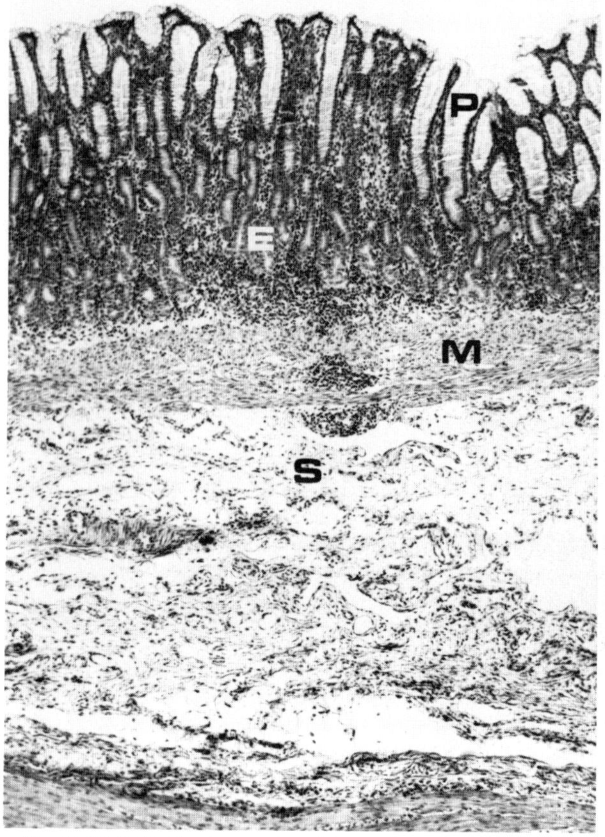

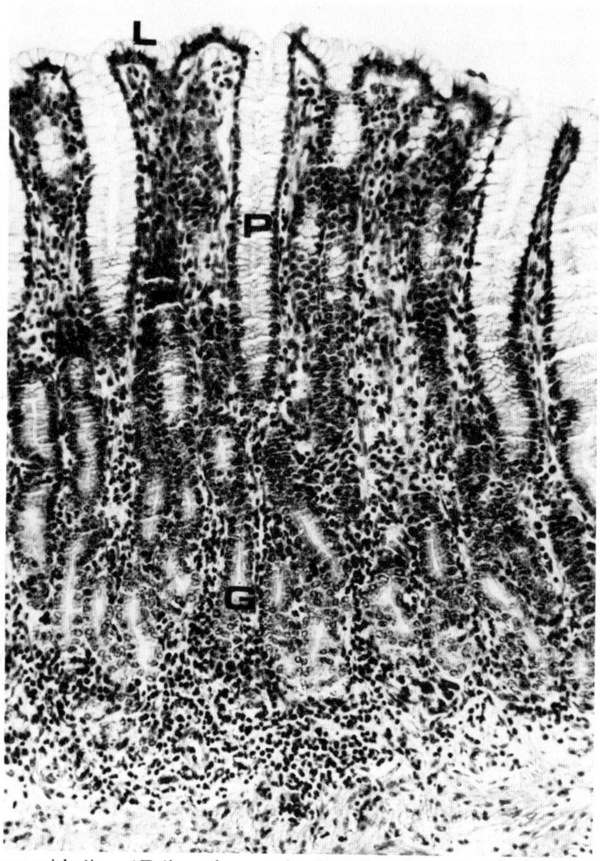

Fig. 17-29 (*left*). Cardiac region of the canine stomach. The columnar epithelium (*E*) lines the gastric pits (*P*) and glands. The lamina muscularis (*M*) and tunica submucosa (*S*) are typical. ×16.

Fig. 17-30 (*right*). Cardiac glands of the canine stomach. The lamina epithelialis is columnar. It lines the surface (*L*), gastric pits (*P*) and cardiac glands (*G*). ×40.

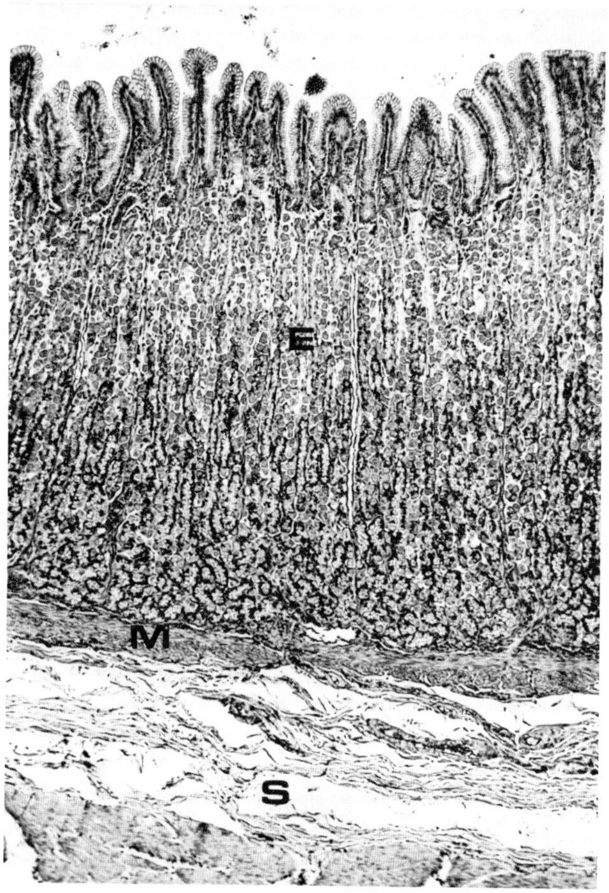

Fig. 17-31. Fundic region of the canine stomach. The lamina epithelialis (*E*) is highly folded. The tunica mucosa is very thick. The lamina muscularis (*M*) and tunica submucosa (*S*) are typical. ×16.

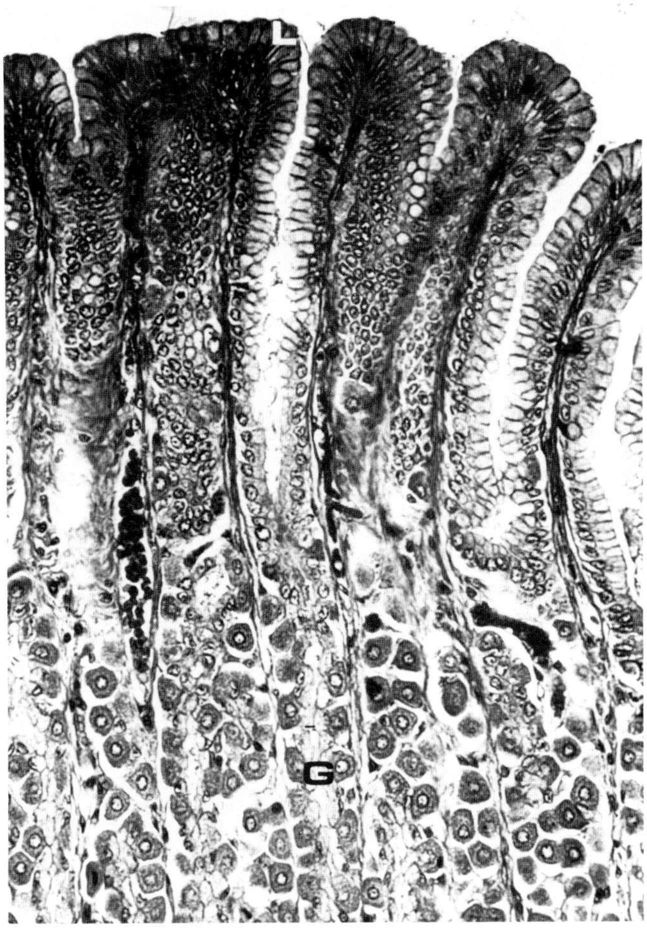

Fig. 17-32. Gastric pits and fundic glands of the canine stomach. The lining epithelium (*L*) is columnar, extends into the gastric pits and is continuous with the lining cells of the fundic glands (*G*). ×63.

Transitional cells are cuboidal cells located in the isthmus which are believed to be responsible for the replacement of lining and glandular epithelium.

Mucous neck cells occupy the constricted neck region of the glands (Fig. 17-33). Although their shape is variable, a cuboidal configuration is not uncommon. The nucleus is flattened and basally located. The apical portion of the cell contains secretory granules which are mucoid. This secretory product, however, is different from that of typical mucous cells.

Chief cells (*zymogen cells*) are the predominant cells in the base of the gland (Fig. 17-34). They are pyramidal cells with a basally positioned round nucleus. In fasting animals, apically positioned secretory granules are present. These cells, however, are quite labile to fixation and the secretory granules may be leeched from the cell leaving an apical foamy appearance. Also, autolysis of these cells is quite common because of the high pH of the stomach. In this instance, the cells may appear foamy. These cells are responsible for the elaboration of the proteolytic and lipolytic enzymes that comprise gastric juice.

The *parietal cell* is easily distinguished from the other cells of this gland because of its bright-staining acidophilic cytoplasm

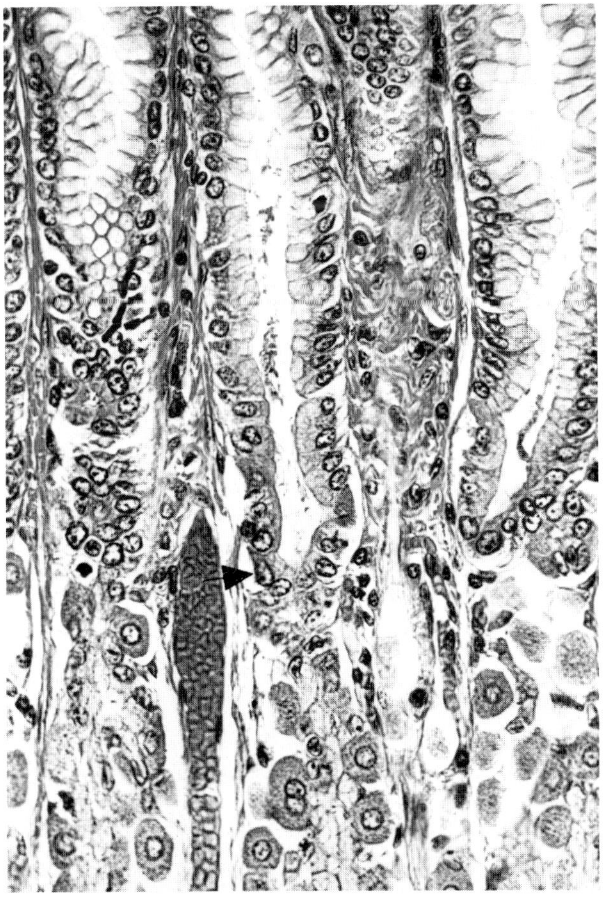

Fig. 17-33. Mucous neck cells of the fundic glands (canine stomach). The neck of the gland is lined by mucous neck cells (*arrow*). Their secretory product is mucoid. ×100.

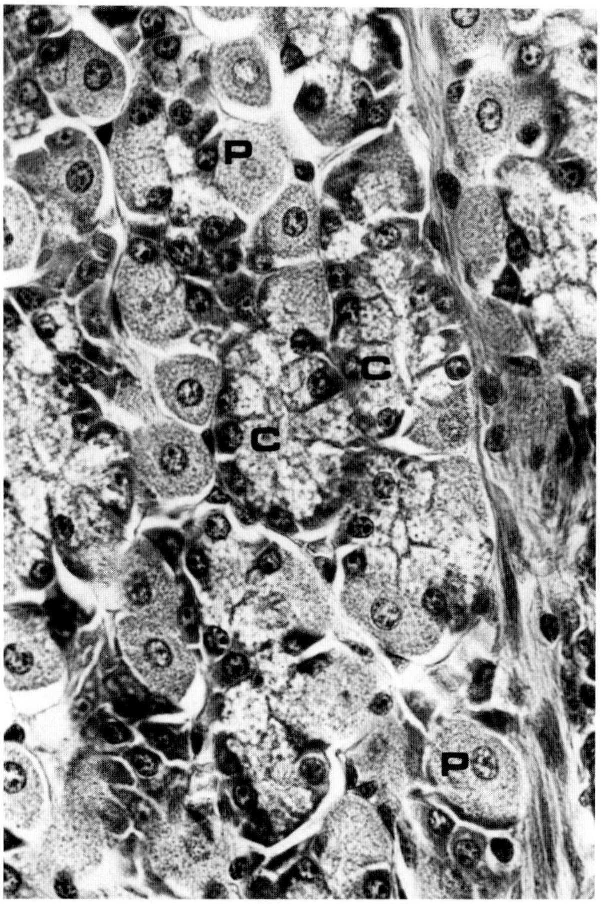

Fig. 17-34. Chief cells and parietal cells of the fundic glands (canine stomach). The chief cells (*C*) have granules along their apical borders. The parietal cells (*P*) are granular and acidophilic. ×160.

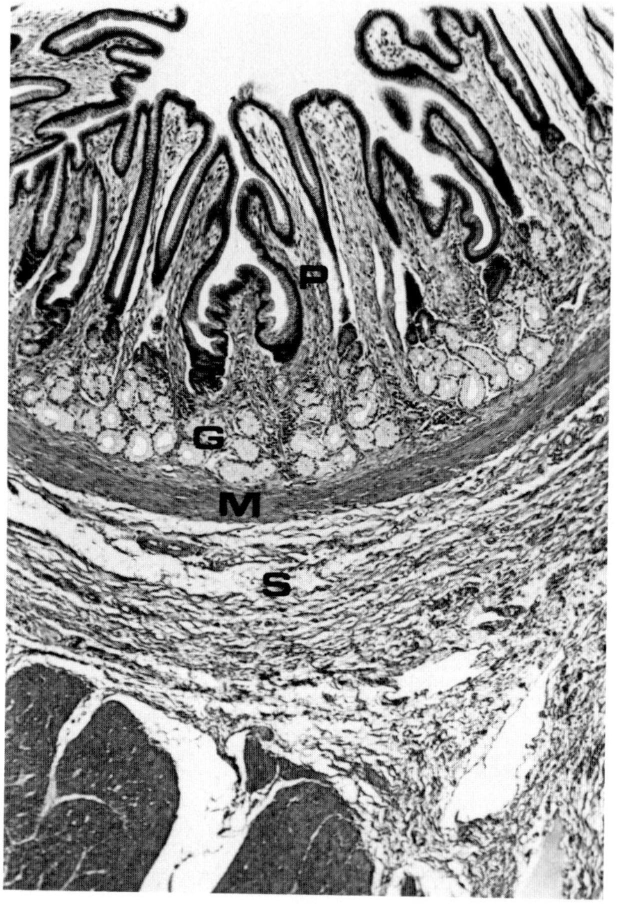

Fig. 17-35. Pyloric region of the canine stomach. The surface and gastric pits are typical. Since the tunica mucosa is not as highly folded as in other areas of the stomach, the lamina propria (*P*) is more clearly visible and contains glands (*G*). The lamina muscularis (*M*) and tunica submucosa (*S*) are typical. ×16.

(Fig. 17-34). They are scattered throughout the length of the gland from neck to base. These cells are elongated or triangular and contain a round nucleus. They appear to be scattered throughout the gland as an afterthought. Although they reside on the basement membrane, some of them reach the luminal surface, while others of them do not. Numerous canaliculi extend from the apical plasmalemma as invaginations into the cytoplasm proper. Apical microvilli extend between the chief cells and reach the luminal surface. Despite the fact that some of them do not reach the surface directly, their secretory product has access to the surface through the canalicular and microvillar system. These cells elaborate hydrochloric acid. They may also be responsible for the elaboration of *intrinsic factor*, a substance necessary for vitamin B_{12} absorption.

Argentaffin cells (*enterochromaffin cells*), although not numerous in the stomach, are scattered throughout the lamina epithelialis of this organ. As their name implies, special silver stains are required to distinguish them definitively. With special silver stains, numerous granules that contain silver are located in an abluminal or infranuclear position. These flattened or pyramidal cells, because of the position of the secretory granules, are believed to deposit their product into the lamina propria. These cells secrete *serotonin*, a vasoconstrictive chemical.

The remaining mural elements are similar to the configuration described for the cardiac region.

Pyloric Gland Region. This region is essentially similar to the cardiac region (Fig. 17-35). The gastric pits are deeper than in other regions of the stomach. The pyloric glands are similar to the cardiac glands (Fig. 17-36). The pyloric glands are short and are simple or branched tubular glands. The predominant cell is a mucus-secreting cell similar to those that occur in the cardiac glands.

The remaining mural elements are present and typical. A striking feature of this region is the well-developed inner circular lamina of the tunica muscularis. This forms the *pyloric sphincter* at the gastroduodenal junction (Fig. 17-37).

Throughout all these regions of the stomach, the lamina propria may contain another zone, the *lamina subglandularis* (Fig. 17-38). An outer zone, adjacent to the lamina muscularis mucosae, the *stratum compactum*, is a condensation of DWFCT. An inner zone, the *stratum granulosum*, consists of numerous fibroblasts. This lamina is especially well-developed in carnivores wherein it may be a protective device against perforation from sharp objects such as bones. It is occasionally observed in the equine stomach.

Compound Stomach

General Remarks. The compound stomach of ruminants consists of four chambers: *rumen*, *reticulum*, *omasum* and *abomasum*. The abomasum is the glandular stomach and is comparable to the simple stomach of nonruminant organisms. The remaining

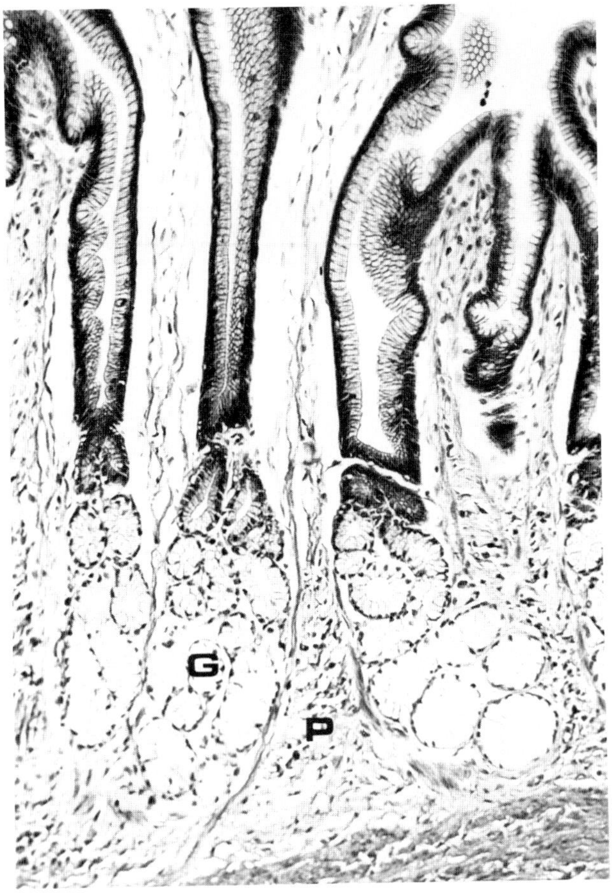

Fig. 17-36. Pyloric glands of the canine stomach. The lining of the gastric pits is continuous with the lining of the pyloric glands (*G*). The lamina propria (*P*) is extensive between the glands and pits. ×40.

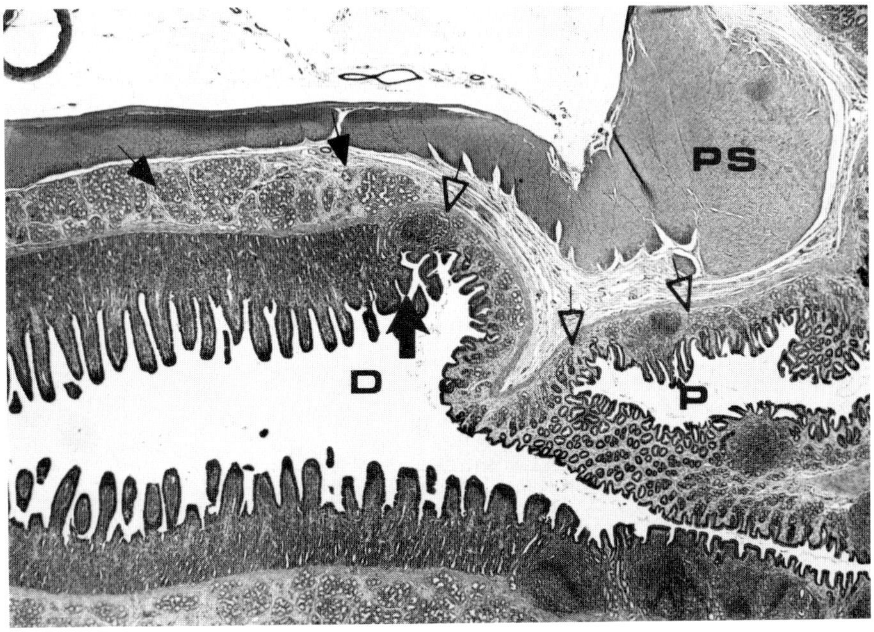

Fig. 17-37. Gastroduodenal junction (canine digestive tract). The pyloric region (*P*) is continuous with the duodenal region (*D*) of the intestine. The tunica muscularis is modified as the pyloric sphincter (*PS*). The pyloric glands (*open arrows*) are similar to the submucosal glands of the duodenum (*small solid arrows*). The latter may be an intestinal continuation of the former. *Larger solid arrow*, actual point of mural reorganization. ×4.

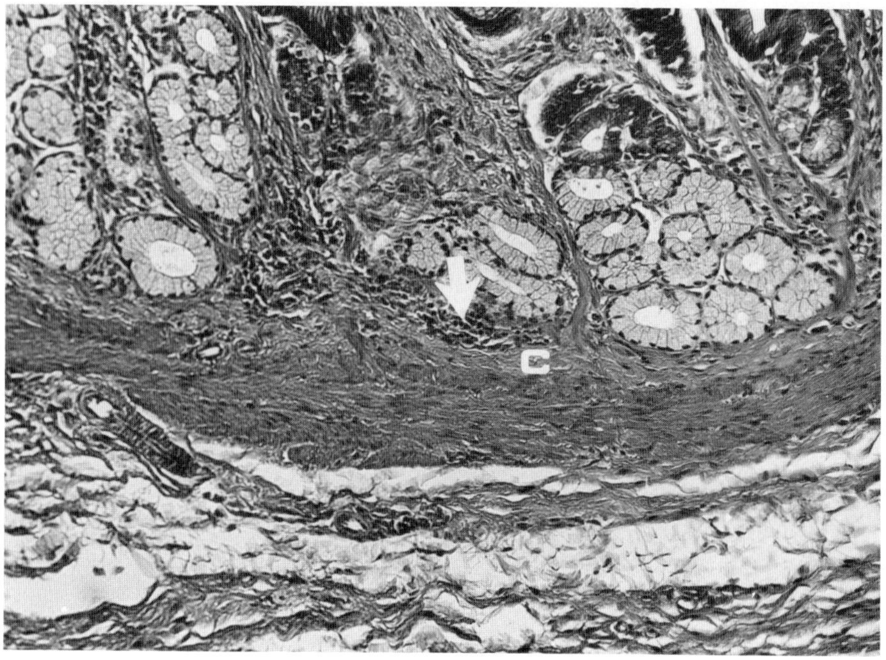

Fig. 17-38. Lamina subglandularis of the canine stomach. This lamina consists of a stratum compactum (*C*) and a stratum granulosum (*arrow*). ×40.

chambers of the compound stomach are modifications of the esophageal region of the stomach. These forechambers facilitate the digestion of plant material (cellulose) through the action of the microorganisms that occupy this region.

Since the abomasum is similar to the glandular stomach described previously, only the chambers of the forestomach will be discussed.

Rumen. The rumen is also referred to as the *paunch* (Fig. 17-39).

The characteristic feature of this chamber is the conical papillae that project into the lumen from the cutaneous mucous membrane. These papillae may be 1 cm long and contain a core of highly vascularized connective tissue composed of fine collagenous and elastic fibers.

The lamina epithelialis is stratified squamous epithelium which is cornified and of variable thickness. The layers of this epithelium are not well-defined. The cells of the stratum corneum are usually swollen or vesiculated. On the apex of the papillae they are typically flattened.

The lamina propria consists of connective tissue identical to that which occupies the papillae. The components, of course, are continuous with each other. A lamina propria, therefore, blends insensibly with the loose connective tissue of the tunica submucosa. A condensation of connective tissue fibers in the deep region of the lamina propria-submucosa extends into the papillae. This area may be similar to the stratum compactum of the lamina subglandularis. This region is sometimes mistaken for the lamina muscularis mucosae. The combined lamina propria-submucosa is generally devoid of lymphatic nodules and is aglandular.

The tunica muscularis is present and typical. The *pillars* of the rumen are extensive folds of the entire wall which contain a core of muscle from the tunica muscularis.

The tunica serosa is present and typical.

The rumen contains numerous microorganisms. Fermentation of cellulose and other carbohydrates by bacteria facilitates ruminant digestive processes. Also, the bacteria synthesize various amino acids and are significant in the synthesis of B-complex vitamins. The ruminal muscular contractions facilitate mechanical breakdown of the foodstuffs, as well as mixture of the entire contents. Papillary absorption of materials reportedly occurs.

Reticulum. The reticulum is also called the *honeycomb* (Fig. 17-40).

The morphology of the reticulum is quite similar to that of the rumen. Only those features that distinguish it from the rumen are presented.

The mucous membrane has numerous *primary folds* which are oriented, upon surface view, as a reticulum or honeycomb. From these vertically projecting folds are numerous *secondary* and *tertiary papillae*. Within the lamina propria of the tips of the primary or *reticular folds* is an isolated mass of smooth muscle of the lamina muscularis mucosae. This mass extends throughout the length of the folds and is continuous with the lamina muscularis mucosae of the esoph-

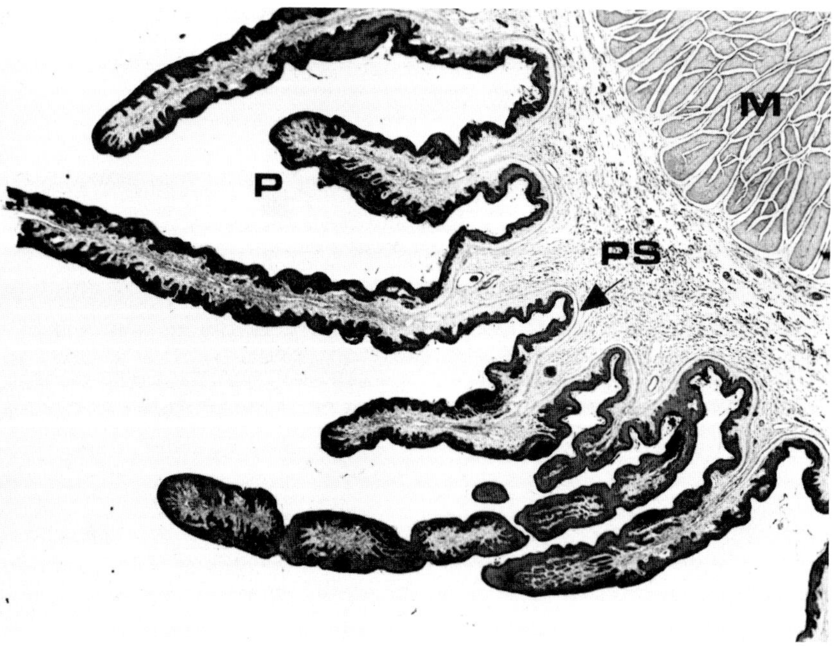

Fig. 17-39. Bovine rumen. Conical papillae (*P*) project from the surface of the organ. A lamina muscularis is not present. The lamina propria-submucosa (*PS*) is typical and adjacent to the tunica muscularis (*M*). A condensation of connective tissue fibers (*arrow*) may be mistaken for the lamina muscularis. ×4.

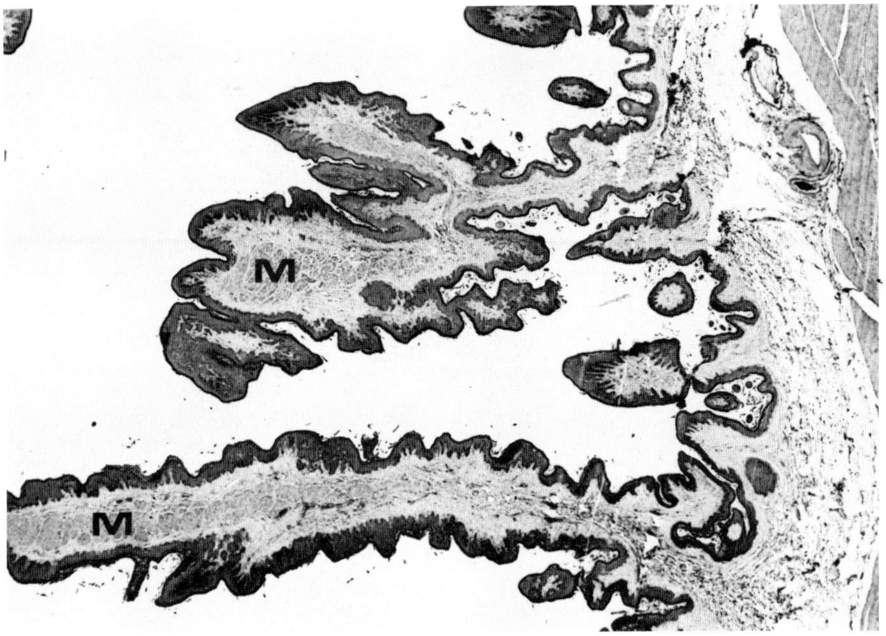

Fig. 17-40. Bovine reticulum. The reticulum consists of primary and secondary papillae projecting from the surface of the organ. A lamina muscularis (*M*) is present, but it is confined to the tips of the papillae. ×4.

agus. The course of the smooth muscle, therefore, is oriented parallel to, but above, the plane of the surface lining. The lamina muscularis mucosae is confined to the aforementioned region in this chamber.

The lamina propria-submucosa, tunica muscularis and tunica serosa are present and typical.

The functions of this chamber are similar to the functions of the rumen.

Omasum. The terms, *many plies* and *book*, are also applied to the omasum (Fig. 17-41).

The keratinized cutaneous mucous membrane has numerous foliate *primary folds* (*laminae*) as well as smaller papillae. The laminae are covered with short, cornified papillae. The lamina muscularis mucosae is present and continuous. The lamina muscularis mucosae forms a double layer of smooth muscle which follows the contour of the laminae as well as that of the unraised surface lining. Another layer of smooth muscle is interdigitated between the smooth muscle of the lamina muscularis mucosae within the laminae. It is continuous with the inner layer of smooth muscle of the tunica muscularis. At the apex of the laminae, the smooth muscle masses fuse into a thickened muscular mass.

The lamina propria, tunica submucosa, tunica muscularis and tunica serosa are present and typical. At the apices of the laminae, however, a mucous connective tissue is present.

Much absorption occurs within the omasum. By extensive muscular contractions the ingesta is reduced to a powder by the abrasive surface before moving to the abomasum.

Abomasum. The abomasum is the glandular portion of the ruminant stomach. The description of the glandular stomach applies to this organ.

Small Intestine

General Remarks. As a continuation of the digestive tube, this region is highly modified for the secretion and absorption of materials. It has numerous modifications to increase the absorptive and secretory surface: *length*, *plicae*, *villi* and *microvilli*. Although there are distinctive features of the various regions of the intestine, these regions share many features in common. The common features will be discussed and then the distinctive features of the specific regions of the intestine will be presented.

At the gastroduodenal junction there is an abrupt change in the character of the mucous membrane. Gastric pits are replaced by finger-like projections, the *villi* of the mucous membrane (Fig. 17-42). Permanent folds, *plicae circulares* (*valves of Kerkring*) are present and have villi projecting from them. These folds also contain portions of the tunica submucosa. At the base of the villi are openings to the *crypts of Lieberkuhn*.

The lamina epithelialis consists of three types of cells: *lining cells*, *goblet cells* and *enterochromaffin cells*.

The *lining cells* are typical columnar epithelial cells. The apical border has numerous microvilli arranged in an orderly

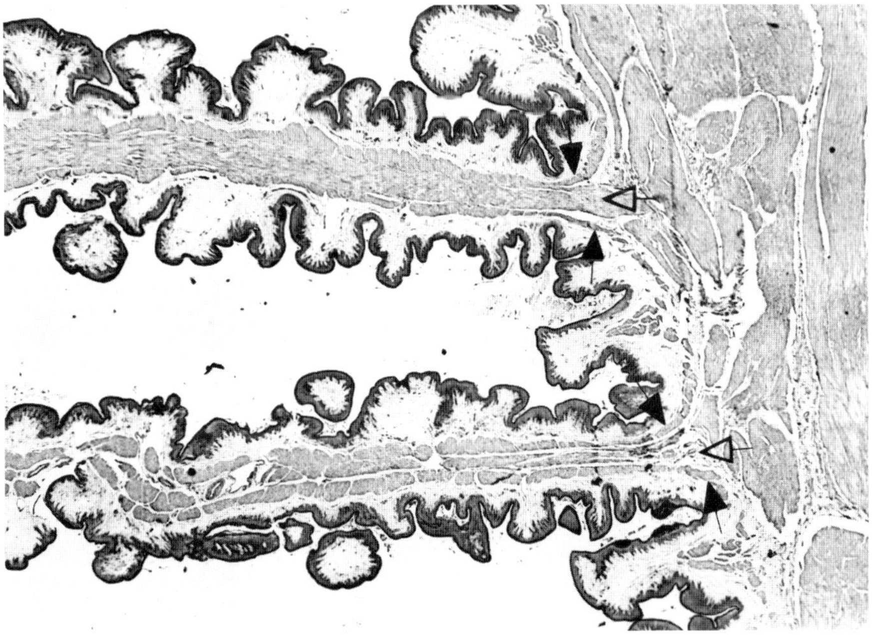

Fig. 17-41. Bovine omasum. This organ has numerous primary papillae with smaller papillae projecting from its surface. Three laminae of smooth muscle occur in the primary papillae. The two peripheral layers are those of the lamina muscularis (*solid arrows*). The center lamina is continuous with the smooth muscle of the tunica muscularis (*open arrows*). ×4.

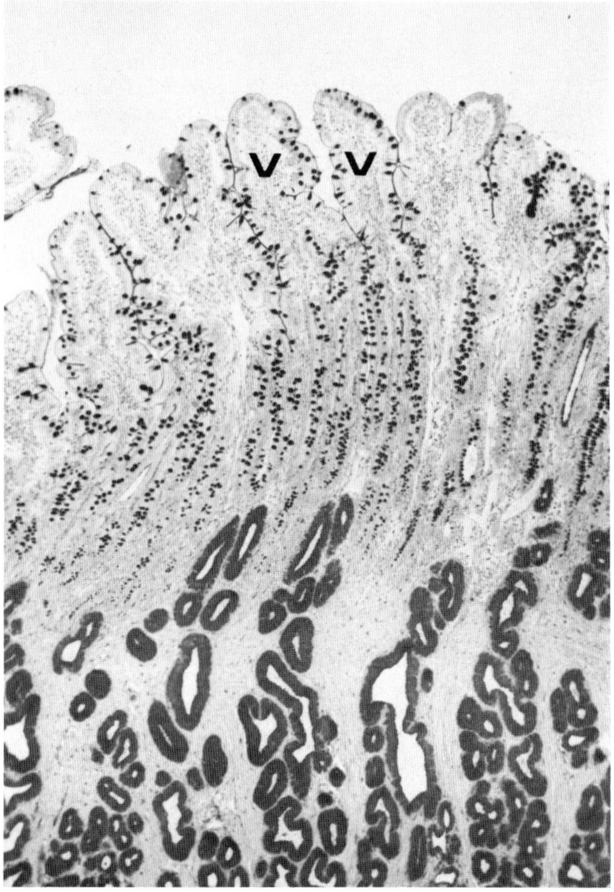

Fig. 17-42. Intestinal villi of the canine duodenum. The villi (*V*) project from the surface of the organ. The dark cells along the apices and lateral margins of the villi are goblet cells. The dark outlines at the base of the intestinal crypts are submucosal glands. ×16. (Alcian blue-periodic acid-Schiff).

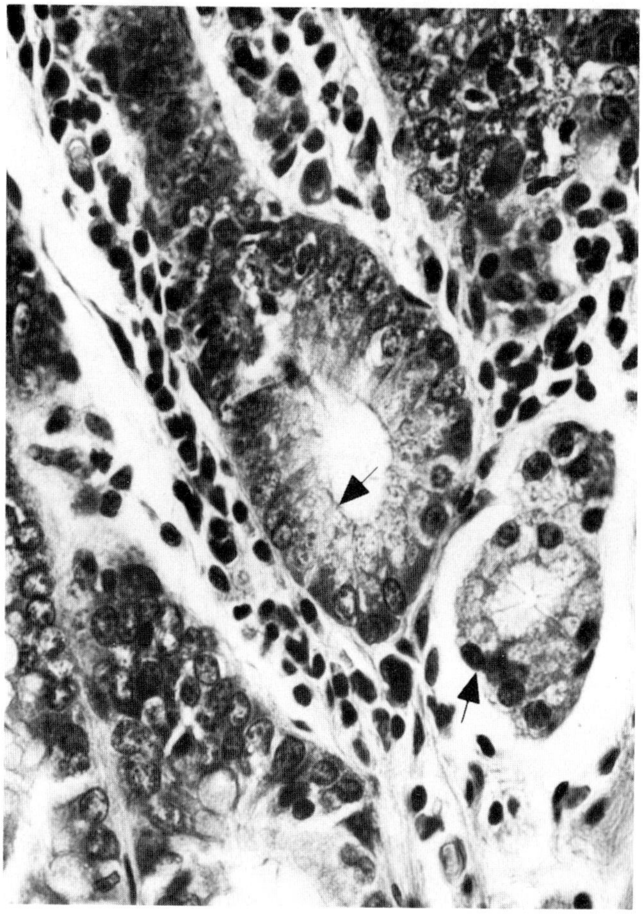

Fig. 17-43. Paneth cells of the intestinal crypts (equine duodenum). These cells are pyramidal cells (*arrows*) with apical granules. ×160.

array as a *striated border*. The finely granular, acidophilic cytoplasm contains the basally displaced, elongated nucleus. These cells are actively engaged in the absorptive process.

The *goblet cells* are typical. They tend to increase in frequency toward the rectum. Their secretory product protects the lining. In the lower intestine, the mucoid layer facilitates the movement of the luminal contents toward the anus.

The *enterochromaffin cells* are typical and have been described with the stomach.

The crypts of Lieberkuhn open at the base of the villi. They are simple, branched tubular invaginations. The epithelium contains *columnar lining cells*, *goblet cells*, *argentaffin cells* and *Paneth cells*.

Paneth cells are the special cells of the intestine (Fig. 17-43). Their precise function is not known. They are absent in the dog and pig. These cells are pyramidal and contain supranuclear acidophilic granules and a basally displaced nucleus. The basal portion of the cell has a basophilic appearance.

The lamina propria mucosae is usually described as areolar. However, the accumulation of reticular fibers, reticular cells, granulocytes and agranulocytes in this tissue has prompted some to classify it as a *reticuloareolar connective tissue*. Crypts of Lieberkuhn and lymph nodules are also present. The crypts of Lieberkuhn may occupy the bulk of this layer. The frequency of lymph nodules, however, increases caudally and may occupy the lamina propria as well as the tunica submucosa, as in the case of *Peyer's patches*.

Besides the aforementioned components, numerous lymphatic vessels (*lacteals*) are present and extend with the connective tissue into the core of the villi.

A lamina subglandularis is present in the initial part of the intestine of carnivores.

The lamina muscularis mucosae is present and typical. Strands of smooth muscle and connective tissue fibers are interdigitated between the crypts of Lieberkuhn and into the cores of the villi.

The tunica submucosa is present and typical. Submucosal glands are simple branched tubuloacinar glands which open into the crypts (Fig. 17-44). They may be mucous (ruminants, dog), mixed (cat) or serous (horse, pig). These glands are variously referred to as *Brunner's glands* or *duodenal glands*. They are most properly referred to as *intestinal submucosal glands*. In carnivores, man and small ruminants, they are confined to the initial or middle portion of the duodenum. In the horse, pig and large ruminants, they extend into the jejunum. These glands may represent a caudal continuation of pyloric glands which have been displaced to the submucosa.

The tunica muscularis with Auerbach's plexus is present and typical. The contraction of this smooth muscle is responsible for peristalsis.

The tunica serosa is present and typical.

Duodenum. This is the fixed portion of the small intestine (Fig. 17-45). The tunica mucosa is highly folded with villi and plicae circulares. Crypts of Lieberkuhn are prominent. Intestinal submucosal glands are of variable occurrence. In man and small ruminants they extend from the initial to the middle portions of the duodenum. In the

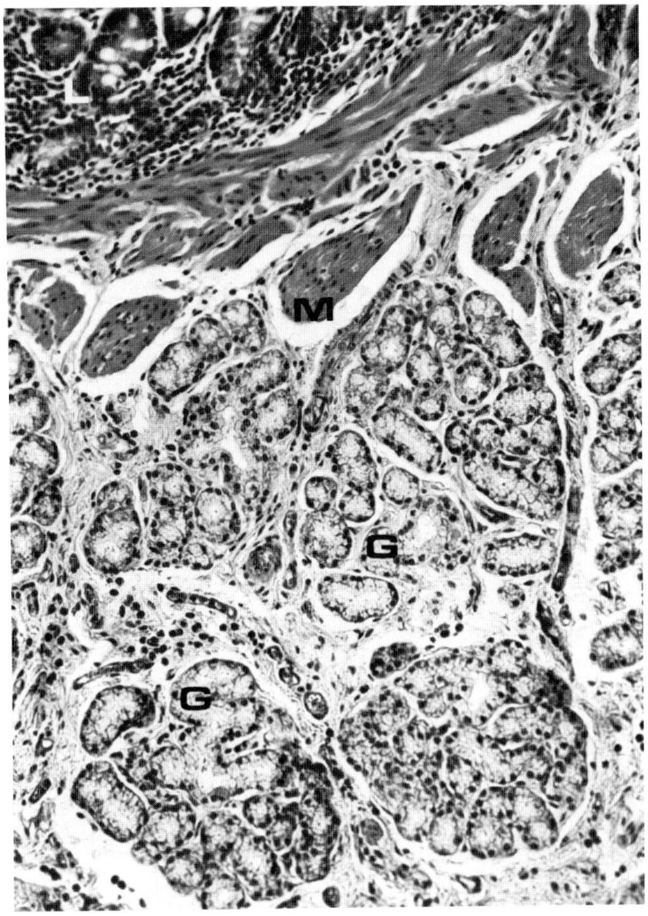

Fig. 17-44. Submucosal glands of the equine duodenum. The submucosal glands (*G*) are located below the lamina epithelialis (*L*) and lamina muscularis (*M*) of the tunica mucosa. These glands, however, are continuous with the intestinal crypts. ×40.

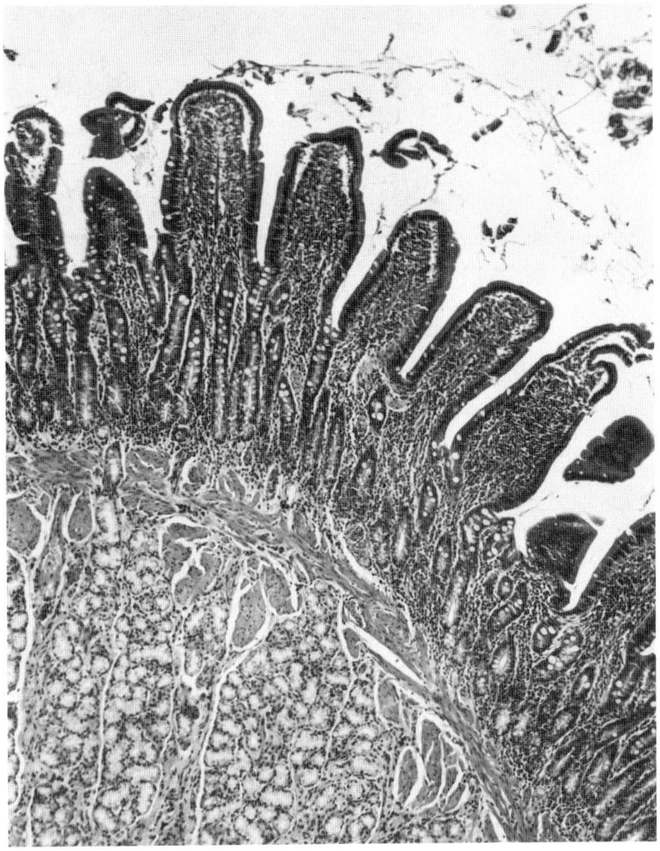

Fig. 17-45. Equine duodenum. The villi are blunt and wide. Submucosal glands are present. ×16.

dog, they are confined to the initial part of the duodenum.

Lymphatic nodules may be present, but they are sparse.

Although variable, the villi tend to be regularly shaped, blunt and wide.

Jejunum. This mesenteric region of the small intestine is essentially similar to the duodenum (Fig. 17-46). Intestinal submucosal glands are confined to the initial portion of the jejunum in some species. The villi are slender, smaller and fewer in number than in the cranial portion of the small intestine. Mucosal-submucosal lymph nodules are present, especially in the pig. The remaining mural elements are present and typical.

Ileum. This region is similar to the jejunum (Fig. 17-47). There is an increasing number of goblet cells. Lymphatic tissue is very prominent in the mucosal-submucosal region. These aggregates are collectively referred to as *Peyer's patches*. These lymphatic nodules may become so prominent that they fill or even obliterate the villi. In such instances, the mucous membrane is flattened and interrupted by crypts. These areas look quite similar to tonsils and their associated crypts and are referred to as *lymph craters*. They are especially prominent in swine. Peyer's patches are located in an antimesenteric position; i.e., they are positioned opposite the point where the tunica serosa is reflected as the mesentery of the organ (Fig. 17-48).

The villi of this region are club-shaped. Plicae are no longer present. Actually, plicae are most prominent in the jejunum and diminish in size orad and aborad.

Large Intestine

General Remarks. The large intestine is generally modified for the absorption of metabolites from the gut and the addition of mucoid secretory materials. In some species, the large intestine is modified for the digestion of plant materials.

Cecum. In herbivores with a simple stomach (horse, rabbit, guinea pig), the cecum is an important intestinal modification for the fermentation of plant materials. No villi are present and intestinal crypts (without Paneth cells) open at the surface (Fig. 17-49). Goblet cells and lymphatic tissue are prominent features of this region. The distribution of lymph nodules is species-variable. The remaining structural features are similar to the small intestine.

Colon. In this region of the gut, intestinal crypts open at the surface because villi are not present (Fig. 17-50). The glands are longer and less coiled than in the small intestine. These crypts do not contain Paneth cells. Plicae are not present. Lymph nodules, although present, are not as frequently encountered as in the small intestine.

The outer layer of the tunica muscularis is thickened, contains numerous elastic fibers and is arranged in longitudinal bands, *taeniae coli*. A thin layer of outer muscle is located between these thickenings. Taeniae occur in the horse, man and pig.

All remaining mural elements are similar to the small intestine.

Rectum. This portion of the gut is similar to other portions of the large intestine with a

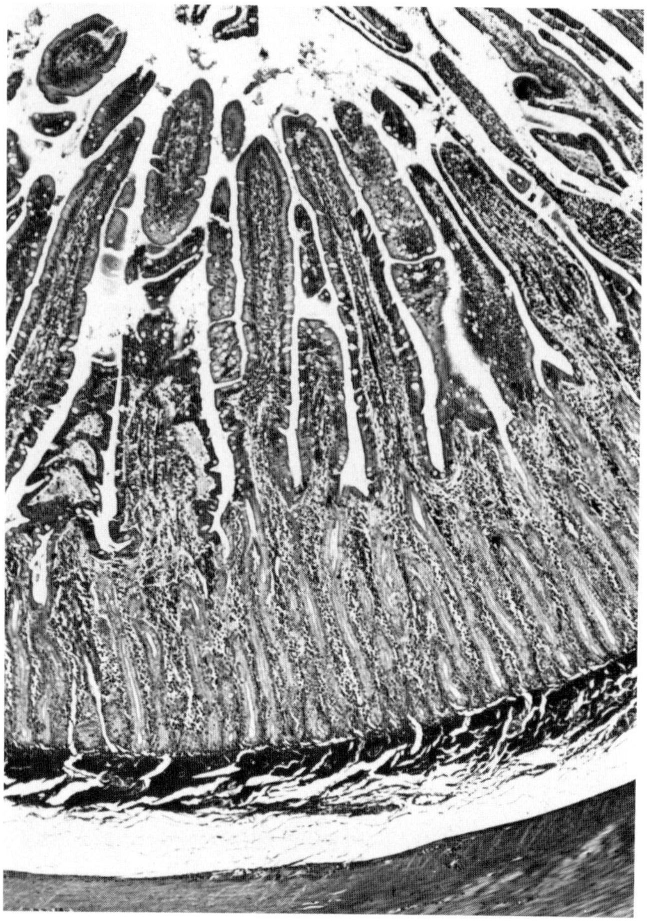

Fig. 17-46. Jejunum of a bushbaby. The villi are slender. ×16.

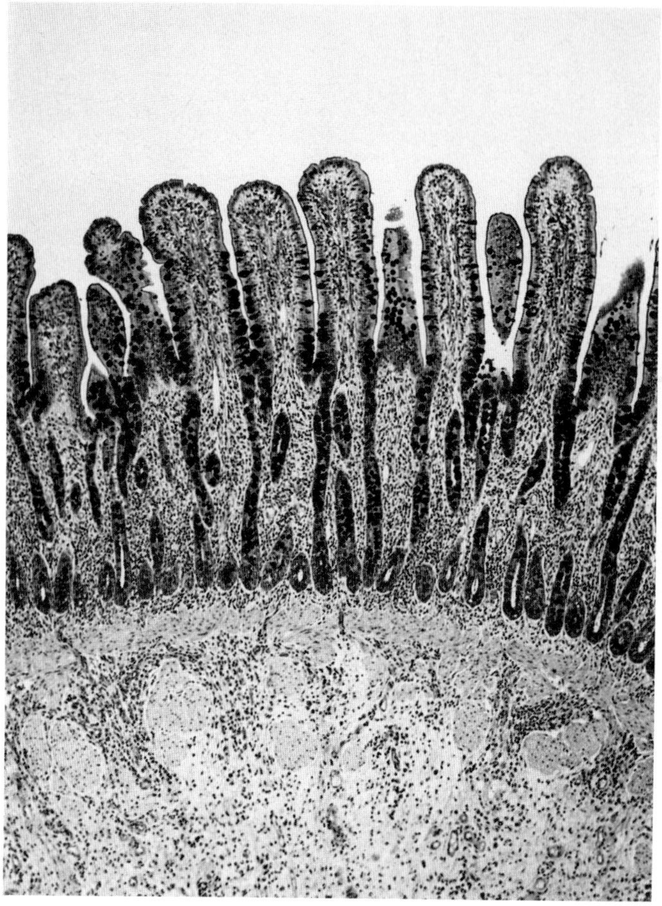

Fig. 17-47. Equine ileum. The villi are club-shaped. ×16.

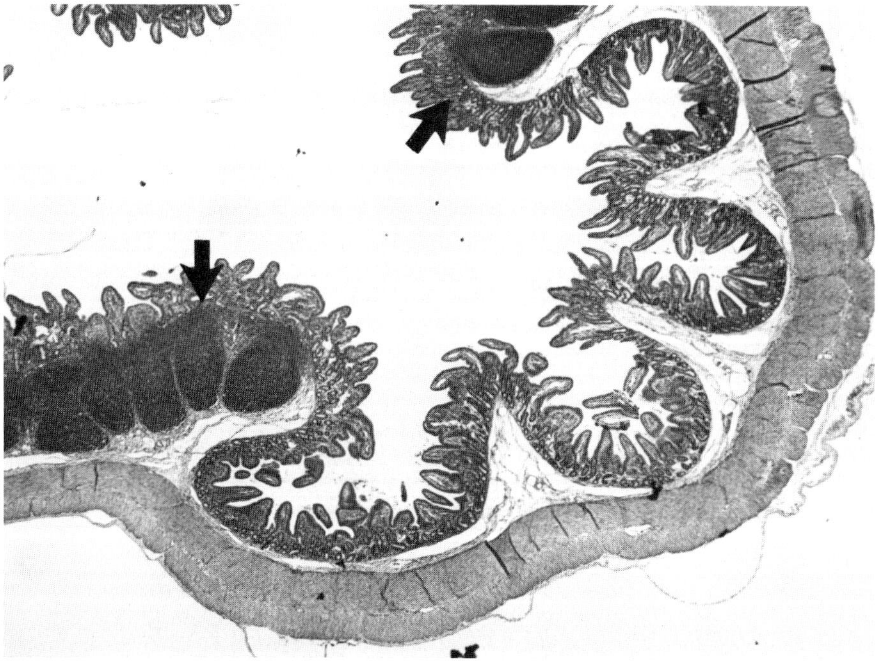

Fig. 17-48. Porcine ileum. Peyer's patches (*arrows*) are located in an antimesenteric position. ×4.

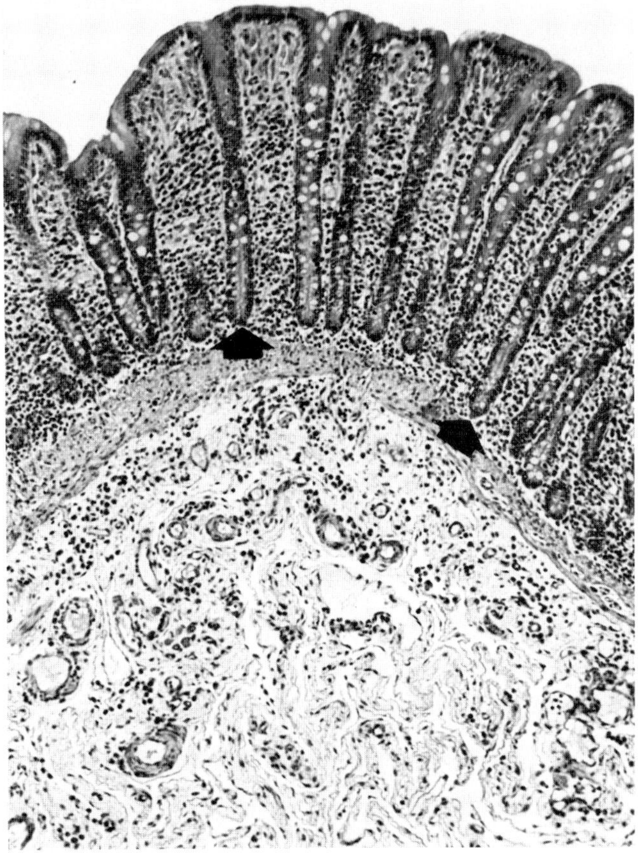

Fig. 17-49. Equine cecum. Villi are absent and intestinal crypts (*arrows*) open at the surface. ×16.

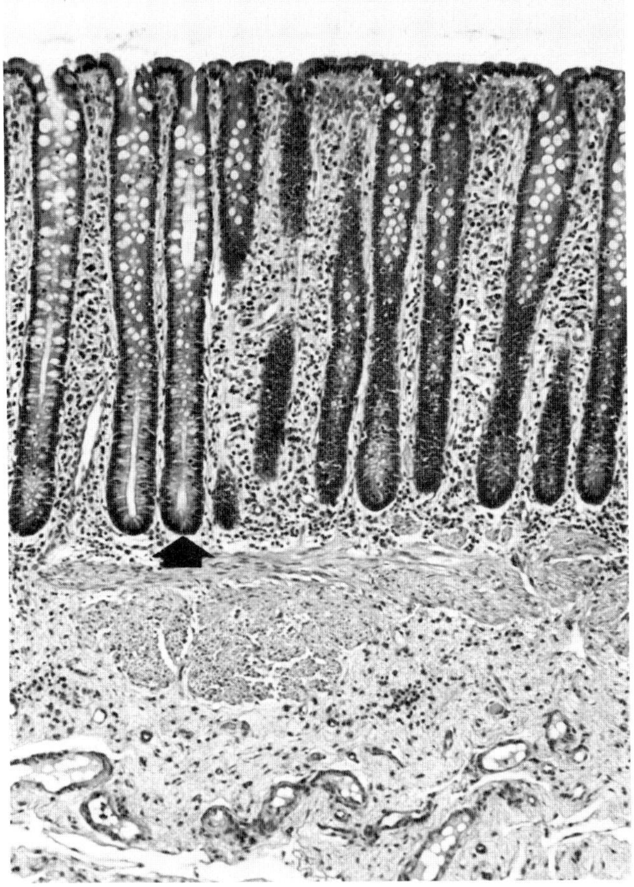

Fig. 17-50. Equine colon. Villi are absent and intestinal crypts (*arrow*) are straight and long. They open at the surface. ×16.

few exceptions. Taeniae coli are absent, but the tunica muscularis is thicker in this region than in the colon. The lining and glandular epithelium contains many goblet cells. Also, a tunica adventitia replaces the tunica serosa. The tunica mucosa has longitudinally oriented folds in which there is a core of erectile tissue within the lamina propria.

The remaining mural elements are present and typical.

Anus. This region of the gut, a mucocutaneous junction, is marked by a transition from columnar epithelium to stratified squamous epithelium at the *rectoanal junction* (Fig. 17-51). The lamina epithelialis is similar to the lining of the buccal cavity.

At the level of the rectoanal junction, the lamina muscularis mucosae and the outer layer of the tunica muscularis end. The inner layer of the tunica muscularis continues and terminates as the internal anal sphincter.

A tunica adventitia is present and blends insensibly with the surrounding connective tissue.

In certain species the anal glands, anal sacs and circumanal glands are associated with the anus (Chapter 16).

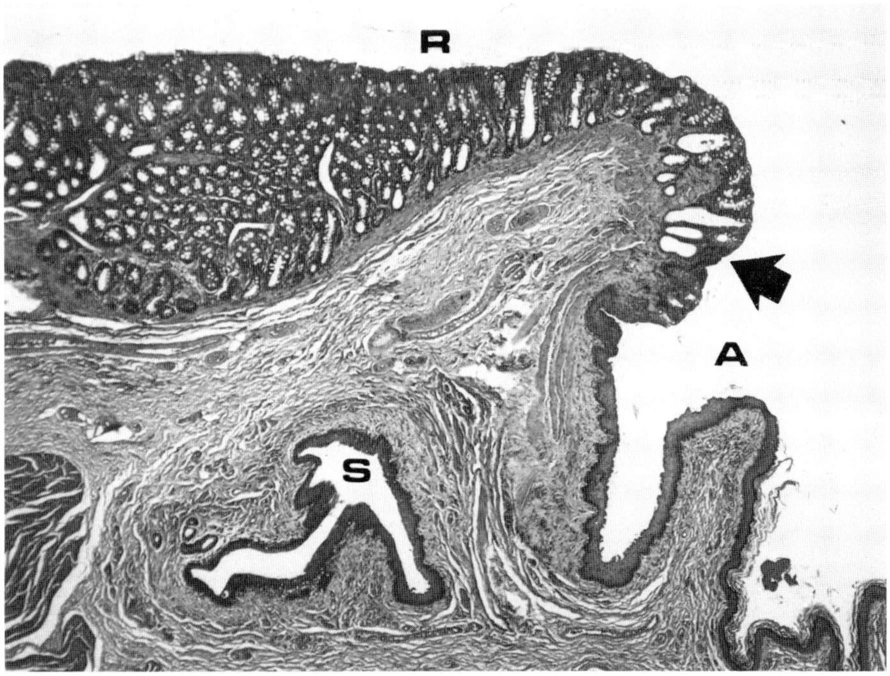

Fig. 17-51. Rectoanal junction (feline). The columnar epithelium of the rectum (*R*) changes to the stratified squamous epithelium of the anus (*A*) at the rectoanal junction (*arrow*). An anal sac (*S*) is apparent in this region. ×10.

Avian Digestive System

Buccal Cavity. The buccal cavity and associated structures are quite different from those observed in mammals generally. Instead of lips and cheeks, a cornified beak is appended to the upper and lower jaw bones. The tongue is narrow, pointed, devoid of taste buds and contains a bone, the *entoglossal bone*. The anterior portion of the bone is continued by hyaline cartilage. The stratified squamous epithelium, which is variously cornified, is continuous with the mucous membrane of the buccal cavity.

Teeth are not present. However, rudimentary tooth buds are present in some birds.

Definitive salivary glands are not present. Instead, the mucosal-submucosal connective tissue of the buccal cavity is well-endowed with simple branched tubular mucous glands (Fig. 17-52). These glands are lined with extremely large cells which conform generally to the morphology of mucous cells.

Esophagus and Crop. The lamina epithelialis of these two structures is a highly cornified stratified squamous epithelium (Fig. 17-53). The lamina propria consists of areolar connective tissue which contains diffuse lymphatic tissue and some lymph nodules. The accumulation of lymphatic tissue is especially prominent caudal to the crop. The mucous membrane is arranged in longitudinal folds. The lamina muscularis mucosae consists of an undulating mass of longitudinally oriented smooth muscle. Simple branched tubuloalveolar mucous glands are present in the esophagus. The tunica submucosa, tunica muscularis, tunica adventitia and tunica serosa are present and typical.

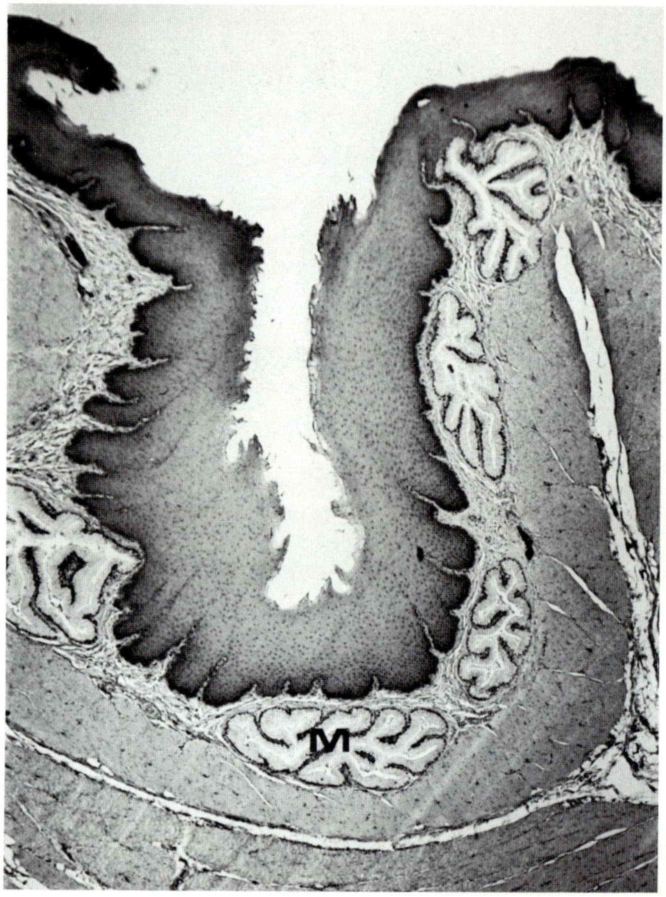

Fig. 17-53. Avian esophagus. The lumen of this structure is lined by stratified squamous epithelium. Mucous glands (*M*) are present. ×10.

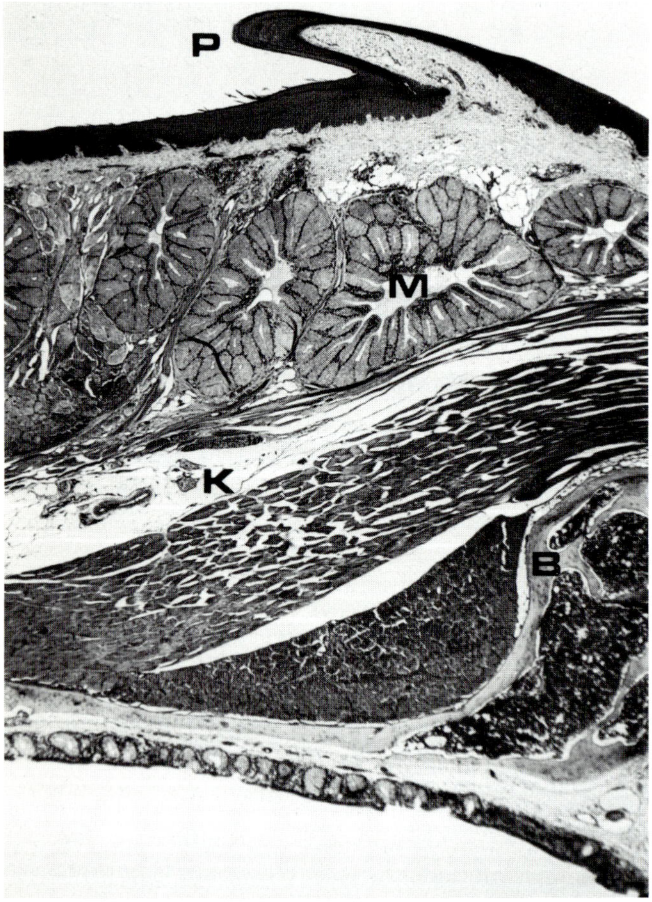

Fig. 17-52. Avian tongue. A papilla (*P*) protrudes from the dorsal surface. The mass of the tongue consists of mucous glands (*M*), skeletal muscle (*K*) and bone (*B*). ×10.

The *ingluvies* or *crop* is an esophageal diverticulum. The lamina epithelialis of the crop is thicker than that of the esophagus. Simple branched tubuloalveolar mucous glands are present in anseriform birds, but they are absent in galliform and columbiform birds. In columbiform birds, the superficial cells of the lamina epithelialis undergo a fatty change to a substance called *crop milk*.

The enlargement of the esophagus serves to moisten foodstuffs through its mucoid secretion as well as to macerate the materials through the muscular contractions of the tunica muscularis.

The remaining tunics of the wall are similar to the esophagus.

Proventriculus. This structure is the glandular stomach of avian species (Fig. 17-54). Its mural structure conforms generally to the pattern that typifies most digestive organs. Its glands, however, are quite different from those which have been encountered thus far.

The tunica mucosa is extensively folded into flattened ridges separated by grooves or sulci. *Mucosal glands* (simple branched tubular glands) open into the base of the sulci. Elevations in the tunica mucosa (papillae) contain the opening of the excretory duct of *submucosal glands* (Fig. 17-54).

The lamina epithelialis consists primarily of columnar cells. These cells extend into the sulci. The lamina epithelialis continues into the mucosal glands as a cuboidal epithelium. The nature of their secretory activity is unknown.

The lamina propria is typical and contains numerous accumulations of diffuse and nodular lymphatic tissue.

The lamina muscularis mucosae consists of an interrupted band of longitudinally oriented fibers, strands of which are interdigitated between the mucosal glands.

The tunica submucosa is typical but is seemingly displaced by the large and numerous *submucosal glands* (Fig. 17-54). These glands are compound, branched tubular glands. The adenomeres radiate 360° around a central excretory duct lined by a tall columnar epithelium which may be simple or pseudostratified. The radially oriented tubular glands are lined by secretory cells which may be cuboidal or pyramidal (Fig. 17-55). The apical portions of the secretory cells are not joined together; thus, a serrated appearance is imparted to the lining. These cells have a granular and acidophilic cytoplasm with a centrally or parabasally positioned nucleus. This is the only cell type in the gland. Since avian gastric juice is similar to the mammalian counterpart, it is assumed that this cell must secrete both zymogenic and acidic secretory products.

The tunica muscularis is slightly modified: inner longitudinal, middle circular and outer longitudinal layers are present.

The tunica serosa is typical.

Ventriculus. This portion of the digestive system, the *gizzard* or *muscular stomach*, is connected to the proventriculus by a narrow isthmus which is devoid of submucosal glands. The luminal surface of this organ is lined by a cornified secretory product that is elaborated by the mucosal glands (Fig. 17-56).

The surface lining of the tunica mucosa consists of low columnar cells with round and basally positioned nuclei (Fig. 17-57). The surface cells continue into the glands and are replaced by a goblet-like cell. The mucosal glands are straight tubular glands.

The lamina propria-submucosa is present and typical. There is no lamina muscularis mucosae.

The tunica muscularis is present, but it is not typical. It consists of smooth muscle and DWFCT. The lateral border of the gizzard consists of regularly arranged DWFCT. From this connective tissue the smooth muscle arises and spreads throughout the muscular tunic.

The tunica serosa is present but thin.

Lower Digestive Tract. The *small intestine* is not divisible histologically into distinct

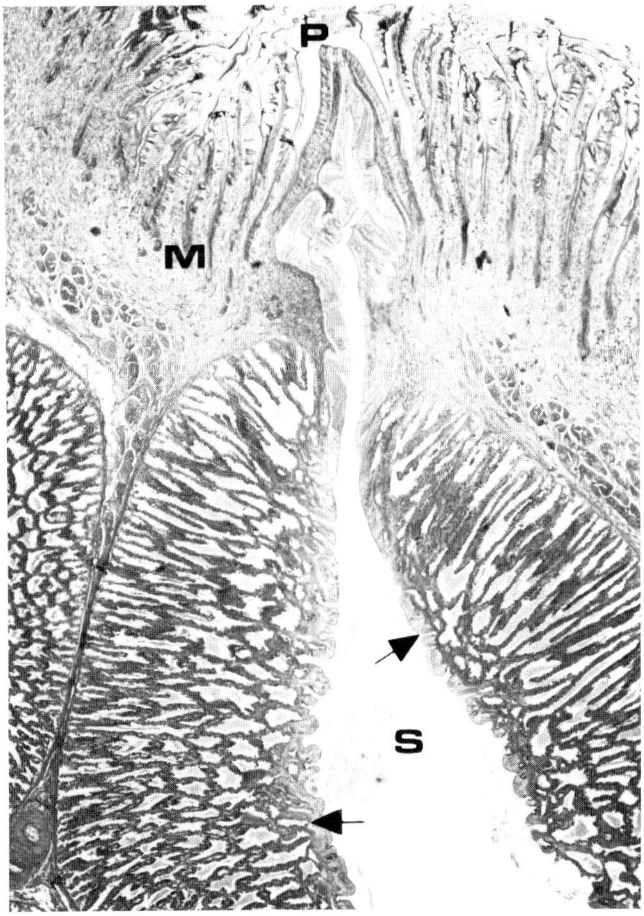

Fig. 17-54. Avian proventriculus. Mucosal glands (*M*) are formed by the grooves or rugae on the surface of the organ. These are referred to as rugosal glands. Submucosal glands (*S*) consist of adenomeres (*arrows*) which radiate from the central excretory duct. These glands, subrugosal glands, open on papillae (*P*) at the surface. ×4.

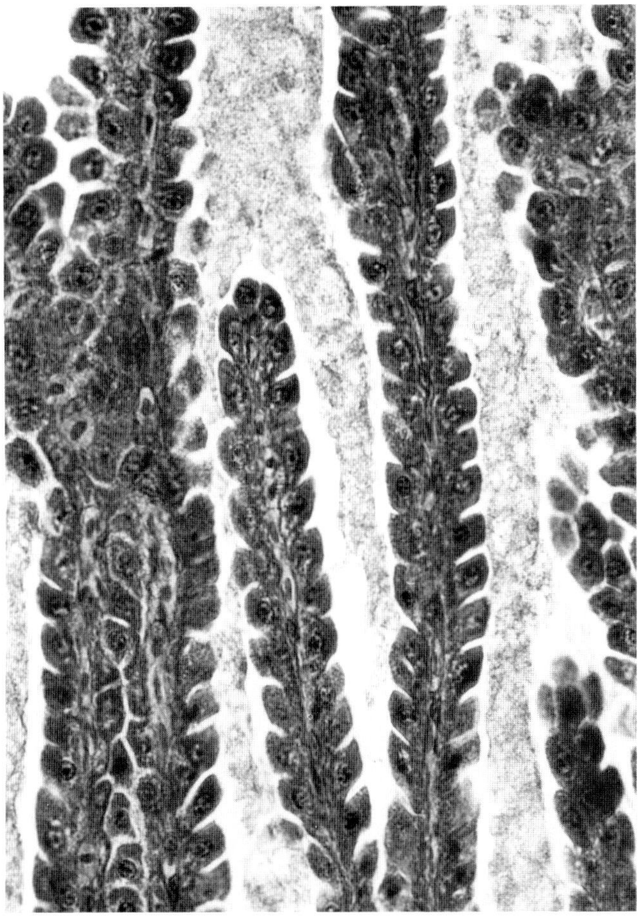

Fig. 17-55. Secretory cells of the avian submucosal glands (proventriculus). The secretory cells are acidophilic. Since their apices are not joined together, they impart a serrated appearance to the lining. ×160.

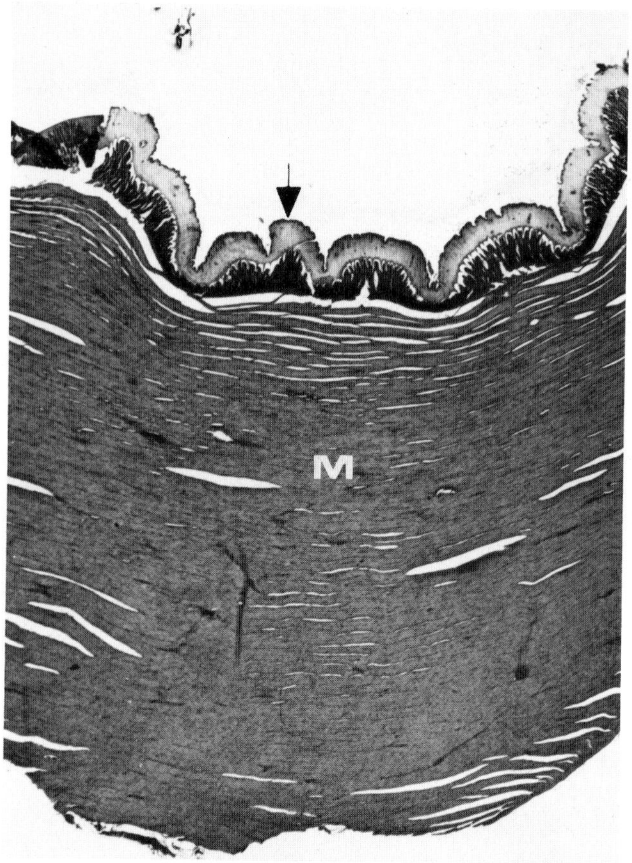

Fig. 17-56. Avian ventriculus. The lining of the ventriculus is a cornified material (*arrow*) which is secreted by the mucosal glands. The tunica muscularis (*M*) is very thick. ×4.

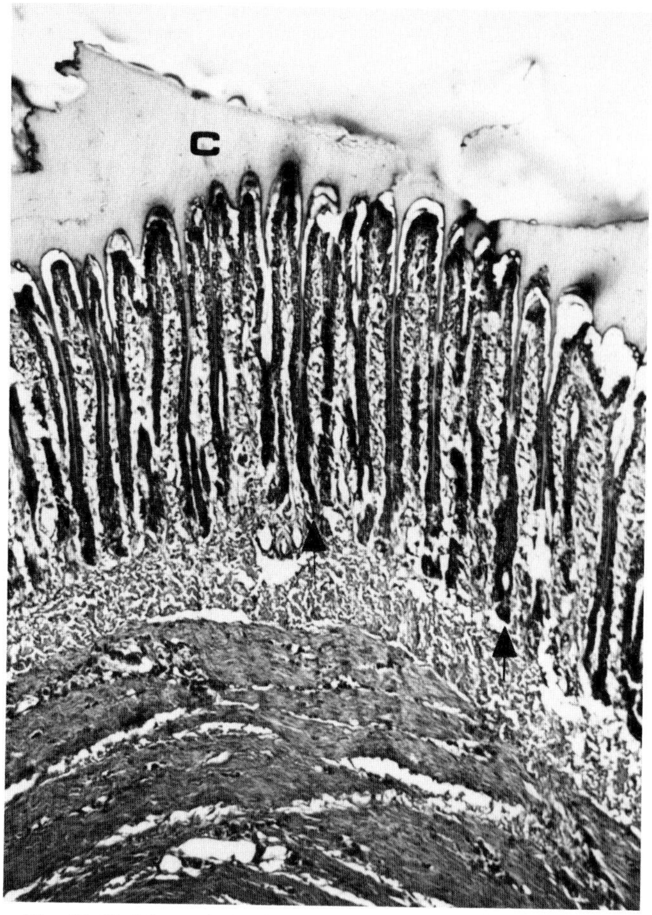

Fig. 17-57. Mucosal glands and lining of the avian ventriculus. The cornified material (*C*) is secreted by the mucosal glands (*arrows*). ×40.

regions. Except for the following exceptions, the small intestine is similar to that of mammals.

The lamina propria and tunica submucosa contain large quantities of diffuse and nodular lymphatic tissue. These may become aggregated in the caudal portion in a manner similar to that of Peyer's patches. A third layer of circular muscle may comprise the inner portion of the tunica muscularis.

The *caeca* are two blind sacs appended to the junction of the small and large intestine. Villi are present at the orifice but diminish and are lost at the end of the organ. The lamina propria and tunica submucosa contain numerous diffuse and aggregated lymphatic tissue. The accumulation of nodules at the caecal orifice is referred to as the *caecal tonsil*. The junction of this organ to the other portions of the intestine is circumscribed by a sphincter from the inner circular mass of the tunica muscularis.

Water absorption occurs in the caeca and some believe that cellulose digestion also occurs.

The *rectum* has short and thick villi and an increased number of goblet cells. Except for those differences, this area is similar to the small intestine.

The *cloaca* is the common orifice for the digestive, excretory and reproductive organs which is divisible into a *coprodaeum*, *urodaeum* and *proctodaeum*. It is lined by a simple columnar epithelium. The tunica mucosa is extensively folded and accounts for the compartmentalization of this structure. Lymphatic tissue is present in the associated connective tissue. The bursa of Fabricius (Chapter 14) is an evagination of the proctodaeum.

The tunica mucosa of the *anus* is highly folded and lined by a stratified squamous epithelium which is cornified. The lamina muscularis mucosae is absent and striated muscle of the tunica muscularis forms the anal sphincter.

Liver

General Characteristics. The liver is the largest single organ in vertebrates and accounts for 2–5% of the total body weight. As a matter of fact, the ratio of liver weight to body weight is usually a constant. The liver is actually a compound tubular gland with exocrine and endocrine functions.

This organ is essential for life. Complete hepatectomy is fatal to the animal. However, the reserve potential of this organ is great. As little as one-third of the organ can be left following hepatectomy without detection of hepatic insufficiency. Moreover, the remaining one-third can totally regenerate itself. Obviously, hepatocytes maintain a fantastic capacity for regeneration.

The liver is an extremely complex and intricate organ. The diverse exocrine and endocrine functions are accomplished by one cell type—the ***hepatocyte***. This, as well as their ability for regeneration, indicates that hepatocytes are rather "unspecialized cells." In other organs, generally, various cells are differentiated to accomplish very specific tasks. This is not true in the liver. Of the numerous and varied functions of the liver, the following are a representative selection to demonstrate the diversity: formation and secretion of bile, glycogenolysis and glycogenesis, protein synthesis, fat metabolism, detoxification of foreign substances, phagocytosis, vitamin production, hemoglobin synthesis, hematopoietic potential and others.

The *Kupffer cell*, a member of the reticuloendothelial system, is present in the liver and accounts for the phagocytic potential of this organ.

Histology of the Liver. The liver is almost completely surrounded by a serous capsule (peritoneum). The fibrous capsule (*capsule of Glisson*) is composed of DWFCT and underlies the serous membrane. The capsular connective tissue is continuous with the septal or interstitial connective tissue which serves as the supportive stroma (Fig. 17-58). The interlobular connective tissue is areolar, while the intralobular connective tissue is reticular.

The parenchyma of the organ consists of *hepatocytes* (Fig. 17-59). These cells are acidophilic and may be binucleated. The appearance of these cells is dependent upon the physiological state of the organism at the time of sampling. In the fasting animal, the cells are small, turbid and indistinctly outlined. Following the ingestion of food, they are well outlined and filled with numerous glycogen and lipid inclusions. In this state they are foamy or honeycombed in appearance.

The cells are arranged as paired plates which are separated by a vast sinusoidal network. The sinusoids are lined by Kupffer cells (Fig. 17-60). These phagocytic cells are stellate and possess a darkly staining, flattened nucleus. The paired plates or laminae of cells are significant in the exocrine function of this organ. Adjacent cell surfaces in the cords have indentations in them that are in register with each other. These indentations have microvilli projecting into them. Although they are small, these *bile canaliculi* are just visible with the light microscope. The cells that contribute to the formation of the bile canaliculi are also secretory. Thus, the canaliculi and adjacent cells may be considered secretory intralobular ducts when compared to other exocrine glands. The canaliculi become confluent with larger ducts that transport bile to the common bile duct and thence to the duodenum.

The larger bile ducts are located in the interstitial areas between adjacent lobules. These ducts are lined by a low cuboidal epithelium which is surrounded by areolar connective tissue. These interlobular bile ducts continue into larger ones that are lined by a columnar epithelium. These larger ducts are surrounded by areolar connective tissue in which smooth muscle and elastic fibers are located. Like other digestive glands studied previously, the epithelium of the duct system blends into, and is actually an extension of, the lamina epithelialis of the duodenum. Of interest, then, is the fact that the small bile canaliculus, located deep in the liver, is actually a space "outside the body."

The interstitial area in which the interlobular bile duct is located is called the *portal area* (Fig. 17-61). It contains three very important structures: *interlobular bile duct*, *hepatic portal vein* and the *hepatic*

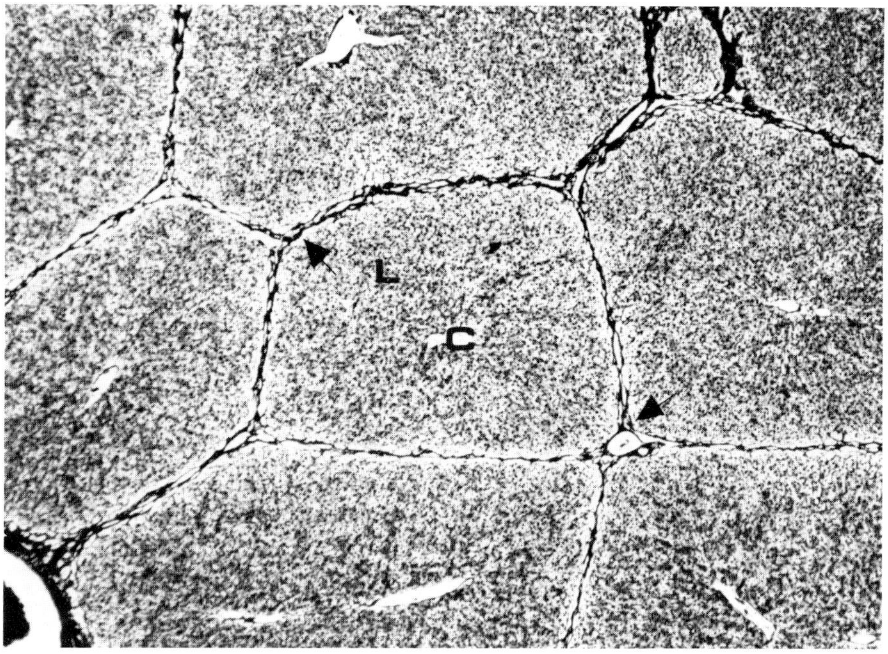

Fig. 17-58. Porcine liver. The lobules (*L*) are well defined by the interlobular connective tissue (*arrows*). A central vein (*C*) is located in the center of each lobule. ×10. (Reticular stain).

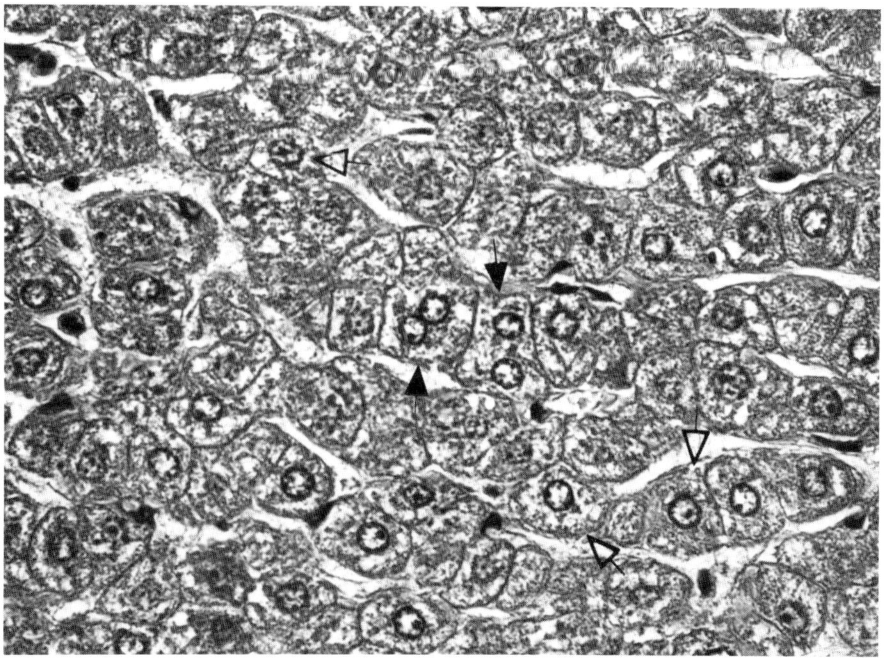

Fig. 17-59. Parenchyma of the liver. The hepatocytes may be uninucleated (*open arrows*) or binucleated (*solid arrows*). ×160.

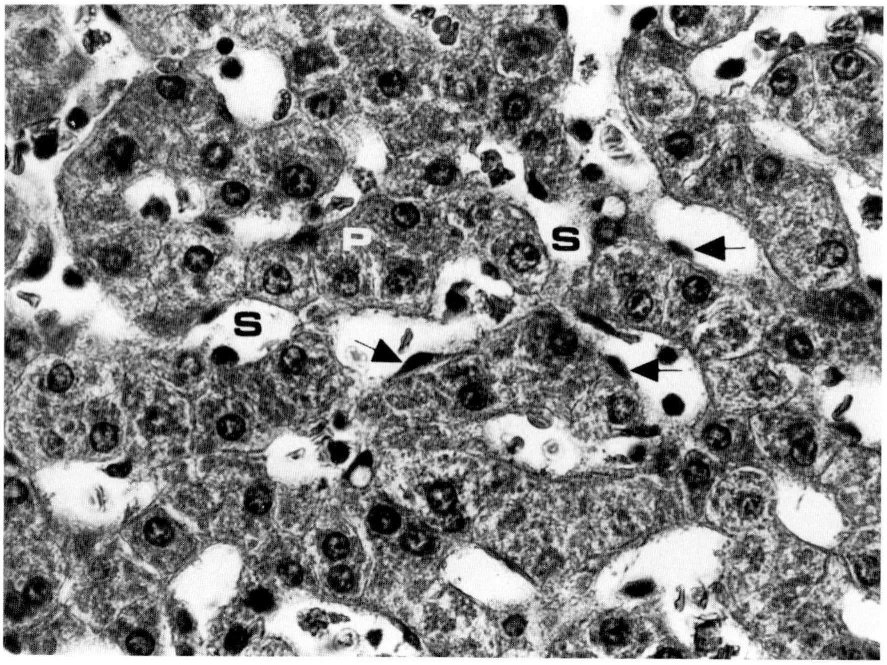

Fig. 17-60. Plates and sinusoids of the liver. The plates of hepatocytes (*P*) are separated from each other by sinusoids (*S*) which are lined by Kupffer cells (*arrows*). ×160.

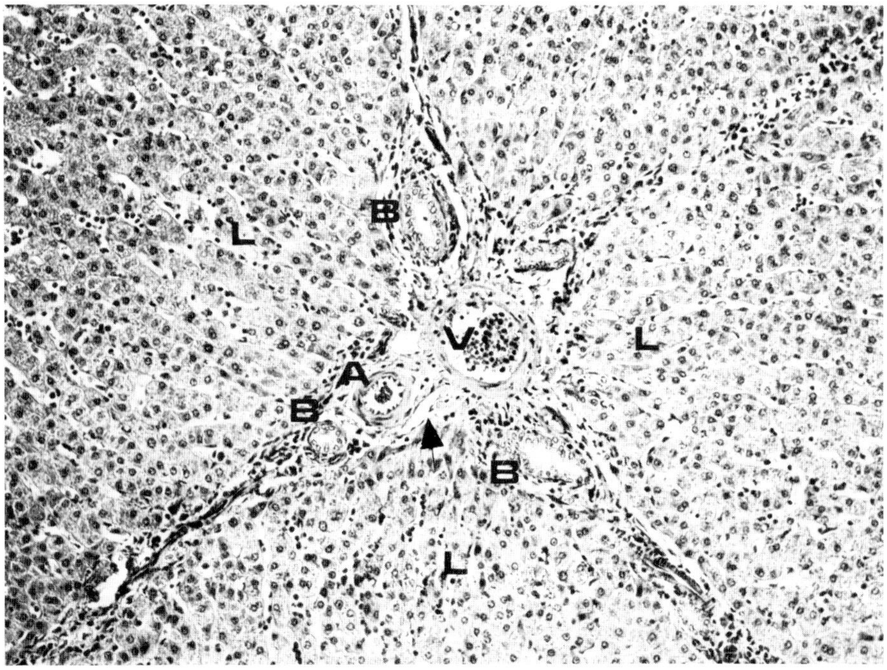

Fig. 17-61. Portal area of the liver. This region is located between lobules (*L*). It contains branches of the bile duct (*B*), hepatic portal vein (*V*) and hepatic artery (*A*). Lymphatic vessels (*arrow*) are present also. ×40.

artery (lymphatics and nerves are also present). Collectively, these structures are referred to as the *portal triad*. The portal triad is an important landmark in the organization of the liver, as well as in the study of the pathology of the liver.

Vascular Relationships. The liver is afforded a dual circulation because of its unique position and function in the body. Its blood supply may be divided into *functional* and *nutritional* units. The nutritional arterial vasculature is supplied by the *hepatic artery*. A branch of this vessel is observed in the portal region. Interlobular arteriolar branches of the hepatic artery send capillaries to the hepatic portal circulation as well as to the hepatic sinusoids. This arteriolar and capillary circulation, naturally, also surrounds the hepatic lobule. The *hepatic portal vein* supplies the functional blood supply to this organ. It contains blood that is laden with nutrients obtained from the intestinal circulation. Smaller branches of this vessel are also observed in the portal area but surround the lobule as well. Inlet veins from this vascular bed also empty into the hepatic sinusoids.

The venous drainage is accomplished by a convergent sinusoidal drainage toward the center of a lobule to a *central vein*. This vessel is oriented perpendicular to the long axis of the lobule and drains into vessels in a sublobular position, the *sublobular veins*. These then become confluent and form branches of the *hepatic veins*.

Lymph flows through the liver and is drained by conspicuous lymphatic vessels. The exact nature of this drainage is not known. It is known, however, that the *hepatic sinusoids*, lined by *Kupffer cells*, are fenestrated. A dialysate of the blood leaves the vascular bed and enters the *space of Disse* (Fig. 17-62). This is a perisinusoidal space which directly bathes the hepatocytes. How the lymph is returned to the main lymphatic circulation has not yet been demonstrated. However, since lymphatic capillaries do arise as blind sacs in connective tissue, the interlobular connective tissue may be the site of pick-up and return. This would make the lymphatic circulation retrograde with respect to the sinusoidal blood flow.

The blood supply to the lobule is composed primarily of venous blood. This would mean that the centrolobular portions of the lobule may be receiving blood extremely deficient in necessary metabolites. This would be consistent with some of the observations which are noted in the pathology laboratory.

Liver Units. The histological unit of the liver is the *hepatic lobule* (Fig. 17-63). In most species this is readily identified, either because of well-developed interlobular connective tissue or by association with the central vein. In the pig, the lobules are especially clear because of the well-

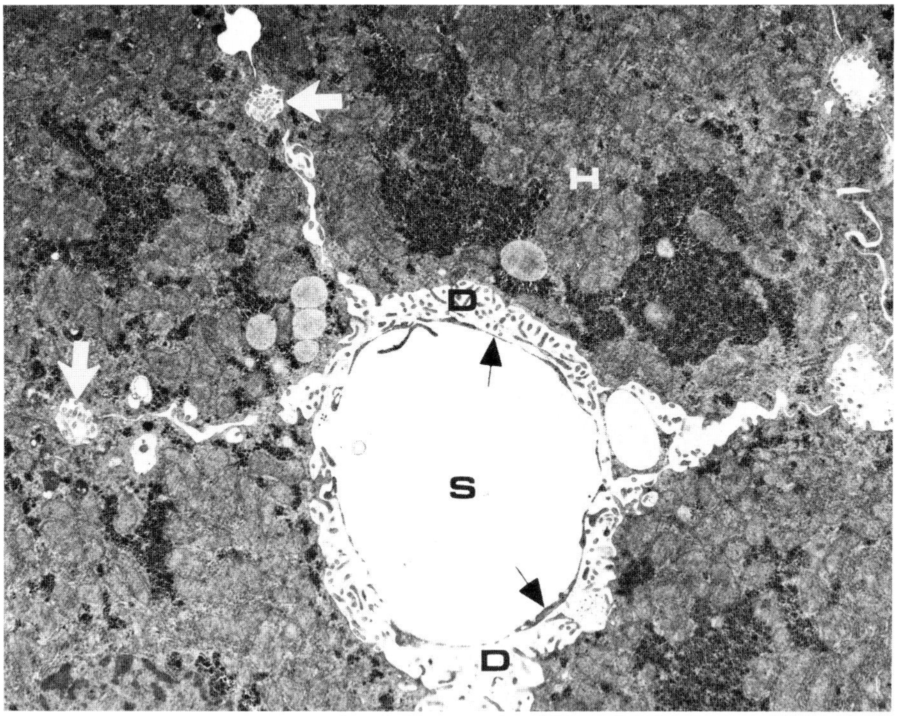

Fig. 17-62. An electron micrograph of the liver. The hepatocytes (*H*) form the bulk of the organ. Portions of their lateral margins are modified as bile canaliculi (*white arrows*). The sinusoids (*S*) are lined by Kupffer cells (*black arrows*) which are separated from the hepatocytes by the space of Disse (*D*). ×6000. (Courtesy of W. Todd).

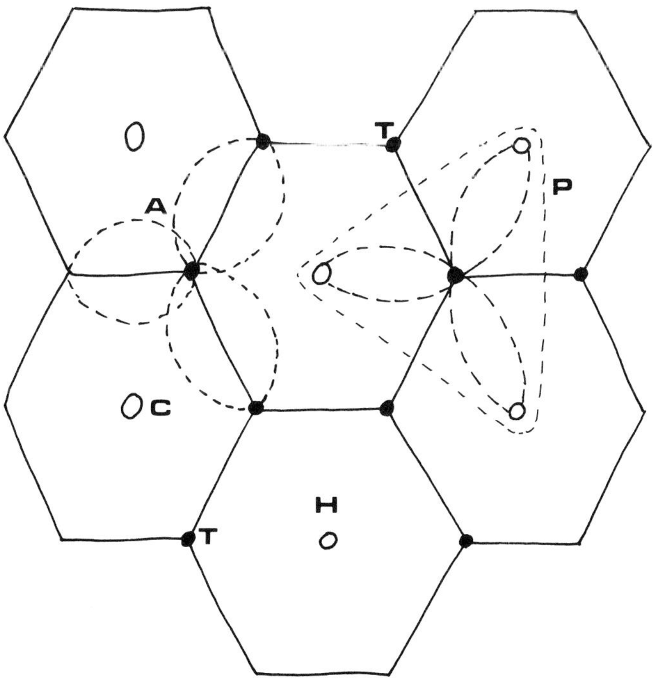

Fig. 17-63. Liver units. *H*, conventional hepatic lobules; *T*, portal triads; *A*, liver acinus; *P*, portal lobule; *C*, central vein.

developed interlobular connective tissue. The concept of the hepatic lobule is based upon two simple relationships: firstly, this organization pattern is structurally obvious; secondly, the drainage pattern of the liver is toward the central vein which is located in the middle of a lobule.

However, the liver is an exocrine gland which has as its adenomeres the plates of cells which empty bile into the canaliculi. These canaliculi then drain to the interlobular bile ducts in the portal region. The liver may be divided, then, into *portal lobules*. This approach considers the secretory activity of the gland as the primary focus.

One may, however, consider the blood supply of the lobules as the focus of functional significance. This being the case, *liver acini* may be recognized on the basis of the vascular supply via the hepatic artery, the venous supply via the hepatic portal vein and the bile and lymphatic drainage via their respective vessels. This concept of liver acini is important in pathology.

Gallbladder

General Characteristics. The *gallbladder* (*cholecyst*) functions as a storage organ for bile. It also concentrates this secretory product of the liver by the absorption of water from its lumen. It is a diverticulum of the common bile duct.

The lamina epithelialis is composed of simple columnar epithelium (Fig. 17-64). The lamina propria-submucosa consists of areolar connective tissue. The tunica muscularis consists of smooth muscle which is not oriented in any particular manner. The tunica serosa is present and typical.

The tunica mucosa is so extensively folded that the invaginations are often misinterpreted as simple glands. However, there are glands in the bile ducts and gallbladder of certain species, notably the ox.

Exocrine Pancreas

General Characteristics. The pancreas is a compound tubuloalveolar gland which, like the liver, is a diverticulum of the epithelium of the gut (Fig. 17-65). It is an exocrine and an endocrine organ. The exocrine structure will be covered in this chapter. The exocrine portion of the organ is very similar to that described for the salivary glands. The main differences in this organ are its special glandular epithelium, the absence of striated ducts, the absence of basket cells and the presence of endocrine tissue.

The cells of the glandular epithelium are conical or pyramidal (Fig. 17-66). Although these cells resemble typical serous cells, the pancreatic glandular cells differ in the basal region. This region possesses radial striations and is basophilic. This is due to the basal accumulation of numerous mito-

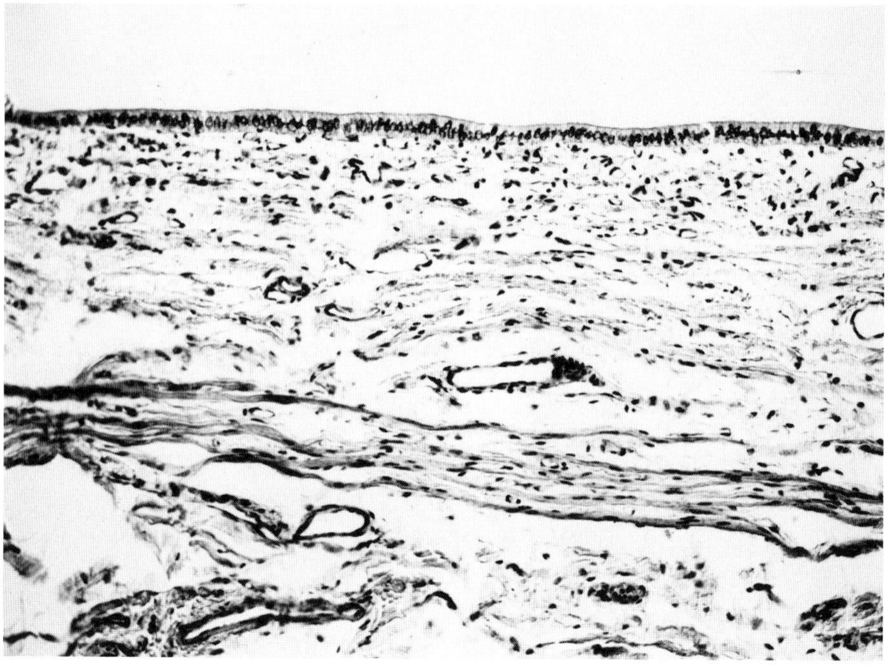

Fig. 17-64. Bovine gallbladder. The columna epithelium is underlaid by a typical lamin propria-submucosa. ×40.

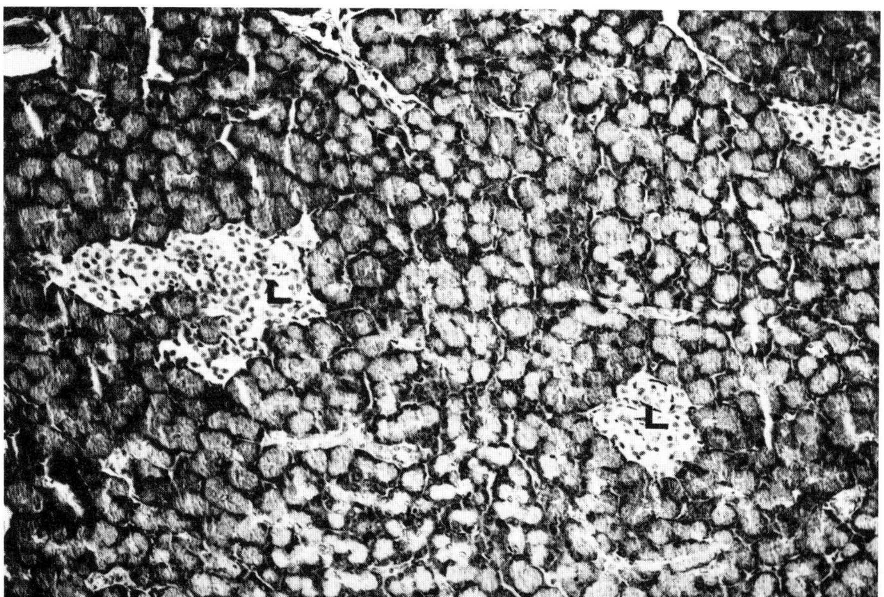

Fig. 17-65. Canine pancreas. The pancreas consists of an endocrine portion, the islets of Langerhans (*L*) and an exocrine portion, pancreatic acini. ×40.

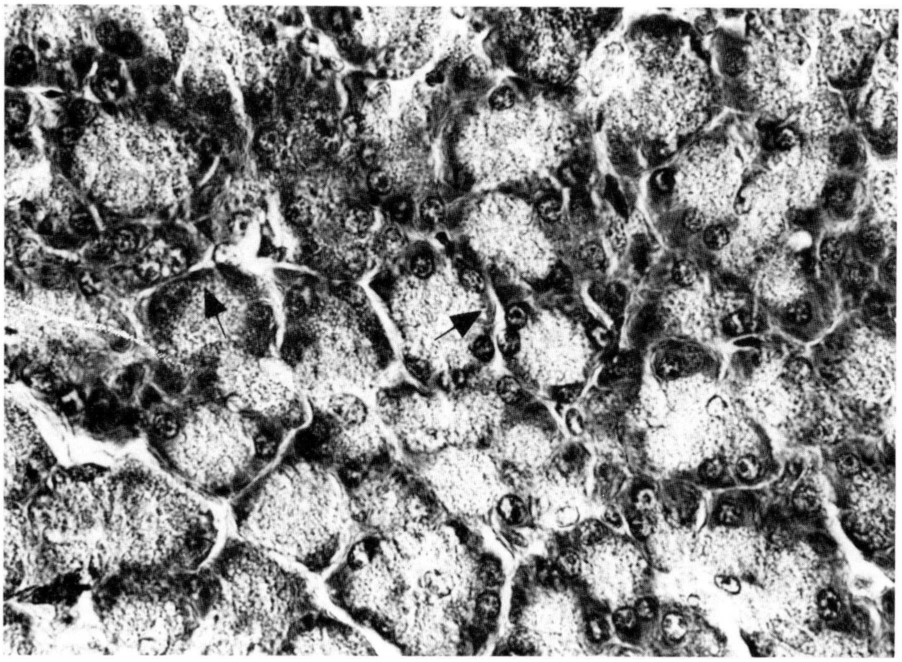

Fig. 17-66. Acini of the canine pancreas. The acini are composed of lining cells (*arrows*) which have an apical acidophilia and a basal basophilia. The apices contain zymogen granules. ×160.

chondria. The nucleus is usually in a parabasal position. A supranuclear pale-staining area (Golgi zone) may be apparent. The acidophilic luminal region is granular and may possess zymogen granules. Their presence or absence is related to the physiological state of the organism. They accumulate during fasting and are extruded during digestion.

The adenomeres open into a small *intercalated duct* which is lined by a squamous or cuboidal epithelium. Rather than the ductular epithelium beginning at the termination of the acinar cells, there is a variable amount of overlap. As such, the lining cells of this duct reside, initially, upon the secretory cells of the acinus. The cells that line this surface are referred to as *centroacinar cells*. These cells do not seem to impair the secretory process, but their significance is not understood.

As the duct system becomes confluent there is a change from cuboidal to columnar epithelium. The epithelium of the larger ducts may contain goblet cells as well as simple branched tubuloaveolar mucous glands.

The DWFCT of the capsule subdivides the gland through the invasion of connective tissue septa. The finest connective tissue is that which is associated with the adenomeres and smaller ducts. It becomes progressively coarse and is continuous with septal connective tissue.

References

Buccal Cavity

Anderes, R. L.: Canine tooth structure, development, blood and nerve supply. North Amer. Vet. *16*: 37, 1935.

Elwood, W. K. and Bernstein, M. H.: The ultrastructure of the enamel organ related to enamel formation. Amer. J. Anat. *122*:73, 1968.

Garlick, N. L.: The teeth of the ox in clinical diagnosis. I. Developmental anatomy. Amer. J. Vet. Res. *15*:226, 1954.

Hand, A. R.: The fine structure of Von Ebner's gland of the rat. J. Cell Biol. *44*:340, 1970.

Kallenbach, E.: Fine structure of rat incisor enamel organ during late pigmentation and regression stages. J. Ultrastruct. Res. *30*:38, 1970.

Lester, K. S. and Boyde, A.: Scanning electron microscopy of developing roots of molar teeth of the laboratory rat. J. Ultrastruct. Res. *33*:80, 1970.

Murray, R. G., Murray, A. and Fujimoto, S.: Fine structure of gustatory cells in rabbit taste buds. J. Ultrastruct. Res. *27*:444, 1969.

Shackleford, J. M. and Wilborn, W. H.: Ultrastructure of bovine parotid glands. J. Morph. *127*:453, 1969.

Tubular Organs

Adkins, R. B., Ende, N. and Gobbel, W. G.: A correlation of parietal cell activity with ultrastructural alterations. Surgery *62*:1059, 1967.

Bonfanti, C.: Duodenal glands in the horse. Rev. Med. Vet. *4*:95, 1952.

Brunser, O. and Luft, J. H.: Fine structure of the apex of absorptive cells from rat small intestine. J. Ultrastruct. Res. *31*:291, 1970.

Cardell, R. R., Badenhausen, S. and Porter, K. R.: Intestinal triglyceride absorption in the rat. An electron microscopical study. J. Cell Biol. *34*:123, 1967.

Demke, D. D.: A brief histology of the intestine of the turkey poult. Amer. J. Vet. Res. *15*:447, 1952.

Elias, H.: Comparison of duodenal glands in domestic animals. Amer. J. Vet. Res. *8*:311, 1947.

Hampton, J. C.: An electron microscopic study of mouse colon. Dis. Colon Rectum *3*:423, 1960.

Johnson, F. R. and Young, B. A.: Undifferentiated cells in the gastric mucosa. J. Anat. *101*:617, 1967.

Leeson, C. R. and Leeson, T. S.: The fine structure of Brunner's glands in the rabbit. Anat. Rec. *159*:409, 1967.

Rubin, W.: Enzyme cytochemistry of gastric parietal cells at a fine structure level. J. Cell Biol. *42*:332, 1969.

Titkemeyer, C. W. and Calhoun, M. L.: A comparative study of the structure of the small intestine of domestic animals. Amer. J. Vet. Res. *16*:152, 1955.

Trier, J. S.: Structure of the mucosa of the small intestine as it relates to intestinal function. Fed. Proc. *26*:1391, 1967.

Large Digestive Glands

Burkel, W. E. and Low, F. N.: The fine structure of rat liver sinusoids, space of Disse and associated tissue space. Amer. J. Anat. *118*:769, 1966.

Caro, L. G. and Palade, G. E.: Protein synthesis, storage, and discharge in the pancreatic exocrine cell. An autoradiographic study. J. Cell Biol. *20*:473, 1964.

Ekholm, R. and Edlund, Y.: Ultrastructure of the human exocrine pancreas. J. Ultrastruct. Res. *2*:453, 1959.

Elias, H. and Sherrick, J. C.: *Morphology of the Liver.* Academic Press, New York, 1969.

Loud, A. V.: A quantitative stereological description of the ultrastructure of normal rat liver parenchymal cells. J. Cell Biol. *37*:27, 1968.

Rappaport, A. M.: The structural and functional unit in the human liver (liver acinus). Anat. Rec. *130*:673, 1958.

Trotter, N. L.: A fine structure of lipid in mouse liver regenerating after partial hepatectomy. J. Cell Biol. *21*:233, 1964.

Yamada, E.: The fine structure of the gallbladder epithelium of the mouse. J. Biophys. Biochem. Cytol. *1*:445, 1955.

18 Urinary System

Kidney

General Characteristics. The kidney and associated urinary passages are designed to ***filter*** the blood, ***remove*** waste materials, ***recover*** useful metabolites, ***store*** the fluid waste and eventually ***transport*** the waste products to the exterior of the body. To accomplish these functions, the following organs are involved: *kidney, ureter, urinary bladder* and *urethra*.

The functions of the urinary system are not confined, however, to the aforementioned aspects. The kidney, specifically, functions as an endocrine organ. A substance called *renin* and a hormone, *erythropoietin*, are secreted. The kidney has been implicated in the metabolism of vitamin D. This involvement in "hormone D" metabolism, in conjunction with other organs, is being described as a new endocrine system.

In mammals, the functional unit of the kidney is the *nephron*. Blood filtration through this unit is accomplished under high pressure; i.e., glomerular filtration is accomplished on the arterial side of the vascular supply. This is not the case in birds because of the involvement of the renal portal system.

The kidney is composed of two distinct morphological regions, an outer *cortex* and an inner *medulla*. This division implies that these regions are composed of different elements that are separated from each other. Actually, a corticomedullary junction is apparent, but elements of one region are found in the other region. There is, however, a quantitative difference in the occurrence of specific elements in the two regions.

The kidney is a compound tubular gland composed of *uriniferous tubules*. The portion that produces the urine is the *nephron*, while that which collects, concentrates and transports this fluid to the renal pelvis is the ***collecting duct system***.

The nephron is composed of a *capsule of* ***Bowman, proximal convoluted tubule, loop of Henle*** and a ***distal convoluted tubule*** (Fig. 18-1). Bowman's capsule and the glomerulus that it encloses constitute a *renal corpuscle*. The tubular portions of the nephron may be present in the medullary region, but the capsule of Bowman and most of the proximal tubules are generally located in the cortex. The *collecting ducts*, which extend into the cortical area, are not randomly scattered throughout the cortex but occur in bands called *medullary rays*. The collecting ducts become progressively larger and eventually terminate as *papillary ducts* in the apices of the *renal pyramids*.

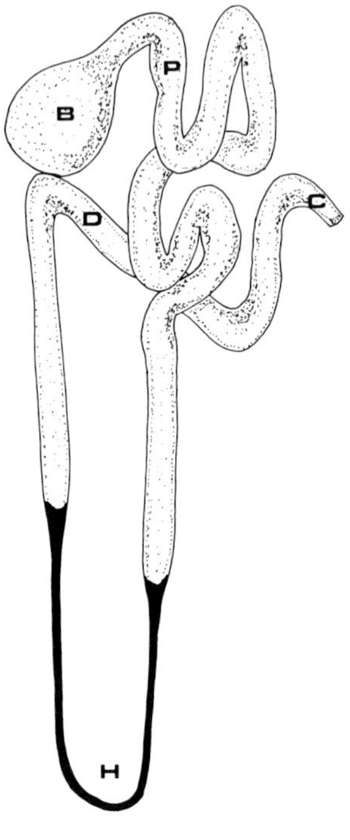

Fig. 18-1. Diagram of a nephron. The expanded bulb, Bowman's capsule (*B*), is continuous with the proximal convoluted tubule (*P*). It continues as the loop of Henle (*H*). The loop of Henle has a descending, thin and ascending segment. The distal convoluted tubule (*D*) continues to the connecting duct (*C*). All light micrographs are the original magnifications. All electron micrographs are the final magnifications.

The kidney, like any compound gland, is divided into lobes and lobules (Fig. 18-2). In some species there is only one lobe, while in others the lobulation may persist or secondarily fuse. A lobe consists of medullary and cortical regions. The medullary portion consists of a *papilla* or pyramid which is composed primarily of collecting ducts. The broad base of the *pyramid* is situated at the corticomedullary junction. The narrow apex of the pyramid projects into the renal pelvis as an individual projection or fused with others to form a *crest*. Among the domestic species, calyces form in the pig and ox.

Cortical lobules are distinguished on the basis of the drainage from the tubules, as well as by the nature of the arterial supply.

Vascular Supply and Drainage. The blood supply for the kidney is obtained from the renal artery which divides into smaller *interlobar arteries*. The *arcuate* or *arciform arteries* are a continuation of the aforementioned in the region of the corticomedullary junction. They follow a course which is parallel to the kidney surface along the corticomedullary junction. The arcuates, which may be branched secondarily, give rise to ascending or perpendicular ***interlobular arteries***. The *afferent arteriole*, an extension of an interlobular artery, may be considered the *intralobular arteriole*. This vessel continues into the renal corpuscle where it divides into a capillary bed. This capillary bed is reconstituted as the *efferent arteriole*. Note: ***The intralobular arteriolar circulation contains a capillary network***. The efferent arteriole in the outer cortical region gives rise to a ***cortical peritubular capillary network***, and a similar arteriole in the juxtamedullary region gives rise to a ***medullary peritubular capillary network***. Arising from the efferent arteriole, the arterioles that supply these capillary beds are referred to as the ***false straight arterioles***. ***True straight arterioles*** may arise from the arcuate or interlobular arteries to supply the peritubular capillary network of the medullary region.

Extensions of the interlobular arteries terminate in a capsular plexus. The venous drainage of the kidney is accomplished through companion vessels to the aforementioned arterial supply. Although the question of lymphatic drainage has not been satisfactorily resolved, it is believed that all regions, except the parenchymatous regions of the cortex, are drained by lymphatics.

The blood supply of the kidney is such that localized changes that arise from vascular disturbances are readily detected. For

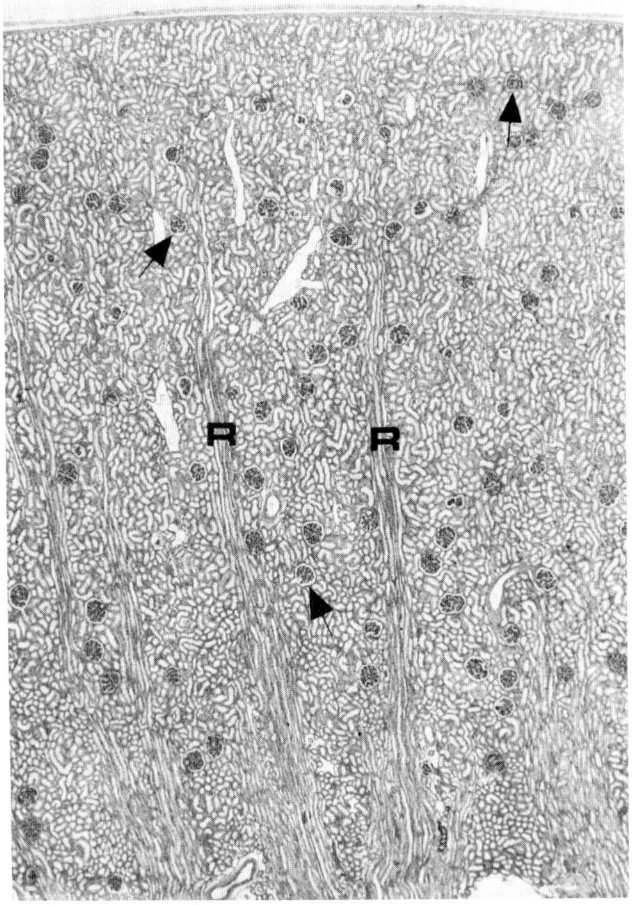

Fig. 18-2. Cortex of the kidney. Numerous glomeruli (*arrows*) are scattered throughout the cortex. The medullary rays (*R*) are prominent. ×4.

represents the capillary bed. The surface of the balloon contacting the finger represents the visceral lining. The space between the "visceral lining" and the outer wall of the balloon ("parietal lining") represents the initial portion of the nephron into which the glomerular filtrate is pushed.

Since the lining of Bowman's capsule is simple squamous epithelium, it is difficult to distinguish the visceral lining from the capillary endothelium. This endothelial lining is fenestrated and covered by a complete basal lamina (Fig. 18-4). The relationship of the visceral lining to capillary endothelium has been clarified with electron microscopy. The body of the lining cells is not in direct contact with the basal lamina. Rather, they are separated from the basal lamina by cytoplasmic processes (Fig. 18-5). The *foot processes* (*pedicles*) are separated from each other by *filtration slits* which are continuous with the urinary space of Bowman's capsule. These cells with foot processes (visceral lining cells) are referred to as *podocytes*. Although the podocytes are aligned along the periphery of the capillaries, the actual barrier to filtration is the basal lamina.

Besides the endothelium and podocytes, a third cell type is usually encountered: *mesangial* or *intercapillary cells*. These stellate cells are located between the capillary loops of the glomerulus. Their precise function is not known.

The squamous cell configuration of the parietal layer of Bowman's capsule is readily apparent. With periodic acid-Schiff

example, if an interlobar artery were occluded, then the infarction would involve an entire lobe. If an interlobular artery were occluded, then the infarction would involve all or portions of a few lobules. An appreciation of this blood supply is essential for the diagnosis and location of specific renal vascular disturbances.

Histology of the Kidney. The kidney is covered by a loosely adherent capsule of dense white fibrous connective tissue (DWFCT). Since the kidney is retroperitoneal in location, only one side of it is covered by a tunica serosa (peritoneum). The capsule of DWFCT in the hilar region is continuous with the adventitial coat of the renal pelvis. The primary supportive stroma of the kidney is a delicate meshwork of reticular connective tissue.

The *renal corpuscle* is composed of a *tuft* or *glomerulus* of capillaries which connects the afferent and efferent arterioles and *Bowman's capsule*, the expanded end of the nephron (Fig. 18-3). The latter consists of a *visceral* and *parietal lining* of squamous epithelium. The glomerular capillaries are interdigitated with the visceral lining. Their relationship to one another is analogous to inserting a finger into a balloon. The finger

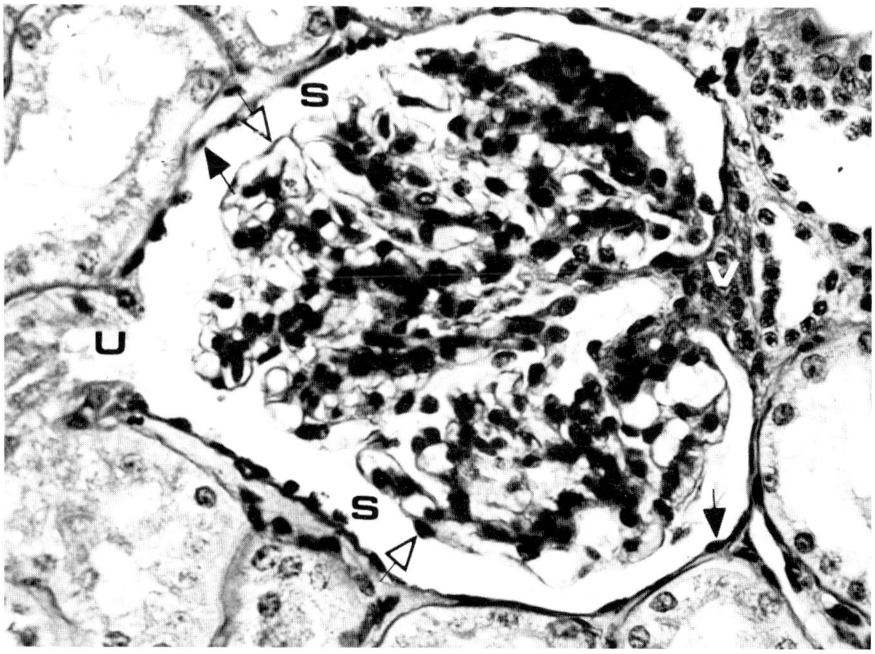

Fig. 18-3. A renal corpuscle. The renal corpuscle consists of Bowman's capsule and a glomerulus. Bowman's capsule is composed of a parietal layer of cells (*solid arrows*) and a visceral layer of cells (*open arrows*) separated by the uriniferous space (*S*). At the vascular pole (*V*) the vessels enter and leave the glomerulus. The parietal layer of Bowman's capsule is continuous with the proximal convoluted tubule at the uriniferous pole (*U*). ×100.

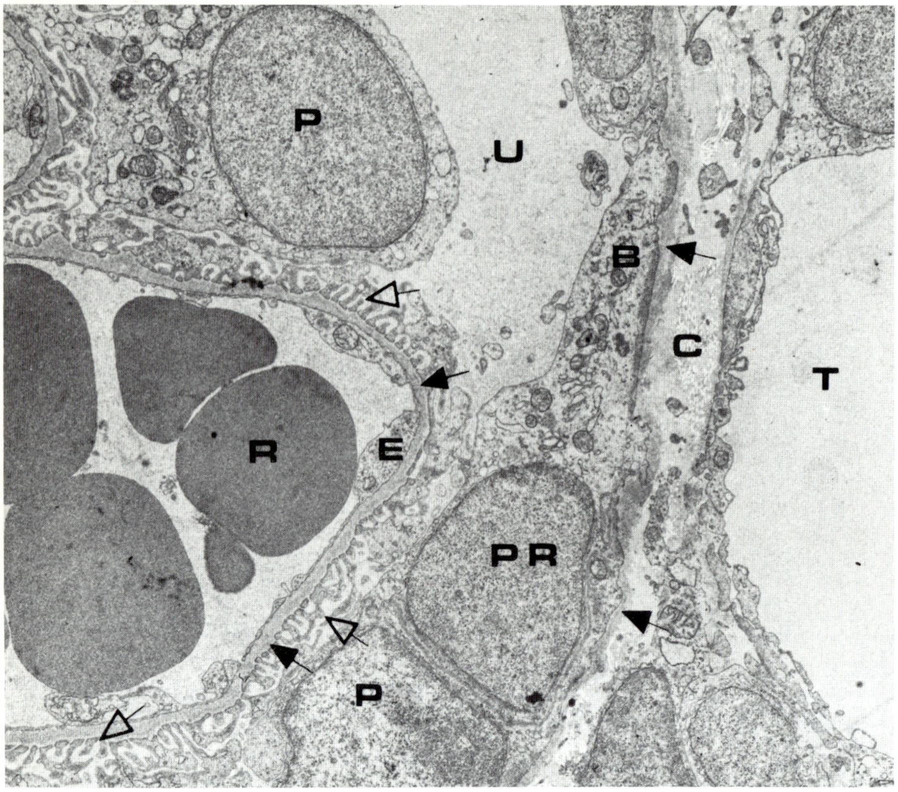

Fig. 18-4. An electron micrograph of a glomerulus. Numerous podocytes (*P*) are in close association with a capillary laden with erythrocytes (*R*). The podocytic processes, pedicles (*open arrows*), are adjacent to a well-developed basal lamina (*solid arrows*). One podocyte (*PR*) is reflected as part of the parietal layer of Bowman's capsule (*B*). The parietal layer is bounded by a basal lamina (*solid arrows*) and connective tissue (*C*). A portion of a uriniferous tubule (*T*) is adjacent to the renal corpuscle. *E*, endothelium. ×6,000.

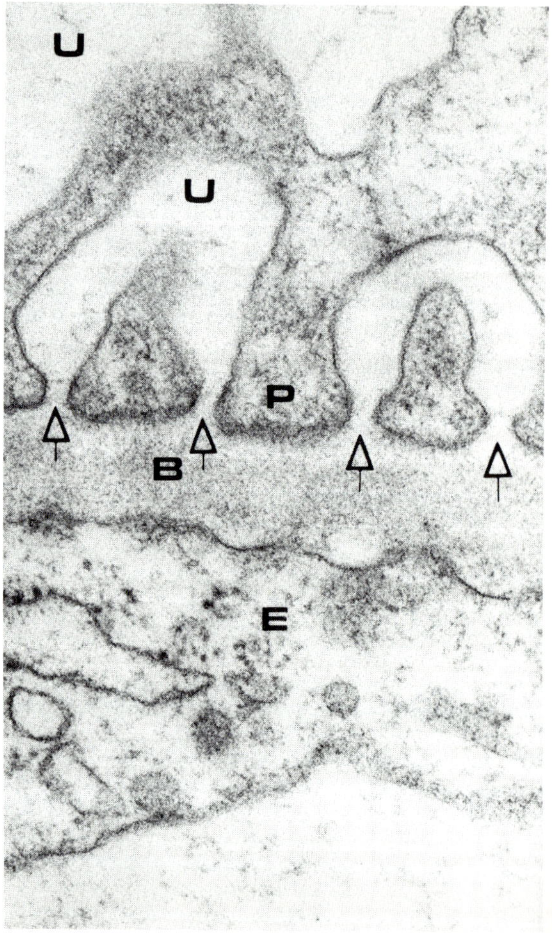

Fig. 18-5. An electron micrograph of the podocytic processes. The pedicles (*P*) are adjacent to the basal lamina (*B*). Materials from the capillary move through the endothelial cell (*E*) and/or its fenestrations, through the basal lamina and into the uriniferous space (*U*) through the filtration slits (*arrows*). ×77,000.

(PAS) staining, the prominent basement membrane surrounding the capsule and glomerulus is readily demonstrated (Figs. 2-39, 2-40). Two distinct regions of the renal corpuscle are apparent in ideal sections: a *vascular pole* and a *urinary pole* (Fig. 18-3). The vascular pole is the region of entry and exit of the arterioles. It is also the region in which the *juxtaglomerular apparatus* is located. The urinary pole is the point of continuity between Bowman's capsule and the proximal convoluted tubule. At this point there is a transition from the squamous epithelium of the parietal layer to the cuboidal epithelium of the proximal tubule.

The *proximal convoluted tubule* is the longest, widest and most highly developed segment of the nephron (Fig. 18-6). Its function is extremely important and is the segment that is easily affected by disease processes and toxic substances. It is lined by cuboidal cells with a well-developed brush border. With routine staining (hematoxylin and eosin), the eosinophilic and granular cytoplasm does not contrast markedly with the brush border. A marked difference, however, is noted with PAS staining. The mucopolysaccharides of the cell coat on the microvilli are strongly PAS-positive. The basal portion of these cells is highly folded and contains numerous mitochondria. The mitochondria contribute to the basal striations which may be apparent. Because the lateral border of cells are highly interdigitated, they are not readily observed in light microscopic sections. The nuclei of these cells are spherical, small and located in a basal or parabasal position. Varying physiological states contribute to an altered morphology of this segment. Generally, however, the luminal size is small and the tube is composed of cells with prominent brush borders

The proximal convoluted tubule continues into the *loop of Henle*. This segment of the nephron is of variable length and the length is indicative of the ability of the organism to conserve water. The loop of Henle consists of three portions: the *straight portion of the proximal tubule (descending limb)*, a *descending and ascending thin segment* and a *straight portion of the distal tubule (ascending limb)*. There are some variations in the loop of Henle. Those nephrons in a juxtamedullary position have long *intermediate segments* (thin segments) the apices of which are deep in the medulla and may extend into the apices of the medullary papillae. Peripherally positioned nephrons (subcapsular) have short loops of Henle which extend a short distance into the medullary region. The transition from the cuboidal epithelium of the descending limb to the squamous epithelium of the *descending thin segment* is abrupt. Since there are numerous capillaries (blood and lymphatic) in this region of the medulla, the microscopist must look carefully to distinguish the thin segments. Usually, the thin segments have larger lumina and more nuclei that protrude into the lumina than the capillaries. The morphology of the actual *loop* (Fig. 18-7) and *ascending thin segment* is similar to the descending thin segment. The transition to the cuboidal epithelium of the *ascending segment* is also abrupt. The straight portion ascends to the region of the vascular pole of the glomerulus and is positioned between the afferent and efferent arterioles. A condensation of cells in part of the wall of this tubule at this point is called the *macula densa*. The tubule continues from this point

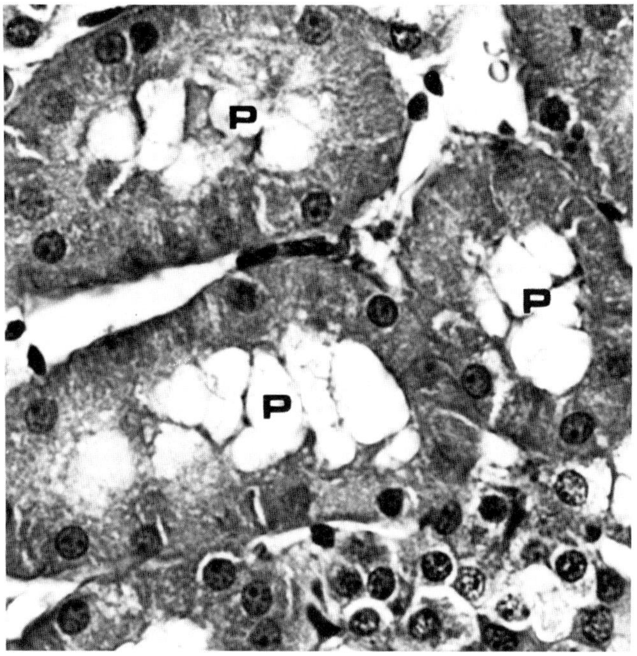

Fig. 18-6. Proximal convoluted tubules of the canine kidney. The tubules (*P*) are lined by cuboidal cells. The brush border is not defined clearly. ×160. (See Fig. 2-47.)

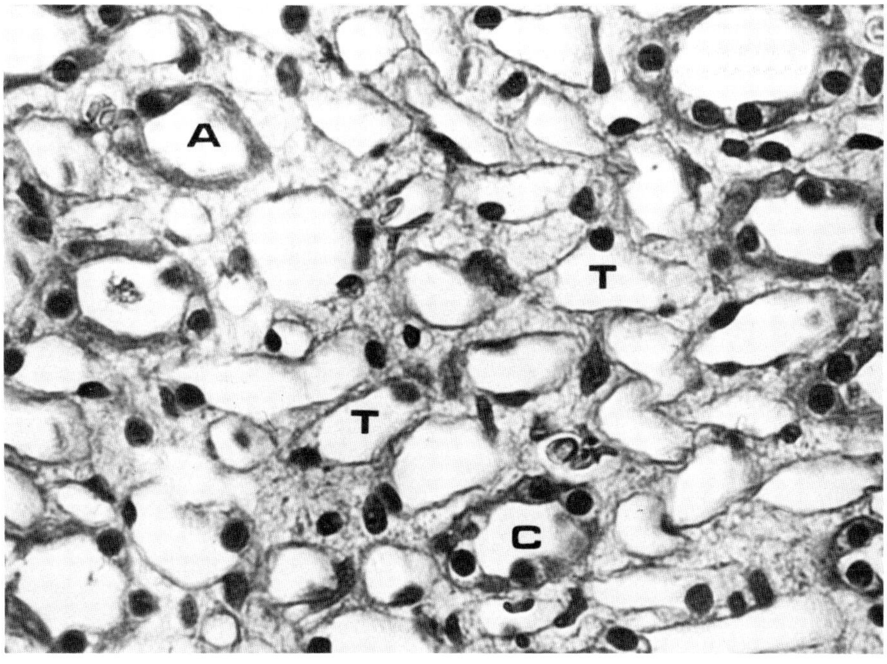

Fig. 18-7. Medulla of the canine kidney. Thin segments of the loop of Henle (*T*), ascending limbs (*A*) and collecting ducts (*C*) are indicated. ×160.

as the *distal convoluted tubule* (Fig. 18-8). The distal tubules are short and are not as frequently encountered in sections as their proximal counterparts. Although distal convoluted tubules are not as large as proximal convoluted tubules, their luminal diameter to mural thickness ratios are greater than the proximal convoluted tubules. More cells line these tubules and their lateral borders are more clearly defined than their proximal counterparts. These cells are less acidophilic than the cells of the proximal tubules. The nuclei of these cells are central to parabasal in position.

The excretory duct system is composed of *connecting tubules*, *collecting tubules* and *excretory ducts*. The *connecting tubules* connect the distal convoluted tubules to the collecting ducts. The former are lined by cuboidal epithelial cells which stain lightly with routine staining techniques. The nucleus is large and the cell borders are distinct.

The *collecting ducts* are similar to the connecting tubules (Fig. 18-9). The collecting duct epithelium is somewhat taller in the medullary region. The *excretory ducts* (*papillary ducts*) are lined by a columnar epithelium (Fig. 18-10). As these ducts open into the renal pelvis, they form an *area cribrosa* on the apical portion of the pyramids. The duct epithelium is reflected on the lining of the renal pelvis as transitional epithelium.

The juxtaglomerular apparatus consists of the ***macula densa, juxtaglomerular cells*** and *mesangial cells*. The macula densa is a modified portion of the distal tubule at the vascular pole of the renal corpuscle (Fig. 18-11). The nuclei of the lining cells adjacent to the renal corpuscle are tightly packed against one another. This portion of the tubule is in contact with Bowman's capsule via an aggregation of small cells with pale nuclei (*polkissen cells*). These may be mesangial cells. The exact function of the macula densa is not established; however, its intimate relationship to the vascular pole and juxtaglomerular cells implies that it is involved in blood flow regulation to the glomerular capillaries.

Juxtaglomerular cells occur in the tunica media of the afferent arteriole. These are modified smooth muscle cells of an epithelioid nature which are in direct contact with the endothelial cells of these vessels and closely positioned to the macula densa. These secretory cells contain granules that are linked to their function. These cells are believed to be responsible for the secretion of ***renin***.

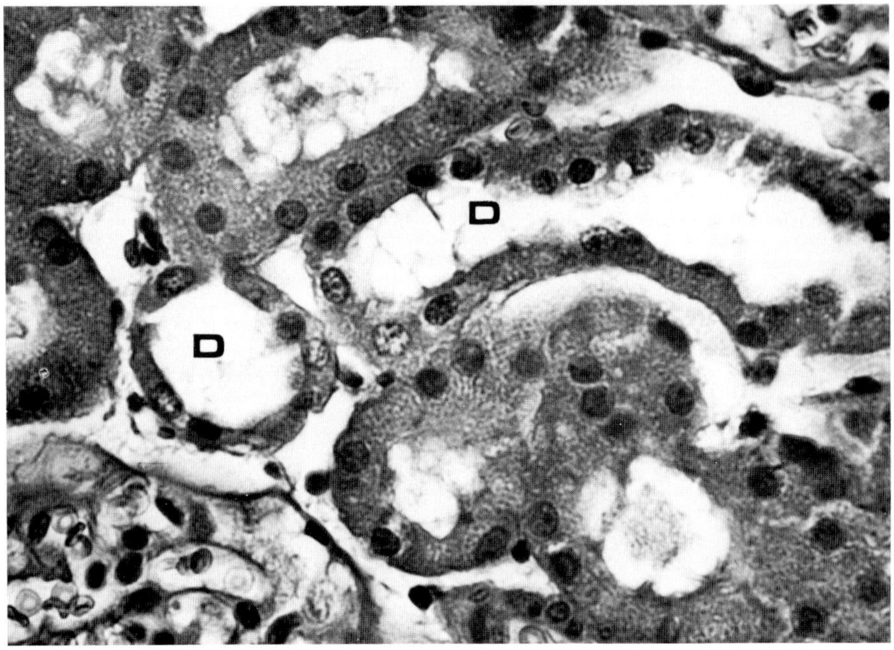

Fig. 18-8. Distal convoluted tubules of the canine kidney. The distal tubules (*D*) are lined by a low cuboidal epithelium. ×160.

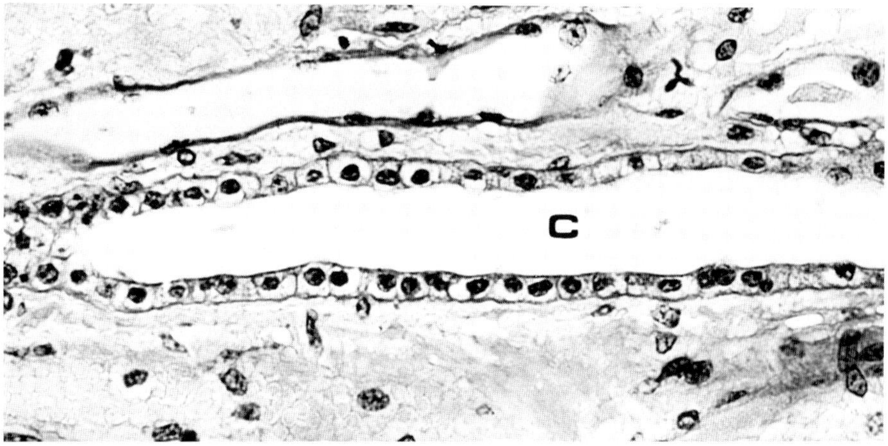

Fig. 18-9. Collecting duct of the equine kidney. The collecting duct (*C*) is lined by cuboidal epithelium. The cytoplasm is clear and the lateral margins are distinct. ×160.

Urinary Passages

Renal Pelvis. The inner surface of the renal pelvis is continuous with the epithelial lining of the papillary ducts. The epithelium becomes a thin transitional lining which becomes thicker toward the pelvis. The lamina propria-tunica submucosa is composed of areolar connective tissue. In equids, branched tubuloalveolar mucous glands occur in this region and extend into the ureter. These glands account for the frothy appearance of the urine of these species. The tunica muscularis may be composed of three layers of muscle which are arranged in bundles. The layers, however, are not always distinct. The contraction of these muscle bundles tends to "milk" urine from the kidney.

Ureters. The ureters are lined by a lamina epithelialis of transitional epithelium (Fig. 18-12). Goblet cells may be present in the horse. The lamina propria-tunica submucosa consists of areolar connective tissue. Mucous glands may be present in some species. The tunica muscularis is present and three layers of muscle may be apparent. The tunica adventitia, also, is present and typical. Part of this structure is covered by a tunica serosa (peritoneum).

Urinary Bladder. The ureters open obliquely into the bladder near the neck and the longitudinal coat of the tunica muscularis continues into the bladder wall. There is very little circularly oriented muscle at this junction. Pressure within the bladder tends to close the orifice. The contractions of the ureteral musculature tend to spurt urine into the bladder.

The mural elements of the bladder are similar to those of the ureter.

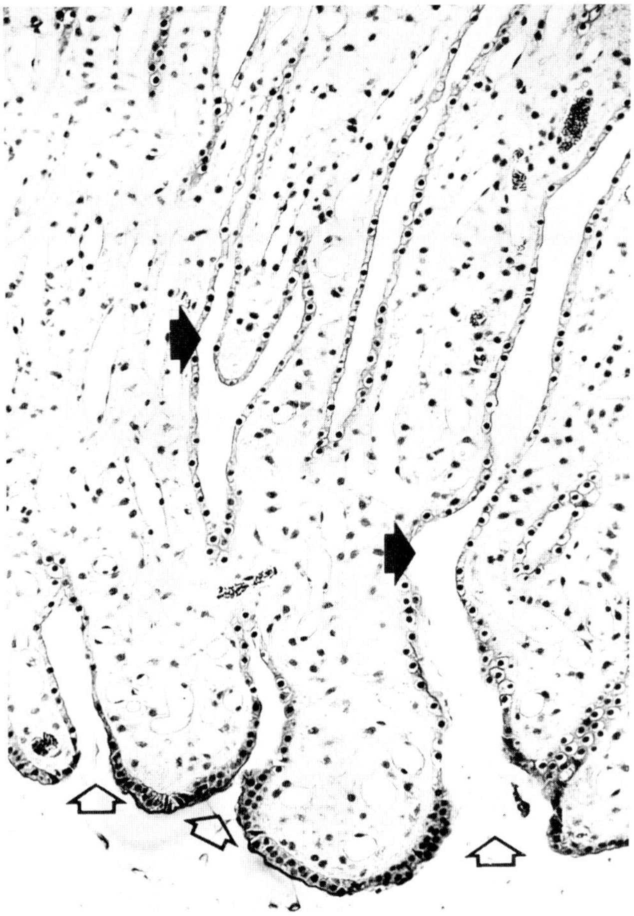

Fig. 18-10. Area cribrosa of the feline kidney. The collecting ducts become confluent as papillary ducts (*solid arrows*). These ducts open into the renal pelvis (*open arrows*) and form an area cribrosa. ×40.

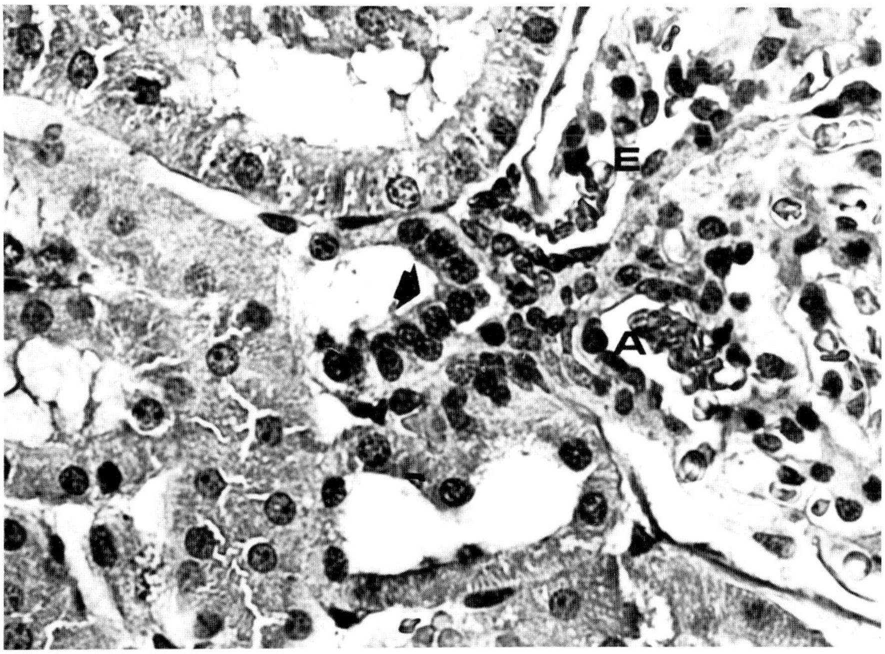

Fig. 18-11. Macula densa. The macula densa (*arrow*) marks the beginning of the distal convoluted tubule. The macula densa is positioned at the vascular pole in close association with the afferent (*A*) and efferent (*E*) arterioles. × 160.

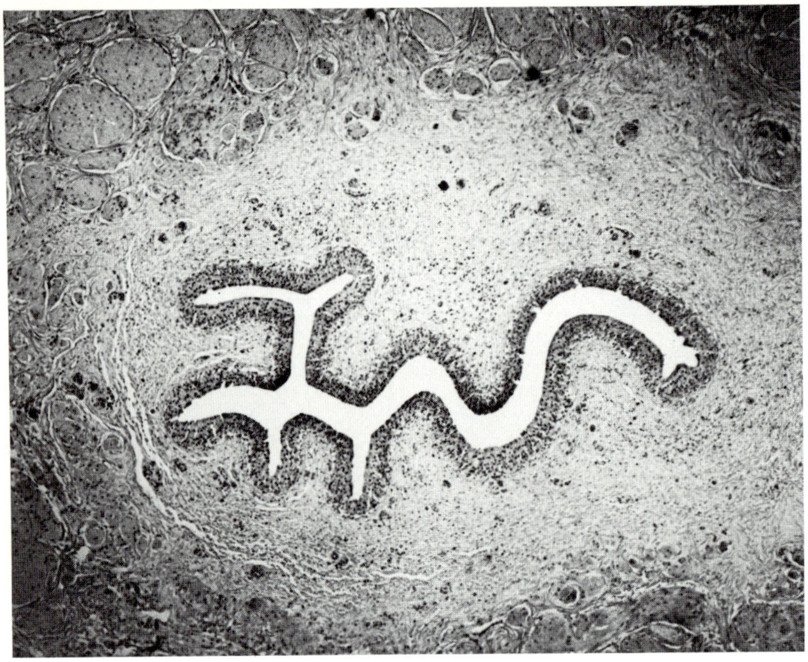

Fig. 18-12. Canine ureter. The ureter is lined by transitional epithelium. The lamina propria-submucosa is extensive. ×10.

The tunica mucosa of the ureters and the bladder may be highly folded. At this time, the lamina epithelialis will be thick (Fig. 2-15). Upon distention of the bladder, the transitional epithelium is reduced in thickness and the mucosal folds are effaced (Fig. 2-16).

The urethrae will be discussed with their respective reproductive systems.

References

Barajas, L.: The ultrastructure of the juxtaglomerular apparatus as disclosed by three dimensional reconstructions from serial sections. J. Ultrastruct. Res. *33*:116, 1970.

Dalton, A. J. and Haguenau, F. (eds.): *Ultrastructure of the Kidney*, Vol. 2. Academic Press, New York, 1967.

Jorgensen, F.: Electron microscopic studies of normal visceral epithelial cells. Lab. Invest. *17*:225, 1967.

Latta, H.: The glomerular capillary wall. J. Ultrastruct. Res. *32*:526, 1970.

Monis, B. and Zambrano, D.: Transitional epithelium of urinary tract in normal and dehydrated rats. Z. Zellforsch. *85*:165, 1968.

Osawa, G., Kimmelsteil, P. and Seiling, V.: Thickness of glomerular basement membranes. Amer. J. Clin. Path. *45*:7, 1966.

Pease, D. C.: Electron microscopy of the tubular cells of the kidney cortex. Anat. Rec. *121*:723, 1955.

19 Respiratory System

General Characteristics

Form and Function. The respiratory system consists of organs that accomplish the primary functions of the *conduction* and *exchange* of gaseous materials. However, numerous ancillary functions are achieved by this system: ***phonation***, ***regulation*** of body temperature, ***excretion*** of certain substances, *olfaction* and others.

The conductive portions of the system include: ***nasal cavity***, ***paranasal sinuses***, ***nasopharynx***, *larynx*, *trachea*, *extrapulmonary bronchi*, *intrapulmonary bronchi* and *bronchioles*. The functional or exchange portion includes various organizational patterns of alveoli in *respiratory bronchioles*, *alveolar ducts* and *alveolar sacs*.

The *lung* is the primary organ of the respiratory system and it contains both conductive and exchange components.

Respiratory Tract—Conductive

General Remarks. The conductive portion of the respiratory tract includes all those structures from the *nares* to the *terminal bronchioles*. Besides the *conduction* of air, this portion of the system is responsible for *cleansing* the air of particulate matter, *humidifying* the air and either *cooling* or *warming* the air. Specific portions of the tract are responsible for *olfaction* and *phonation*.

Nasal Cavity. The nasal cavity is divisible into three histologically distinct regions: *vestibular region*, *respiratory region* and *olfactory region*.

The extent of the *vestibular region* is species-variable. It does represent, however, the point of reflection of the integument as the mucous membrane of the nasal cavity. The lamina epithelialis is stratified squamous epithelium which is nonkeratinized. Pigment cells may be present. The lamina propria-tunica submucosa is coarse areolar connective tissue which blends with the underlying fascia of muscle or the fibrous layer of the associated investments of bone or cartilage. Hairs (vibrissae), sweat glands and sebaceous glands occur in the cutaneous part. Branched tubuloalveolar glands (serous and mixed) may also be present. These glands assist in humidifying the inspired air.

The mucous membrane of the vestibular region gradually changes to the mucous membrane of the *respiratory region* (Fig. 19-1). The latter comprises the bulk of the nasal cavity. The lamina epithelialis is a pseudostratified ciliated columnar epithelium which contains goblet cells. Together, these cells both humidify and cleanse the air. The lamina propria-tunica submucosa is areolar connective tissue. Numerous branched tubuloalveolar mixed glands, the *nasal glands*, which are predominantly serous, are scattered throughout this layer. *Erectile tissue* may also be present in this area. Erectile tissue consists of cavities which are lined by endothelium and are continuous with the blood vessels of a particular area. Although they are usually collapsed, they become engorged with blood under proper nervous stimulation. The glandular tissue humidifies the air, while the engorged erectile tissue cools or warms it by using the mucous membrane as a heat transfer device. The connective tissue of this region is continuous with the underlying connective tissue associated with the bone or cartilage.

The *paranasal air sinuses* are continuous with the nasal cavity. These are spaces within the maxillary, frontal, ethmoid and sphenoid bones of the skull. The epithelium varies from cuboidal and squamous to thin pseudostratified ciliated columnar. Goblet cells and nasal glands occur less frequently than in the nasal cavity proper. Erectile tissue is not present. The remaining connective tissue and bone relationships are similar to those of the nasal cavity proper. Because of the intimate relationship of the mucosa to the underlying bone, these structures are referred to collectively as a ***mucoperiosteum***.

The *olfactory region* is a specialized area for olfaction which is positioned on the

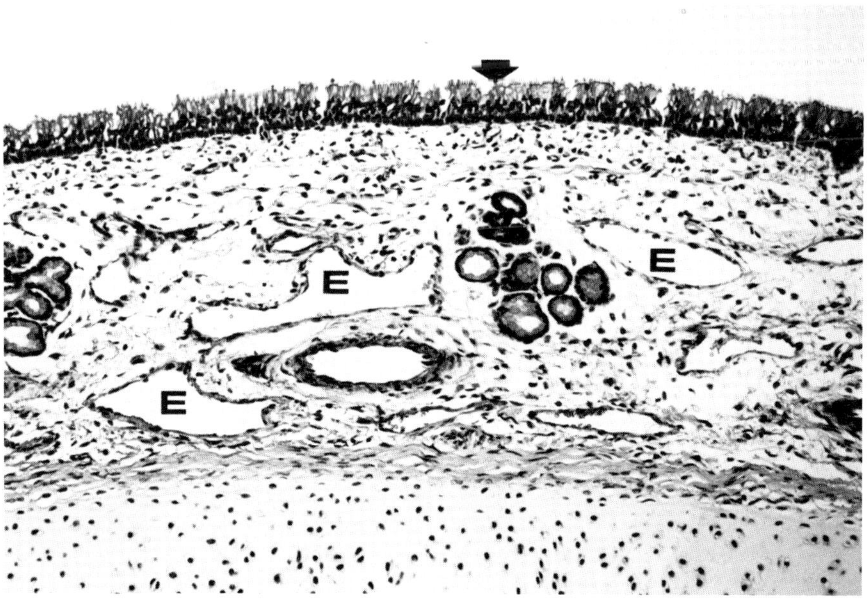

Fig. 19-1. Respiratory mucosa. The lamina epithelialis (*arrow*) is pseudostratified ciliated columnar epithelium with goblet cells. The lamina propria-submucosa contains serous glands and erectile tissue (*E*). This connective tissue is continuous with the perichondrium of the underlying cartilage. ×40. All light micrographs are the original magnifications. All electron micrographs are the final magnifications.

ethmoturbinates, adjacent dorsal turbinates and nasal septum (Fig. 19-2). Grossly, it may be yellow, brown, gray or black due to the accumulation of pigment. The lamina epithelialis consists of nonciliated pseudostratified columnar epithelium. It is a very thick lamina and as many as 15 strata of nuclei may be apparent. This region consists of three cell types: *sustentacular cells*, *basal cells* and *olfactory cells*. The *sustentacular cells* are tall cells with broad apices and narrow bases. The oval, vesicular nuclei are positioned toward the apex of the cell. Pigment granules responsible for the color of this region are contained within these cells. The *basal cells* are typical of those that occur in this type of epithelium. The *olfactory cells* are modified neurons, the basal processes of which continue to the brain as axons of the first cranial nerve. The apex of the cell is modified as a bulblike projection, the *olfactory vesicle*, from which modified cilia, *olfactory hairs*, project. The hairs are the receptors for olfactory stimuli. The round, vesicular nucleus is positioned centrally or basally. The underlying lamina propria is typical and contains branched tubuloalveolar serous glands (*Bowman's glands*). These are responsible for the cleansing of the olfactory surface, as well as solubilizing odor-producing substances.

Nasopharynx. The *nasopharnyx* is that portion of the pharynx above the soft palate. It connects the nasal cavity with the oropharynx.

The lamina epithelialis consists of pseudostratified ciliated columnar epithelium. Goblet cells are present. The lamina propria-tunica submucosa consists of areolar connective tissue with numerous diffuse and aggregated lymphatic tissue and tonsils. Elastic fibers are prominent in the connective tissue space. Branched tubuloalveolar glands (mucous, serous and mixed) occur throughout this region. The tunica muscularis is composed of skeletal muscle in various orientations. The tunica adventitia is continuous with the fascia of this area.

Larynx. The larynx is that portion of the respiratory tract which connects the pharynx with the trachea. It is an irregularly shaped, muscular tube which is reinforced with cartilage (Fig. 19-3).

The lamina epithelialis varies with specific foci within the larynx. It may be stratified squamous or pseudostratified ciliated columnar epithelium. Taste buds may be present in the epiglottic region of some species (carnivores, swine, ruminants, man).

The lamina propria-tunica submucosa consists of areolar connective tissue with various numbers of elastic fibers. Diffuse and nodular lymphatic tissue is present. Branched tubuloalveolar glands are predominantly mucoid, but serous and mixed glands are present also.

The tunica muscularis does not consist exclusively of striated muscle fibers. Rather, cartilage replaces some of the muscle mass in a specific manner which accounts for the recognition of specific laryngeal cartilages and muscle masses at the gross level of examination. Although hyaline cartilage predominates, elastic cartilage is present also.

The tunica adventitia is typical loose connective tissue.

Trachea. This tubular organ continues from the larynx and terminates at the primary bronchi (Fig. 19-4).

The lamina epithelialis is composed of pseudostratified ciliated columnar epithelium with goblet cells. The number and distribution of the latter are subject to species variation.

The lamina propria-tunica submucosa is areolar connective tissue. Elastic fibers are prominent and are believed to replace the lamina muscularis mucosae in the deeper layers. Mucosal glands of the branched, coiled tubuloalveolar mucous type are present and extend into the depths of the submucosal region between and peripheral to the cartilage that is present.

The tunica muscularis is reduced to a transversely oriented mass of smooth muscle (*trachealis muscle*) which extends between the open ends of the horseshoe-shaped cartilage. The actual attachment of the muscle to the cartilage is species-variable. The smooth muscle mass may also be interrupted by the mucosal glands.

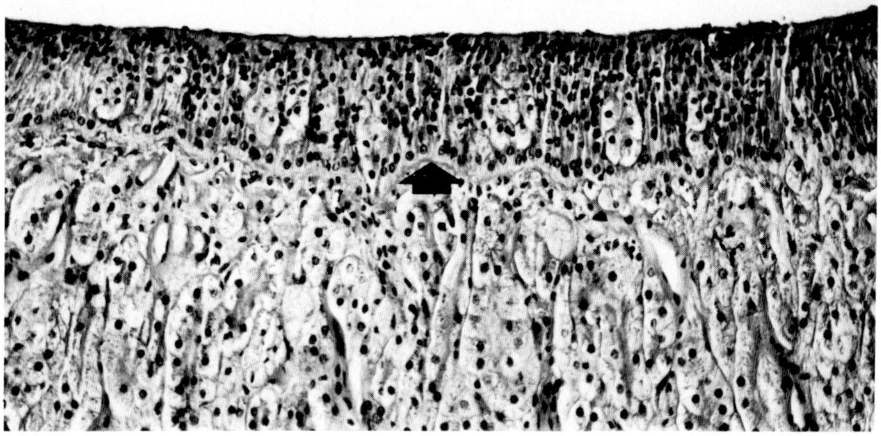

Fig. 19-2. The olfactory mucosa (*arrow*) is a lamina of very thick pseudostratified columnar epithelium which contains olfactory cells. ×50.

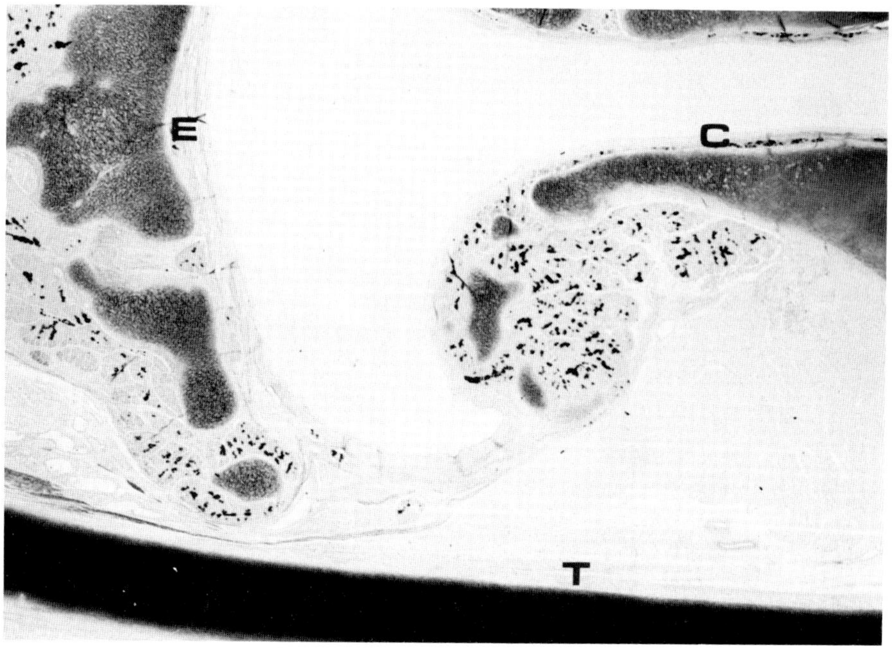

Fig. 19-3. Frontal section of the larynx. The dark tissue is the epiglottic (*E*), cricoid (*C*) and thyroid cartilage (*T*). ×4. (Aldehyde fuchsin).

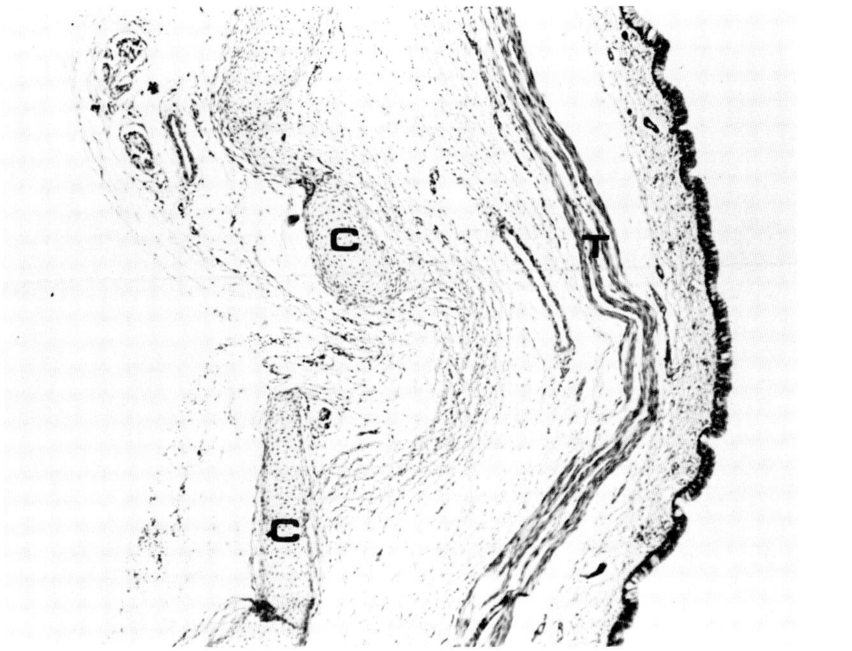

Fig. 19-4. Canine trachea. The cartilage rings (*C*) are incomplete and connected by connective tissue. The trachealis muscle (*T*) is internal to the cartilage. ×16.

The tunica adventitia is areolar connective tissue which blends with the surrounding fascia.

Extrapulmonary Bronchi. The *extrapulmonary* or *primary bronchi* arise at the bifircation of the trachea and are structurally similar to it.

Lung

General Remarks. Structurally, the lung may be considered a compound tubuloalveolar gland. Its excretory product, carbon dioxide, is "secreted" across the alveolar surface in exchange for the uptake of oxygen. This exchange is facilitated by the elastic properties of the lung. An extensive network of elastic fibers accounts for part of its contractility in response to an alteration in the size of the thoracic cavity. The latter is controlled by the expansion and contraction of the diaphragm and thoracic cage.

The lung consists of two *half-lungs*. Each half-lung, often referred to simply as a lung, is subdivided into various numbers of *lobes* (species variable). Lobes are subdivided into *lobules*. In ruminants and the pig the lobular subdivisions are readily apparent on the lung surface. In the horse and man the lobular subdivisions are less distinct. In the dog and cat the lobular subdivisions are not present. In man the lobular subdivisions are apparent because of the deposition of particles in the interlobular spaces.

The lung is covered by a serous membrane (*visceral pleura*). The subserosal connective tissue, often referred to as the capsule of the lung, consists of a thin layer of coarse areolar connective tissue which is rich in elastic fibers (Fig. 19-5). This serous membrane follows the surface contours of the lobes. The interlobular connective tissue is loose connective tissue which is also rich in elastic fibers. The intralobular or interstitial space is occupied by reticular connective tissue. Elastic fibers may also be present.

The embryological development of the lung requires contributions from the endoderm and mesoderm. The endoderm gives rise to the lining of the conductive and alveolar portions, while the mesoderm is responsible for all interstitial elements. There are three distinct but continuous stages of pulmonary development: *glandular*, *canalicular* and *alveolar* stages. The *glandular stage* is characterized by an extensive arborization of the airways. The *canalicular stage* is characterized by the initial attenuation of the lining cells and the differentiation of two lining cells. The *alveolar stage* represents the achievement of the functional blood-air barrier.

Intrapulmonary Bronchi. The intrapulmonary duct system is a modification of the extrapulmonary bronchi. The elastic fibers of extrapulmonary bronchi, positioned in the area normally occupied by the lamina muscularis mucosae, become closely associated with the lamina membrana propria in the intrapulmonary bronchi. The smooth muscle fibers of the trachealis muscle become positioned as the lamina muscularis mucosae. The cartilage, however, remains in the position normally occupied by the tunica muscularis.

Intrapulmonary bronchi may be subdivided into *primary*, *secondary* and *tertiary bronchi* on the basis of their branching, luminal size and mural constituents. There is a gradual continuum of change from the primary to the tertiary bronchi. The intrapulmonary primary bronchi are continuations of the extrapulmonary primary bronchi. Their mural constituents are similar (Fig. 19-6). The lamina epithelialis is a pseudostratified ciliated columnar epithelium which contains numerous goblet cells. The lamina propria, which is continuous with the connective tissue of the *hilus*, is areolar. It contains numerous elastic fibers. The lamina muscularis mucosae is present

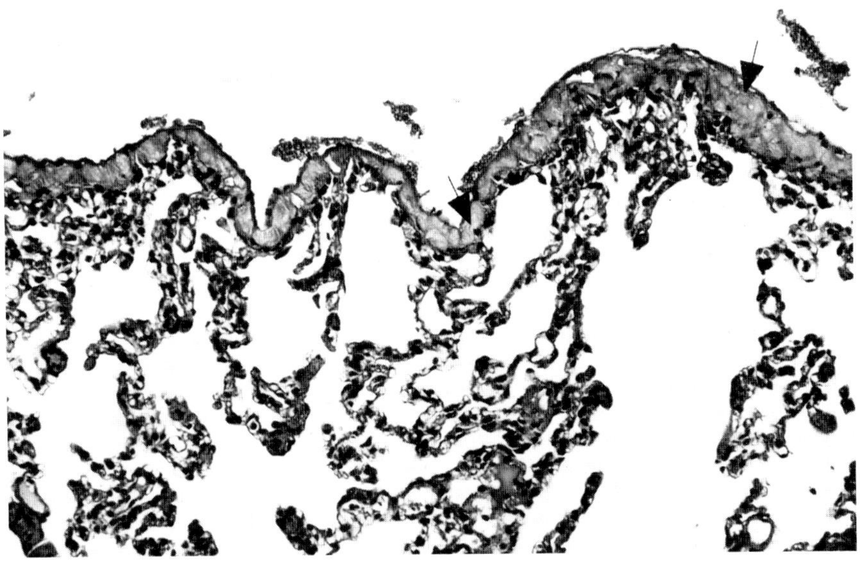

Fig. 19-5. Capsule of the feline lung. The capsule (*arrows*) is covered by a layer of mesothelium. ×40.

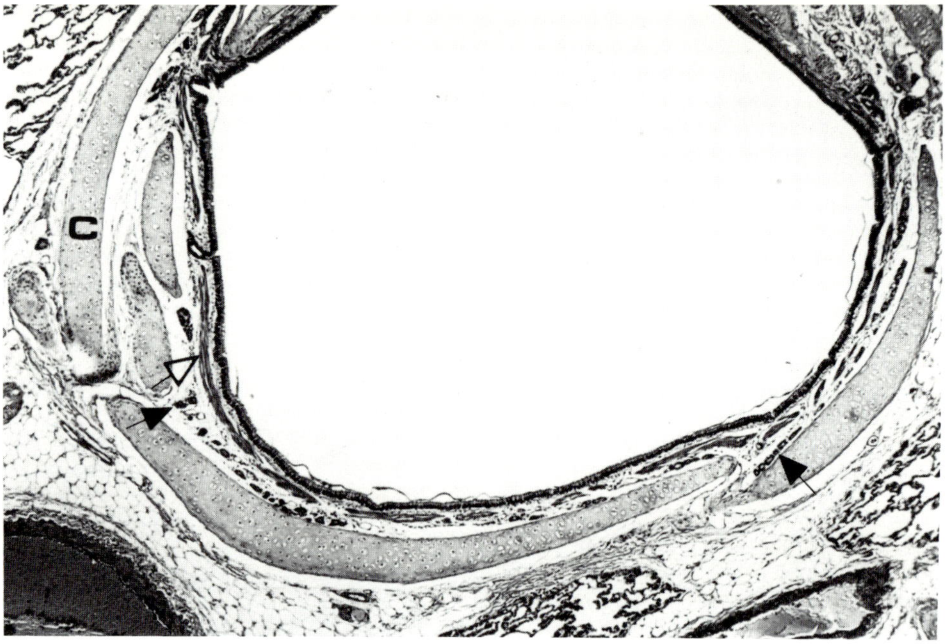

Fig. 19-6. Primary bronchus (feline lung). The cartilage (*C*) is disposed as plates. A lamina muscularis (*open arrow*) and mucous glands (*solid arrows*) are present. ×10.

and disposed in a manner similar to that of the elastic fibers. The spiral configuration of these components results in a highly folded tunica mucosa. The tunica submucosa also consists of areolar connective tissue and contains branched, coiled tubuloalveolar mucous glands. Usually, these glands diminish in number toward the tertiary bronchi. In the cat, however, they may extend into the primary bronchioles. In some species, they are present only in the extrapulmonary bronchi or may extend only a short distance into the lung. The cartilaginous rings of the larger bronchi diminish in size, become cartilaginous plaques and are missing at the transition to primary bronchioles (Fig. 19-7). The peripheral connective tissue is areolar and is continuous with that of the interstitial space.

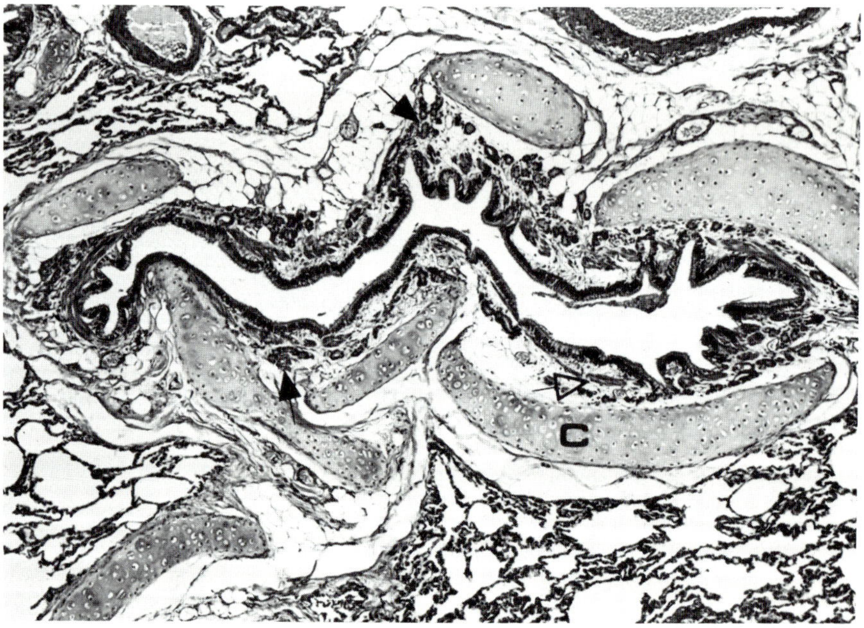

Fig. 19-7. Small bronchi (feline lung). Cartilaginous plates (*C*), mucous glands (*solid arrow*) and smooth muscle are present, but the luminal diameter is reduced. ×16.

Bronchioles. The bronchioles are the smallest divisions of the nonrespiratory or conductive portions of the lung (Fig. 19-8). The lamina epithelialis consists of simple columnar or cuboidal cells and is devoid of goblet cells. The lining cells are ciliated in the *primary bronchioles*. The cilia diminish in the more distal bronchioles and are lost in the tertiary bronchioles. Importantly, cilia extend further down the respiratory tree than do glands. The lamina propria consists of fine collagenous and elastic fibers. The lamina muscularis mucosae is present and continuous. The peripheral connective tissue is similar to the lamina propria but is not extensive. No cartilage is present. The tertiary or terminal bronchioles are the primary conducting supply to a secondary lobule and divide into several respiratory bronchioles.

Respiratory Bronchioles. The *respiratory bronchioles* are the initial portion of the lung responsible for the exchange of gases (Fig. 19-9). The lamina epithelialis consists of cuboidal cells, some of which may be ciliated (Fig. 19-10). The cuboidal cells are not a continuous lining but are interrupted by alveoli which outpocket from the walls of this bronchiole (Fig. 19-11). The lamina propria is indistinct, but fine collagenous and elastic fibers support the lining cells. Smooth muscle is present, but it is loosely organized beneath the cuboidal epithelium.

Respiratory bronchioles are not equally developed, nor are they present in all species. They are infrequently observed in ruminants and swine, poorly developed in horse and man, well-developed in monkey and carnivores and absent in the mouse. In those species in which they are absent, the terminal bronchioles open directly into several alveolar ducts.

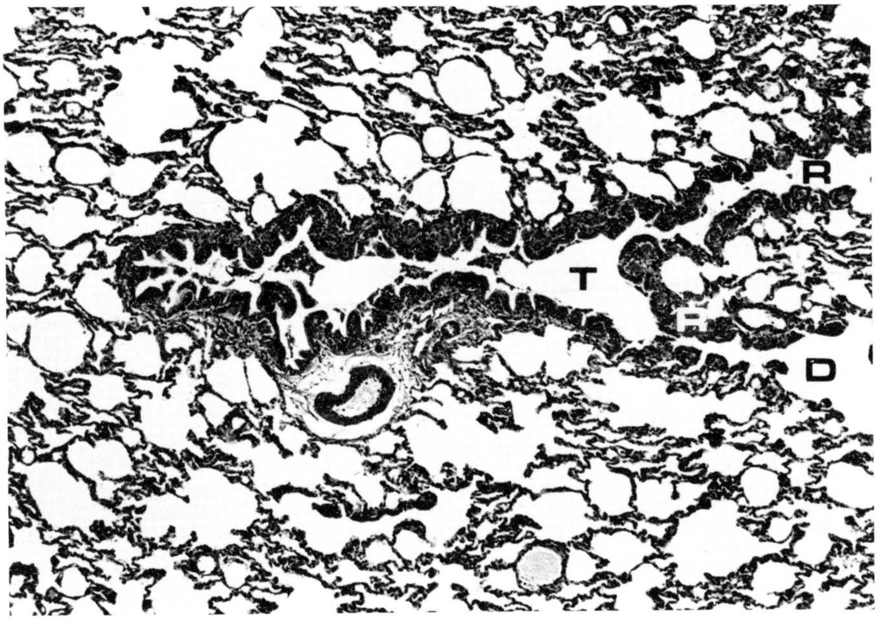

Fig. 19-8. Bronchioles of the feline lung. The wall is devoid of cartilage. The terminal bronchiole (*T*) divides into two respiratory bronchioles (*R*). An alveolar duct (*D*) is present also. ×16.

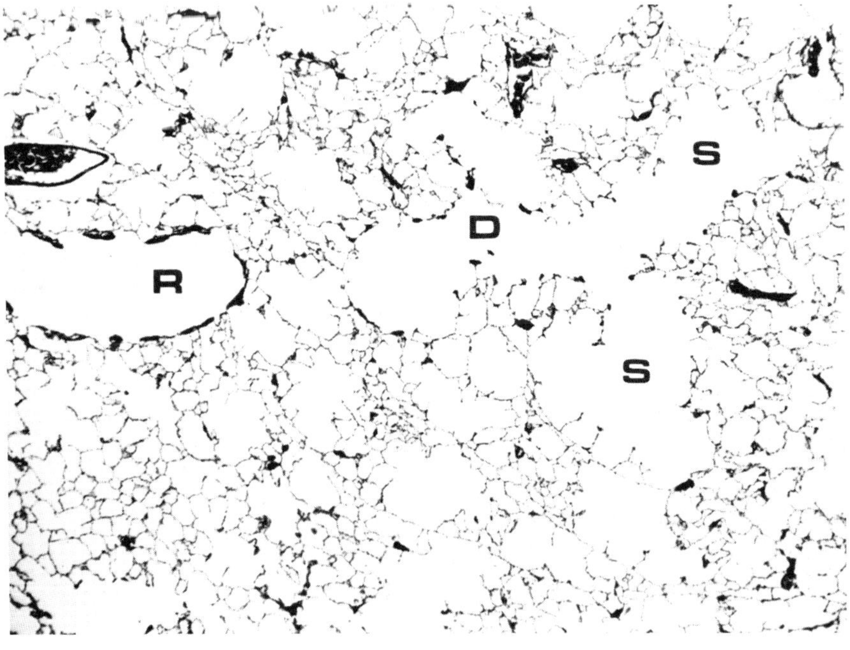

Fig. 19-9. Distal pathways of the canine lung. A respiratory bronchiole (*R*) continues as an alveolar duct (*D*) which divides into two alveolar sacs (*S*). ×40.

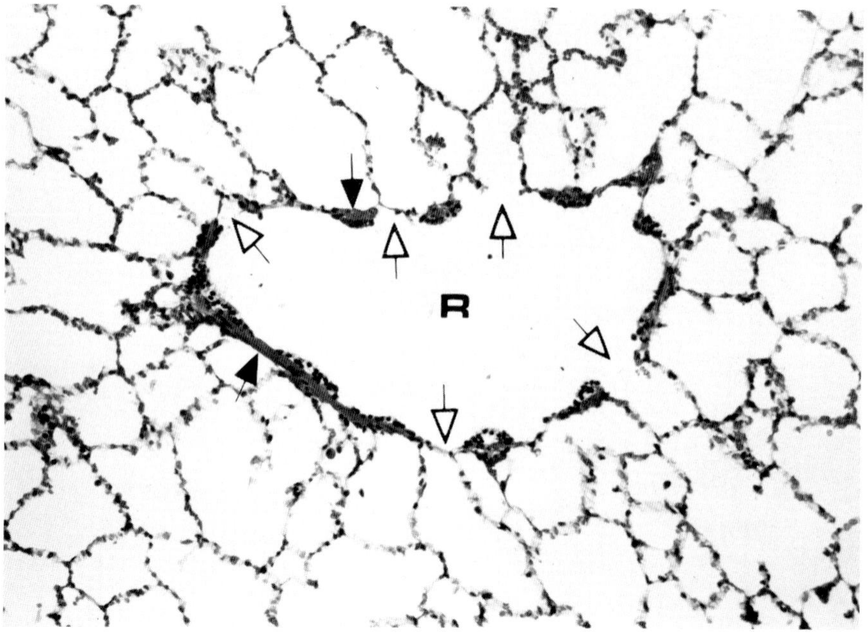

Fig. 19-10. Respiratory bronchiole (*R*) (canine lung). The lamina epithelialis is underlaid by smooth muscle (*solid arrows*). The epithelial lining is interrupted by alveoli (*open arrows*). ×40.

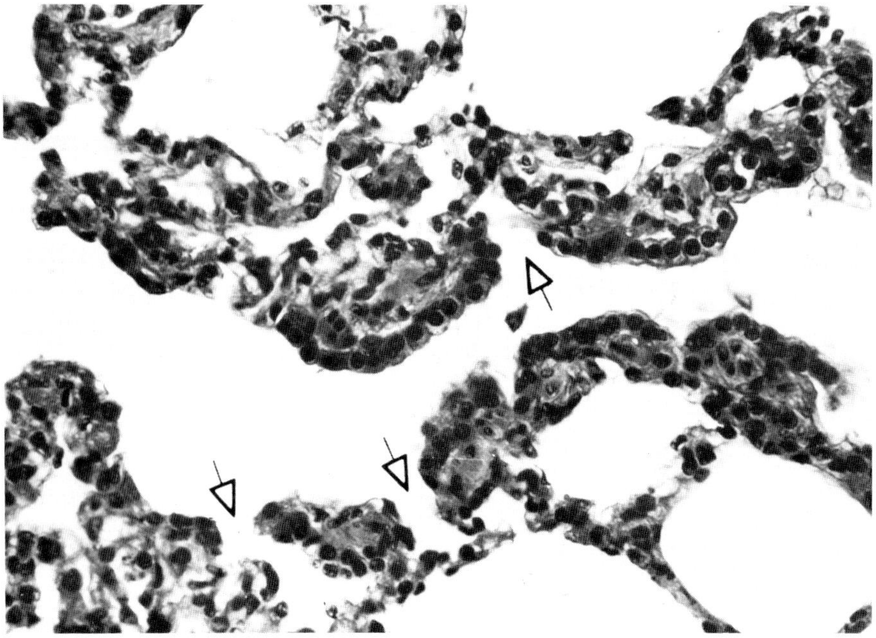

Fig. 19-11. Lining of feline respiratory bronchiole. The cuboidal epithelium is interrupted by alveoli (*arrows*). ×100.

Some of the cuboidal cells of these bronchioles, *Clara cells*, have been implicated in the metabolism of *surface-active substance* (*surfactant*). Although originally proposed as being responsible for its production, other cells now have been demonstrated as being responsible for the production of surfactant. The role of the Clara cell, therefore, is not clarified.

Alveolar Ducts, Saccules and Atria. The respiratory bronchiole of a lobule or the terminal bronchiole of a lobule, divide into numerous *alveolar ducts* (Fig. 19-12).

These tubules are completely lined by alveoli. Smooth muscle may be present along the luminal border at the apices between adjacent alveoli. Alveolar ducts divide and expand peripherally into *saccules* (sacs) which are completely lined by alveoli (Fig. 19-13). The common opening of the saccules is referred to as the *atrium*.

Pneumonocytes and Alveoli. The lining of the alveoli consists of two types of cells: *membranous pneumonocytes* (*type I pneumonocytes*) and *granular pneumonocytes* (*type II pneumonocytes, alveolar giant cells, dust cells*).

The *membranous* (*agranular*) *pneumonocyte* is the primary constituent of the alveolar lining (Fig. 19-14). It is an endothelial-like cell with an attentuated cytoplasm which is reduced to the limit of resolution of the light microscope. Its nucleus is apparent and protrudes into the alveolar lumen. Examination of alveoli with the electron microscope supplied the first conclusive evidence that the alveoli were in fact lined by cells (Fig. 19-15).

The *type II pneumonocyte* has been, until recently, the subject of much controversy. Although the cell was thought originally to be a macrophage, current evidence supports the secretory role of this cell. It is the cell responsible for the elaboration of *surfactant* material. Surfactant is a detergent-like material which reduces alveolar surface tension and prevents alveolar collapse during expiration. Despite the numerous synonyms given for this cell, the most precise names for this cell are *type II pneumonocyte* or *granular pneumonocyte* (Fig. 19-16). This cell is of variable occurrence; the numbers may vary from one to several per alveolus. These are cuboidal or rounded cells which intermittently line the alveolar surface. Their cell bodies are foamy and project into the alveolar lumina. Tight junctions connect the cytoplasmic processes of these cells with those of the membranous pneumonocytes. Osmiophilic, *lamellar bodies* are the diagnostic features of these cells at the electron microscopic level (Fig. 19-17).

A third lining cell, the *alveolar brush cell*, has been described in the alveoli of rats. This type III pneumonocyte is covered by a thin process of the type I cell. The alveo-

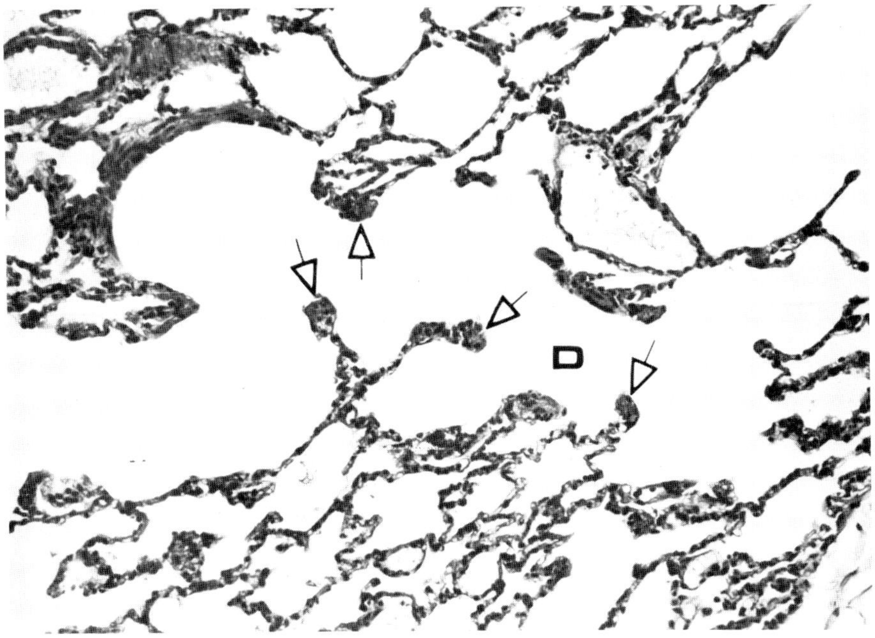

Fig. 19-12. Alveolar duct of the feline lung. The alveolar duct (*D*) is lined by alveoli. Smooth muscle and attenuated lining cells occupy the apices of septa between adjacent alveoli (*arrows*). ×40.

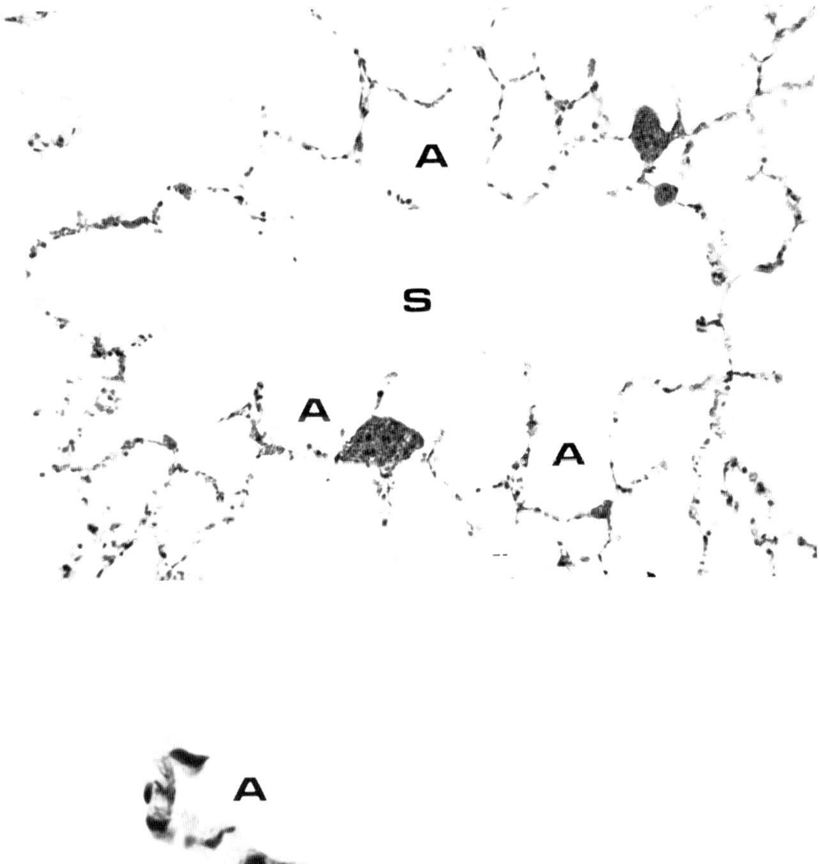

Fig. 19-13. Alveolar sac of the canine lung. The alveolar sac (*S*) is surrounded by alveoli (*A*). The septa are devoid of smooth muscle. ×40.

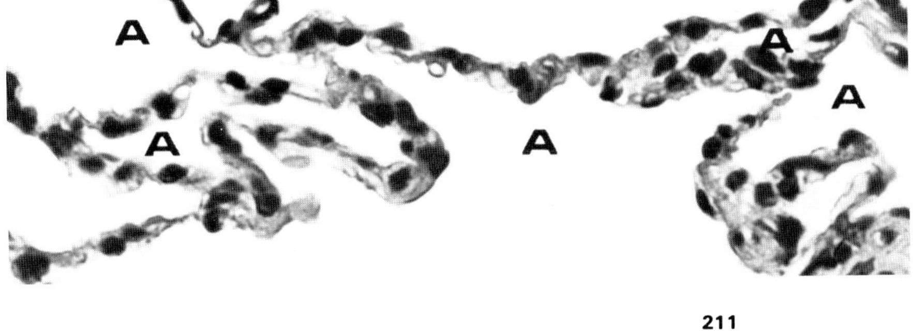

Fig. 19-14. Alveoli. Alveoli (*A*) are adjacent to each other. They are separated by capillaries and a minimal amount of connective tissue. ×160.

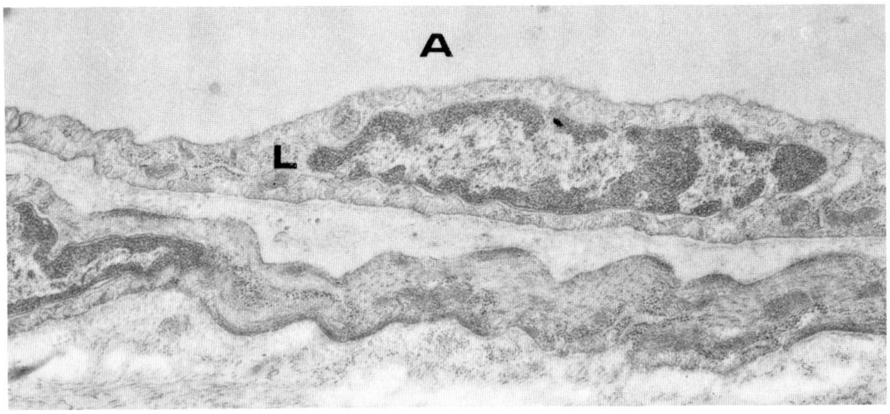

Fig. 19-15. An electron micrograph of a membranous (agranular) pneumonocyte (bovine). The squamous cell (*L*) lines the alveolus (*A*). A fibroblast is subjacent to the lining cell. ×18,000. (Courtesy of G. P. Epling).

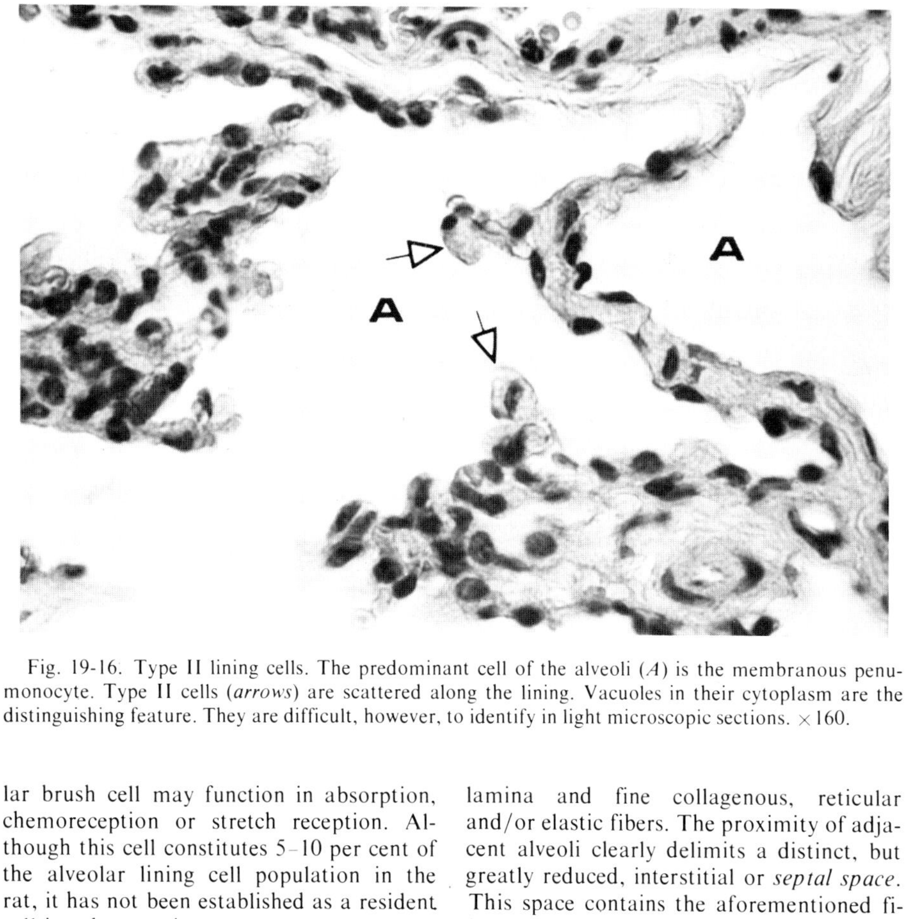

Fig. 19-16. Type II lining cells. The predominant cell of the alveoli (*A*) is the membranous penumonocyte. Type II cells (*arrows*) are scattered along the lining. Vacuoles in their cytoplasm are the distinguishing feature. They are difficult, however, to identify in light microscopic sections. ×160.

lar brush cell may function in absorption, chemoreception or stretch reception. Although this cell constitutes 5–10 per cent of the alveolar lining cell population in the rat, it has not been established as a resident cell in other species.

Adjacent alveoli are sometimes connected by pores, called *alveolar pores of Kuhn*. These pores are believed to distribute equally the gases and resulting pressure among alveoli. They may also serve for the interalveolar transmission of fluids, particulate matter, bacteria and alveolar macrophages.

Blood-Air Barrier. These cells, both type I and type II, are supported by a basal lamina and fine collagenous, reticular and/or elastic fibers. The proximity of adjacent alveoli clearly delimits a distinct, but greatly reduced, interstitial or *septal space*. This space contains the aforementioned fibers, fibroblasts, macrophages and blood capillaries.

The blood-air barrier (blood-air pathway) consists of the following elements: *alveolar lining cell, alveolar basal lamina, septal space, endothelial-associated basal lamina* and *endothelial cell* (Fig. 19-18). The thickness of the barrier, however, is variable. Minimally, it is composed of the *alveolar lining cell, fused basal laminae* and *endothelial cell*. This is the thinnest and most efficient diffusion pathway. The least efficient and thickest would involve an expansion of the septal region.

Since the lung is exposed to inspired foreign materials, various methods are utilized to cleanse the air—goblet cells, cilia and macrophages. Macrophages are the primary mediators of this activity in the lower portion of the respiratory tree (Fig. 19-19). Transalveolar migration of these cells (histiocytes) from the septal areas as well as from the blood (monocytes) is probable. They may protrude into the alveolar lumina between the lining cells, reside on the lining cells or be free in the lumina. They are rarely observed as a constituent of the lining in residence upon the basal lamina. These and associated cells comprise the *transient alveolar cell population*, while the pneumonocytes comprise the *resident alveolar cell population*.

Vascular Supply and Drainage. The vascular supply to the lung is achieved by two arterial systems: the *pulmonary artery* and *bronchial artery*. This type of dual circulation is not unique to the lung, but it does represent a division of functional and nutritional blood supply, respectively. The pulmonary artery and its peripheral subdivisions follow the distribution of the airways to the level of the respiratory bronchioles at which point they are continued as an extensive capillary bed associated with the alveoli. In carnivores and the monkey, this artery also supplies the pleura. In ruminants, swine, horse and man the bronchial artery supplies the pleura.

The position of the pulmonary veins is species variable. In some species the pulmonary vein is interlobular in position and thus receives blood from adjacent lobules. In others, it is intralobular and requires that each lobule has its own pulmonary vein.

The bronchial arteries, which may supply the pleura (horse, man, ruminants and swine) as well as the alveoli (horse), are the primary blood supply for the walls of the bronchi and bronchioles. Although bronchial veins are present, most of the bronchial arterial blood is returned to the heart via the pulmonary veins. The pulmonary vein of the ox is unique. The tunica media is very thick and disrupted. This imparts a sphincter-like appearance to the vessel when it is cut in cross-section.

Avian Respiratory System

Upper Respiratory Tract. The upper respiratory tract of birds includes all those structures described for mammals with the addition of the syrinx. These organs function in a manner similar to those in mammals.

The *nasal cavity* is lined by the same types of epithelia characteristic of the mammal. The vestibular region is lined by a

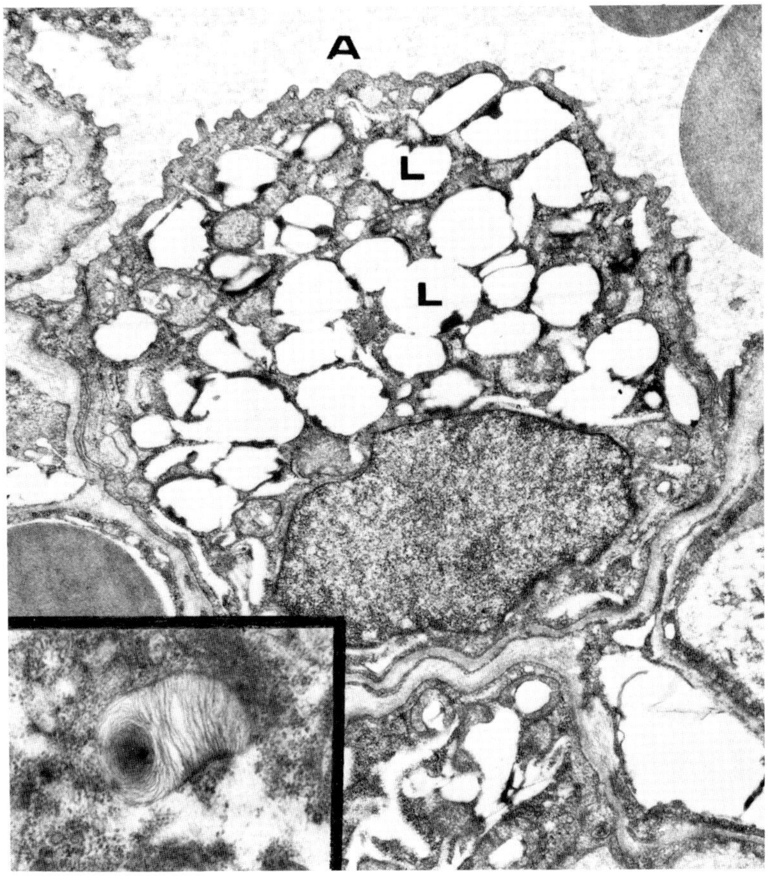

Fig. 19-17. An electron micrograph of a granular pneumonocyte. The cytoplasm protrudes into the alveolus (*A*). Pale areas (*L*) are lamellar bodies. The lamellar bodies, however, have been dissolved due to the method of preparation. ×14,000. (Courtesy of G. P. Epling). *Inset:* A typical lamellar body of a granular penumonocyte. ×17,000.

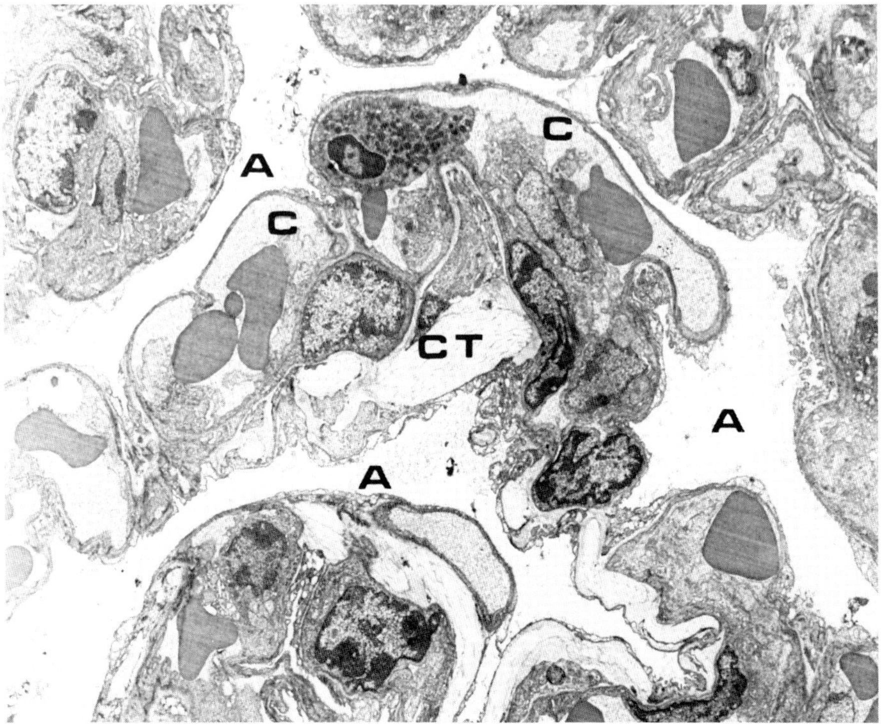

Fig. 19-18. An electron micrograph of the lung. Capillaries (*C*) are juxtaposed to alveolar lining cells. These components constitute the blood-air barrier. Alveoli (*A*) are collapsed. Small amounts of connective tissue (*CT*) comprise the septal areas. ×4000. (Courtesy of G. P. Epling).

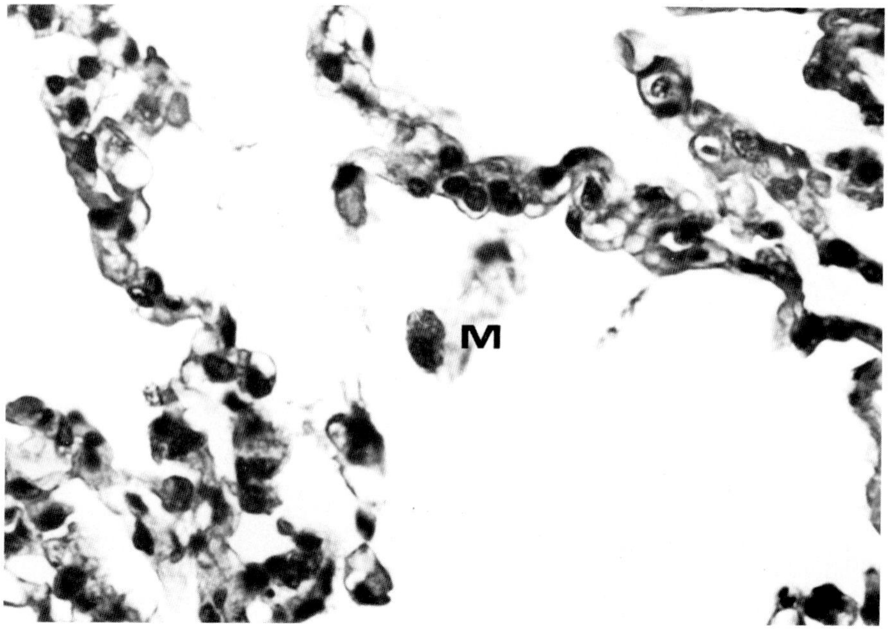

Fig. 19-19. An alveolar macrophage. An alveolar macrophage (*M*) is free in the lumen of the alveolus. ×160.

stratified squamous epithelium which, from surface view, has a beaded appearance. The basal and intermediate cell layers are vertically oriented. They consist of large cells with centrally located nuclei. These rows are covered by a thin double layer of cornified cells. The remaining respiratory and olfactory epithelium is typical. Intraepithelial glands typify the respiratory epithelium (Fig. 2-18). The lamina propria is areolar connective tissue with diffuse and aggregated lymphatic tissue. It is continuous with the underlying connective tissue investments of bone or cartilage.

The *trachea* of the bird is similar to that of the mammal. The following differences are apparent. The typical epithelium contains intraepithelial mucous glands which may protrude slightly into the typical lamina propria. Mucosal and submucosal glands are of variable occurrence. The cartilaginous rings are complete and alternate in size. Ossification of these supportive rings is common in some species (goose, duck). Longitudinally oriented striated muscle is located at the periphery of the trachea in a lateral position.

The primary bronchi are similar in structure to the trachea. The cartilaginous rings, however, are gradually replaced by dense white fibrous connective tissue, and smooth muscle may connect the free surfaces of the cartilage.

The *syrinx* is located at the junction of the trachea and bronchi. It is an inverted Y-shaped structure. At the bifurcation of the trachea, a cartilaginous bar with a mucosal-submucosal fold constitutes the *median vocal fold*. By drawing the bronchi toward each other, two *lateral vocal folds* are produced at the level of the median vocal fold. The combination of these folds is responsible for phonation.

The lamina epithelialis of the syrinx consists of either a bistratified squamous or a columnar epithelium. Mucosal glands as well as diffuse and nodular lymphatic tissue are present in the lamina propria.

Lung. The lungs of birds are very different from the lungs of mammals. Compared to the size of the thoracic cavity, the lungs are extremely small. Moreover, they do *not* change volume during inhalation and exhalation. The structures that do change volume are the air sacs, which are continuous with the duct system of the lung.

The duct system bears no similarity to the one in mammals (Fig. 19-20). The *primary bronchi* enter the lung and expand as the *vestibulum*. This continues through the lung as the *mesobronchus* and is connected to the *abdominal air sac*. *Secondary bronchi* and air sacs arise from the vestibulum and mesobronchus. Secondary bronchi are described as *dorsal bronchi*, *ventral bronchi* or *lateral bronchi* on the basis of their gross orientation. Secondary bronchi give rise to *tertiary bronchi* (*parabronchi*) which are then continuous with other secondary bronchi. Thus, a complete air-conducting loop is formed. The parabronchi are analogous to the alveolar ducts of mammals. *Air vesicles* (*atria*) project radially from the parabronchi. These atria are continuous with the *air capillaries* (*air cells*). These air capillaries are continuous loops that open back into the atria. These are the moieties responsible for the actual exchange of gases with the closely associated vascular capillaries.

The air sacs associated with the avian lung aid in the movement of air through the lung. They are membranous structures which do not contribute to the exchange of gases. Most birds have nine air sacs: *unpaired interclavicular*, *paired claviculars*, *paired cranial thoracics*, *paired caudal thoracics*, *paired abdominals*. The air sacs occur free in the body cavities and send diverticula into the bones with which they are associated. *Recurrent bronchi* extend from the air sacs and attach to the parabronchi. *Recurrent bronchi* are involved in the return of the air from the air sacs to the lung proper.

Histology of the Lung and Associated Structures. The *intrapulmonary primary bronchi* are extensions of the bifurcated trachea and are similar in structure to their extrapulmonary counterparts. The lamina epithelialis consists of pseudostratified ciliated columnar epithelium with goblet cells and intraepithelial mucous glands. The lamina propria is areolar connective tissue with numerous diffuse and aggregated lymphatic tissue. Lymph nodules, however, are rarely present. The lamina muscularis mucosae is disposed primarily as a circularly or spirally oriented mass of muscle with some longitudinal bundles as well. Cartilaginous rings are present in the initial portions of these

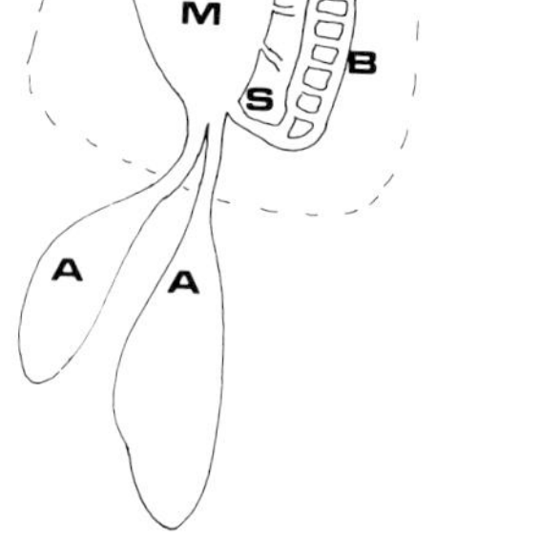

Fig. 19-20. Avian lung. *T*, trachea; *P*, primary bronchus; *V*, vestibulum; *M*, mesobronchus; *A*, air sacs; *S*, secondary bronchi; *B*, parabronchi. (Modified and redrawn from Sturkie, P.D.: *Avian Physiology*, 2nd ed. Cornell University Press, Ithaca, N.Y., 1965).

bronchi but are replaced by plaques of cartilage. The latter are lost within the vestibulum. The tunica adventitia blends with the surrounding interstitial connective tissue.

The mural elements of the *vestibulum*, except for the previously mentioned differences in the cartilage, are similar to those of the intrapulmonary primary bronchi. The vestibulum, however, is an enlarged portion of the primary conductive pathway through the lung which is continued caudally by the *mesobronchus*. The latter is a continuation of the primary conductive pathway. Its morphology is similar to the vestibulum. The luminal diameter of this tubule, however, is smaller than those described previously.

Secondary bronchi, whether they are lateral, dorsal or ventral, have a similar morphology (Fig. 19-21). The lamina epithelialis is composed of columnar or cuboidal cells and is devoid of goblet cells. The lamina propria is composed of areolar connective tissue which is usually devoid of lymphatic tissue. The lamina muscularis mucosae is interrupted and multidirectionally oriented. Cartilage is not present. Numerous interruptions of the mural elements are commonly encountered due to the occurrence of parabronchi and, in some areas, air vesicles. Because of the latter, portions of the secondary bronchi may be considered analogous to mammalian respiratory bronchioles.

The mucosal lining of *parabronchi* is interrupted by the laterally projecting air vesicles (Fig. 19-22). Between the interruptions, the parabronchi are lined by a cuboidal or squamous epithelium. The reduced lamina propria is composed of a fine areolar connective tissue. The lamina muscularis mucosae is confined to the area beneath the ridges of the lamina epithelialis as separate bundles of smooth muscle.

The *air vesicles* are lined by a simple squamous epithelium and are supported by a fine interstitial connective tissue (Fig. 19-23). The epithelium of the air vesicles is continuous as a simple squamous lining of the *air capillaries*. The air capillary-blood capillary relationship is similar to that described for mammals.

The ventilation of the avian lung has not been satisfactorily determined. The configuration of the lung and air sacs permits a double ventilation of the air capillaries. Since the bird is an abdominal breather, the abdominal and caudal thoracic air sacs are subject to alterations of volume. These air sacs, therefore, may establish the necessary currents to facilitate the double ventilation and exchange of gases. The flow, however, during inspiration and expiration is unidirectional; i.e., it appears always to follow a mesobronchial-dorsal bronchial-parabronchial-ventral bronchial-mesobronchial pattern.

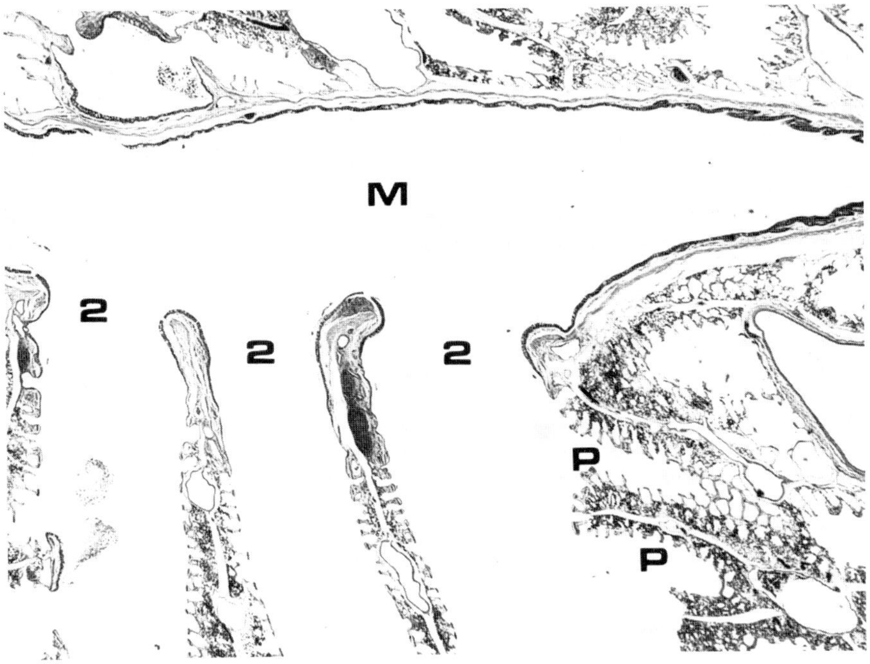

Fig. 19-21. Avian lung. The mesobronchus (*M*) is continuous with secondary bronchi (*2*). Parabronchi (*P*) radiate from secondary bronchi. ×4.

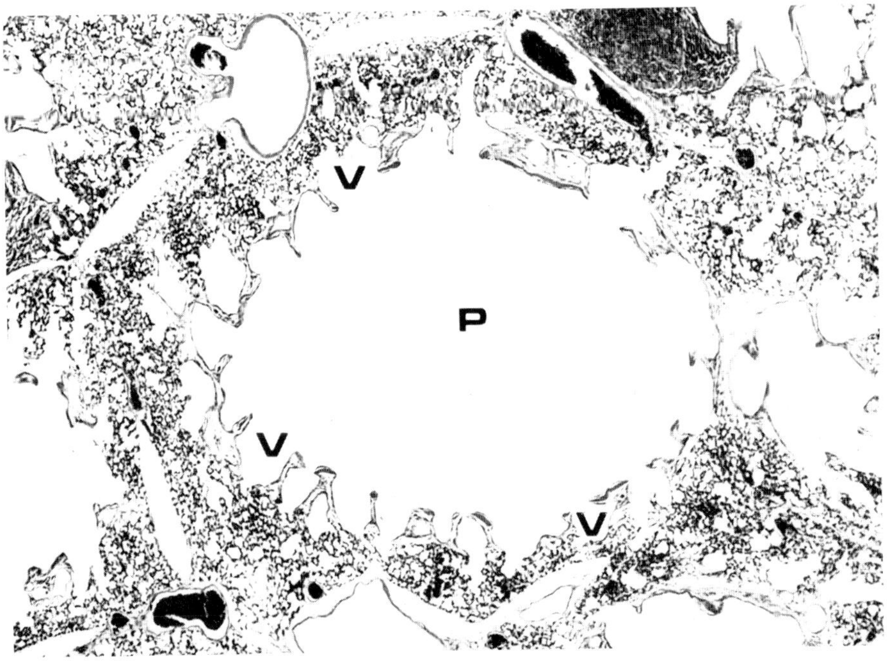

Fig. 19-22. A parabronchus of the avian lung. The parabronchus (*P*) has numerous air vesicles (*V*) in its wall. ×16.

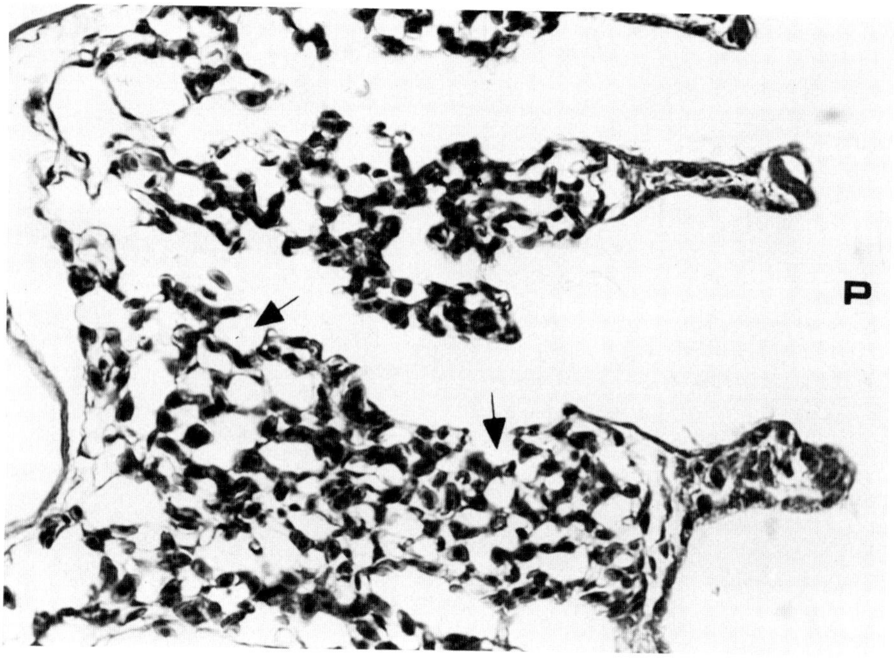

Fig. 19-23. Air vesicles of the avian lung. The walls of parabronchi (*P*) have numerous air vesicles. These are composed of air capillaries (*arrows*) and blood capillaries. ×100.

References

Respiratory Tract—Conductive

Ali, M. Y.: Histology of the human nasopharyngeal mucosa. J. Anat. *99*:657, 1965.

Amoare, J. E., Johnston, J. W. and Rubin, M.: The stereochemical theory of odor. Sci. Amer. *210*:43, 1964.

Baradi, A. F. and Bourne, G. H.: Gustatory and olfactory epithelia. Int. Rev. Cytol. *2*:289, 1953.

Bojsen-Moller, F.: Topography and development of the anterior nasal glands in pigs. J. Anat. *101*:321, 1967.

Frisch, D.: Ultrastructure of mouse olfactory mucosa. Amer. J. Anat. *121*:87, 1967.

Hansell, M. M. and Moretti, R. L.: Ultrastructure of the mouse tracheal epithelium. J. Morph. *128*:159, 1969.

Rhodin, J. and Dalhamn, T.: Electron microscopy of the tracheal ciliated mucosa in rat. Z. Zellforsch. *44*: 345, 1956.

Mammalian Lung

Banks, W. J., Jr. and Epling, G. P.: Differentiation and origin of the type II pneumocyte: An ultrastructural study. Acta Anat. *78*:604, 1971.

Bertalanffy, F. D.: Respiratory tissue: structure, histophysiology and cytodynamics. I. Review and basic cytomorphology. Int. Rev. Cytol. *16*:233, 1964.

Bowden, D. H., Adamson, I. Y. R., Grantham, G. and Wyatt, J. P.: Origin of the lung macrophage: Evidence derived from radiation injury. Arch. Pathol. *88*:540, 1969.

Epling, G. P.: Electron microscopy of the bovine lungs: Lattice and lamellar structures in the alveolar lumina. Amer. J. Vet. Res. *25*:1424, 1964.

Karrer, H. E.: The ultrastructure of mouse lung. The alveolar macrophage. J. Biophys. Biochem. Cytol. *4*:693, 1958.

Krahl, V. E.: Current concept of the finer structure of the lung. Arch. Intern. Med. (Chicago) *96*:342, 1955.

Krahl, V. E.: Anatomy of the Mammalian Lung. In *Handbook of Physiology. Sect. 3, Respiration.* Vol. 1, Chapter 6, edited by W. O. Fenn and H. Rahn. American Physiological Society, Washington, D.C. Williams & Wilkins, 1964.

Krahl, V. E.: *The Human Lung* (translation of *Die Menschliche Lunge* by H. von Hayek, Springer Verlag, Berlin, 1953). Hafner, New York 1960.

Loosli, C. G. and Potter, E. L.: Pre- and postnatal development of the respiratory portion of the human lung. Amer. Rev. Resp. Dis. *80*:5, 1959.

Low, F. N.: Electron microscopy of the rat lung. Anat. Rec. *113*:437, 1952.

Meyrick, B. and Reid, L.: The alveolar brush cell in rat lung—a third pneumocyte. J. Ultrastruct. Res. *23*:71, 1968.

Miller, W. S.: *The Lung*. C. C Thomas, Springfield, Ill., 1937.

Avian Lung and Associated Structures

Akester, A. R.: The comparative anatomy of the respiratory pathways in the domestic fowl, pigeon and domestic duck. J. Anat. *94*:488, 1960.

Cover, M. S.: The gross and microscopic anatomy of the respiratory system of the turkey. I. The nasal cavity and infraorbital sinus. Amer. J. Vet. Res. *14*:113, 1953.

Cover, M. S.: The gross and microscopic anatomy of the respiratory system of the turkey. II. The larynx, trachea, syrinx, bronchi and lungs. Amer. J. Vet. Res. *14*:230, 1953.

Cover, M. S.: Gross and microscopic anatomy of the respiratory system of the turkey. III. The air sacs. Amer. J. Vet. Res. *14*:239, 1953.

McLeod, W. M. and Wagers, R. P.: The respiratory system of the chicken. J. Amer. Vet. Med. Assoc. *95*: 59, 1939.

Sturkie, P. D.: *Avian Physiology*. 2nd ed. Cornell University Press, Ithaca, N.Y., 1965.

20 Endocrine System

General Characteristics

Form and Function. The glands that comprise the endocrine system are those structures described as *ductless glands* or *glands of internal secretion.* Although they are derived from all the germ layers, they do not maintain anatomical contacts with these layers (Fig. 2-19). Furthermore, the glands may be a distinct organ (pituitary, adrenals, thyroid, etc.) or they may be parts of other organs (islets of Langerhans, interstitial cells of the testes, follicles and corpora lutea of the ovary).

The organization of these glands is simple. They may be encapsulated, lack an extensive stroma, are highly vascularized and possess cells in varied configurations. The configurations may include *single cells, cell clusters, cell cords* or *cell follicles.* Whatever their configuration, they are intimately associated with an extensive vascular supply (capillaries or sinusoids) into which they secrete their products.

The *hormones* that these glands secrete are variable. They may be proteins, glycoproteins, polypeptides, steroids or catecholamines. One gland may secrete one hormone, while other glands may secrete several hormones. These hormones may be synthesized and immediately secreted (adrenal cortex), synthesized and temporarily stored as presecretory granules (islets of Langerhans) or synthesized and stored in a follicle (thyroid). Once these products have been secreted into the blood stream, they may have an effect upon the entire organism, selected organs or a specific organ. Although the entire organism may be affected, one organ or group of organs may respond specifically. The latter are termed the *target organ* or *target organs*; i.e., some organs have a sufficiently low threshold to a specific hormonal stimulation that their response is readily measured.

The endocrine system consists of organs with an exclusive endocrine function (pituitary, pineal, thyroid, parathyroid, adrenal), as well as organs with an endocrine and exocrine function (pancreas, gonads, kidneys, liver, stomach, intestines, placenta). Except for the islets of Langerhans of the pancreas, only those organs with an exclusive endocrine function are included in this section. The others have been or will be discussed in other sections of the presentation.

Hypophysis Cerebri

General Remarks. Scheme 20-1 represents the organizational pattern of the hypophysis cerebri (*pituitary gland*). The *pars tuberalis* and *pars distalis* constitute the *anterior lobe* or *anterior pituitary* (Fig. 20-1). The *pars intermedia* and the *infundibular process* constitute the *posterior lobe* or *posterior pituitary.* The *pars tuberalis* and the *infundibular stalk* are referred to as the *hypophyseal stalk.* The terms anterior and posterior pituitary are not totally applicable to all mammalian species (Fig. 20-2). In some species, the posterior pituitary is actually dorsal to the anterior pituitary, while in other species the anterior pituitary totally surrounds the posterior pituitary.

hypophysis cerebri

- adenohypophysis (glandular lobe)
  - pars tuberalis
  - pars distalis
  - pars intermedia
- neurohypophysis (neural lobe)
  - median eminence
  - infundibular stalk
  - infundibular process

Scheme 20-1.

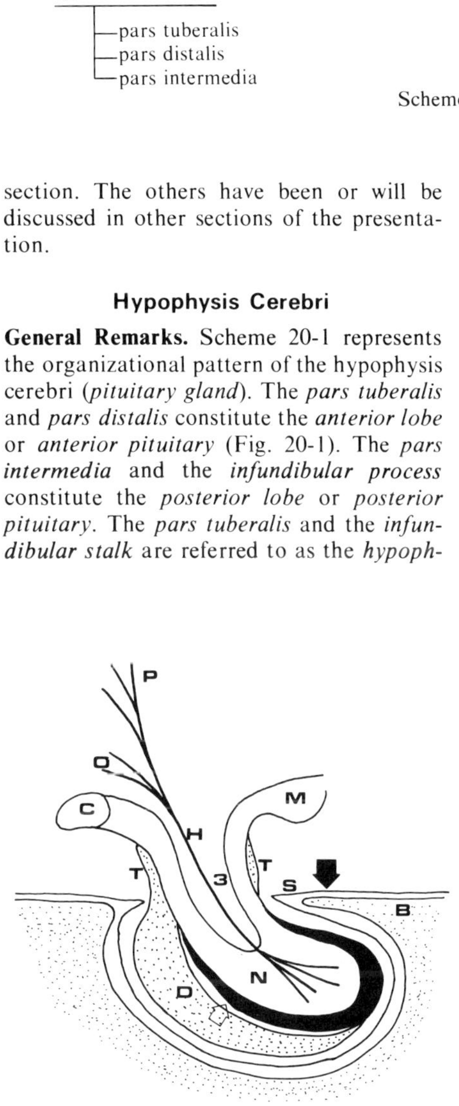

Fig. 20-1. Hypophysis cerebri of the pig. *B*, sphenoid bone; *S*, sella turcica; *D*, pars distalis; *T*, pars tuberalis; *M*, mammillary body; *C*, optic chiasma; *N*, pars nervosa; *H*, hypothalamico-hypophyseal tract; *O*, supraoptic area; *P*, paraventricular area; *3*, third ventricle; *solid arrow*, dura mater; *open arrow*, residual lumen. All light micrographs are the original magnifications.

The development of the pituitary gland is dependent upon contributions from the buccal cavity (ectoderm) and the floor of the diencephalon (neuroectoderm). *Rathke's pouch*, an outgrowth of the roof of the oral cavity, grows toward the base of the brain. This pouch is responsible for the differentiation of the *adenohypophysis.* As it grows and contacts the infundibulum from the floor of the diencephalon, its connection with the oral cavity is lost. That portion of Rathke's pouch that contacts the neurohypophysis differentiates into the pars intermedia. The rostral portion becomes the pars distalis, while the dorsal extension of the pars distalis that comes in contact with the infundibular stalk becomes the pars tuberalis. The *residual lumen* of Rathke's pouch may be persistent and separates the anterior from the posterior pituitary.

The infundibular stalk is an outgrowth of the median eminence. The median eminence is the ventral boundary of the third ventricle in this region. As the infundibular stalk grows, part of the third ventricle is carried with it as the *infundibular recess.* In most species, the recess is confined to the region of continuity of the infundibular stalk with the median eminence (Fig. 20-2). In others (pig and cat especially), the infundibular recess extends into the infundibular process.

Adenohypophysis. The constituents of the adenohypophysis are the *pars distalis, pars intermedia* and *pars tuberalis.*

The *pars distalis* comprises the greatest bulk of the adenohypophysis (Fig. 20-3). It

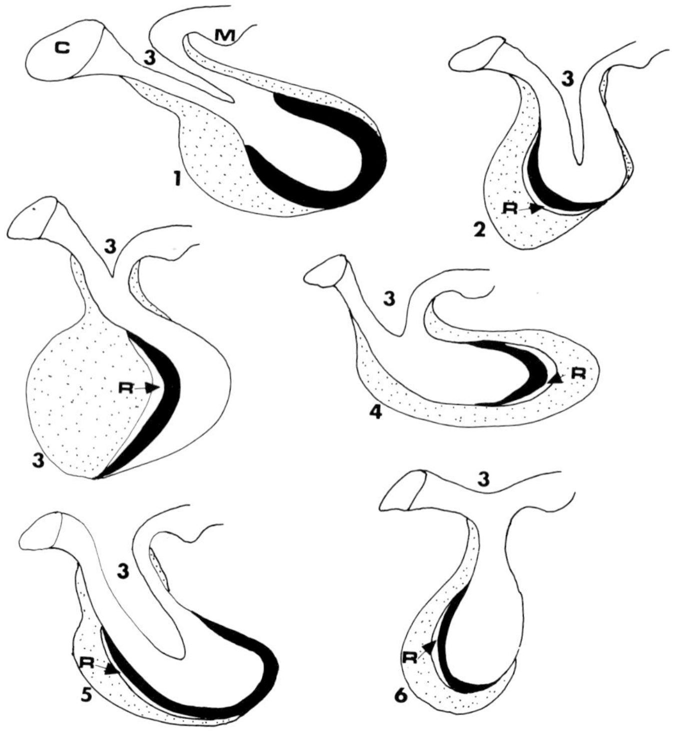

Fig. 20-2. The hypophysis cerebri of selected species. *1*, horse; *2*, cat; *3*, large ruminant; *4*, dog; *5*, pig; *6*, man; *stipple*, adenophypophysis; *white*, neurohypophysis; *black*, intermediate lobe; *C*, optic chiasma; *M*, mammillary body; *R*, residual lumen; *3*, third ventricle. (Redrawn, modified and supplemented from Krolling, O. and Grau, H., *Lehrbuck der Histologie und vergleichenden mikroskopischen Anatomie der Haustiere*. Paul Parey, Berlin, 1960).

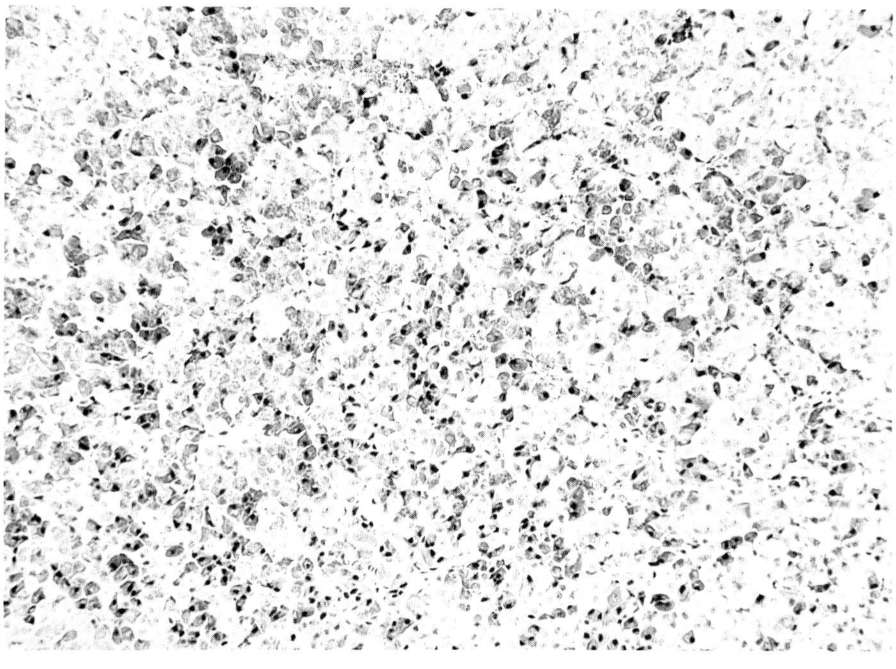

Fig. 20-3. Feline pars distalis. Cords and clumps of variously stained cells are intimately associated with sinusoids. ×10.

is covered by a fibrous capsule of dense white fibrous connective tissue (DWFCT) which is continuous with the reticular fibers which comprise the stroma of the organ. The parenchyma consists of cords or clusters of cells which are intimately associated with sinusoids. The cells of the pars distalis may be divided into two groups: *chromophobic cells* and *chromophilic cells*.

The *chromophobic cells* are also referred to as *chief cells*, *principal cells*, *reserve cells*, *C cells* or *gamma cells*. These small round cells have little cytoplasm which is usually devoid of granules (Fig. 20-4). As their name chromophobe implies, they have very little affinity for stains. These cells are usually clustered and may form the center of a cord of cells. The exact nature of these cells has not been clarified. They may be reserve cells that are capable of differentiating into chromophilic cells, or they may be cells in the process of degranulation.

The *chromophils* are initially divisible into *acidophils* and *basophils*. The acidophils include *alpha cells* and *epsilon cells*. Although these cells contain granules which are periodic acid-Schiff (PAS)-positive, the granules also stain with eosin, acid fuchsin, orange G and azocarmine. *Acidophils*, generally, are much larger than chromophobes, possess a granular cytoplasm which is acidophilic and may be polarized (Fig. 20-4). Specific staining techniques permit the subdivision of the acidophils into two distinct groups. The alpha cell has granules about 300 nm in diameter. These granules also stain positively with orange G; thus, they are also referred to as *orangeophils*. The *epsilon cells*, however, have granules which range between 100 and 900 nm. These granules specifically stain with the azocarmine dye. These cells are referred to as *carminophils*.

The *basophils* contain granules which are especially PAS-positive because of the glycoprotein nature of the secretory products (Fig. 20-4). They are larger cells than the acidophils. The granules of the basophils range from 150 to 200 nm in diameter. Although all of the basophilic granules are strongly PAS-positive, the cells are further subdivided on the basis of specific staining reactions accordingly: *beta cells* and *delta cells*. The granules of *beta cells* are alcianophilic and aldehyde fuchsin-positive. The delta cells have granules that are fast green-positive.

With routine staining (hematoxylin and eosin) only three cell types are identifiable: *chromophobe* (agranular and unstained), *acidophils* (granules which are eosinophilic) and *basophils* (granules with an affinity for hematoxylin). The proportion of cell types varies according to the age, species, sex, physiological condition, etc. Generally, 50 per cent are chromophobes 40 per cent are acidophils and 10 per cent are basophils.

The *pars tuberalis* is composed of cuboi-

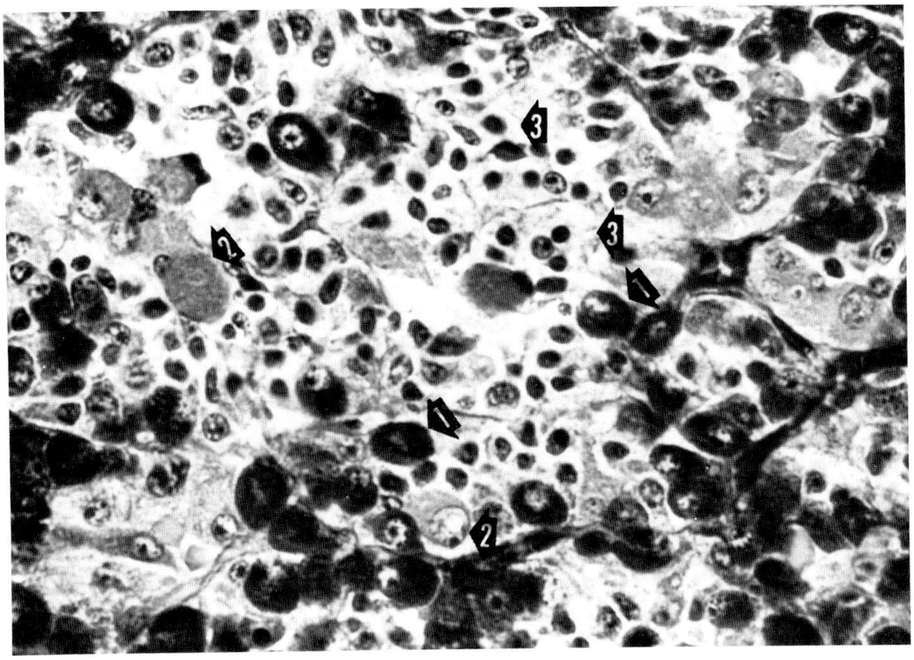

Fig. 20-4. Equine pars distalis. With this Azan stain, three cell types are easily identified: acidophils (*1*), basophils (*2*) and chromphobes (*3*). Fine connective tissue septa delineate the clumps of cells. ×160. (Azan).

dal cells which are weakly basophilic (Fig. 20-5). Granules, if present, are small. The cells are disposed in cords or clusters or as follicles. The function of the pars tuberalis has not been established.

The *pars intermedia* is not well-developed in man, but it is well-developed in domestic animals (Fig. 20-6). This portion of the pituitary is adjacent to, but separated from, the neurohypophysis by a connective tissue sheath which is discontinuous. Migration of cells of the pars intermedia into the pars nervosa is common. The predominant cell type of this area is a nonspecific basophil (Fig. 20-7). Although these cells are usually disposed as cords or clusters of cells, follicles are commonly encountered.

Hormones of the Adenohypophysis. Specific hormones have been associated with specific cells of the pars distalis.

Somatotrophic hormone (*STH*) is secreted by the *alpha cells*, those cells that stain with orange G (*orangeophils*). This hormone is responsible for general body growth and is especially influential at the growth plate of bones. An oversecretion during adolescence causes *gigantism*, while an undersecretion in adolescence causes *dwarfism*. Following the closure of the growth plates, an oversecretion of this hormone results in *acromegaly*.

The *epsilon cells* (*carminophils*) are responsible for the secretion of *luteotrophic hormone* (*LTH*, *lactogenic hormone*, *prolactin*). This hormone causes the secretion of milk following mammary gland development. It is also responsible, with other hormones, for the development of the mammary gland. It also stimulates the corpus luteum to secrete progesterone. In columbiform birds, it is responsible for the secretory activity of the crop associated with the formation of crop milk.

The *chromophobe* is believed to be responsible for the secretion of *adrenocorticotrophic hormone* (*ACTH*). This hormone increases the glucocorticoid secretory activity of the adrenal cortex and also stimulates melanocytes.

The remaining hormones of the pars distalis are secreted by specific *basophils*. These include *follicle-stimulating hormone* (*FSH*), *thyrotrophic hormone* (*TSH*) and *luteinizing hormone* (*LH*). There is some evidence that *ACTH* may also be secreted by a basophil.

Follicle-stimulating hormone (*FSH*) is responsible for the growth and development of ovarian follicles. It also activates the testes to produce spermatozoa. In the female, the combined activities of FSH and LH are responsible for maturation of ova, ovulation and the development of the corpus luteum.

Thyrotrophic hormone (*TSH*, *thyroid-stimulating hormone*) is responsible for the stimulation and maintenance of the secretory activity of the thyroid gland.

Luteinizing hormone (*LH*) promotes the conversion of the ruptured follicle into the corpus luteum. It is, therefore, responsible for progesterone secretion. In conjunction with FSH, it is responsible for ovulation. In the male, LH is referred to as *ICSH* (*interstitial cell-stimulating hormone*). It stimulates the secretion of testosterone from the *cells of Leydig*.

The only other hormone which has been identified in the adenohypophysis is *intermedin*. Intermedin or *melanocyte-stimulating hormone* (*MSH*) is responsible for the dispersion of melanin in melano-

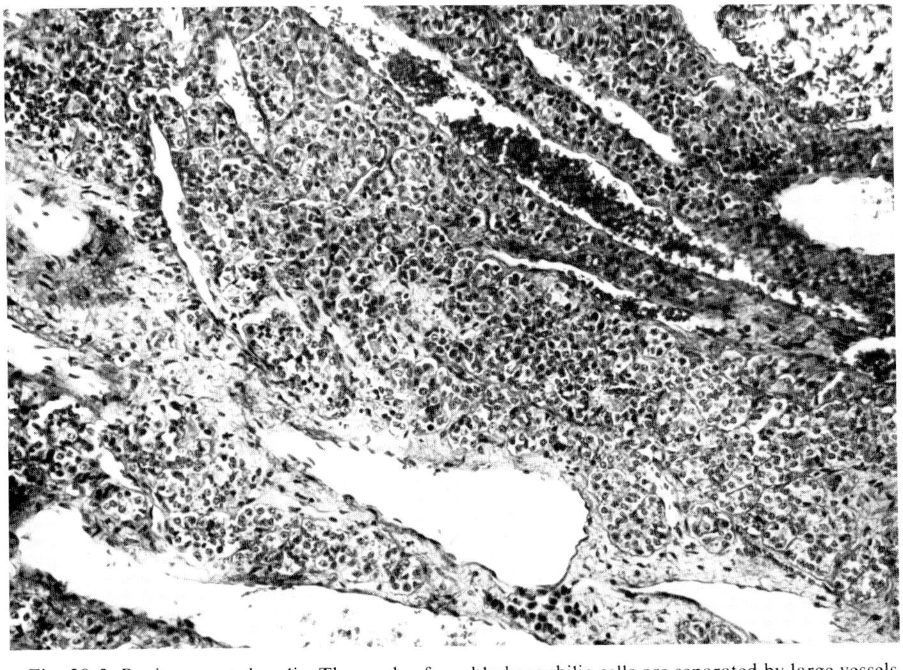

Fig. 20-5. Bovine pars tuberalis. The cords of weakly basophilic cells are separated by large vessels. ×40.

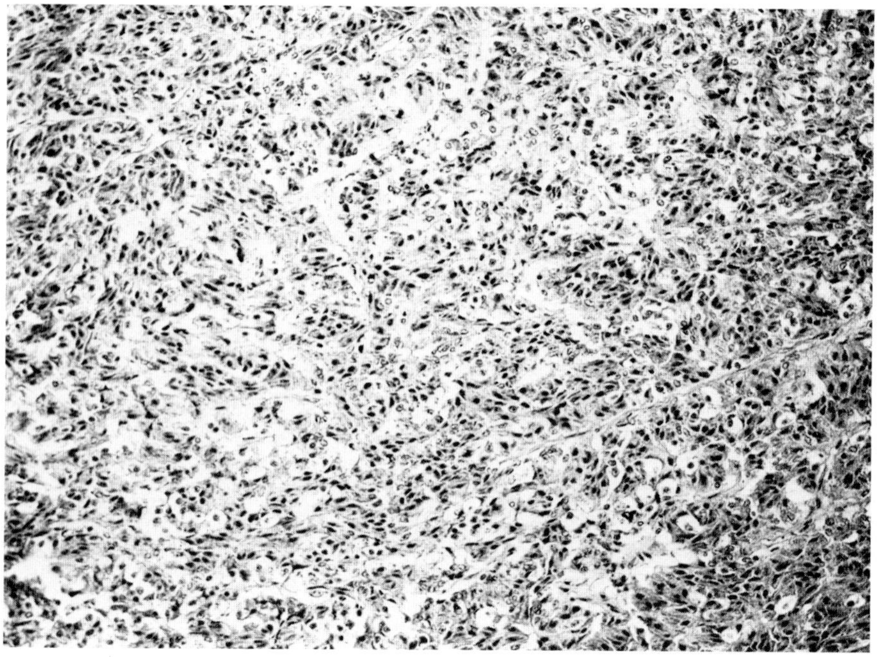

Fig. 20-6. Bovine pars intermedia. The nonspecific basophils are disposed as cords and clumps closely associated with vessels. ×40.

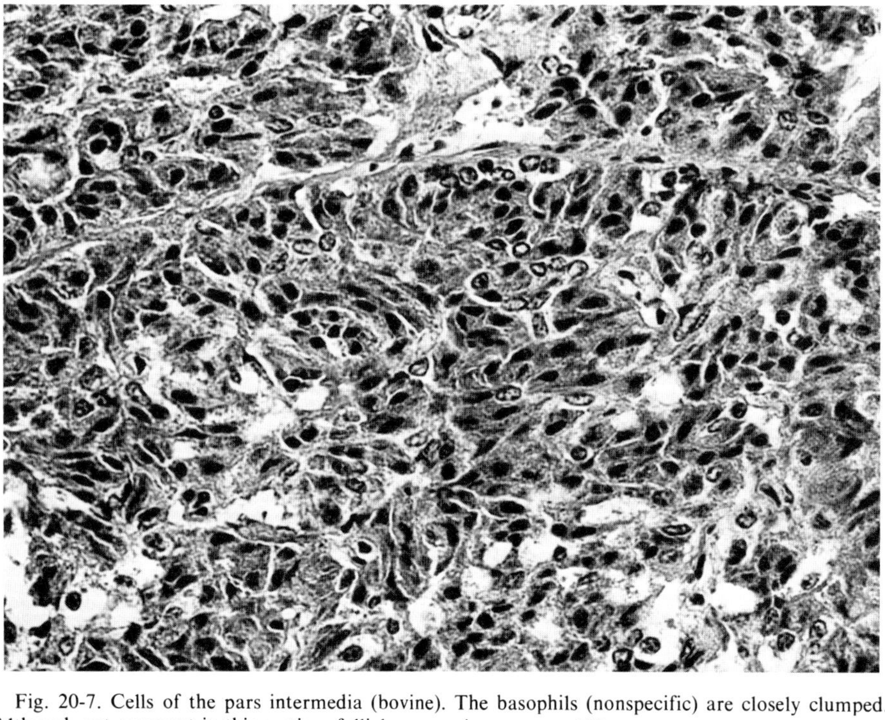

Fig. 20-7. Cells of the pars intermedia (bovine). The basophils (nonspecific) are closely clumped. Although not apparent in this section, follicles may also occur. ×100.

cytes. This activity is well established in lower vertebrates (amphibians) and may be applicable in higher vertebrates.

Regulation of the Adenohypophysis. The regulation of the adenohypophysis is mediated through a negative feedback system which involves the hypothalamic region of the diencephalon. This system operates through the *hypothalamohypophyseal portal system*. Specific hypothalamic neurons are sensitive to a deficiency in the blood of the secretory products of target organs or other changes. Due to a change in the blood, a releasing factor in the form of a neurosecretory substance passes into the blood capillaries of the median eminence. It then drains to the capillary bed of the pars distalis via the portal circulation. Appropriate cells are activated to secrete their trophic hormones. The trophic hormones increase the specific output of the target gland. The increased blood level of the target gland hormone reduces the activity of the sensitive hypothalamic neurons. Their reduced activity, in turn, reduces the activity of the corresponding cells of the pars distalis.

Neurohypophysis. The *neurohypophysis* is a ventral evagination of the hypothalmic region of the diencephalon. It includes the *median eminence* of the *tuber cinereum*, *infundibular stalk* and *infundibular process* (Fig. 20-8). This region, therefore, is very similar to typical nervous tissue. It includes numerous unmyelinated neurons as part of the *hypothalamohypophyseal tract*. The cell bodies of these fibers are located in the supraoptic and paraventricular nuclei of the hypothalamus. These neurons are neurosecretory. Their *neurosecretions* move along the axons and are stored in the terminal parts as *Herring bodies* (Fig. 20-9). Numerous *pituicytes* and neuroglial elements are scattered among the nerve fibers.

The neurosecretory substances that comprise the hormonal content of this part of the pituitary gland are *oxytocin* and *vasopressin* (*antidiuretic hormone, ADH*). The Herring bodies represent the stored, perhaps altered, form of these hormones prior to release into the capillary bed of the inferior hypophyseal artery.

Oxytocin is produced within the paraventricular nuclei and affects uterine smooth muscle. During or shortly after copulation, its effects facilitate the ascent of spermatozoa to the oviduct. During pregnancy its release increases the rate of uterine contractions which facilitate parturition. Milk flow is also mediated by the effects of this hormone on the myoepithelial cells of the mammary gland.

Vasopressin, which is produced within the supraoptic nuclei, manifests its antidiuretic properties on the lining cells of the collecting ducts wherein water is recovered by the vascular system from the kidney tubules.

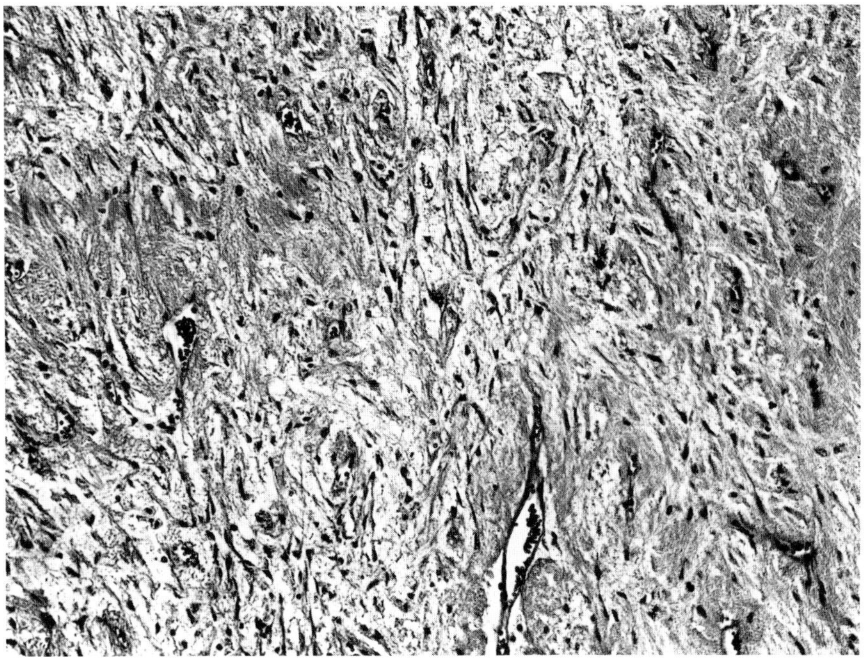

Fig. 20-8. Bovine neurohypophysis. It appears as typical nervous tissue. ×40.

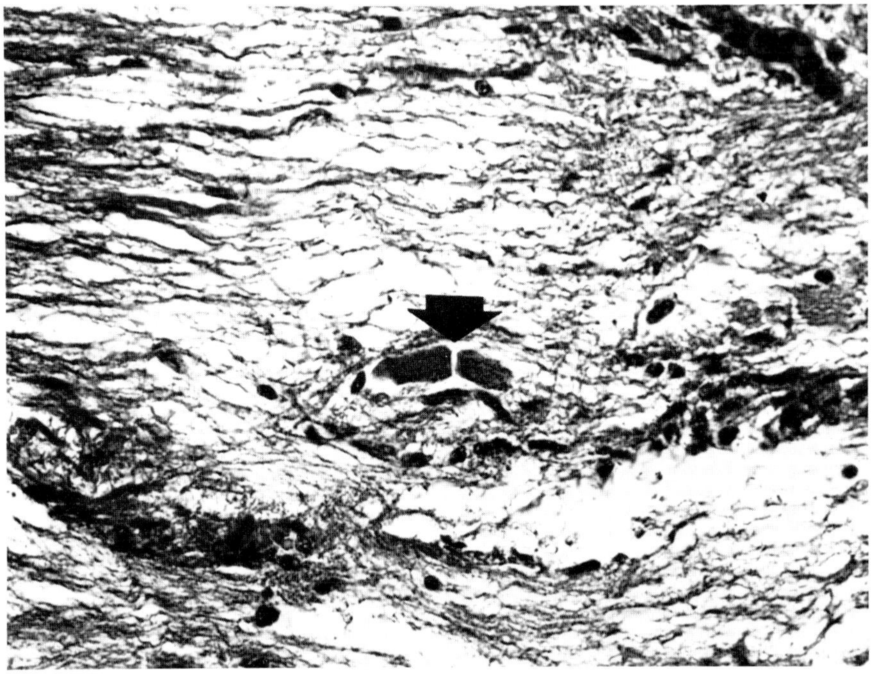

Fig. 20-9. Herring bodies. The neurosecretory products of specific hypothalamic nuclear regions are transported down axons and stored as Herring bodies (*arrow*). ×100.

Epiphysis Cerebri

General Remarks. This organ is also referred to as the *pineal gland*. It is a dorsal evagination of the roof of the diencephalon.

An understanding of the functional significance of the pineal body has been slow to evolve. In lower vertebrates, it is a photoreceptor organ, the *third eye* or *pineal eye*. Its position in the mammalian cranium, however, would appear to preclude a light-sensitive function. In fact, despite its position in the cranium, it is a light-sensitive organ. Information from the optical system is carried to the midbrain and thence to the thoracic region of the spinal cord wherein sympathetic nerves carry the information to the apex of the pineal body.

Melatonin and *serotonin* have been identified as secretory products of this gland. Under continuous light stimulation, the pineal gland decreases in activity, melatonin production decreases and gonadal activity increases. Melatonin, therefore, has an inhibitory effect on gonadal development. This is consonant with the observation that pineal body tumors result in delayed puberty. It is not clear, however, whether the pineal gland mediates its influence through the hypothalamus (releasing factors), pars distalis, or directly upon the gonads.

The gland is sensitive to indirect stimulation from light and does affect the gonads. It is probably the biological clock which sets circadian rhythms associated with estrous cycles and seasonal breeding characteristics of some species.

Histology of the Epiphysis Cerebri. The pineal body is covered by the connective tissue of the pia mater (Fig. 20-10). Septation and lobulation of the organ is accomplished by invasion of the connective tissue elements. The primary cellular components are *astrocytes* and *pinealocytes* (epithelioid cells). Typical connective tissue cells (plasma cells, fibroblasts, mast cells and macrophages) may also be present.

The *pinealocytes* (*chief cells*) are large cells with a large, round and open nucleus set in an acidophilic cytoplasm (Fig. 20-11). The *astrocytes* are typical and are interdigitated between the vascular supply and the pinealocytes. These are often referred to as *interstitial cells*.

The pineal body gradually undergoes retrogressive changes following puberty which involve the stromal elements. Increased connective tissue and the presence of *acervuli* (*brain sand*, *corpora arenacea*) are common changes.

Thyroid Gland

General Remarks. The thyroid gland is an outgrowth from the floor of the buccal cavity which subsequently loses its cellular connection (*thyroglossal duct*) with the pharyngeal endoderm. This glandular mass

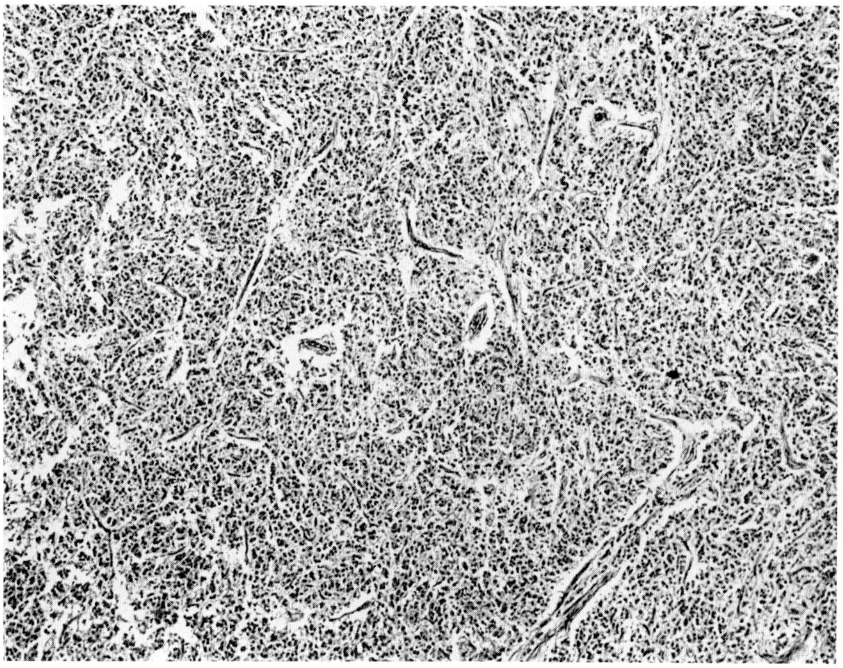

Fig. 20-10. Epiphysis cerebri (ovine). ×16.

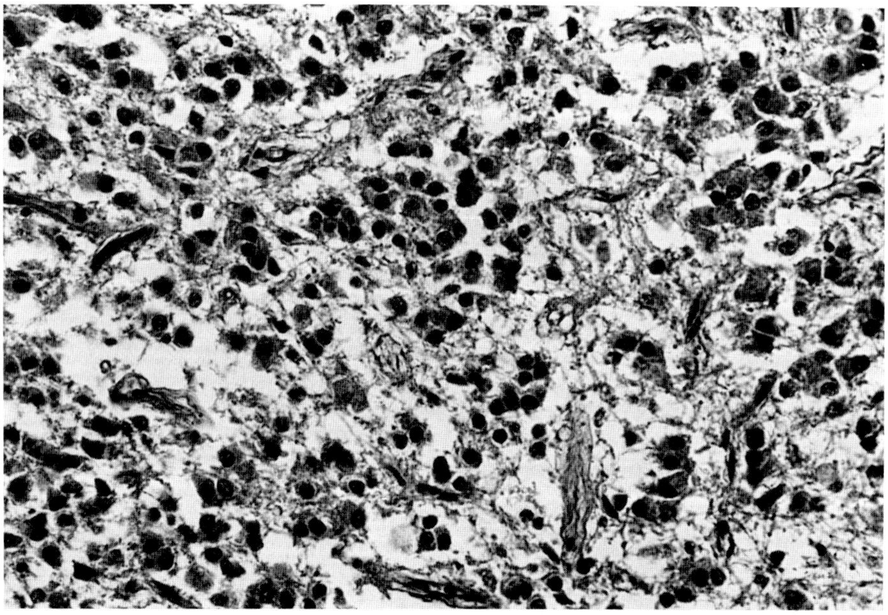

Fig. 20-11. Cellular components of the pineal body (ovine). ×90.

fuses with cellular masses from each fifth pharyngeal pouch (*ultimobranchial body*). Endodermal evaginations from the third and fourth pharyngeal pouches (parathyroid glands) also become intimately associated with or are embedded within the mass of thyroid tissue. The thyroid gland eventually assumes an anterolateral relationship with the trachea in the region of the larynx.

Histology of the Thyroid Gland. The capsule of the two lobes of the thyroid gland consists of areolar connective tissue. Connective tissue septa of similar tissue support the organ. Perifollicular connective tissue consists of extensive quantities of reticular fibers.

The structural unit of the thyroid gland is the *thyroid follicle* (Fig. 20-12). Follicles are hollow spheres which are variable in size. Individual follicular size is a function of the activity of the lining cells. The center of the follicle is filled with a gel-like material called *colloid*. This is the storage form of the follicular epithelial secretory products. The lining epithelium varies from low cuboidal to high columnar (Fig. 20-13). The height of the cells within a given follicle, however, is uniform.

The follicular lining actually consists of two cell types: *follicular lining cells* which comprise at least 90 per cent of the cellular population and *light cells* (*parafollicular cells*, *C cells*). The *follicular lining cells* are acidophilic with a basally positioned nucleus (Fig. 20-13). A pale-staining Golgi area may be seen in a supranuclear position. There may be colloid droplets adjacent to the luminal surface. The *parafollicular cells* may occur in a parafollicular position as the name implies, or they may occur within the lining of the follicle wherein they occasionally reach the luminal surface (Fig. 20-14). In either instance, they are surrounded by the basal lamina which delimits the follicle from the connective tissue space. They are cells with a pale-staining cytoplasm. The parafollicular cells have an entirely different function than the lining cells of the follicle.

Colloid, which contains proteins, glycoproteins and enzymes, is usually acidophilic. The glycoprotein component imparts a strong PAS-positive reaction. In an active follicle, the colloid has peripheral irregularities and vacuoles as well as a strong acidophilia. In an inactive follicle, the colloid is slightly basophilic or even acidophilic. The periphery has a smooth profile and vacuoles are not present. The size of the follicles as well as the height of the epithelium are also indicators of follicular or glandular activity. The activity of a follicle is approximately inversely proportional to the diameter of the follicle. Small follicles usually have a high epithelium (and the appropriate colloid characteristics) and are active. Large follicles usually have a low epithelium (and the appropriate colloid characteristics) and are

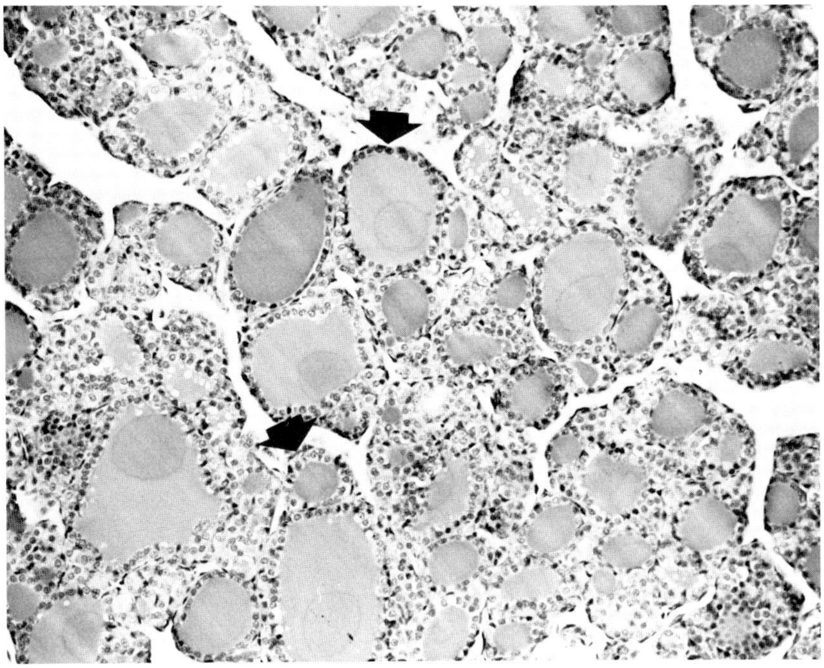

Fig. 20-12. Thyroid gland. The parenchyma of the organ is disposed as follicles (*arrows*) surrounding acidophilic colloid. ×40. (PAS).

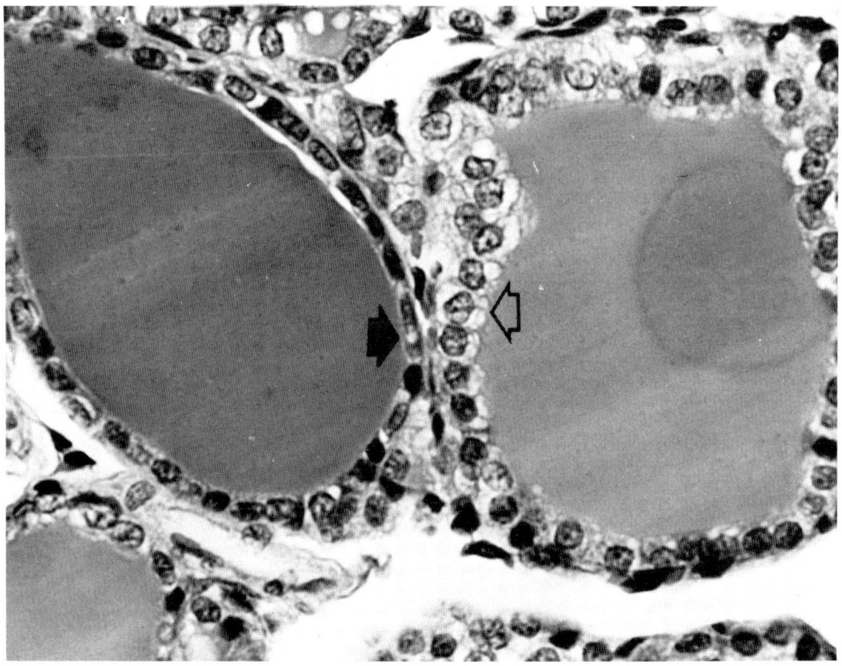

Fig. 20-13. Follicular epithelium. The lining cells may vary from low cuboidal (*solid arrow*) to columnar (*open arrow*). ×160. (PAS).

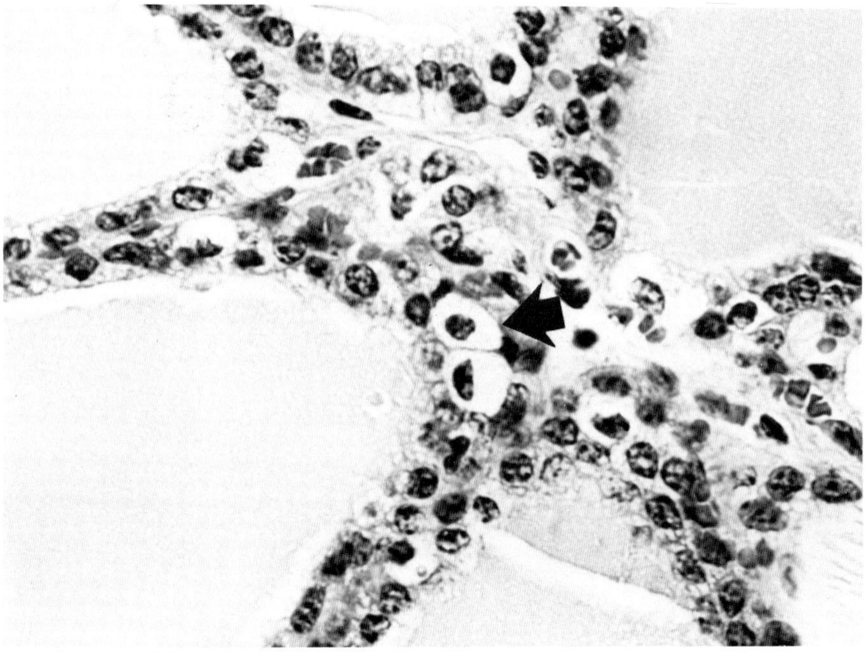

Fig. 20-14. Parafollicular cells. These cells (*arrow*) are light-staining cells positioned at the edges of the follicles. ×160. (PAS).

less active. In inactive follicles, the follicular epithelium may even be squamous.

Secretory Activity of the Thyroid Gland. The simplicity of thyroid follicular morphology is only barely indicative of the complex mechanisms involved in the synthesis, secretion and mobilization of its hormonal products.

The uptake of iodide from the juxtaposed capillary network is accomplished by the basal region of the follicular cells. They not only concentrate the iodide but oxidize it to iodine. At the same time as this occurs, the smooth endoplasmic reticulum, rough endoplasmic reticulum and Golgi apparatus are involved in the synthesis, packaging and export of *thyroglobulin*, a glycoprotein. The thyroglobulin is released into the follicular space at which point the iodination of tyrosine (an amino acid component of thyroglobulin) occurs. These steps account for the synthesis and secretion of the storage product.

The release or mobilization of thyroglobulin is dependent upon the presence of hydrolytic enzymes within the colloid which probably respond to activation, directly or indirectly, from TSH. The hydrolysis of thyroglobulin yields four significant products: *monoiodotyrosine*, *diiodotyrosine*, *triiodotyrosine* and *tetraiodotyrosine* (*thyroxine*). Two of these substances are picked up at the luminal surface, probably transported through the cell and deposited in the adjacent capillary bed (triiodotyrosine and thyroxine). The remaining tyrosyl moieties are dehalogenated and recycled for use in the synthesis of thyroglobulin. The synthesis, secretion, iodination, hydrolysis and mobilization of these moieties occur simultaneously in the follicles.

The *parafollicular cells* are responsible for the elaboration of a polypeptide hormone called *thyrocalcitonin* (*calcitonin*).

Thyroxine has numerous effects on the body's tissues. It is responsible for calorigenesis and thus the maintenance of body temperature in homiotherms. This is accomplished by increasing the energy production and oxygen consumption of mitochondria in the orthodox conformation. This hormone is also involved in general electrolyte and water balance, as well as both anabolic and catabolic aspects of protein metabolism. In conjunction with energy requirements, thyroxine has an influence on fat mobilization and degradation. It is also a hyperglycemic factor as well as being a synergist with somatotrophic hormone (STH). Triiodotyrosine is even more active than thyroxine.

Calcitonin is a hypocalcemic factor which tends to reduce blood calcium levels. It is, therefore, an antagonist for parathyroid hormone.

Parathyroid Glands

General Remarks. The parathyroid glands are derived from the third (*external parathyroids*) and fourth (*internal parathyroids*) pharyngeal pouches. The position of the external parathyroids may vary from cranial to the thyroids to the level of the thoracic inlet. The internal parathyroids may be missing (bird, pig) or may be embedded within, upon or close to the thyroid gland.

Histology of the Parathyroid Glands. The capsule of the external parathyroids is areolar connective tissue which blends with the surrounding fascia. The internal parathyroids do not have a capsule per se but are surrounded by the areolar connective tissue of the interstices of the thyroid gland.

The parenchyma of the organ consists of cords, clusters, strands, sheets or rosettes of secretory cells. Occasionally, follicles may be present (Fig. 20-15). These cells are supported by a fine stromal network of

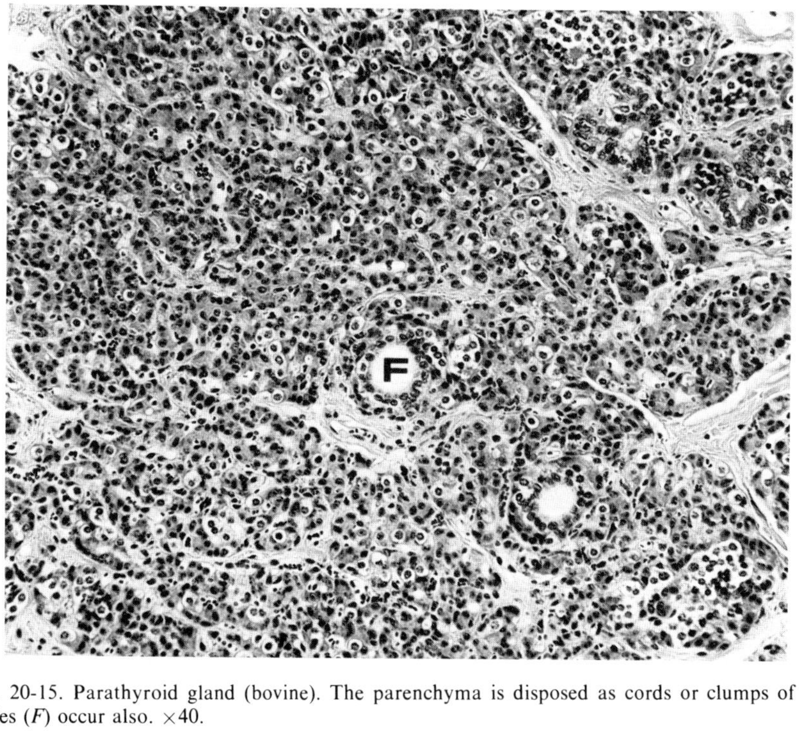

Fig. 20-15. Parathyroid gland (bovine). The parenchyma is disposed as cords or clumps of cells. Follicles (*F*) occur also. ×40.

reticular fibers with numerous capillaries in close association with the parenchyma. The primary cell types of the organ include *chief cells* and *oxyphil cells*. The *chief* or *principal cells* may be subdivided into *clear* or *light chief cells* and *dark chief cells*. Chief cells are more abundant than the oxyphilic cells.

The dark and light chief cells may represent different physiological states of the same cell. The *light chief cell* is a small cell with a large, vesicular nucleus (Fig. 20-16). Its cytoplasm is acidophilic, agranular and has lipid and glycogen inclusions. The *dark chief cell* has an acidophilic cytoplasm which contains argyrophilic granules. The nucleus is vesicular but smaller than that of the light chief cell. The dark chief cell contains less glycogen and lipid than its lighter counterpart. Dark chief cells produce parathormone.

The *oxyphil cells* occur in the ox, the horse and man, but they do not occur regularly in other domestic species. They are large cells with a granular, acidophilic cytoplasm (Fig. 20-16). Their nuclei are small and dark-staining. These cells usually occur in small clusters. It is presumed that chief cells give rise to these cells. The precise function of these cells has not been determined.

Parathyroid Hormone. The secretory product of the chief cells of the parathyroid glands is the polypeptide hormone, *parathormone*. This is a hypercalcemic factor which is antagonistic to thyrocalcitonin. Ionic calcium levels in the blood are maintained at a homeostatic level of 10 mg per 100 ml. A lowering of this level results in the release of parathormone. Although it was thought that this hormone resulted in the differentiation and increased activity of osteoclasts, current experimental evidence indicates otherwise. The delayed differentiation of osteoclasts from exogenous administration of parathormone is too slow to maintain homeostatic calcium levels and preclude the occurrence of tetany from hypocalcemia. It is currently hypothesized that the action of this hormone in the mobilization of mineral from bone is mediated through the combined activity of osteoblasts and osteocytes.

Adrenal Glands

General Remarks. The *adrenal glands* or *suprarenal glands* are small organs situated at the cranial poles of the kidneys. Embryologically, the adrenal glands are derived from two germ layers: *mesoderm* and neural crest *ectoderm*. The adrenal cortex develops from a thickening of coelomic mesothelium in close association to the kidneys and gonads. The neural crest ectoderm migrates to this region and invades the cortex as adrenal medullary tissue. In mammals a distinct cortex and medulla are apparent despite the striking interdigitations that may occur (Fig. 20-17). In birds, the cortical and

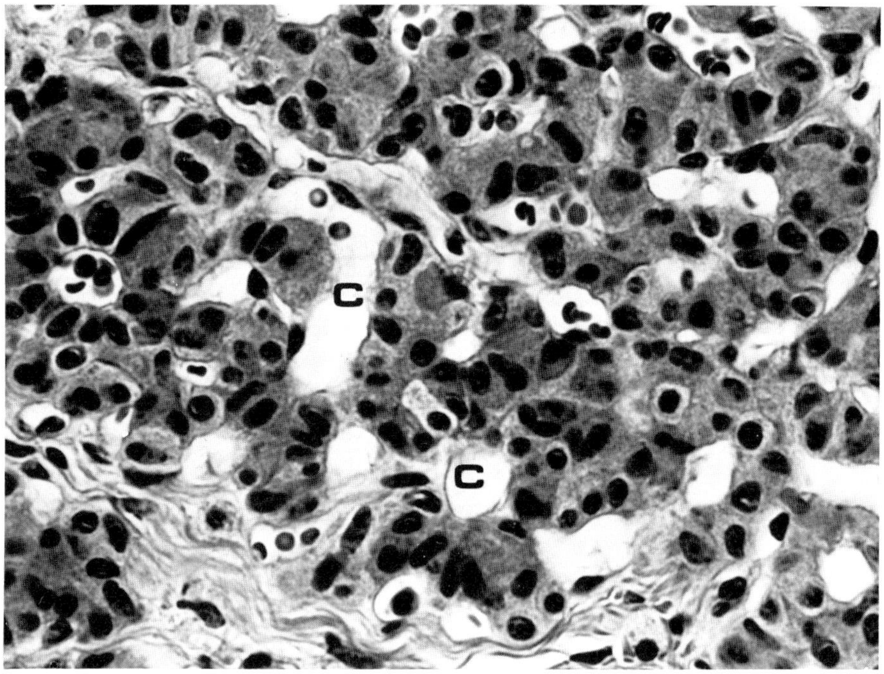

Fig. 21-16. Cells of the parathyroid (bovine). The cells are disposed as cords or clumps of cells in close association to capillaries (*C*). ×160.

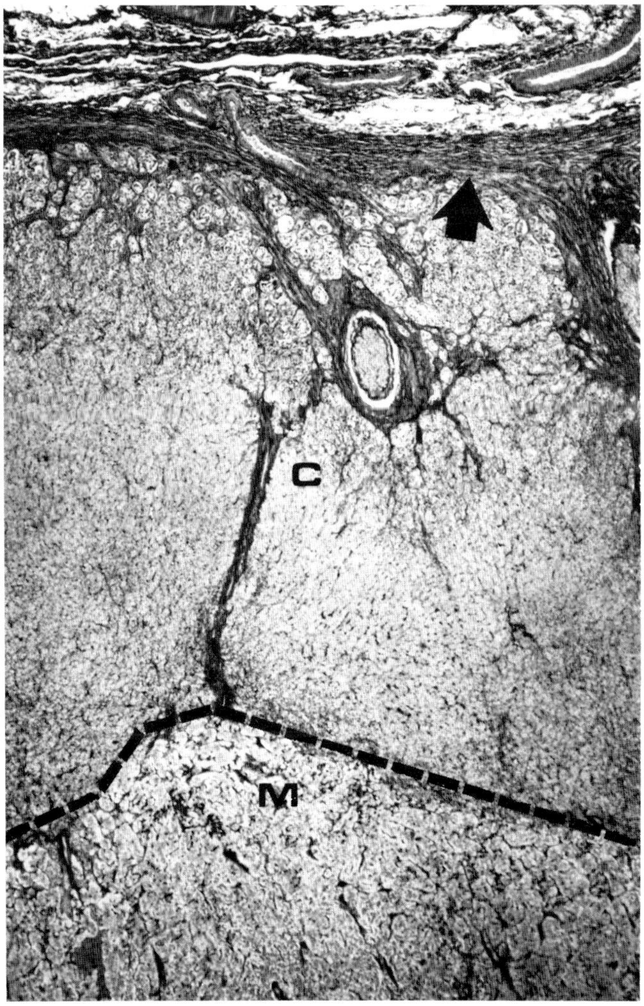

Fig. 20-17. Adrenal gland (bovine). The adrenal gland is covered by a capsule (*arrow*). It is divided into a cortex (*C*) and medulla (*M*) which are clearly delimited (*dashed line*). ×10. (Azan).

medullary tissue is intermixed (Fig. 20-18). Auxiliary cortical adrenal tissue is a common occurrence in some species. In some rodents, auxiliary adrenal tissue is contained within the epididymis.

The organ is enclosed within a capsule of DWFCT. The trabeculae of areolar connective tissue invade the parenchyma to the level of the medulla. The supportive stroma consists of fine collagenous and reticular fibers.

Adrenal Cortex. The adrenal cortex consists of polyhedral secretory cells which are organized into cords, usually two cells thick, which are oriented radially from the medullary region (Fig. 20-19). The orientation of the cords and some cytological differences permit the identification of cortical subdivisions: *zona glomerulosa*, *zona fasciculata*, *zona reticularis*.

The *zona glomerulosa* is also referred to as the *zona arcuata* and the *zona multiformis* (Fig. 20-20). This subcapsular zone (Fig. 20-21) consists of curved cords or arcades (horse, carnivores, pig), or clustered groups or glomeruli (ruminants, man). The cells of this zone are columnar (man, horse, carnivores, pig) or polyhedral (other species) (Fig. 20-22). The parenchyma, despite its spatial arrangement, is closely associated with an extensive vascular network. The cytoplasm is more evenly acidophilic and less foamy than the cells of the adjacent zone. The nuclei of the cells of the zona glomerulosa are smaller and darker than those of the adjacent zone. The occurrence of fine lipid inclusions is usually linked with an increased cellular activity. In man and ruminants, basophilic granules may be observed in the cytoplasm.

The *zona fasciculata* is the widest zone of the cortex (Fig. 20-23). It consists of cuboidal or polyhedral cells which are arranged in radial cords. Each cord consists of one or two cells separated from adjacent cords by an extensive sinusoidal network. The large cells of the outer two-thirds of this zone contain a large, vesicular nucleus (binucleations are common) within a very foamy cytoplasm. These cells are often referred to as *spongiocytes* (Fig. 20-24). The inner third of this zone contains cells that are free of lipids and have a more basophilic cytoplasm.

The *zona reticularis* consists of cells that are disposed as freely anastomosing cords (Fig. 20-25). The cells are very similar to the cells of the zona fasciculata. The cells contain less lipid than the cells of the peripherally adjacent zone. Their nuclei and cytoplasm are dark-staining. Lipofuscin pigments are commonly encountered.

Initially, it was thought that the zonation of the adrenal cortex represented a centripetal differentiation process. Mitosis occurs in all zones, however.

The aforementioned zonation is predi-

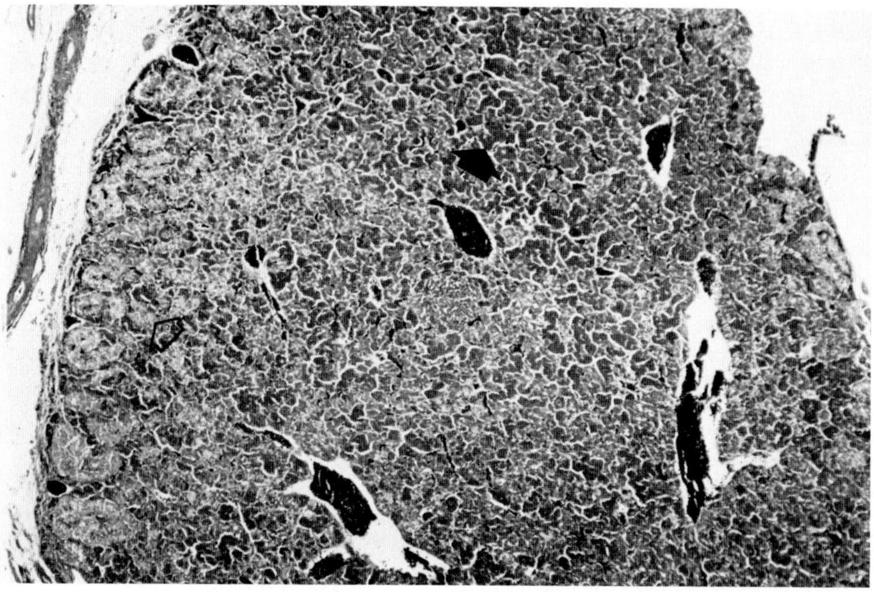

Fig. 20-18. Avian adrenal gland. This gland is not divided into a distinct cortex and medulla. The medullary tissue (*solid arrow*) is dark, while the cortical tissue is light (*open arrow*). ×9. (Azan).

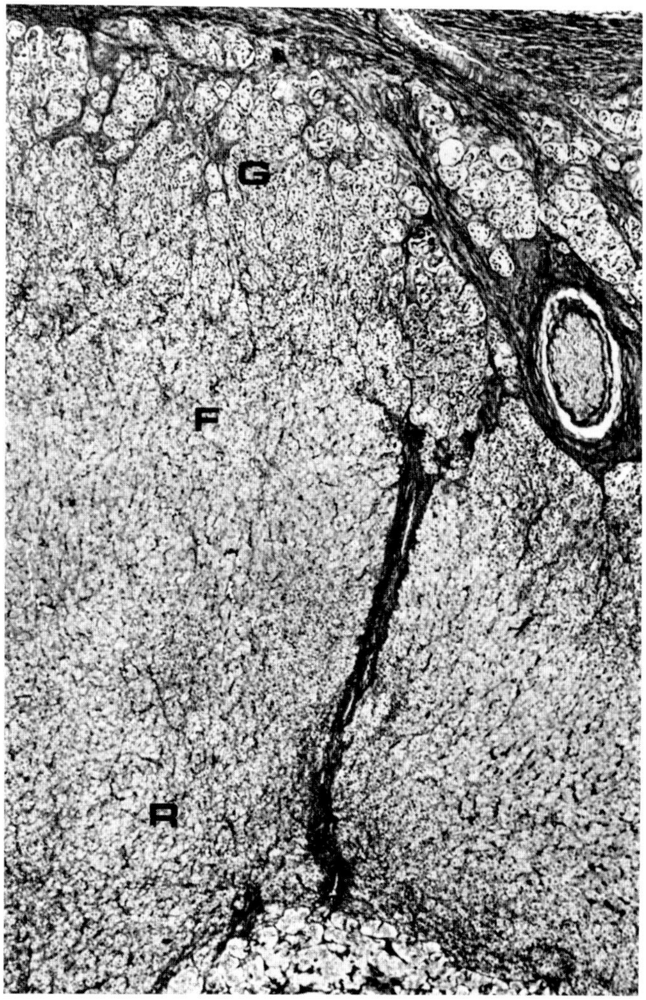

Fig. 20-19. Adrenal cortex (bovine). The cortex consists of a zona glomerulosa (*G*), zona fasciculata (*F*) and zona reticularis (*R*). ×16. (Azan).

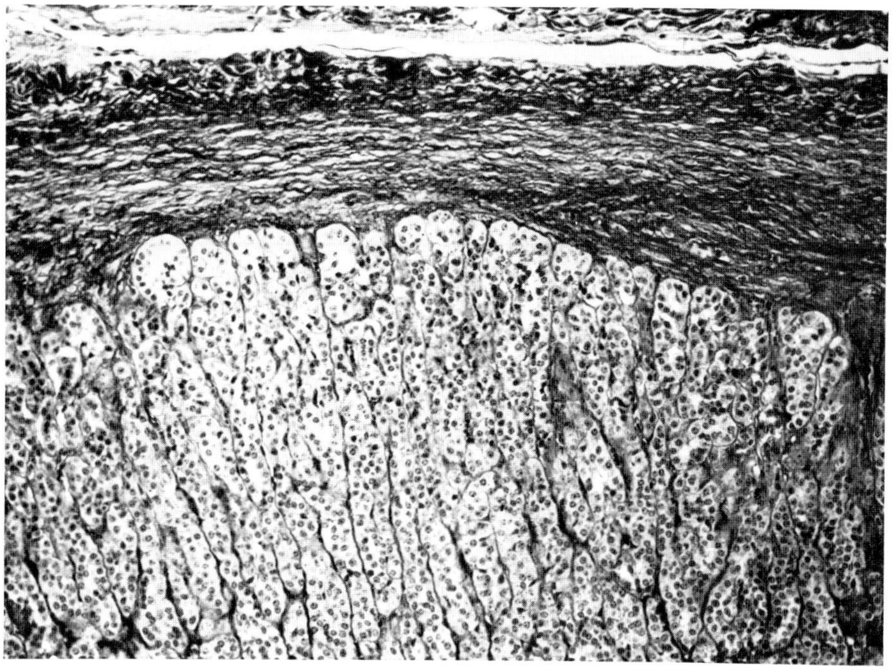

Fig. 20-20. Zona glomerulosa (bovine). The cells of this zone are clustered as glomeruli. ×40. (Azan).

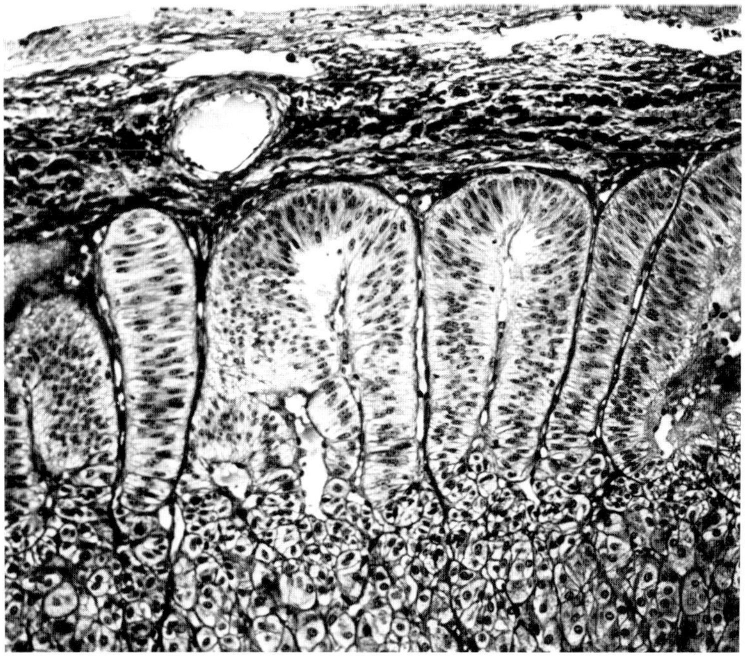

Fig. 20-21. Zona arcuata (equine). The cells of this zone are lustered as arcades. ×40. (Azan).

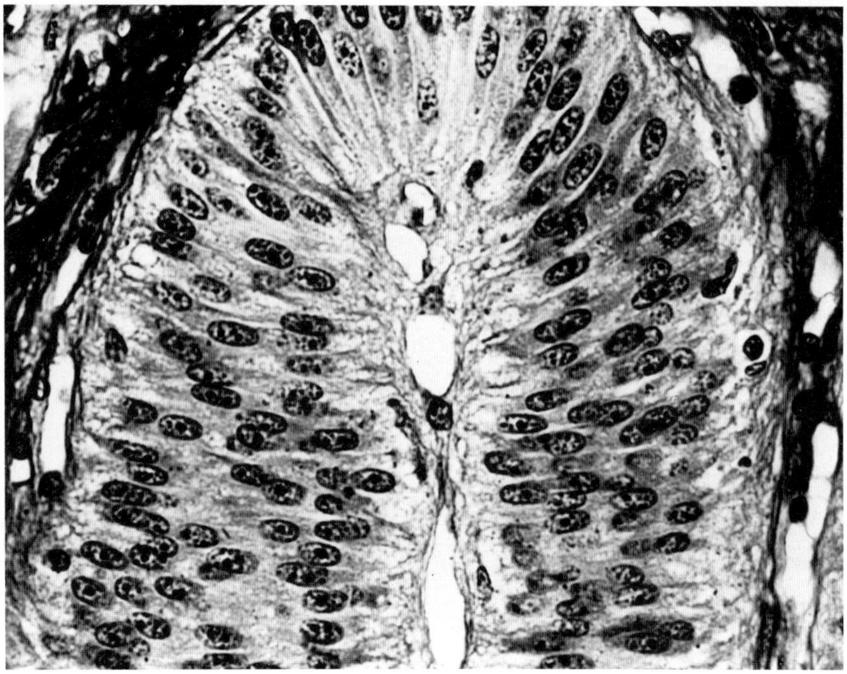

Fig. 20-22. Cells of the zona arcuata (equine). The cells of this zone are columnar. ×160. (Azan).

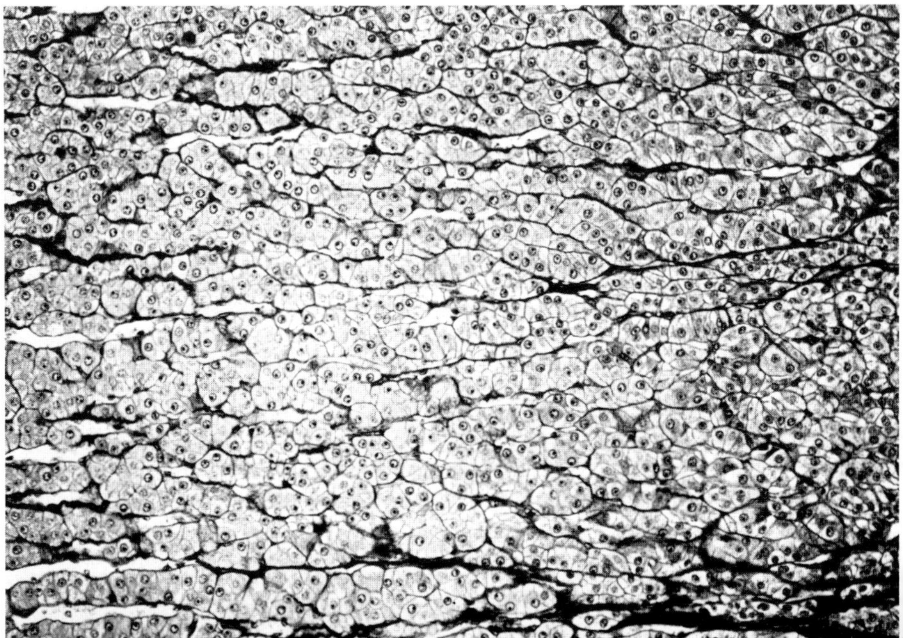

Fig. 20-23. Zona fasciculata (equine). The polyhedral cells are arranged as cords. ×40. (Azan).

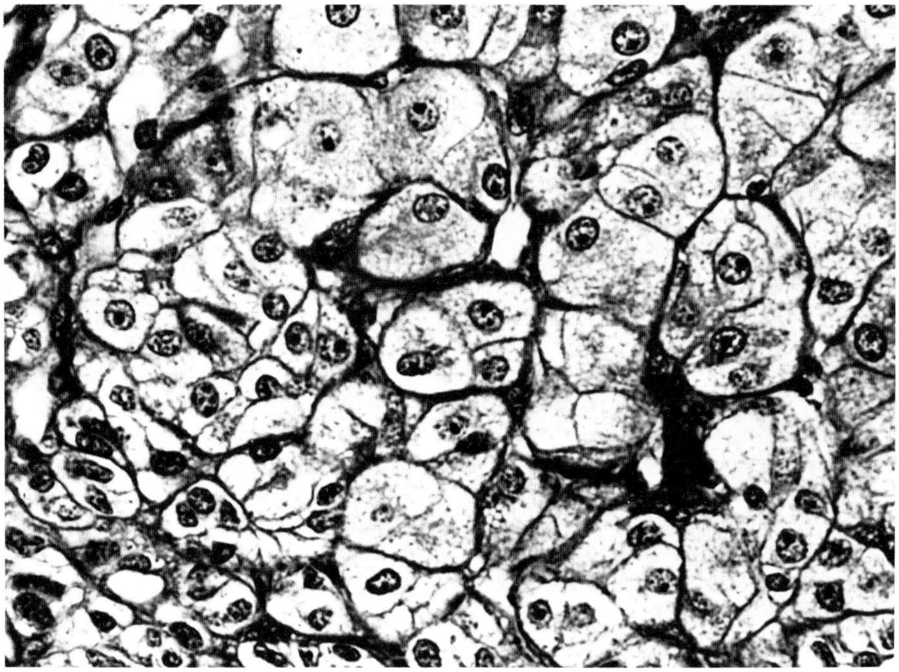

Fig. 20-24. Spongiocytes of the outer zona fasciculata (equine). These are large cells with a foamy cytoplasm and vesicular nucleus. ×40. (Azan).

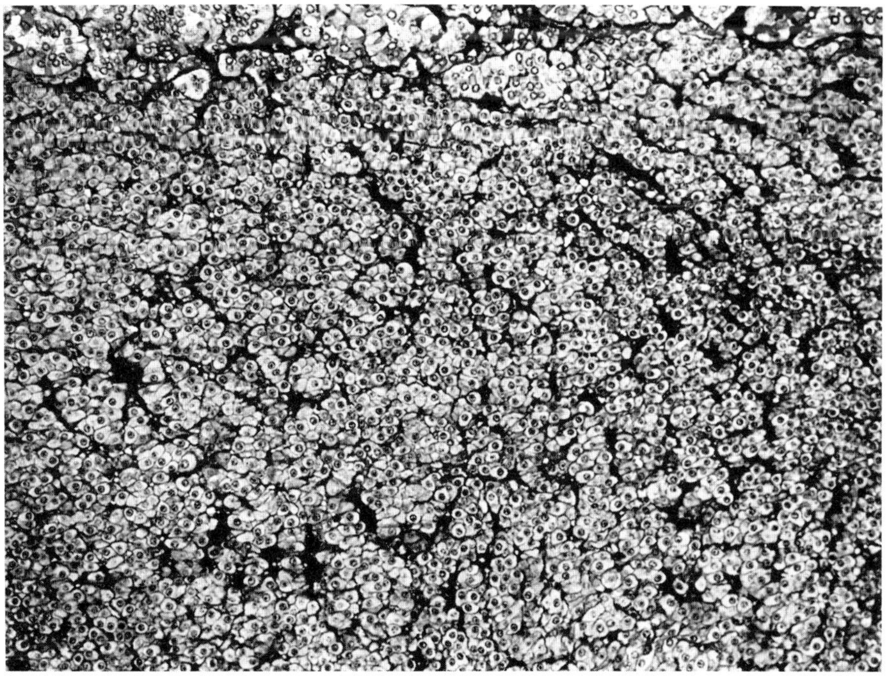

Fig. 20-25. Zona reticularis (equine). The cells are disposed as freely anastomosing cords. ×40. (Azan).

cated upon the organizational pattern of the cells. On the basis of cytological and cytochemical features, some authors divide the adrenal cortex into five zones: *zona glomerulosa, outer part of the zona fasciculata, inner part of the zona fasciculata, outer part of the zona reticularis* and the *inner part of the zona reticularis* adjacent to the adrenal medulla.

Hormones of the Adrenal Cortex. The adrenal cortex is required for life because its hormones influence numerous essential somatic processes. Although numerous steroid hormones have been isolated from the cortical tissues, they are readily grouped accordingly: *mineralocorticoids*, *glucocorticoids* and *sex hormones*.

The mineralocorticoids (*aldosterone* and *deoxycorticosterone*) are secreted by the zona glomerulosa apart from the influence of ACTH. These hormones are required for electrolyte and water balance in the body. The release of aldosterone is mediated by the renin-angiotensin axis which is responsive to the decreased blood pressure associated with a sodium deficiency.

The *glucocorticoids* are secreted from the zona fasciculata and zona reticularis under the influence of the trophic hormone, ACTH. The glucocorticoids include *cortisone*, *hydrocortisone* and *corticosterone*. These hormones are influential in carbohydrate metabolism because they facilitate protein catabolism and gluconeogenesis. They enhance the immediate immune response by releasing gamma globulins from lymphocytes. They do so, however, at the expense of the lymphocytes.

Adrenal Medulla. The corticomedullary junction may be a sharply delineated junction or may be highly interdigitated (Fig. 20-26). The primary constituents of the medulla include *glandular cells*, *ganglion cells*, *venules* and *capillaries*. The aforementioned cells are derived from neural crest ectoderm.

The *glandular cells* are large columnar or polyhedral cells which possess a large, vesicular nucleus (Fig. 20-27). The cells are polarized: one pole is opposed to a capillary; the other is opposed to a venule. The cytoplasm is basophilic and contains fine, chromaffin-positive granules (Fig. 20-26). The resulting pigments are sometimes referred to as *adrenochromes*. As a result of this chromaffin reactivity, the glandular cells are also called *chromaffin cells* or *pheochrome cells*. This reactivity is due to the presence of the *biogenic amines* (catecholamines), *epinephrine* and *norepinephrine*. The reaction of the catecholamines with chromic acid produces a brown reaction product. The chromaffin cells secrete one or the other of the catecholamines. In most species, these cells are randomly distributed throughout the medulla. In the ox, however, an outer lamina of epinephrine-producing

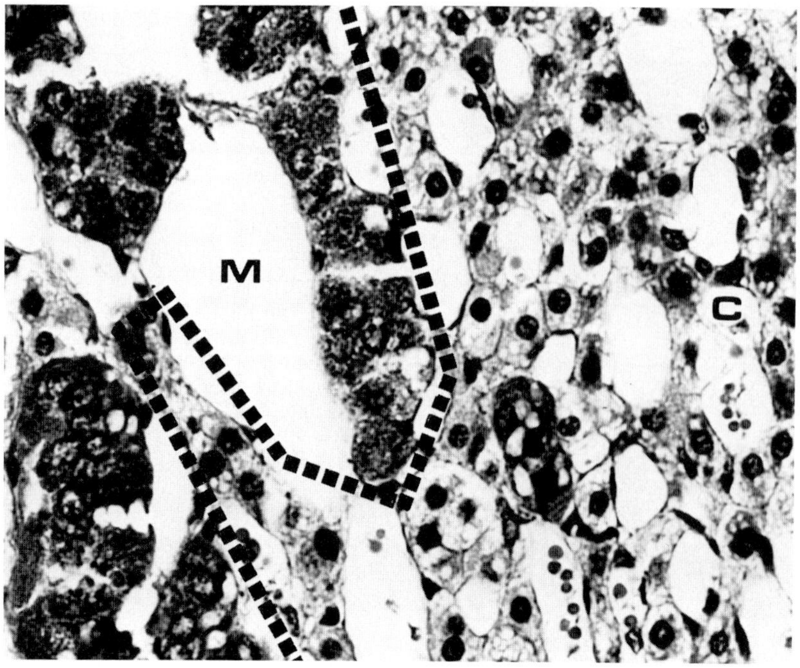

Fig. 20-26. Adrenal medulla and zona reticularis (porcine). The corticomedullary junction (*dashed line*) is irregularly defined. The medulla (*M*) consists of dark cells, while the zona reticularis of the cortex (*C*) consists of light cells. ×160. (chromaffin stain).

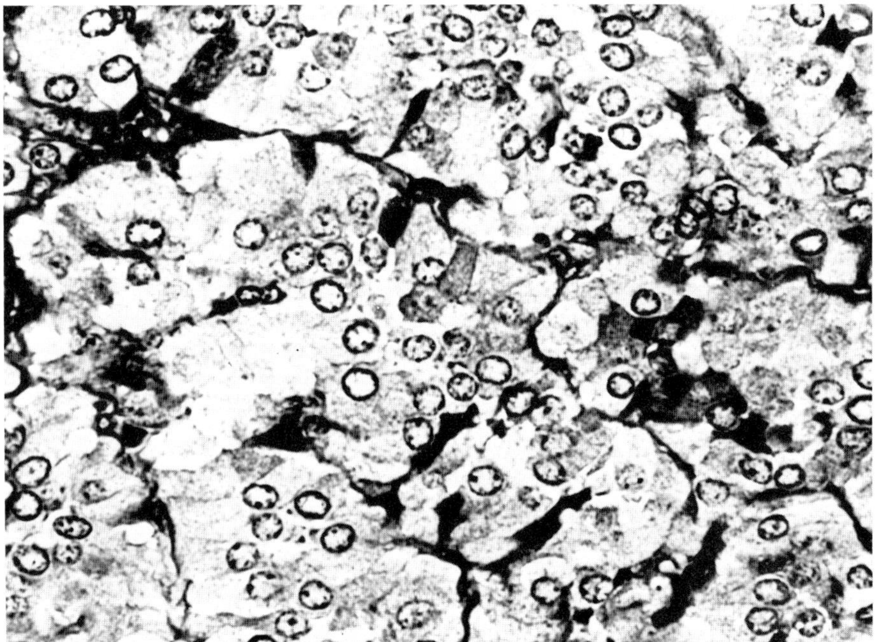

Fig. 20-27. Cells of the adrenal medulla (bovine). The large, columnar cells are polarized. ×160. (Azan).

cells is distinct from an inner lamina of norepinephrine-producing cells.

Sympathetic ganglion cells are randomly scattered throughout the medulla.

Hormones of the Adrenal Medulla. The synthesis and release of norepinephrine and epinephrine is achieved synaptically by the termination of preganglionic fibers on the glandular cells. Epinephrine has a general somatic effect which includes increased cardiac output, increased cellular respiration and oxygen consumption, glycogenolysis and the release of glucose for increased metabolic needs. Epinephrine, therefore, is the hormone of "fight or flight."

Norepinephrine is a neurotransmitter substance which increases blood pressure by peripheral vasoconstriction.

The adrenal medulla is not essential for life.

Chromaffin System. Besides the occurrence of chromaffin cells in the adrenal medulla, there are numerous small bodies (*paraganglia*) associated with the abdominal aorta in a retroperitoneal position. The paraganglia include two large bodies, the *glands of Zuckerkandl*. The paraganglia contain chromaffin-positive granules. The paraganglia plus the adrenal medulla comprise the chromaffin system.

Endocrine Pancreas

General Remarks. The organization of the pancreas reflects its duplicity of function as an exocrine and endocrine organ. The endocrine portion of the organ develops from the duct system. The endocrine portions are the *islets of Langerhans* which are randomly scattered throughout the organ.

Islets of Langerhans. The islets are scattered masses of pale-staining cells which are supported by reticular connective tissue (Fig. 20-28). Large sinusoids separate the cords or clusters of cells. The basic cell types of the islets are: ***alpha cells*** and ***beta cells***. *C cells* and *delta cells* have been identified also.

The *alpha cells* are polygonal cells with a nucleus which has a coarse distribution of heterochromatin. The granules of the alpha cells are insoluble in alcohol, stain pink or red with the Gomori aldehyde fuchsin technique and stain red with the Mallory-Azan stain.

The *beta cells* are structurally similar to the alpha cells. Their granules, however, are soluble in alcohol, stain dark purple with the Gomori aldehyde fuchsin technique and stain orange with the Mallory-Azan stain.

C cells do not contain granules. Delta cells stain blue with the Mallory-Azan technique. The function of these cells is unknown. It is likely, however, that they may represent different physiological states of alpha and beta cells. The C cells may be a resting, undifferentiated or exhausted form

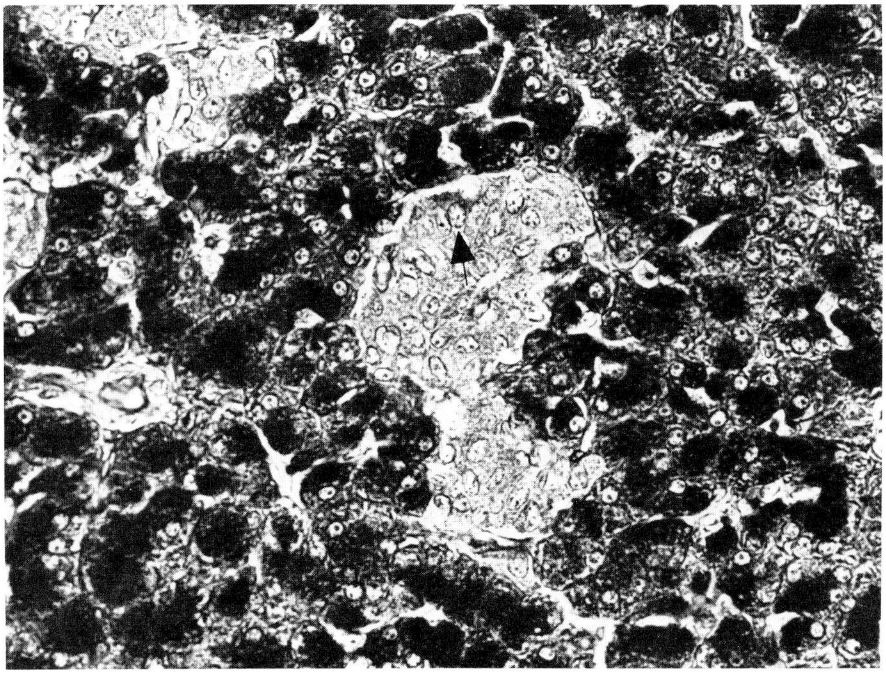

Fig. 20-28. Pancreatic islets. The light cells are alpha cells. The dark cell (*arrow*) is a beta cell. ×100. (Gomori aldehyde fuchsin).

of the alpha and beta cells, while the delta cell may be an altered alpha cell. Delta cells are rare in domestic species. Alpha cells comprise approximately 25 per cent of the cell population, while the beta cells comprise about 75 per cent of the cell population in canine islets of Langerhans.

Hormones of the Pancreas. The hormones of the pancreas are *insulin* and *glucagon*. Insulin is produced by the beta cells and is a *hypoglycemic factor*. Glucagon, a product of the alpha cells, is a *hyperglycemic factor* that stimulates glycogenolysis.

Miscellaneous Endocrine Glands

Scattered Glands and Their Products. Numerous endocrine glands, besides those covered in this section, are included in the endocrine system. The endocrine nature of the *ovary*, *testis* and *placenta* will be discussed in subsequent sections.

The duodenal mucosa secretes hormones (*secretin*, *cholecystokinin*, *enterogastrone*) that stimulate the flow of pancreatic juice, contraction of the gallbladder and the inhibition of gastric secretory activity and motility, respectively.

The gastric mucosa secretes a hormone, *gastrin*, which stimulates the secretion of gastric juice.

Numerous other hormones, including blastokinin, bradykinin, prostaglandins and 1,25-dihydroxycholicalciferol are secreted by various other tissues of the body.

References

Pituitary Gland

Brahms, S.: The development of the hypophysis of the cat (*Felis domestica*). Amer. J. Anat. *50*:251, 1932.

Conklin, J. L.: The identification of acidophilic cells in the human pars distalis. Anat. Rec. *156*:347, 1966.

Goldberg, R. C. and Chaikoff, I. L.: On the occurrence of six cell types in the dog anterior pituitary. Anat. Rec. *112*:265, 1953.

Harris, G. W. and Donovan, B. T. (eds.): *The Pituitary Gland*, University of California Press, Berkeley, 1966.

Herlant, M.: The cells of the adenohypophysis and their functional significance. Int. Rev. Cytol. *17*:299, 1964.

Lederis, K.: An electron microscopical study of the human neurohypophysis. Z. Zellforsch. *68*:847, 1965.

Zambrano, D.: Ultrastructural changes of the neurohypophysis of the rat after castration. Z. Zellforsch. *86*:14, 1968.

Pineal Body

Herbert, J.: The pineal gland and light-induced oestrus in ferrets. J. Endocr. *43*:625, 1969.

Jordan, H. E.: The histogenesis of the pineal body of the sheep. Amer. J. Anat. *12*:249, 1911.

Wurtman, R. J., Axelrod, J. and Kelly, D. E.: *The Pineal*. Academic Press, New York, 1968.

Thyroid Gland

Ekholm, R.: Thyroglobulin biosynthesis in the rat thyroid. J. Ultrastruct. Res. *20*:103, 1967.

Ekholm, R. and Ericson, L. E.: The ultrastructure of the parafollicular cells of the thyroid gland in the rat. J. Ultrastruct. Res. *23*:378, 1968.

Kingsbury, B. E.: Ultimobranchial body and the thyroid gland in the fetal calf. Amer. J. Anat. *56*:445, 1935.

Sobel, H. J.: Electron microscopy of I-irradiated thyroid. Arch. Path. *78*:53, 1964.

Welsch, U., Flitney, E. and Pearse, A. G. E.: Comparative studies of the ultrastructure of the thyroid parafollicular C cells. J. Microscop. *89*:83, 1969.

Parathyroid Glands

Capen, C. C. and Rowland, G. N.: The ultrastructure of the parathyroid glands of young cats. Anat. Rec. *162*:327, 1968.

Gaillard, P. J., Talmage, R. V. and Budy, A. M. (eds.): *The Parathyroid Glands*. University of Chicago Press, Chicago, 1965.

Godwin, M. C.: The development of the parathyroids in the dog with emphasis upon the origin of accessory glands. Anat. Rec. *68*:305, 1937.

Nakagami, K., Yamazaki, Y. and Tsunoda, Y.: An electron microscopic study of the human fetal parathyroid gland. Z. Zellforsch. *85*:89, 1968.

Adrenal Glands

Bloodworth, J. M. B., Jr. and Powers, K. L.: The ultrastructure of the normal dog adrenal. J. Anat. *102*: 457, 1968.

Brenner, R. M.: Fine structure of adrenocortical cells in adult male rhesus monkeys. Amer. J. Anat. *119*: 429, 1966.

Elfvin, L. G.: The development of the secretory granules in the rat adrenal medulla. J. Ultrastruct. Res. *17*: 45, 1967.

Hopwood, D.: Adrenal medullary basophilia in ox, pig and sheep: A histochemical, immunohistochemical and cell fractionation study. Histochemie *11*:268, 1967.

Rhodin, J. A. G.: The ultrastructure of the adrenal cortex of the rat under normal and experimental conditions. J. Ultrastruct. Res. *34*:23, 1971.

Whitehead, R. H.: The histogenesis of the adrenal in the pig. Amer. J. Anat. *2*:349, 1903.

Wood, J. G.: Identification of and observations on epinephrine and norepinephrine containing cells in the adrenal medulla. Amer. J. Anat. *112*:285, 1963.

Endocrine Pancreas

Greider, M. H., Howell, S. L. and Lacy, P. E.: Isolation and properties of secretory granules from rat islets of Langerhans. J. Cell Biol. *41*:162, 1969.

Lacy, P. E.: Electron microscopy of the beta cells of the pancreas. Amer. J. Med. *31*:851, 1961.

Like, A. A.: The ultrastructure of the islets of Langerhans in man. Lab. Invest. *16*:937, 1967.

Machino, M.: On the substructure of secretory granules of the chick beta islet cell. J. Ultrastruct. Res. *31*: 199, 1970.

21 Male Reproductive System

General Characteristics

Form and Function. The male reproductive system consists of various organs which subserve a variety of functions. Most of the functions complement the primary function of reproduction. These include production and transportation of spermatozoa, contribution to semen by the secretory activity of numerous accessory glands, as well as the placement of semen in the female tract. The intermittent copulatory organ also functions in the transport of urine to the external environment. This system subserves an endocrine function also. The organs that comprise this system include *testes*, *epididymidis*, *deferent ducts*, *ampullary glands*, *vesicular glands*, *prostate gland*, *bulbourethral glands*, *urethral glands* and *penis*.

Testes and Associated Structures

General Remarks. These organs are contained within a specialized pouch of the skin, the *scrotum*, which contains the usual epidermal and dermal constituents, as well as smooth muscle (*tunica dartos*), fascia and peritoneum.

The testes are combined exocrine and endocrine organs. The exocrine portion is a compound, coiled tubular gland which produces cells, spermatozoa, as its secretory product. The endocrine portion is represented by the interstitial *cells of Leydig* and the sustentacular *cells of Sertoli*.

The testes are enclosed by a capsule, the *tunica albuginea*, which is composed of dense white fibrous connective tissue (DWFCT) (Fig. 21-1). This capsule is covered by mesothelium, the *visceral layer of the tunica vaginalis*, and is separated from the *parietal layer of the tunica vaginalis* by a portion of the peritoneal cavity. Both these membranes are typical serous membranes, but the areolar connective tissue of the visceral layer of the tunica vaginalis blends insensibly with the connective tissue of the tunica albuginea. The retroperitoneal development of the testes within the abdominal cavity and their subsequent migration to the scrotum accounts for the presence of serous membranes and coelomic space associated with the testes.

A *stratum vasculare*, or vascular layer, is present in the tunica albuginea of most species. It is superficial in the dog and ram, and it is deep in the stallion and boar. Smooth muscle fibers may be present in the tunica albuginea of the horse.

The tunica albuginea is continuous with the areolar connective tissue of the *mediastinum testis*, in most species, at the anterior pole of the testis (Fig. 21-1). It surrounds the *rete testis*. In the stallion, the mediastinum and rete testis are absent and are replaced by a vast interconnected network of connective tissue, vessels and ducts. The latter combine in the anterior pole and become confluent with the *ductuli efferentes*.

The tunica albuginea also gives rise to areolar connective tissue of the *septuli testis* (Fig. 21-1). These septa vary in thickness and completeness, extend from the tunica albuginea to the mediastinum testis and effectively divide the testis into lobules, called *lobuli testis*. The tubules of the lobule, *tubuli contorti* and *tubuli recti*, are surrounded by a delicate network of areolar connective tissue which contains numerous reticular fibers. The interstitial cells of Leydig are located within this connective tissue space.

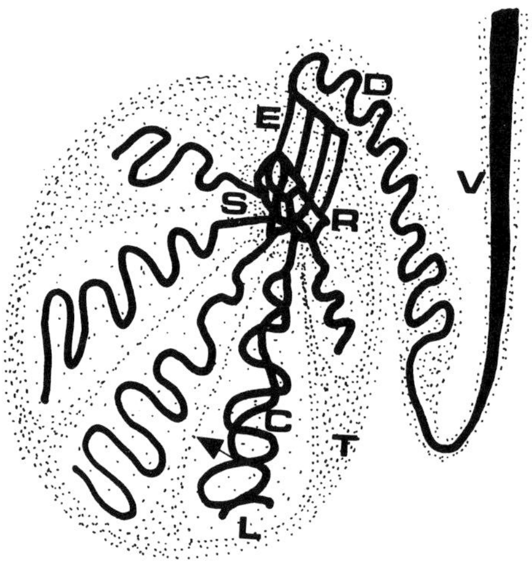

Fig. 21-1. Testis and associated. The testis is covered by the tunica albuginea (*T*). Septa (*arrow*) arise from it and divide the testis into lobules (*L*). The connective tissue is continuous with the mediastinum. The tubuli contorti (*C*) continue as tubuli recti (*S*). These continue through the mediastinum as the rete testis (*R*). Ductuli efferentes (*E*) connect the rete testis with the ductus epididymidis (*D*). The latter is continued as the ductus deferens (*V*). All light micrographs are the original magnifications.

Seminiferous Tubules. The parenchyma of the organ consists of the lining cells of the seminiferous tubules and their ducts, as well as the *cells of Leydig*.

The *seminiferous tubules* (*tubuli contorti*) are the exocrine portions of the gland (Fig. 21-2). They radiate from the mediastinum testis as coiled, tubular adenomeres. The tubules are lined by a stratified epithelium which consists of basal, intermediate and superficial zones (Fig. 21-3). The presence as well as the constituents of the zones is dependent upon the spermatogenic activity of the tubules. Although the epithelium is stratified, it is not similar to the stratified epithelia thus far encountered. The stratified cells consist of *spermatogonia*, *primary spermatocytes*, *secondary spermatocytes*, *spermatids*, and *spermatozoa*. The developmental sequence of these cells will be presented in a subsequent section on *spermatogenesis*.

The other parenchymatous components of the testes are the *Leydig cells* (Fig. 21-4). These cells are the endocrine portion of the testes and are responsible for the elaboration of *testosterone*. The cells, which are located in the connective tissue between the tubuli contorti, are polyhedral with a large spherical nucleus and a distinct nucleolus. Their acidophilic cytoplasm contains numerous lipid droplets and granules, but these are lost during routine processing. As a result, they are foamy (similar to the spongiocytes of the zona fasciculata of the adrenal cortex). These cells are especially abundant in the boar and the ox.

Tubuli Recti and Rete Testes. The seminiferous tubules are continuous with the *straight tubules* (*tubuli recti*) and the passages of the *rete testis* (Fig. 21-5). These areas are lined by a squamous, cuboidal or columnar epithelium. In the bull, the rete testis may be lined by a bistratified cuboidal epithelium. These two regions are similar to each other and are best identified by position within the testis. Whereas the tubuli recti are straight tubules, the rete testis consists of randomly anastomotic tubules

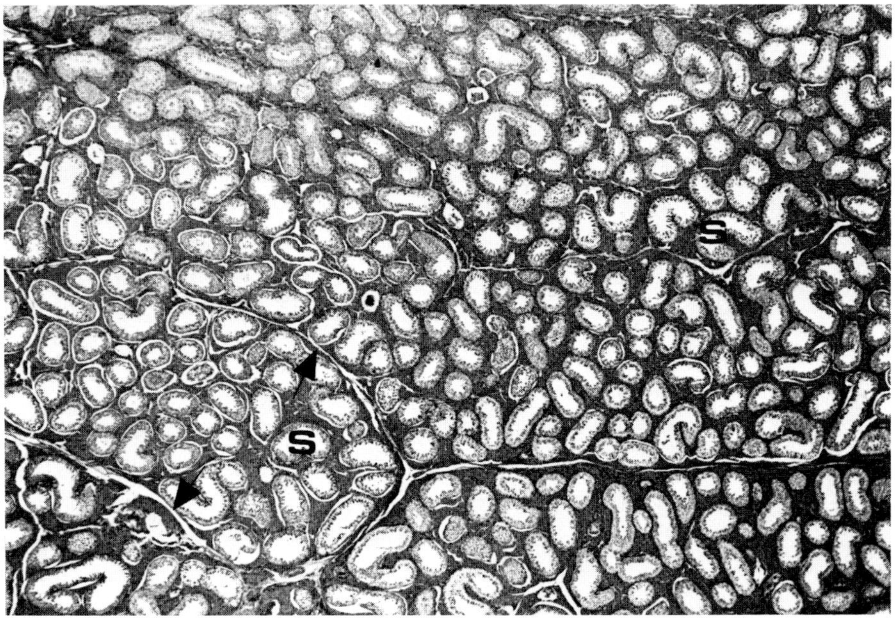

Fig. 21-2. Organization of the testis. The seminiferous tubules (*S*) are contained within lobules which are separated from one another by connective tissue septa (*arrows*). × 4.

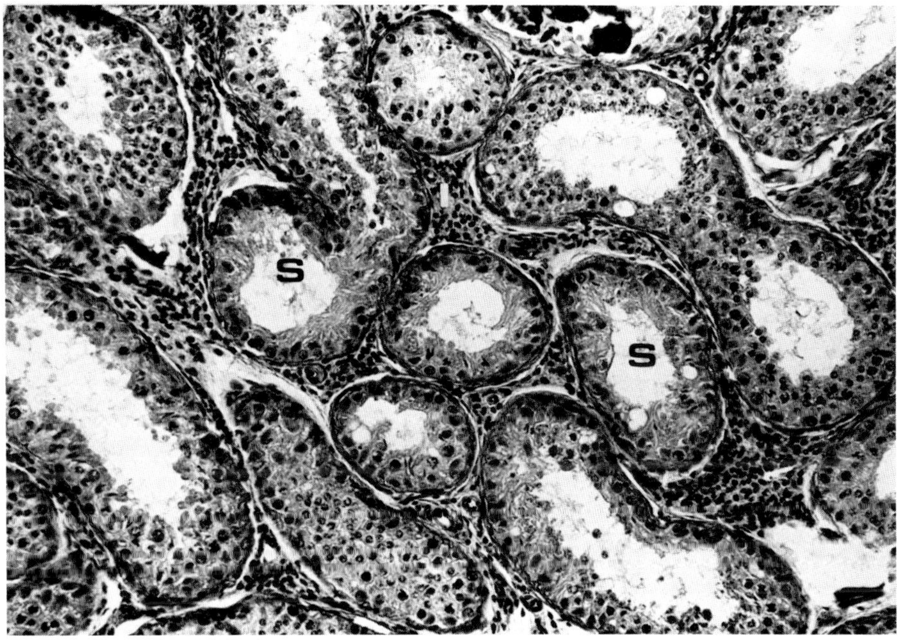

Fig. 21-3. Seminiferous tubules of a cervine testis. The seminiferous tubules (*S*) are separated by connective tissue and interstitial cells (*I*). ×40.

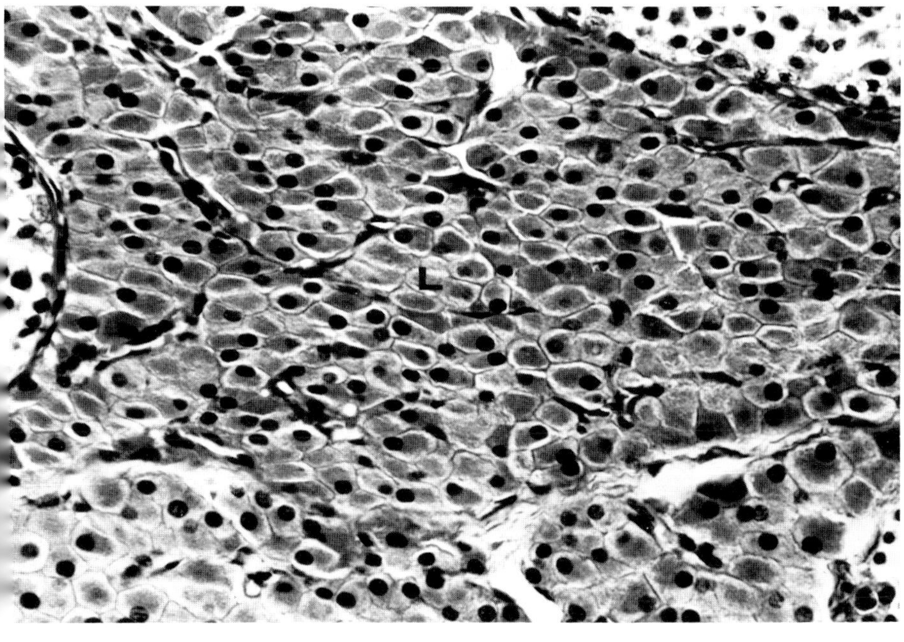

Fig. 21-4. Interstitial cells of the porcine testis. The Leydig cells (*L*) have an acidophilic and foamy cytoplasm. ×100.

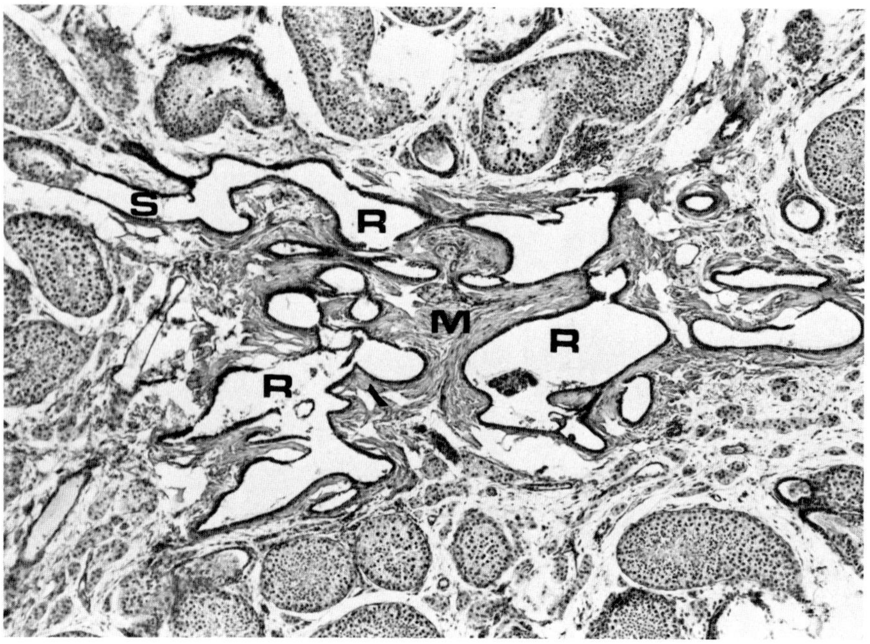

Fig. 21-5. Mediastinum testis. The mediastinum (*M*) contains the rete testis (*R*). Straight tubules (*S*) connect this region with the seminiferous tubules. ×10.

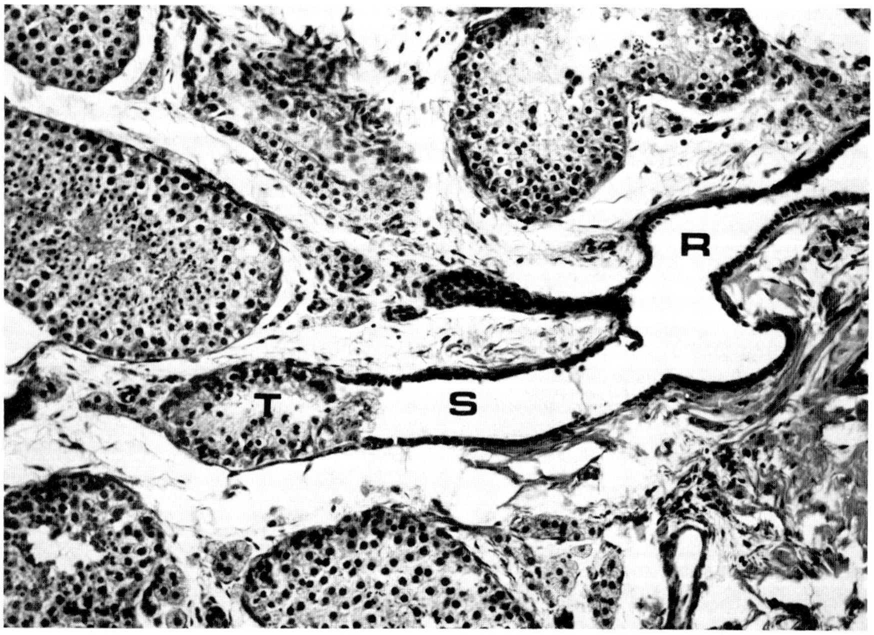

Fig. 21-6. Rete testis and tubuli recti. The tubuli contorti (*T*) are connected to the rete testis (*R*) by the tubuli recti (*S*). ×40.

(Fig. 21-6). In the boar, the apical borders of the lining cells may possess blebs which have been interpreted as apocrine secretory activity. Some believe that the lining cells of these regions actually represent a continuation of the Sertoli cell population of the tubuli contorti.

Ductuli Efferentes. The *ductuli efferentes* connect the rete testis with the ductus epididymidis (Fig. 21-7). The efferent ductules vary from 6 to 20 coiled ducts. These ductules, on the basis of their tortuous path and increasing diameter, are also referred to as *coni vasculosi*. They are lined by intermittently kinociliated columnar epithelium (Fig. 21-8). The current created by the movement of the cilia assists in the movement of spermatozoa toward the larger ducts. The nonciliated cells possess secretory blebs at their apical surface, but the significance of this secretory product is not understood. The surrounding lamina propria blends with the other connective tissue of the area and some smooth muscle cells are present. The widened and tightly convoluted portions of these tubules which connect with the ductus epididymidis constitute the head of the organ.

Ductus Epididymidis. This is the coiled tube which, with associated connective tissue and muscle, forms the *head*, *body* and *tail* of the epididymis (Fig. 21-9). The latter continues as the ductus deferens.

The lamina epithelialis consists of pseudostratified stereociliated columnar epithelium (Fig. 21-10). The basal cells contain lipid droplets, while the columnar cells are long and slender, contain lipids and have apical modifications in the form of stereocilia (Fig. 21-11). These processes are nonmotile and serve to increase the absorptive and/or secretory surface of the lining. They are usually heavily matted together by their secretory products. The nature and significance of these products is not known. The lamina propria consists of a highly vascularized areolar connective tissue. The lamina muscularis is arranged in a circular array and becomes thicker toward the tail of the epididymis. The tunica submucosa is areolar connective tissue centrally and DWFCT peripherally which is continuous with the tunica albuginea. Numerous spermatozoa are stored within the lumen of the ductus epididymidis during which time they mature.

Ductus Deferens. The ductus deferens is the continuation of the ductus epididymidis (Fig. 21-12). The lamina epithelialis consists of a pseudostratified columnar epithelium. There is, however, a gradual transition from the lining epithelium of the ductus epididymidis to that of the ductus deferens. The lamina propria-submucosa consists of areolar connective tissue. The tunica mucosa-submucosa is highly folded. The tunica muscularis is very thick and varies from two distinct inner and outer layers to inter-

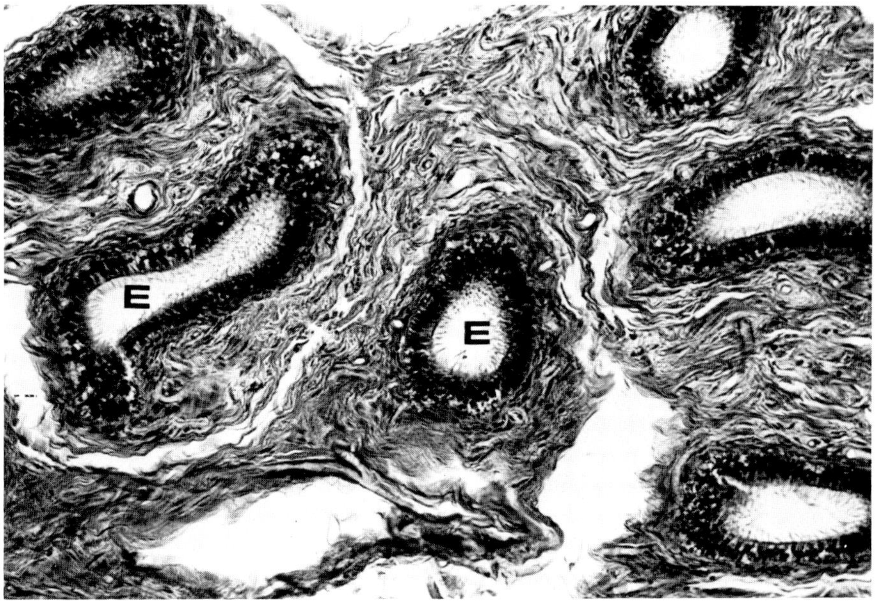

Fig. 21-7. Ductuli efferentes. These tubules (*E*) connect the rete testis to the ductus epididymidis. ×40.

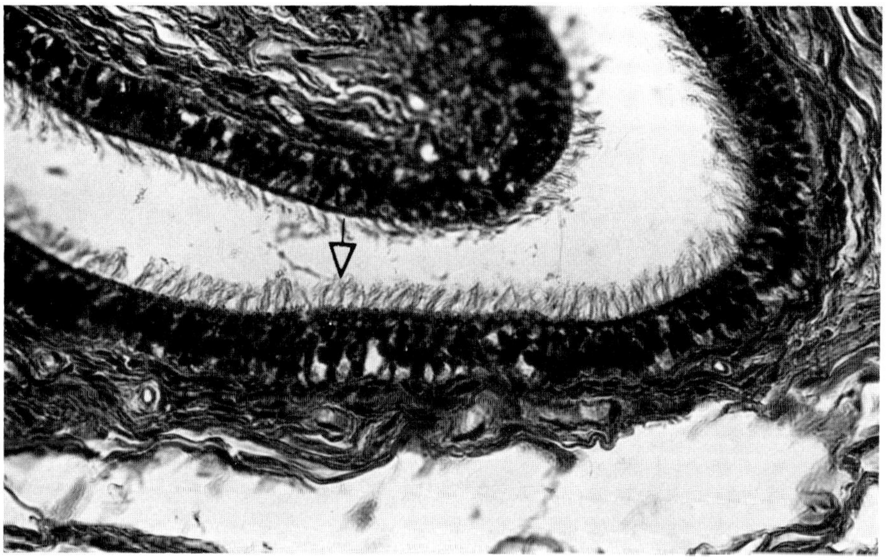

Fig. 21-8. Lining of the efferent ducts. The lining of these ducts is columnar epithelium which is kinociliated (*arrow*). ×100.

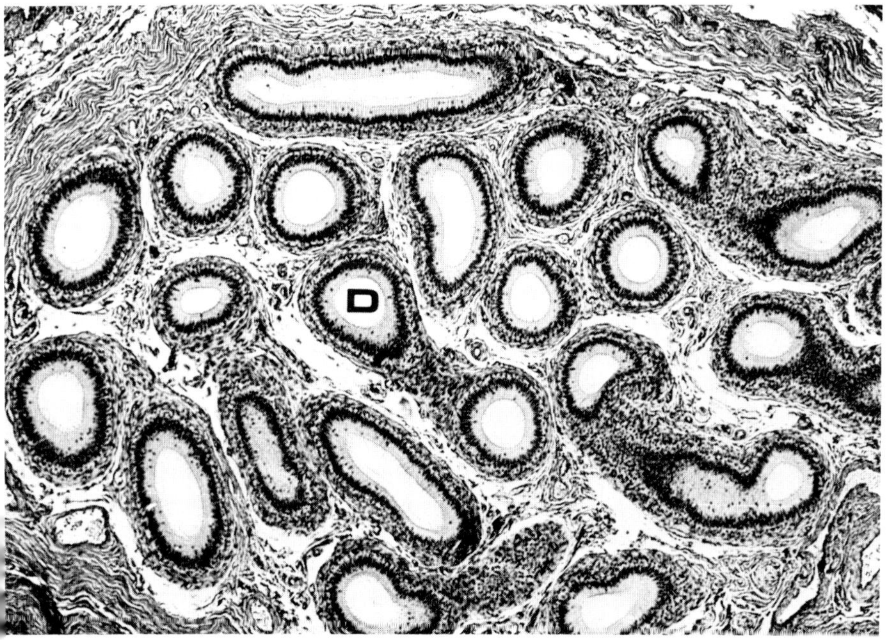

Fig. 21-9. Ductus epididymidis. This is a coiled tube (*D*) which partially forms the epididymis. ×20.

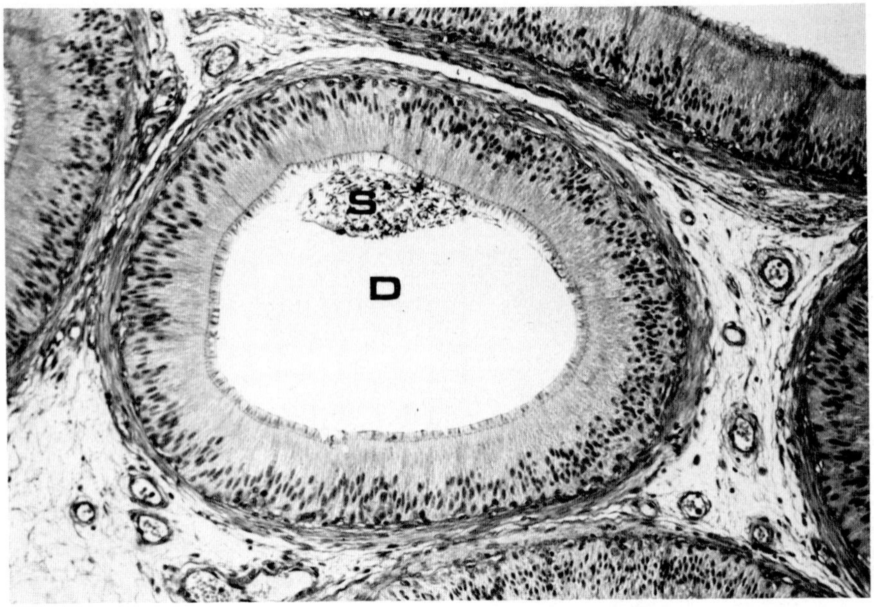

Fig. 21-10. Lining of the ductus epididymidis. The tubules (*D*) contain spermatozoa (*S*) and are lined by a pseudostratified stereociliated epithelium. ×10.

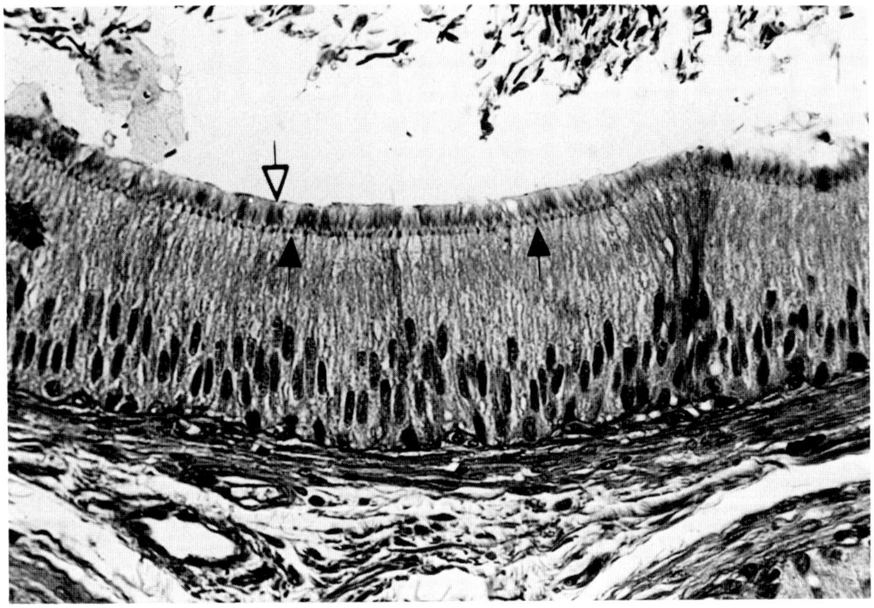

Fig. 21-11. Stereocilia of the ductus epididymidis. The pseudostratified epithelium is stereociliated (*open arrow*). Terminal bars (*solid arrows*) are apparent. ×100.

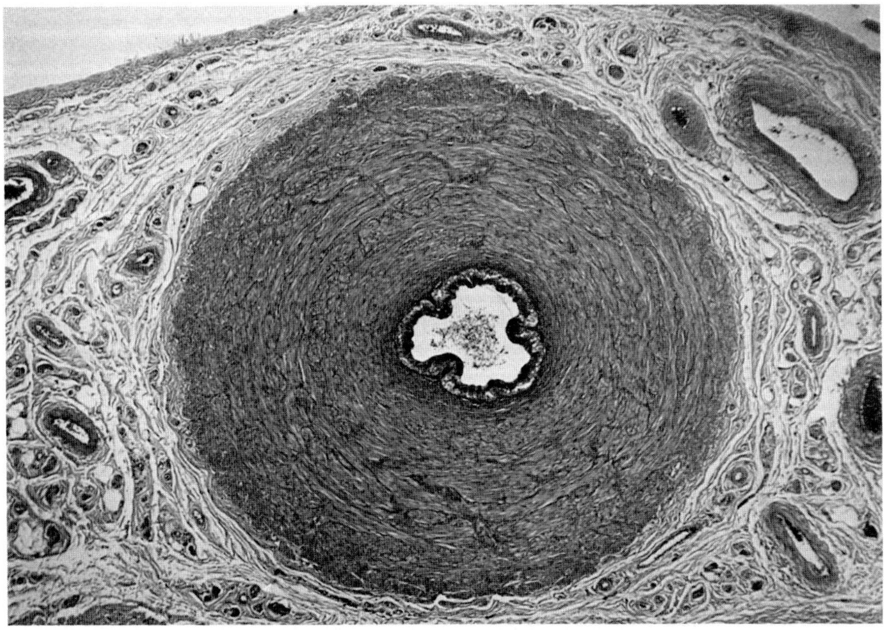

Fig. 21-12. Ductus deferens. This duct is a continuation of the ductus epididymidis. ×10.

mingled fibers. The tunica serosa is present and typical.

Spermatogenesis

General Remarks. *Spermatogenesis* occurs within the tubuli contorti and the ductus epididymidis. The former is responsible for the actual production of the male gametes, while the latter aids in their maturation process. The sequence of events involves a series of nuclear and cytoplasmic changes that result in haploid cells which are highly motile and suited to survive for short periods outside the body. The progression begins with *spermatogonia* and terminates with *spermatozoa*. These cells, with *Sertoli cells*, comprise the stratified seminiferous tubular lining. The most primitive cells are located near the periphery of the tubule (near the basement membrane), while the more advanced cells are located on the luminal border. In the case of the spermatozoa, they eventually occur within the lumina.

Three distinct periods are characteristic of the spermatogenic process: *mitotic*, *meiotic* and *metamorphic*. Not all seminiferous tubules will be in the same period of activity, nor will different portions of the same tubule possess cells with the same degree of differentiation. Although there are species variations, the spermatocytogenic process is described as occurring in helical waves down the tubule contorti to the straight tubules.

The *Sertoli cells* of these tubules function as sustentacular or nurse cells for the developing gametes (Fig. 21-13). These are columnar or tall triangular cells the cytoplasm of which is difficult to distinguish. The adjacent spermatogenic cells are encircled by cytoplasmic processes of the Sertoli cells. This encirclement reduces the concentrated mass of the cytoplasm. These cells, however, are readily identified by their nuclear morphology. The nucleus is positioned basally, vesicular and has a distinct nucleolus. The pyramidal nucleus has an invagination which is not usually visible with light microscopy.

The extensive contact of the Sertoli cell with the basal lamina implies that it is readily exposed to the extracellular fluid. The encirclement of the spermatogenic cells implies that this cell may function as a metabolic regulator. This relationship implies that they not only physically support the spermatogenic cells, but they may regulate the process of differentiation. These cells are also estrogenic. Also, Sertoli cell tumors are common in the dog. This type of tumor in any species may lead to the development of secondary female sex characteristics in the male.

Stage of Multiplication. The *stage of multiplication* or *mitotic stage* is characterized by an increase in the number of spermatogonia. Through successive mitotic divisions numerous spermatogonia undergo changes which result in spermatozoa—all derived from one cell. If one spermatogonium differentiated into subsequent cell types, then only four haploid gametes would be produced. As a result of the mitotic stage, the number of spermatogonia is increased greatly. Accordingly, the number of potential spermatozoa increases also. Just as importantly, however, not all spermatogonia differentiate. Some are retained as stem cells for future differentiation. If complete differentiation were to occur, it is obvious that the potential for gamete production would diminish rapidly and eventually terminate.

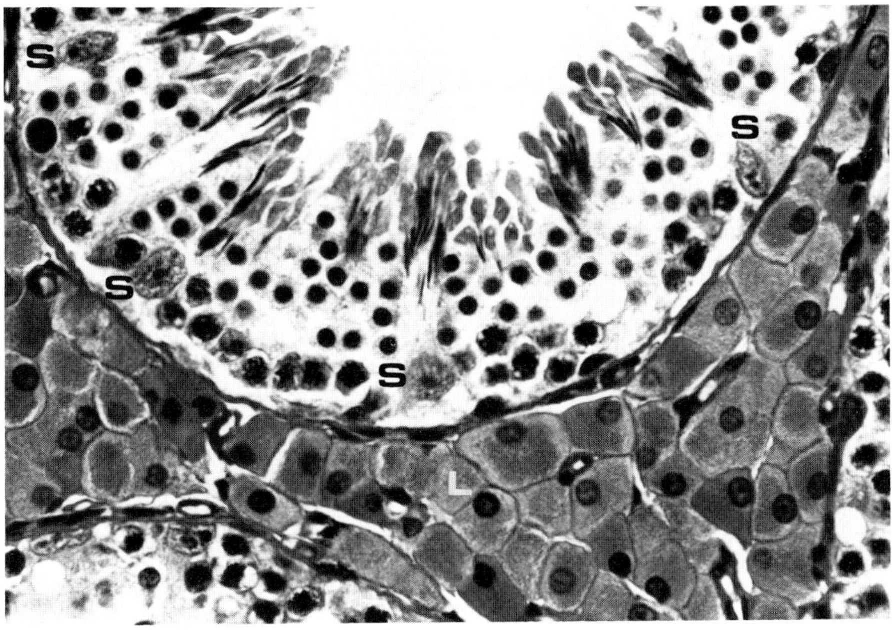

Fig. 21-13. Sertoli cells of the porcine testis. The Sertoli cells (*S*) are triangular cells with triangular nuclei which are positioned basally. The developing spermatozoa are intimately associated with these cells. Leydig cells (*L*) are visible. ×160.

Spermatogonia actually represent many generations of cells. These include: A cells, intermediate cells (I_1 and I_2), and B cells. The *A spermatogonia* are the stem cells for this process. The cell is round with a large, round nucleus which contains finely dispersed chromatin and an eccentrically positioned nucleolus. Upon mitotic division, one cell remains as a stem cell while the other divides and its progeny differentiate into *intermediate (I) spermatogonia*. I spermatogonia are oval with an oval nucleus. The nucleus contains peripheral coarsely clumped chromatin and two or three nucleoli. Subsequent divisions of intermediate spermatogonia give rise to *B spermatogonia*. These cells are round and small. The oval nucleus contains coarsely clumped chromatin. Subsequent division of these spermatogonia leads to the differentiation of *primary spermatocytes*. As many as eight primary spermatocytes may be derived from a single A spermatogonium. Incomplete cytokinesis is characteristic of the mitotic process that results in B spermatogonia.

Importantly, spermatogonia occur adjacent to the basement membrane, either singly or in clusters. They do not form a complete basal layer and may be difficult to find.

Spermatocytogenesis. This stage of the spermatogenic process involves the *spermatocytes*. These are the largest cells of the spermatogenic epithelium which comprise the intermediate zone. Type B spermatogonia differentiate into *primary spermatocytes*. These cells have rather long lifetimes (approximately 16 days in the bull) and usually are easy to find and identify. Although their interphase nuclei contain a fine chromatin network, they are often observed in the first division of meiosis. They also have a long premeiotic prophase. Therefore, the nucleus may be coarsely granulated or chromosomes may be visible.

The end of the first division of meiosis marks the differentiation of the *secondary spermatocytes*. These cells are still diploid (2N number of chromosomes). These cells are smaller than primary spermatocytes and are difficult to find. Their life-span varies from minutes to one hour. The division of these cells results in the formation of *spermatids*. Throughout these divisions cytokinesis is incomplete and the cells are joined by numerous intercellular bridges.

Spermiogenesis. The *spermatids* that result from the division of the secondary spermatocytes are haploid (1N number of chromosomes). These cells, spermatids, comprise the most developed, most numerous and largest layer of the seminiferous tubular epithelium. This luminal zone is referred to as the *zone of metamorphosis*. The process by which spermatids are converted to spermatozoa is referred to as *metamorphosis* or *spermiogenesis*. As spermatogenesis ensues the spermatids move in a centrifugal direction (toward the basement membrane) then in a centripetal direction toward the lumen.

The primary organelles involved in the spermiogenic process are the nucleus, Golgi apparatus and centrioles (Fig. 21-14).

Small granules (*proacrosomal granules*) appear in the vesicles of the Golgi apparatus. These small vesicles coalesce to form a single large *acrosomal vesicle* which contains the *acrosome*. The acrosome results from a coalescence of proacrosomal vesicles. The acrosomal vesicle migrates to the nucleus and contacts the outer nuclear membrane at the acrosome.

The acrosomal vesicle enlarges and extends itself over half the nucleus and collapses to form the *head cap*. At the same time, the centrioles migrate to the periphery of the cell in a position opposite the acrosome. Residual Golgi apparatus also migrates to this general region.

The acrosome becomes indistinguishable from the head cap. The nucleus becomes dense and begins to elongate. At this time, the centrioles and developing *flagellum* migrate toward and come in contact with the nuclear membrane. A *caudal sheath* or *manchette* develops at the caudal edge of the head cap. This sheath is composed of microtubules. At the same time, the spermatid elongates.

A small dense ring condenses around the proximal centriole. This *annulus* is attached to the inner lamina of the plasmalemma. It slides down the flagellum. At the same time, the mitochondria orient themselves in a helical pattern between the proximal centriole and the annulus. Nine longitudinal fibers develop in a position between the flagellar doublets and the mitochondria. This structure comprises the *middle piece*.

The *principal piece* is composed of a flagellar core, dense fibers and a fibrous sheath.

The irregularly arranged flagellar microtubules comprise the *endpiece*.

As the formation of these entities occurs, the remaining cytoplasm is displaced distad along the tail and eventually lost as the *residual body*.

The mature spermatozoon, therefore, consists of the following: *head, neck, middle piece, principal piece* and *endpiece* (Fig. 21-15). The *head* is covered by the head cap on the rostral and lateral surface and the calyx on the lateral and caudal surface. The *neck* has a depression (fossa) in which the centriole is located. Longitudinally segmented columns connect the head to the tail. The *middle piece* consists of a flagellar core in a 9 + 2 arrangement, fibers which are continuous with those of the neck, a helical arrangement of mitochondria and an annulus which is attached to the plasmalemma. The *principal piece* contains a flagellar core in a 9 + 2 arrangement, fibers of various sizes that end in this segment and a fibrous sheath. The *endpiece* consists of a flagellar 9 + 2 core that terminates in a random fashion. Naturally, the entire spermatozoon is enclosed with a plasmalemma.

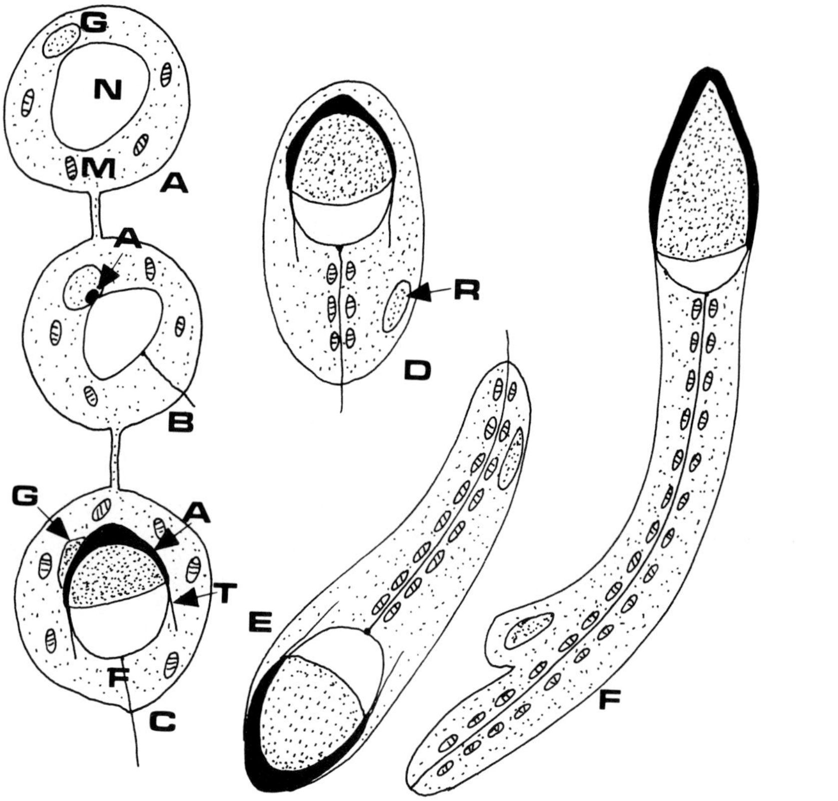

Fig. 21-14. Progressive development of spermatids (external *A* to *F*). *G*, Golgi apparatus; *N*, nucleus; *M*, mitochondria; *A*, acrosome; *T*, caudal tube; *R*, residual Golgi apparatus; *F*, flagellum. (Redrawn and modified from Clermont, Y. and Leblond, C. P.: Amer. J. Anat. *96*:229, 1955.)

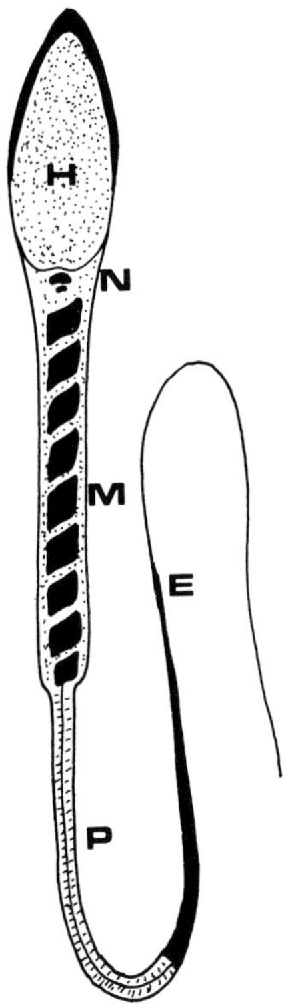

Fig. 21-15. The structure of a mature spermatozoon. *H*, head; *N*, neck; *M*, middle piece; *P*, principal piece; *E*, endpiece.

Spermatogenic Cycle. As mentioned previously, not all seminiferous tubules or regions of the same tubule are in the same stage of development (Fig. 21-16). The activity is cyclic, may occur in a helical pattern within a seminiferous tubule and is referred to as a *spermatogenic wave*. Various combinations of cells are always associated with each other during the developmental process. In the bull, for example, eight stages have been identified. Stage 1, from basal to luminal border would include the following: *spermatogonia, pachytene primary spermatocytes* and *round spermatids*. Stage 8, however, would include: *spermatogonia, zygotene primary spermatocytes, secondary spermatocytes, round spermatids* and *spermatozoa*. The six re-

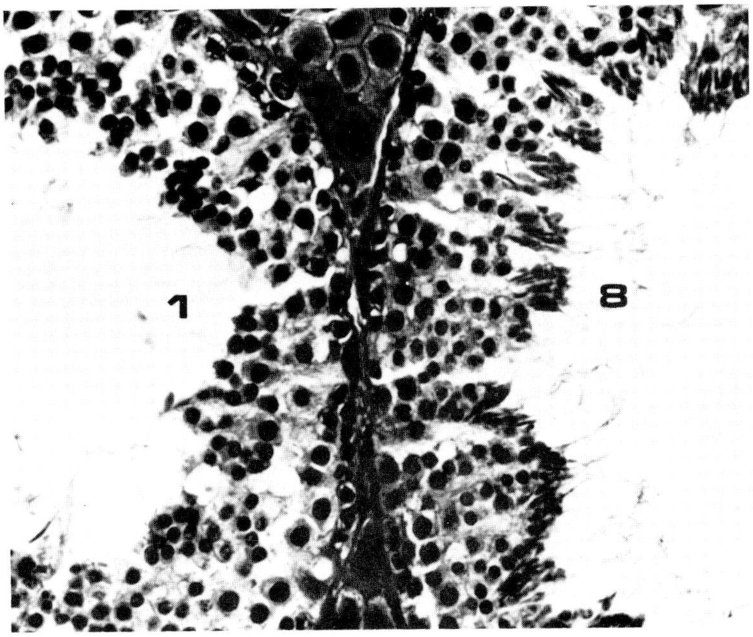

Fig. 21-16. Different developmental stages in adjacent tubules. Stages 1 and 8 represent different degrees of development of spermatozoa. ×100.

maining stages would involve other permutations of the basic cell types. Various stages, the number of stages, as well as the overall duration of the stages are species variable. The *spermatogenic wave* or *cycle*, therefore, is the sequence of cellular events that occur between two successive identical stages.

In some species, from a spermatogenic point of view, the male is always capable of spermiation; i.e., the ejection of viable sperm from the testes. In seasonal breeders, the epithelium of the seminiferous tubules is incapable of producing spermatozoa except during specific periods of the year, the breeding season (Fig. 21-3). Examination of tubuli contorti during the nonbreeding season would reveal the presence of scattered spermatogonia and Sertoli cells. Few other tubules would be present. Also, the tubules would be involuted and replaced by connective tissue.

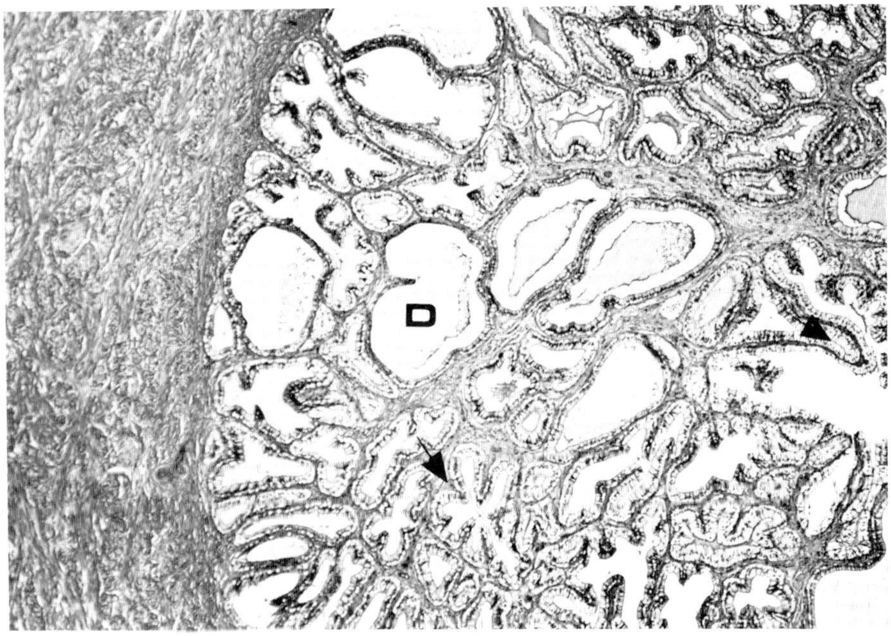

Fig. 21-17. Bovine ampullary glands. These are branched (*arrows*), tubular glands with saclike dilations (*D*). ×10.

Accessory Glands

General Remarks. The accessory genital glands of the male include *ampullary glands*, *vesicular glands*, *prostate gland*, *bulbourethral glands* and *urethral glands*. They elaborate serous and mucous excretory products that subserve various functions. Together these secretory products may serve to nourish the spermatozoa, activate the spermatozoa, clear the urethral tract prior to ejaculation, serve as a vehicle for the transport of the spermatozoa within the female tract, as well as plugging the female organs to help ensure fertilization.

All of the glands are generally described as branched tubular or branched tubuloalveolar glands which are arranged into lobular units. Each lobular unit may drain into a dilated collecting sinus. These sinuses are not present in all the glands of all species, however. They are absent in equine vesicular glands and in porcine and ruminant pars disseminata prostatica. The glandular epithelium and that of the collecting sinus (when present) consist of a simple columnar lining which is continuous with the pseudostratified or transitional epithelium of the excretory ducts. The glands of a given species may be readily distinguished from one another, but extreme care must be taken when making interspecific comparisons. There is much variation among the domestic species.

Ampullary Glands. The *ampulla* is an enlargement of the terminal portion of the ductus deferens. This enlargement is not present in the tom and boar. Whether or not this portion is enlarged, glands are usually present. They are, however, absent in the tom and minimally developed in the boar. They are present in the canine ampullae and are best developed in the bull and stallion.

The glands are branched, tubular structures with saclike dilations (Fig. 21-17).

Some authors describe them as branched tubuloalveolar glands. These glands are lined by a simple columnar epithelium (Fig. 21-18). In the bull, basal accumulations of lipid droplets may be apparent. There is no special excretory duct system.

The ampullary glands elaborate a white serous fluid product by the merocrine method. Its function, however, is not known, but the product is similar to the secretory product of the vesicular glands.

Vesicular Glands. The *vesicular glands* are also referred to as the *seminal vesicles* (Fig. 21-19). The glands are absent in carnivores. They are truly vesicular outpocketings in the stallion and compact organs in the bull and boar.

The glandular epithelium is simple columnar (Fig. 21-20). Infranuclear lipid droplets may be apparent in the bull. The main excretory ducts are lined by a stratified columnar epithelium. The overall configuration of the gland is that of a pinnately arranged structure; i.e., a central duct is present from which radially branching secretory endpieces emanate. Lobular subdivisions are present.

The lamina propria-submucosa consists of areolar connective tissue. The tunica muscularis may consist of inner circular and outer longitudinal layers or may be entirely intermingled. A tunica adventitia or a tunica serosa may be present. They are typical.

Seminal fluid, as well as the products of other glands, may provide a vehicle for transport of the spermatozoa. In some rodents, this gelatinous secretory product aids in the formation of the vaginal plug. The secretory product contains high quantities of fructose. Of the 60 to 90% of the fluid volume of semen that comes from the accessory glands, the vesicular glands account for a major portion of it. The precise function of these glands, however, is not known.

Prostate Gland. This organ consists of two parts, the *corpus prostatae* and *pars disseminata*. These regions, however, are not equally developed in all species. The body of the prostate, which is located peripheral to and completely surrounds the pelvic urethra, is particularly well-developed in carnivores and the stallion. The disseminate portion is better developed than the body in the bull and boar, while there is no distinct body in the ram.

The gland is a compound tubuloalveolar structure which is lined by secretory cells in a cuboidal or low columnar configuration (Figs. 21-21 and 21-22). Secretory cells have apical blebs which indicate an apocrine-type secretory activity. Acidophilic granules and lipid droplets may be present. The duct system, initially lined by a cuboidal or columnar epithelium, is lined by transitional epithelium at the entrance to the urethra.

The body of the gland is surrounded by a capsule of DWFCT which is continuous

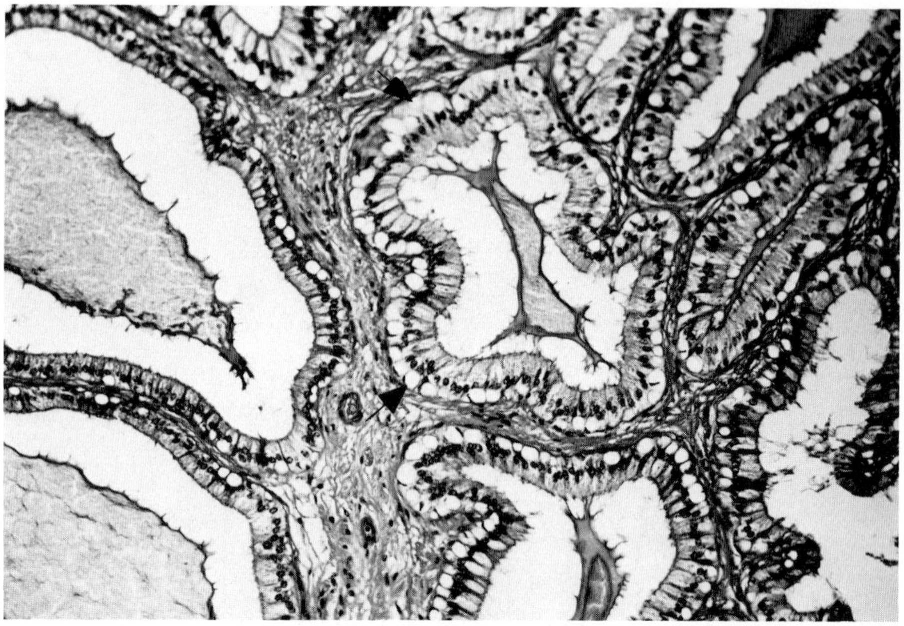

Fig. 21-18. Lining of bovine ampullary gland. Columnar epithelium contains basal lipid deposits (*arrows*). ×40.

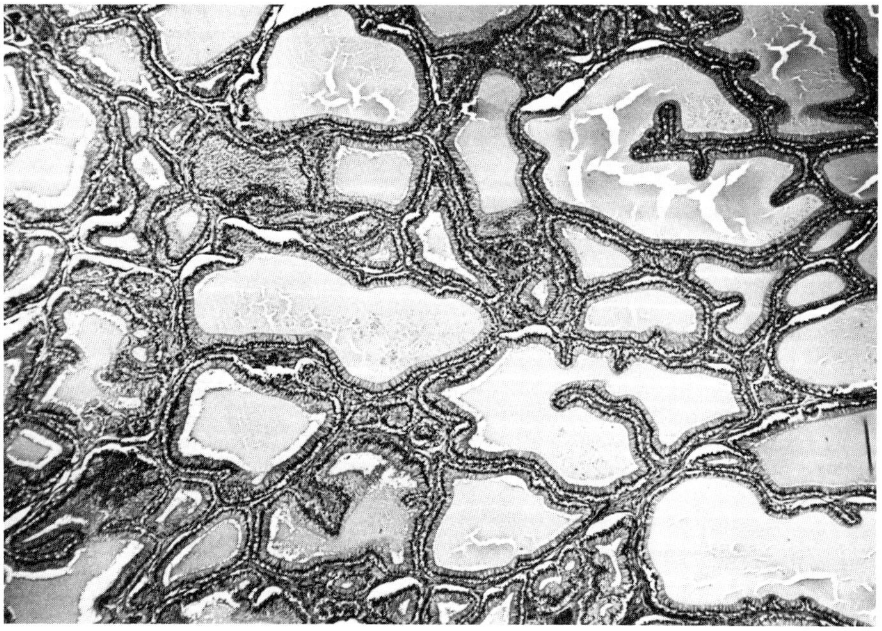

Fig. 21-19. Bovine seminal vesicle. ×10.

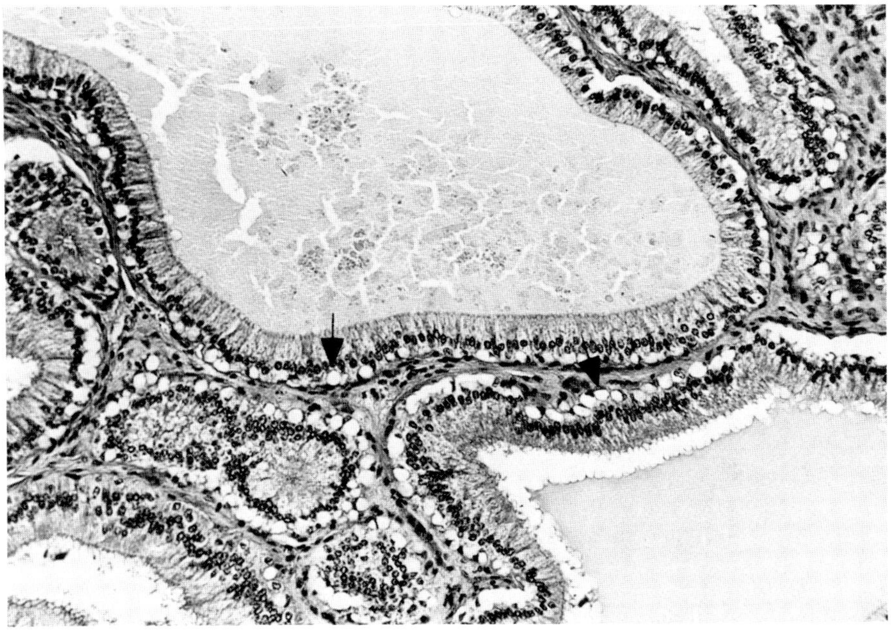

Fig. 21-20. Lining of the bovine seminal vesicle. The columnar cells have infranuclear lipid deposits (*arrows*). ×40.

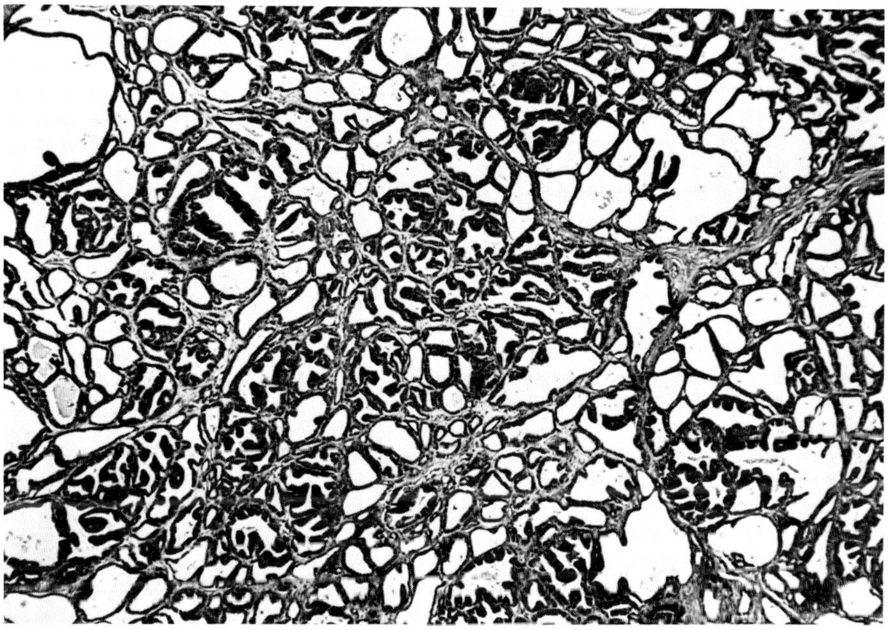

Fig. 21-21. Canine prostate gland. ×10.

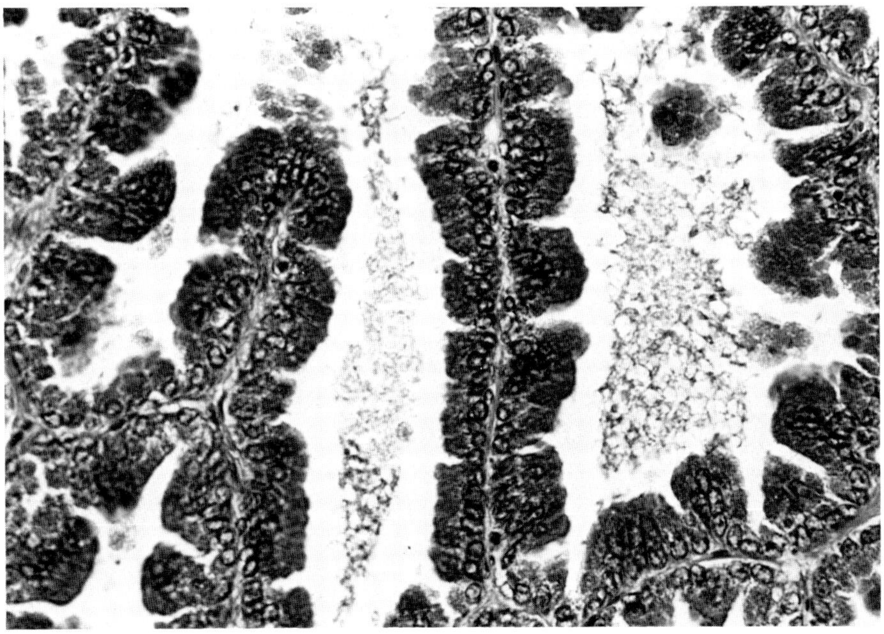

Fig. 21-22. Lining of the canine prostate gland. The lining epithelium is columnar. ×100.

with the areolar connective tissue of the lamina propria-submucosa in which the adenomeres are located. The disseminate portion is surrounded by the areolar connective tissue of the lamina propria-submucosa.

The pars disseminata is best developed along the dorsal surface of the urethra and extends laterad and ventrad to totally encompass the urethra. The disseminate portion is continuous with both laterally oriented lobes of the body of the gland. Although the disseminate portion is usually confined to the pelvic urethra, *it is not unusual to find isolated portions of the gland in the wall of the penile urethra.*

The gland is basically a serous gland with occasional mucous endpieces. Concretions of these secretory products may be found in the alveoli and duct system. Its secretory activity is known to increase the motility of spermatozoa, as well as contribute to the formation of the vaginal plug. In the bull, the secretory fluid contains high quantities of fructose and citric acid. Little else is known of the functional significance of this secretory product.

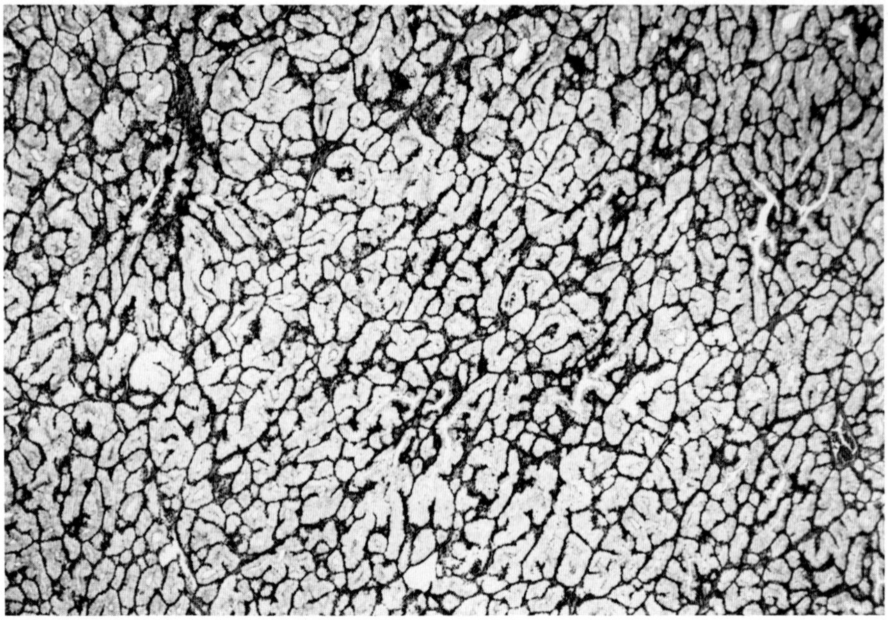

Fig. 21-23. Bovine bulbourethral gland. ×10.

Bulbourethral Glands. These glands are also referred to as *Cowper's glands*. These glands are paired structures which are located dorsolateral from the pelvic urethra. They are not present in the dog. The bulbourethral glands are compound tubuloalveolar glands (Fig. 21-23). The lining cells of the adenomeres are columnar or pyramidal (Fig. 21-24). They have a basophilic cytoplasm and a basally displaced nucleus which is rounded or flattened. The duct system is lined by columnar, pseudostratified or transitional epithelium.

The capsule of the organ is DWFCT which may contain some smooth muscle. Striated muscle from the bulbocavernosus and urethralis muscle is associated with the capsule. The capsular connective tissue is continuous as septal components (areolar connective tissue) of the lamina propria-submucosa. Diffuse and nodular lymphatic tissue is commonly encountered.

The mucus secreted by these glands serves to clear the urethra of urine and to lubricate the urethra and vagina with a preejaculatory fluid.

Urethra

General Remarks. The male urethra is the continuation of the duct system which arises at the urinary bladder and opens to the outside. It serves the dual function of transporting urine as well as semen and spermatozoa. Secretory products involved in reproduction gain access to the pelvic urethra at the *colliculus seminalis* which is the apex of the *urethral crest*. It is in this region that the *deferent ducts*, *vesicular glands* and some *prostatic ducts* gain access to the urethra. The urethra is divided into *pelvic* and *penile portions* which contain erectile tissue along

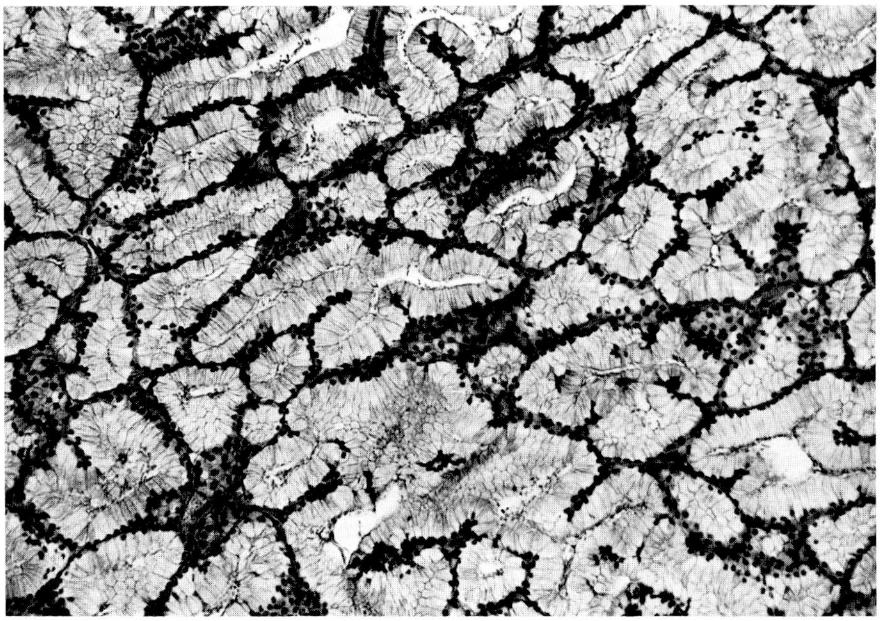

Fig. 21-24. Lining of the bovine bulbourethral gland. The lining cells are columnar and basophilic. Nuclei are positioned basally. ×40.

the entire length. The urethra also contains branched tubular mucous glands, *glands of Littré* or *urethral glands*, along its length. The occurrence and distribution of these glands, however, is species-variable. They are obliquely oriented and are especially numerous along the dorsal surface of the urethra.

Pelvic Urethra. The pelvic urethra is lined by a transitional epithelium. The surrounding lamina propria-submucosa consists of areolar connective tissue, numerous glandular elements and erectile tissue (*stratum cavernosum*). A tunica muscularis with three muscle layers is present in the neck of the bladder, but these are rapidly replaced by a striated *urethral muscle*. However, an inner and outer layer (superficial and deep to the musculus urethralis) may be present throughout the extent of the pelvic urethra. A tunica adventitia is present. This portion of the urethra generally has more glands but less erectile tissue than the penile urethra.

Penile Urethra. The penile urethra is lined by a transitional epithelium as well (Fig. 21-25). This, however, may change to stratified squamous epithelium prior to or at the urethral opening in some species. Glands may be present in the lamina propria-submucosa, especially in the stallion and boar. The tunica muscularis returns to being composed of smooth muscle. Cavernous tissue (*corpus cavernosum urethrae*) is also present in the subepithelial connective tissue space.

Copulatory Organ

Penis. The penis is the organ that serves as the common outlet for urine and the copulatory ejaculate (semen and spermatozoa). It is, therefore, a part of the urinary system as well as serving as an intermittent copulatory organ.

Although the histological components of the penis are similar among most mammalian species, the organizational differences are too numerous to be able to cite a configuration as being absolutely typical. Moreover, a section from one part of this structure may differ appreciably from a section through a different part. This variability is due to the differential distribution of some component parts along the length of the organ.

The following description applies to the general configuration and component parts. The penis is divided into: *roots*, *body*, and *glans*. The structure of each root and the body of the penis are similar. The body consists of a capsule, erectile tissue (*corpora cavernosa penis*, *corpus cavernosum urethrae* or *corpus spongiosum*), smooth muscle (*retractor penis muscle*), skeletal muscle (*bulbocavernosus muscle*) and urethra (Fig. 21-26).

The body of the penis is enclosed by the DWFCT of the tunica albuginea which is

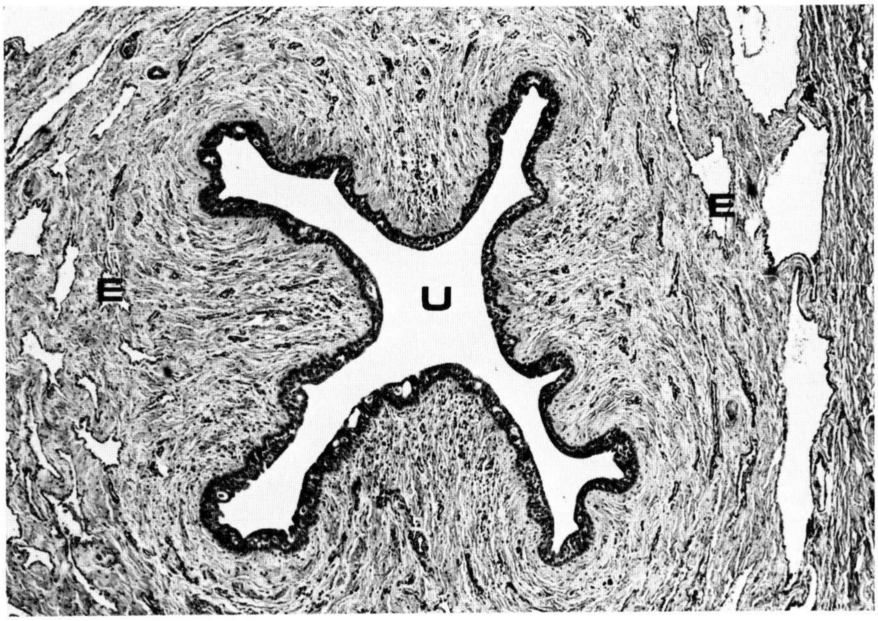

Fig. 21-25. Canine penile urethra. The urethra (*U*) is lined by transitional epithelium. Erectile tissue (*E*) is peripheral to the lumen of the urethra. ×16.

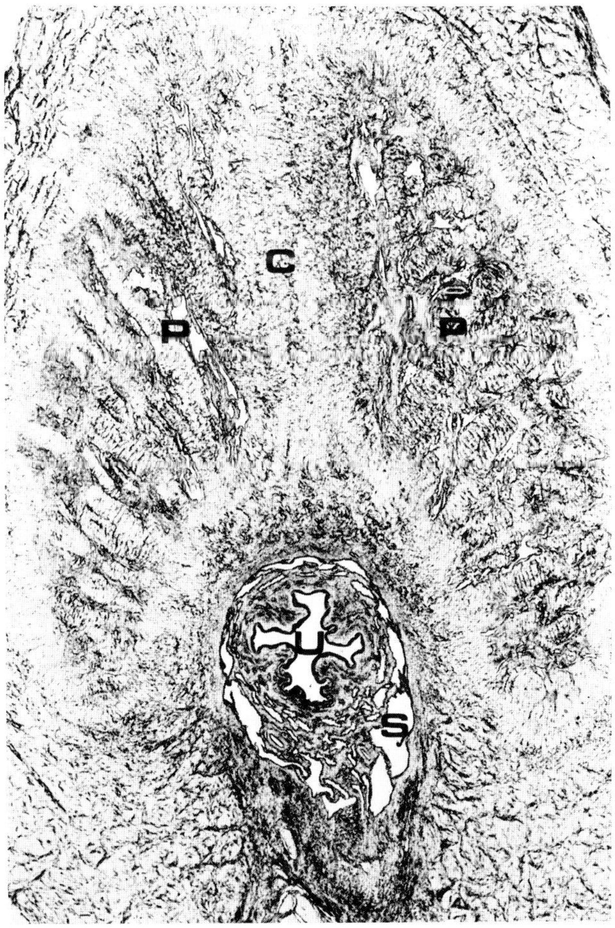

Fig. 21-26. Section through the canine penis. The urethra (*U*) is surrounded by erectile tissue of the corpus spongiosum (*S*). Dorsally, the two corpora cavernosa penis (*P*) are separated by connective tissue (*C*) continuous with the tunica albuginea. ×4.

especially well-developed in those species with a fibrous-type penis (boar, carnivores, ruminants). Connective tissue septa originate from the capsule and continue as the fibrous coverings of the erectile tissue components. These components may include elastic fibers and smooth muscle.

The erectile tissue consists of DWFCT rich in elastic fibers and sinuses. These are capable of being engorged with blood during erection. In the vascular-type penis (horse, man), this erectile tissue is well-developed.

The glans penis is well-developed in primates, the stallion and the dog. It is covered by the penile portion of the prepuce, which is actually a reflection of the integument. The reflected portion is, therefore, a mucous membrane. The glans penis may contain erectile tissue (vascular type), bone (*os penis* of carnivores), cartilage and DWFCT (bull). The bulk of this portion of the penis consists of highly vascularized areolar connective tissue.

The free portion of the penis is covered by stratified squamous epithelium.

Erectile Mechanism. The primary blood supply of the penis, under erotic stimulation, is directed through *helicine arteries* which open into the cavernous tissue. These vessels, as well as the cavernous tissue, become engorged with blood. The peripherally located, thin-walled veins are occluded against the tunica albuginea. This further enhances rigidity. The cavernous tissue of the corpus spongiosum (corpus cavernosum urethrae) is not as thickly encapsulated as the other cavernous tissue. This permits expansion without occluding the urethra.

During the period of *detumescence*, the helicine arteries contract and regain their initial tone. The resulting diminution of blood supply results in a decreased pressure against the compressed veins. The blood is gradually removed from the erectile tissue and normal blood flow through the penis is resumed.

References

Testes and Associated

Belt, W. D. and Cavazos, L. F.: Fine structure of the interstitial cells of Leydig in the boar. Anat. Rec. *158:* 333, 1967.

Christensen, A. K. and Fawcett, D. W.: The fine structure of the interstitial cells of the mouse testis. Amer. J. Anat. *118:*551, 1963.

Elftman, H.: Sertoli cells and testis structure. Amer. J. Anat. *113:*25, 1963.

Fawcett, D. W. and Burgos, M. H.: Studies on the fine structure of the mammalian testes. II. The human interstitial tissue. Amer. J. Anat. *107:*245, 1960.

Kretser, D. M. D.: The fine structure of the testicular interstitial cells in men of normal androgenic status. Z. Zellforsch. *80:*594, 1967.

Ladman, A. J.: The fine structure of the ductuli efferentes of the opossum. Anat. Rec. *157:*559, 1967.

Spermatocytogenesis

Clermont, Y.: The cycle of the seminiferous epithelium in man. Amer. J. Anat. *112:*35, 1963.

Goldzvieg, S. A. and Smith, A. U.: The fertility of male rats after moderate and after severe hypothermia. J. Endocr. *14:*40, 1956.

Heller, C. G. and Clermont, Y.: Kinetics of the germinal epithelium in man. Recent Progr. Hormone Res. *20:* 545, 1964.

Kehlstrom, J. E.: A sex cycle in the male. Experientia *22:* 630, 1966.

Rattner, J. B. and Brinkley, B. R.: Ultrastructure of spermiogenesis. J. Ultrastruct. Res. *32:*316, 1970.

Roosen-Runge, E. C.: The process of spermatogenesis in mammals. Biol. Rev. *37:*343, 1962.

Swiestra, E. E. and Foote, R. H.: Duration of spermatogenesis and spermatozoan transport in the rabbit based on cytological changes, DNA synthesis and labeling with tritiated thymidine. Amer. J. Anat. *116:*401, 1965.

Accessory Glands

Bharadwaj, M. and Calhoun, M. L.: Histology of the bulbourethral gland of the domestic animals. Anat. Rec. *142:*216, 1962.

Brandes, D.: The fine structure and histochemistry of prostatic glands in relation to sex hormones. Int. Rev. Cytol. *20:*207, 1966.

Fisher, E. R. and Jeffrey, W.: Ultrastructure of human normal and neoplastic prostate. Amer. J. Clin. Path. *44:*119, 1965.

Hirsch, E. W.: Comparative anatomy of prostate gland. J. Urol. *25:*669, 1931.

Kainer, R. A., Faulkner, L. C. and Abdel-Raouf, M.: Gland associated with the urethra of the bull. Amer. J. Vet. Res. *30:*963, 1969.

McDonald, L. E.: *Veterinary Endocrinology and Reproduction.* Lea and Febiger, Philadelphia, 1969.

Riva, A.: Fine structure of human seminal vesicle epithelium. J. Anat. *102:*71, 1967.

Young, W. C. (ed.): *Sex and Internal Secretions.* Williams & Wilkins, Baltimore, 1961.

Penis and Associated

Bharadwaj, M. and Calhoun, M. L: The histology of the urethral epithelium of domestic animals. Amer. J. Vet. Res. *20:*841, 1959.

Bharadwaj, M. B. and Calhoun, M. L.: Mode of formation of the preputial cavity in domestic animals. Amer. J. Vet. Res. *22:*764, 1961.

Hart, B. J. and Kitchell, R. L.: External morphology of the erect glans penis of the dog. Anat. Rec. *152:*193, 1965.

22 Female Reproductive System

General Characteristics

Form and Function. The female reproductive system includes, as its male counterpart, various organs that contribute directly to or complement the primary function of reproduction. Among the varied functions are *production* of ova, *transport* of male and female gametes for fertilization, *accommodation* and *nourishment* of the developing organism, *parturition* at the appropriate time and *secretion* of hormones. Portions of the system also complement the function of the urinary system. The organs of this system include *ovary*, *oviduct*, *uterus*, *vagina* and *vulva*. Although the mammary gland was included with the integument, this gland is also considered part of the reproductive system.

Cyclic activity is an integral part of female reproductive organs. These changes are much more pronounced in the female and have an effect on more organs than in the male. These changes are especially notable in the ovaries, oviducts and uterus throughout the estrous cycle as well as during pregnancy. A general structural organization of these organs will be presented. The structures will be subsequently related to the various stages of the estrous cycle.

Ovary

General Remarks. The ovaries are paired structures which are the female counterparts of the testes. The ovary performs an endocrine as well as an exocrine function. The former involves the production of estrogen and progesterone, while the latter is concerned with the production of the *female gametes*, the *ova*.

The ovary is covered by a *surface epithelium* which is a modification of the visceral peritoneal covering of the ovary and is continuous with the *mesovarium*. During early developmental stages of the ovary and oogenesis, the epithelium is cuboidal. It changes with age to a squamous lining. Underlying the germinal epithelium is a capsule of dense white fibrous connective tissue (DWFCT) which may have a lamellar configuration—the *tunica albuginea ovarii*. It is similar to the male counterpart, but it is thinner than that associated with the testis.

The ovaries of most animals, the mare excepted, consist of two distinct zones: an outer *cortex* or *zona parenchymatosa* and the inner *medulla* or *zona vasculosa* (Fig. 22-1).

The cortex contains numerous *follicles* in various stages of development, *corpora lutea* as well as interstitial cells and stromal elements. Although the connective tissue fibers of the tunica albuginea are continuous with the stromal connective tissue, the connective tissue of the cortex must be considered a specialized tissue. Various cells typical of areolar connective tissue are present. However, this tissue is very cellular and dense aggregates of "fibroblasts" are present. They may be parallel to the surface or in an orderly arrangement around the follicles or vessels with which they are associated. The "fibroblasts" of this region are not ordinary fibroblasts. They are extremely adaptive and pleomorphic. They are readily converted to macrophages and even assume epithelioid characteristics as follicular sheath cells in association with developing follicles. In the latter instance, they perform a nutritive and secretory function. These epithelioid cells are readily converted back to stromal "fibroblasts."

The ovarian cortex is the target organ for some trophic hormones of the pars distalis [follicle-stimulating hormone (FSH), leuteinizing hormone (LH)]. The production of ovarian hormones in response to these trophic hormones is responsible for the cyclic activity of the ovary. This includes differentiation of ova, development and atresia of follicles, ovulation and formation and degeneration of corpora lutea.

The *medulla* is characterized by large vessels, lymphatics, nerves and some embryonic remnants. It is an areolar connective

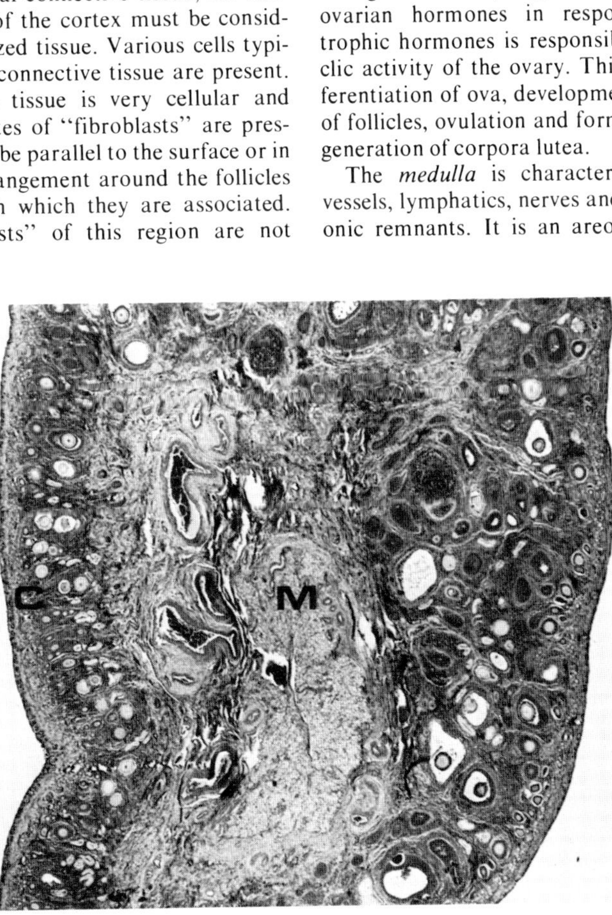

Fig. 22-1. Canine ovary. The ovary has a distinct cortex (*C*) and medulla (*M*). ×4. All light micrographs are the original magnifications.

tissue which is rich in elastic and reticular fibers. The medullary constituents are continuous with the mesovarial attachment. The embryonic remnants are parts of the *rete ovarii*, the female homologue of the rete testis. They are short, solid cords of epithelial cells.

Ovarian Cycle. The ovary undergoes cyclic changes which are influenced by the previously mentioned trophic hormones. The cycle includes the following periods: *differentiation of ova*, *development of follicles*, *ovulation*, *formation of the corpus luteum* and *degeneration of follicles*, and *corpus luteum*. The differentiation of ova and the subsequent development of follicles occurs in two stages that are similar to the development of the male gametes: *stage of mitosis* and *stage of meiosis*.

During the stage of mitosis or multiplication, *oogonia* proliferate from primordial sex cells which had migrated to the germinal ridges from the yolk sac endoderm. These oogonia divide and give rise to several generations of these cells. In some species (man, ruminants, rodents and swine), this differentiation occurs in the fetus, long before parturition. In others (carnivores and lagomorphs), this differentiation is prolonged into the immediate postnatal period.

The subsequent development of *oocytes* is intimately associated with the development of follicles. Terminal oogonia develop into *primary oocytes* which are large round cells with a vesicular nucleus and a prominent and eccentrically placed nucleolus. The cytoplasm is pale-staining. Independent of when these primary oocytes are differentiated, they are arrested in the diplotene stage of the first meiotic division until sexual maturity is achieved.

Concomitant with the differentiation of primary oocytes, a single layer of flattened mesodermal cells, *follicular cells*, surrounds the primary oocyte. At this stage, the complex is referred to as a primordial follicle. A *primordial follicle*, therefore, contains a *primary oocyte*. These are also referred to as *quiescent follicles* (Fig. 22-2). They are located in the periphery of the cortex in clusters or evenly distributed.

The activation of the primordial follicle results in a *primary follicle* (Fig. 22-3). This activation involves alterations in the ovum, follicular cells and other stromal elements. An accumulation of yolk granules is noted within the ovum. The follicular cells become cuboidal. *The primary follicle still contains a primary oocyte*.

When two or three layers of cuboidal cells are proliferated the structure is termed a *secondary follicle* (Fig. 22-4). These cells are now referred to as the *membrana granulosa*. They are separated from the ovum by a periodic acid-Schiff-positive, amorphous material, the *zona pellucida*. This is actually a very thick basal lamina. Stromal cells

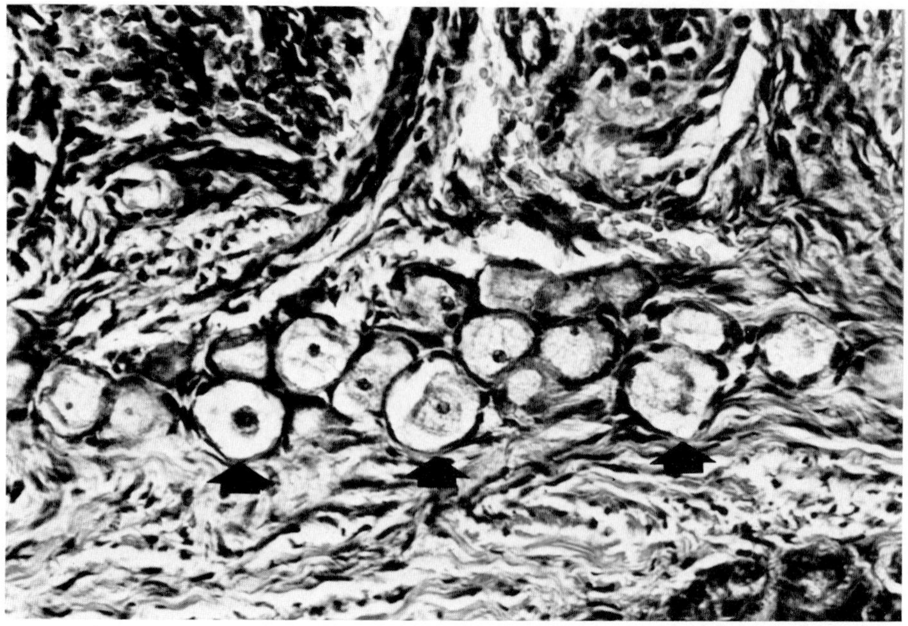

Fig. 22-2. Primordial follicles of the canine ovary. A single layer of flattened follicular cells surrounds the primary oocyte. These comprise the primordial follicle (*arrows*). ×100.

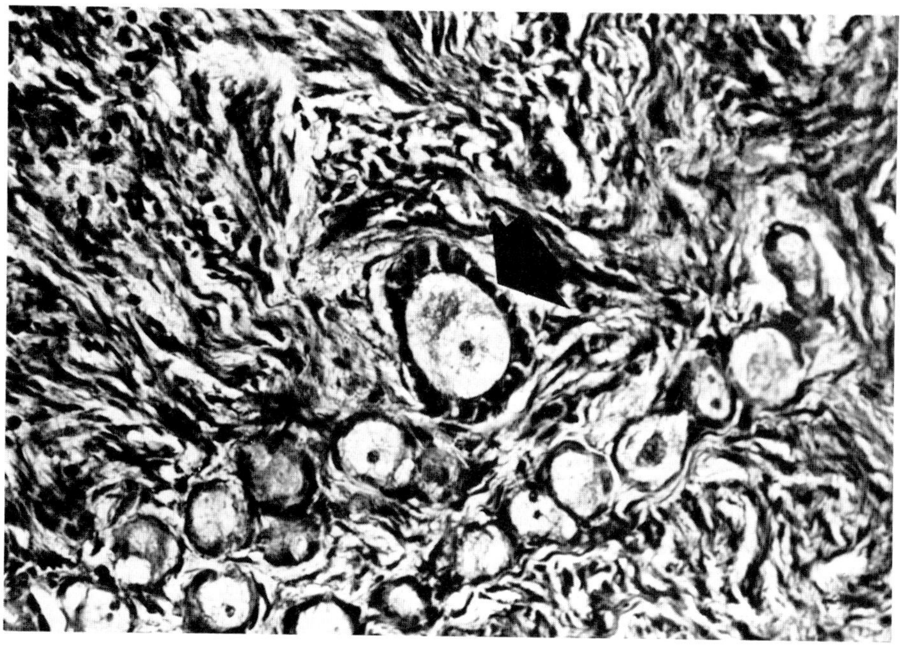

Fig. 22-3. Primary follicle of the canine ovary. The primary follicle (*arrow*) is surrounded by a layer of cuboidal follicular cells. Primordial follicles are in the same area. ×100.

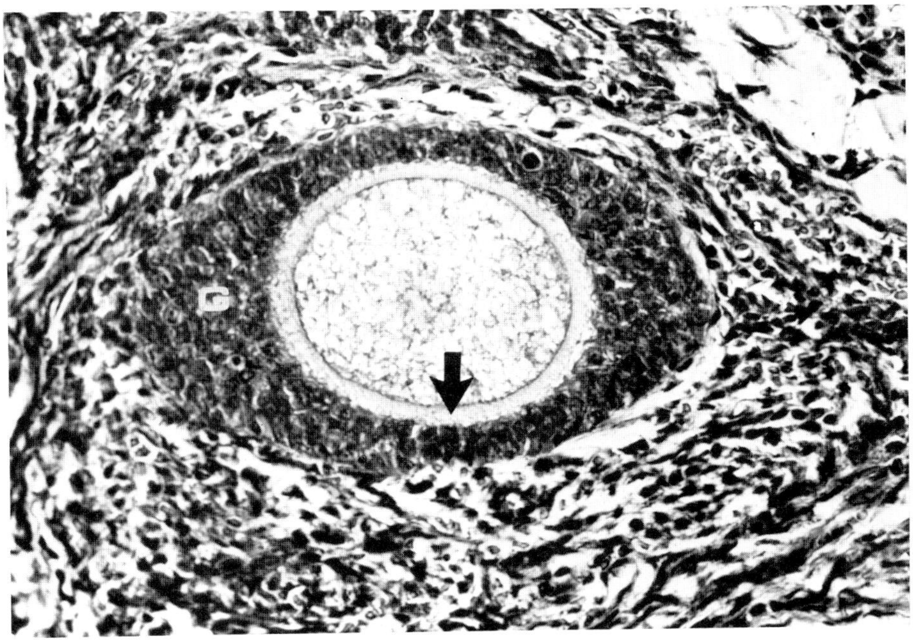

Fig. 22-4. Secondary follicle of the canine ovary. The layer of follicular cells has become thicker. Now they are referred to as the membrane granulosa (*G*). These cells are separated from the oocyte by the zona pellucida (*arrow*). ×100.

differentiate into two layers: *theca folliculi interna* and *theca folliculi externa*. The thecal cells are separated from the membrana granulosa cells by a basement membrane, the *glassy membrane*. The theca folliculi interna consists of large, epithelioid cells and an extensive vascular network. These cells secrete estrogens. The theca folliculi externa is a fibroblastic layer of cells.

The development of a *secondary follicle* (*vesicular follicle*) results from the secretory activity of the granulosa cells (Fig. 22-5). Intercellular clefts develop, become confluent and form the *follicular antrum* filled with *liquor folliculi*. This is accompanied by a continued growth of the follicle. The ovum is still surrounded, however, by a cluster of granulosa cells which is continuous with the peripherally displaced membrana granulosa. This mound of cells is referred to as the *cumulus oophorus*. Granulosa cells of the cumulus oophorus immediately adjacent to the ovum comprise the *corona radiata*. These cells have cytoplasmic processes which penetrate the zona pellucida and contact microvilli from the ovum. *Despite the development of a vesicular follicle, it still contains a primary oocyte arrested in the first meiotic prophase.*

The *mature follicle* (*Graafian follicle*) is a greatly enlarged structure (Fig. 22-6). It extends from a protrusion at the surface to the depths of the cortex. The antrum is large and its attenuated wall still consists of the previously mentioned cellular and intercellular components.

Ovulation is achieved by a rupture of the mature follicle. Although the precise mechanism has not been clarified, a reduced blood flow may produce a focal necrosis which results in the follicular rupture at the ovarian surface. The extruded "egg" consists of a primary or secondary oocyte, zona pellucida and corona radiata. The first meiotic division and the resulting *first polar body* formation are usually achieved after ovulation in nearly all domestic species. The second meiotic division and *second polar body* formation is not achieved usually until after penetration of the spermatozoon into the egg cell within the oviduct. Either a primary or secondary oocyte is ovulated. The term, ovum, is loosely applied to the extruded cell.

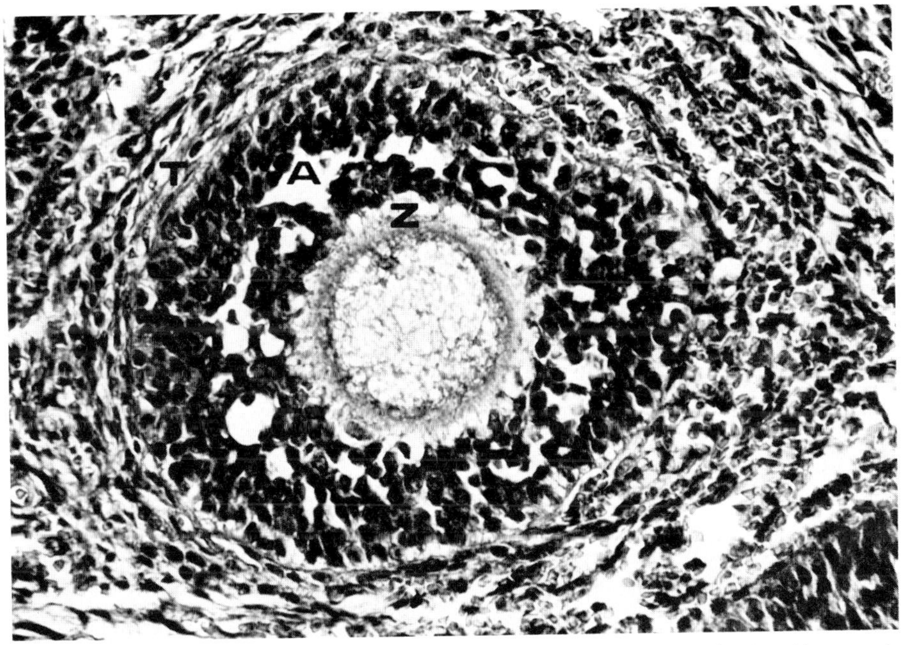

Fig. 22-5. A growing secondary follicle of the canine ovary. Intercellular clefts developed between the membrana granulosa cells. Their confluence will result in the formation of the antrum (*A*). The zona pellucida (*Z*) and theca cells (*T*) are apparent. ×100.

Follicular Atresia. The degeneration of follicles may occur at any point in their developmental sequence (Fig. 22-7). During the primordial follicular stage, the dissolution of the ovum and granulosa cells is not characterized by remaining scar tissue (extensive connective tissue fiber development). It simply disintegrates. Polyoocytic follicles are common and are invariably destined to become atretic.

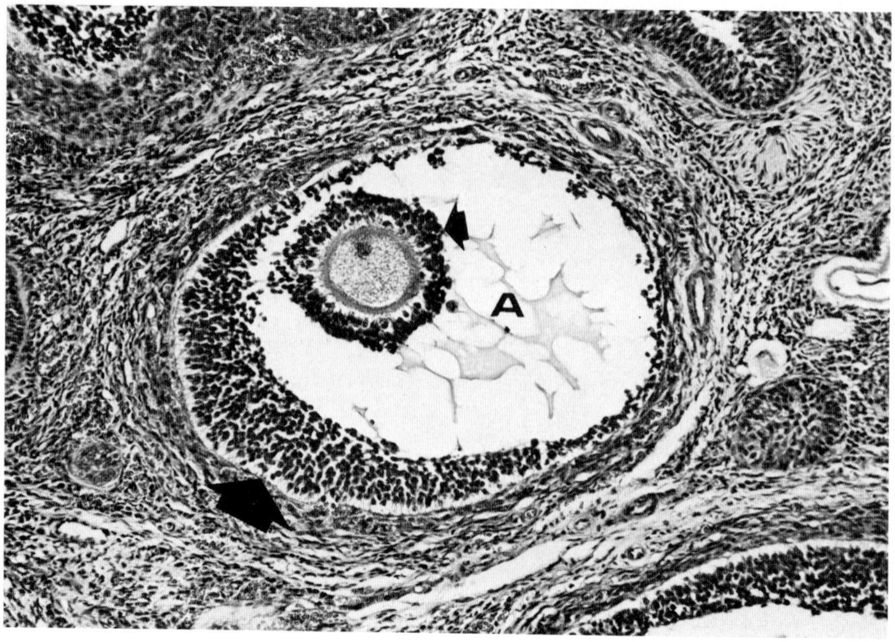

Fig. 22-6. A vesicular follicle from the canine ovary. The antrum (*A*) is formed and some membrana granulosa cells remain attached to the oocyte as the corona radiata (*small arrow*). The entire mound of cells is the cumulus oophorus. The glassy membrane (*large arrow*) delimits the vesicular follicle from the surrounding theca cells. ×40.

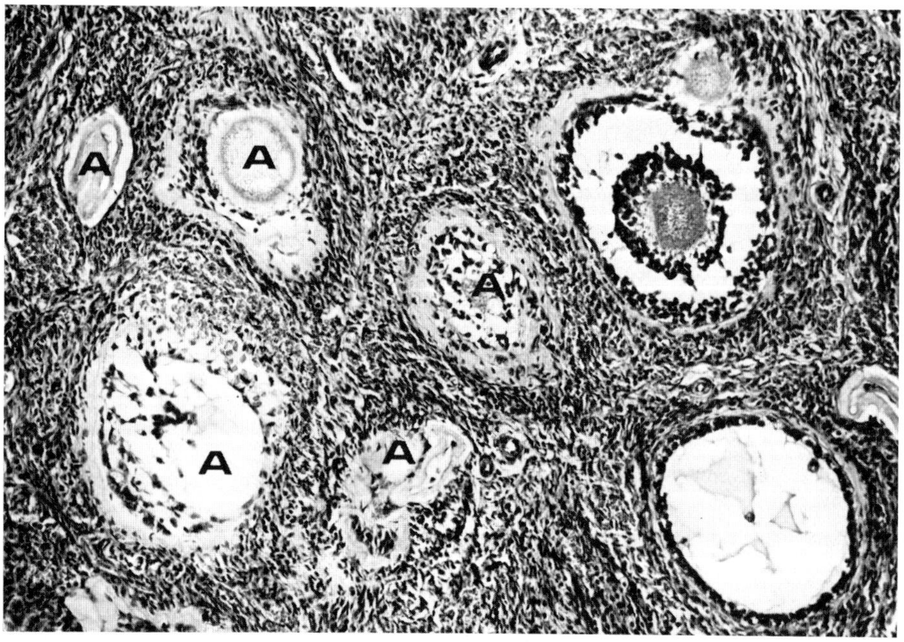

Fig. 22-7. Atretic follicles (canine ovary). Not all follicles reach maturity. Some undergo atresia (*A*). ×40.

In the more advanced stages of follicular development, degeneration results in the formation of a scar, the *corpus atreticum*. The walls of the follicle collapse and the membrana granulosa cells degenerate. This is accompanied by a connective tissue and vascular invasion of the follicular antrum. The glassy membrane thickens and the cells of the theca folliculi interna may hypertrophy and undergo changes similar to their conversion to theca lutein cells (see corpus luteum). At this stage the atretic follicle may be considered a temporary gland. The follicular cells are arranged as cords around the degenerating ovum. Phagocytic activity from associated histiocytes and fibrotic activity from fibroblasts completes the transition to a corpus atreticum.

Corpus Luteum. Following the rupture of the ovarian wall and associated mural elements of the follicle, the ovum is ejected and passes into the oviduct. The remaining portions of the follicle do not degenerate but undergo pronounced changes which lead to the formation of the corpus luteum (Fig. 22-8).

The follicular walls collapse upon themselves and the granulosa cells protrude into the residual lumen. The hemorrhage which accompanies ovulation clots and the resulting transitory structure is referred to as a *corpus hemorrhagicum*. The granulosa cells proliferate, hypertrophy and are transformed into *granulosa lutein cells* (Fig. 22-9). In the mare, cow, bitch, queen and human, the accumulation of a yellow lipid pigment (*lutein*) and other lipids marks the transition to granulosa lutein cells. Although lutein does not accumulate in the ewe and sow, the accumulation of other lipids marks the transition from membrana granulosa cells to granulosa lutein cells.

The invasion of this region by stromal cells and vasculature removes the clot, results in reticular fiber deposition and converts this area into a highly vascularized gland.

The cells of the theca folliculi interna are also converted to lipid-producing cells, the *theca lutein cells*. These cells are smaller than the granulosa lutein cells and are dispersed peripherally or as septal-like clusters intimately associated with the other cell type which is predominant. In some species (ox), two types of lutein cells cannot be distinguished.

Whether lutein is present or absent, the resulting structure is referred to as the *corpus luteum* (*yellow body*).

The fate of the corpus luteum is dependent upon the reproductive success or failure of the individual.

If fertilization does not occur, the *corpus luteum spurium* slowly degenerates and is replaced by connective tissue. It is, therefore, converted to a *corpus albicans* or *corpus fibrosum*.

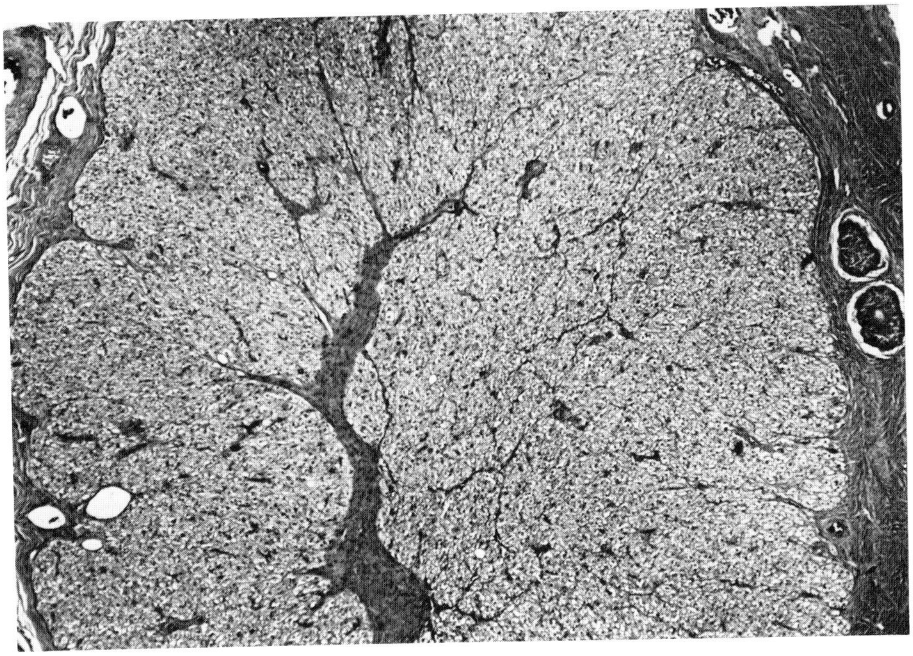

Fig. 22-8. Canine corpus luteum. This cellular mass results from the transformation of membrana granulosa cells and theca interna cells. ×10.

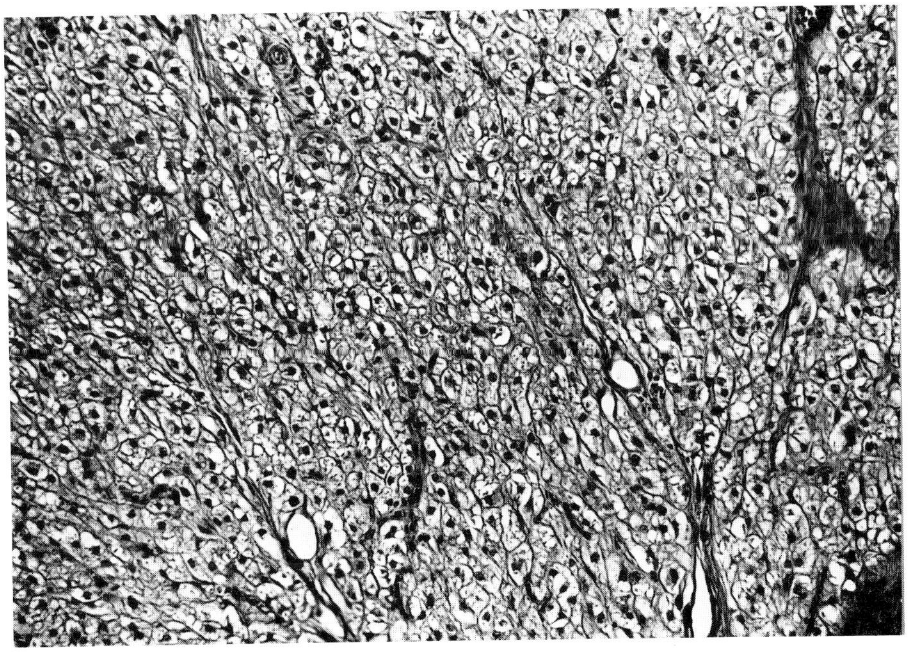

Fig. 22-9. Cells of the corpus luteum (canine ovary). The large, clear cells are granulosa lutein cells. ×40.

If fertilization does occur, the *corpus luteum verum* is persistent and active for a variable amount of time throughout the pregnancy. Retrogressive changes similar to the aforementioned characterize the degeneration of this structure. In some species, the corpus luteum verum is required throughout the entire pregnancy. In others, it may be removed at various time periods without any detrimental effects upon the gravid uterus.

Uterine Tubes

General Remarks. The uterine tubes are extensions of the uterus which serve for the transport of the male and female gametes. Fertilization occurs within the oviducts. Grossly, this structure is subdivided into *infundibulum*, *ampulla* and *isthmus*.

Histology of the Oviduct. The lamina epithelialis consists of intermittently ciliated columnar cells in most species (Fig. 22-10). In the sow and cow, however, it may be pseudostratified intermittently ciliated columnar epithelium. Kinocilia are especially prominent in the cranial portion of the oviduct wherein they assist in the movement of ova along the highly folded tunica mucosa (Fig. 22-11). The secretory cells may nourish the ova as well as capacitate the spermatozoa for fertilization.

The lamina propria-submucosa consists of areolar connective tissue and is devoid of glands. The tunica muscularis is best developed in the isthmus wherein it consists of inner longitudinal, middle circular and outer longitudinal layers. Craniad, it is typical. The tunica serosa is present and typical.

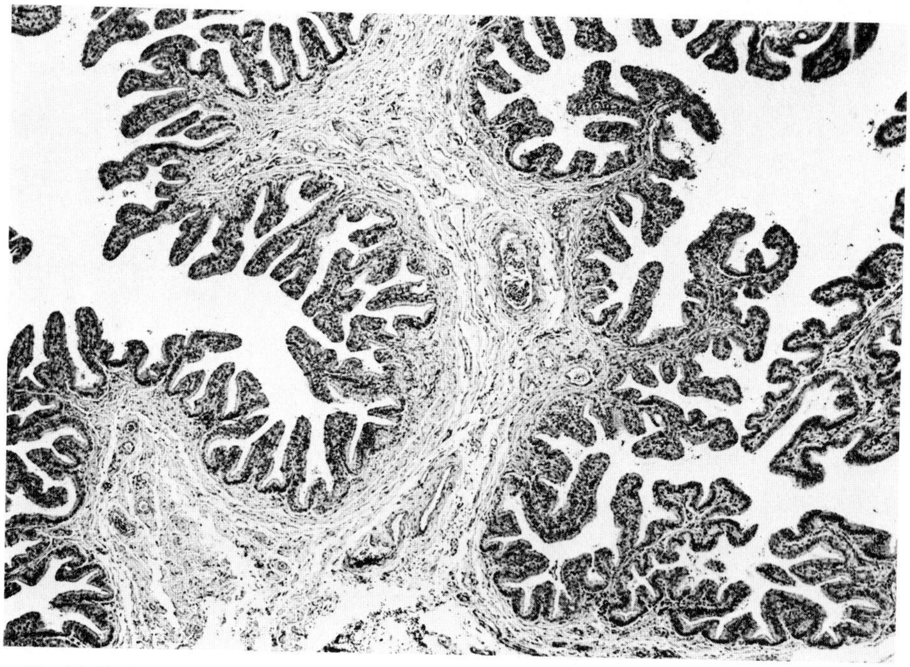

Fig. 22-10. Equine oviduct. The lining is intermittently ciliated columnar epithelium. ×16.

Uterus and Associated Structures

General Remarks. The uterus and its associated structures subserve a variety of functions. These include development of the embryo and fetus, transportation of spermatozoa, accommodation of the copulatory organ and excretion. Those structures that are part of the uterus include *body of the uterus* and *cervix*. Those structures associated with the uterus include *vagina*, *vulva* (*vestibule*, *labia*, *clitoris*) and *urethra*.

Uterus. The form of the uterus is species-variable. Most domestic species have a *bicornuate uterus*, while primates have a *simplex uterus*. Lagomorphs, monotremes and marsupials have a *duplex uterus*.

The wall of the uterus, by convention, is divisible into three distinct regions: *endometrium*, *myometrium*, and *perimetrium* (Fig. 22-12). Although the terminology is different, the mural elements are similar to those encountered in other tubular viscera. The morphology of the uterus varies with the stages of the estrous cycle. The following is a general description of the uterus.

The *endometrium* includes the tunica mucosa (Fig. 22-13). The lamina epithelialis mucosae is simple columnar epithe-

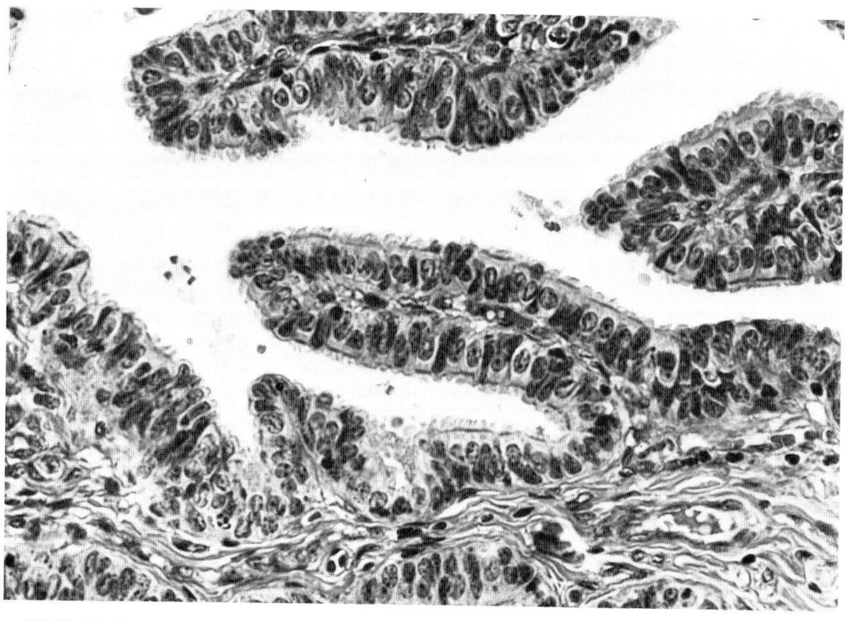

Fig. 22-11. Lining of equine oviduct (infundibulum). ×100.

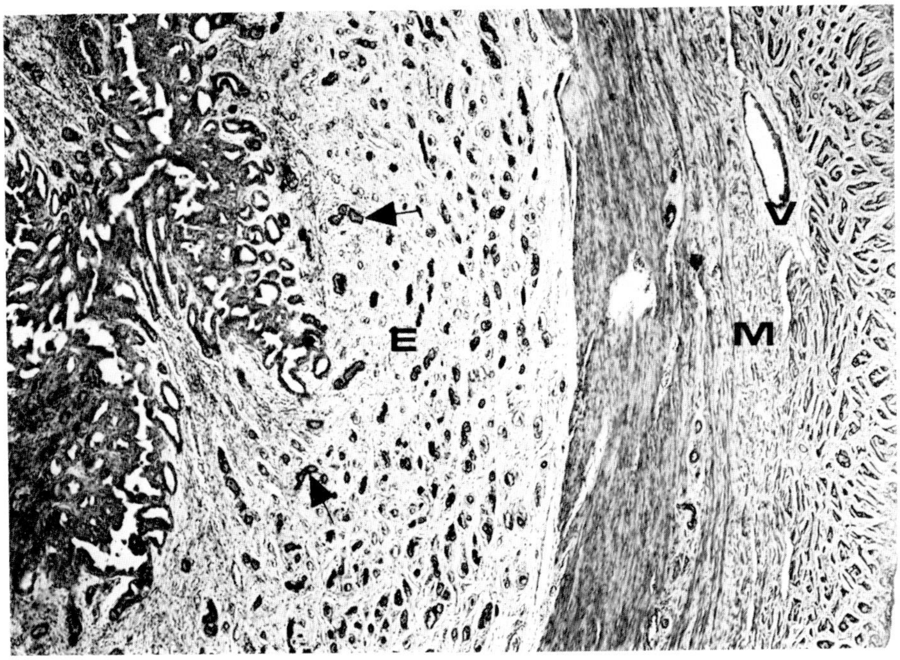

Fig. 22-12. Gravid uterus (canine). The tubular glands (*arrows*) are branched and coiled. ×40. *E*, endometrium. *M*, myometrium. *V*, vessels of the stratum vasculare.

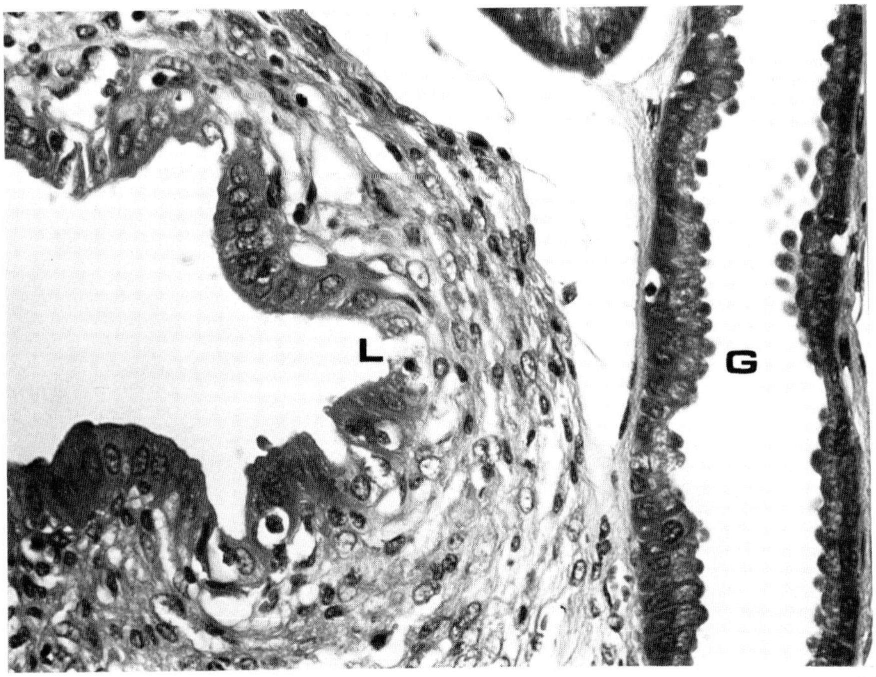

Fig. 22-13. Lining and glands of bovine uterus (metestrus). The lining (*L*) is columnar. The cells of the gland (*G*) have apical blebs. ×100.

lium. Patches of pseudostratified columnar epithelium may be encountered in the sow and cow. Isolated foci of cuboidal epithelium may occur also. *Uterine glands* are simple or branched tubular glands (Fig. 22-14). Their distal ends have a variable degree of coiling which is species-dependent. The secretory products of the lining and glandular epithelia include mucus, lipids, glycogen and proteins. These glands extend into the lamina propria.

The lamina propria is a very cellular areolar connective tissue. In ruminants, an area of the lamina propria is highly vascularized and devoid of glands. These *caruncles* are devoid of uterine glands and are the eventual sites at which the maternal tissues make contact with the extraembryonic membranes (Fig. 22-15). Although there is no tunica submucosa, the peripheral connective tissue is less cellular than that which is subepithelial.

The endometrium is subject to changes during the estrous cycle.

The *myometrium* consists of a thick inner circular and thinner, outer longitudinally oriented coat which continues into the mesometrium. A *stratum vasculare* occurs between the two layers of smooth muscle.

The *perimetrium* or tunica serosa is typical, although a large number of lymphatic vessels may be present.

The *cervix uteri* serves as a valve to close off the uterine lumen from the vagina. In the bitch, it may possess glands similar to those which occur in the uterus. In other domestic species, it is usually glandless. In the sow, it is a thin-walled structure, while in the cow it is extremely well-developed. The lining cells of the cervix of the cow are highly glandular. Its secretory activity varies with the stages of the estrous cycle and pregnancy. A clear mucus is secreted during estrus and a thick cervical seal is produced during pregnancy. Numerous longitudinal folds impart the impression that it is glandular.

The lamina epithelialis mucosae of the endocervical canal is composed primarily of goblet-like cells, but some kinociliated columnar cells may be present. The lamina propria-submucosa varies from loose connective tissue to DWFCT during various stages of the estrous cycle. The tunica muscularis is well-developed and rich in elastic fibers.

Vagina. The lamina epithelialis mucosae is a stratified squamous lining which is usually nonglandular (Fig. 22-16). In the cow, isolated foci of goblet cells are present in the cranial portion of the organ. In the bitch, intraepithelial glands have been observed during estrus. The tunica mucosa and tunica submucosa are highly folded.

The underlying DWFCT of the lamina propria-submucosa possesses scattered lymphatic nodules.

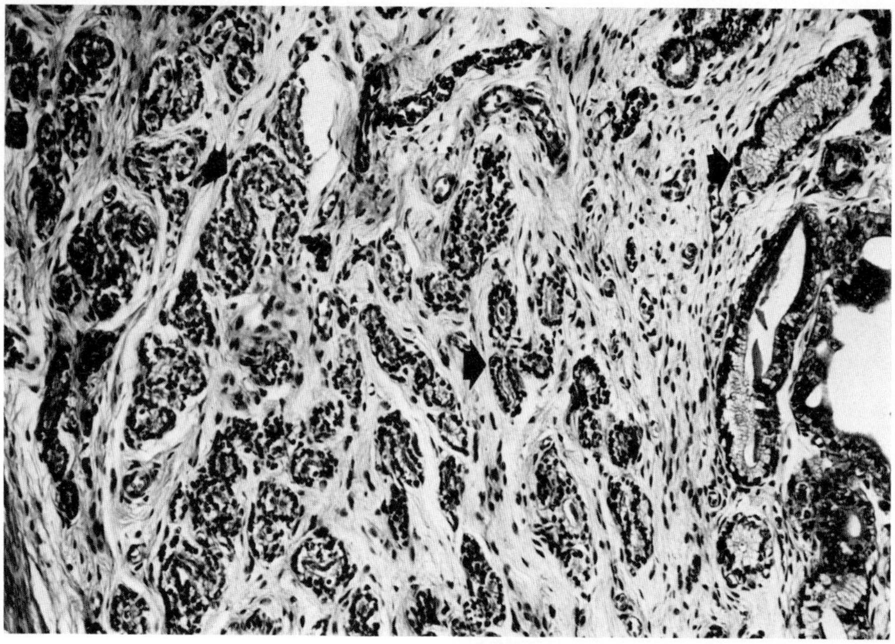

Fig. 22-14. Uterine glands of the gravid uterus (canine). The tubular glands (*arrows*) are branched and coiled. ×40.

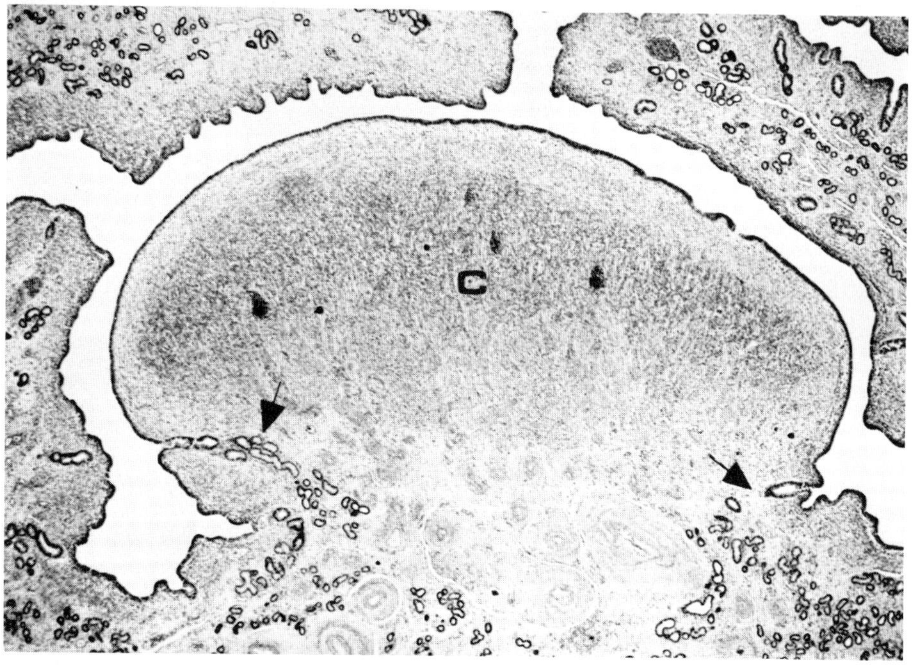

Fig. 22-15. A bovine caruncle. The caruncle (*C*) is devoid of uterine glands (*Arrows*) ×5.

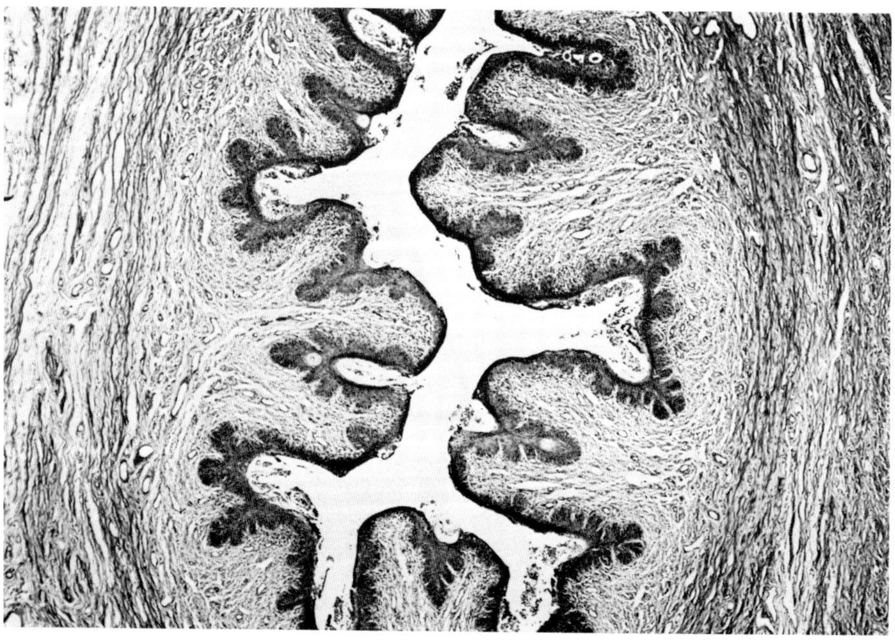

Fig. 22-16. Feline vagina. The tunica mucosa is highly folded and covered by stratified squamous epithelium. ×10.

The tunica muscularis consists of two or three layers: an inner longitudinal (variable), middle circular and an outer longitudinal. A tunica serosa is present cranially and is continued caudad as a tunica adventitia. Some smooth muscle (*muscularis serosae*), as a continuation of that of the broad ligament, may also be observed in the subserosal space.

Vulva. The vulva consists of the *vestibule* and *labia*. The *clitoris* is part of the vestibule and the *urethra* opens into the vestibule.

The structure of the *vestibule* is similar to the caudal portion of the vagina. There is nonkeratinized stratified squamous epithelium with an extensive lymphocytic infiltration. The lamina propria-submucosa consists of loose and dense connective tissue which is rich in elastic fibers. *Vestibular glands* (compound tubuloalveolar mucous glands) are present. *Major vestibular glands* (ewe, cow, queen) are embedded within the constrictor vestibuli muscle. *Minor vestibular glands* (queen, bitch, ewe, sow and mare) are scattered throughout the vestibule. In the cow, they are concentrated near the clitoris.

The tunica muscularis consists of an inner longitudinal and outer circular layer. The outer layer comprises two distinct muscles, *constrictor vestibuli* and *constrictor vulvae*. The tunica adventitia is typical.

The *clitoris* is homologous to the male penis. It consists of a body, glans and preputial covering. The body or *corpus clitoridis* contains cavernous tissue, adipose tissue and smooth muscle which is surrounded by a sheath of DWFCT. The *glans clitoridis* may contain cavernous tissue (bitch, mare) or areolar connective tissue which is highly vascularized. The *preputial* covering is an aglandular and hairless reflection of the cutaneous mucous membrane of the vestibule which is rich in sensory nerve endings.

The female *urethra* is lined by transitional epithelium which is continuous with the mucous membrane of the vestibule. Branched tubular mucous glands, *glands of Littré*, may be present. The lamina propria-submucosa is areolar connective tissue which contains cavernous sinuses. The tunica muscularis is composed of two or three layers of smooth muscle.

The *labia* are folds of the integument which are comprised of typical integumentary structures.

Cyclic Changes of the System

General Remarks. The female reproductive tract is subject to a greater periodicity than that associated with the male. Moreover, female cyclic activity is manifested microscopically and grossly, as well as behaviorally. These various states of morphology, function and behavior are directly related with the estrous cycle. The estrous cycle, or period of varying reproductive activity, is under the influence of the trophic hormones of the adenohypophysis. This cycle is subdivided into five distinct but continuous stages: *proestrus*, *estrus*, *metestrus*, *diestrus* and *anestrus*. *Proestrus* is that period of the cycle characterized by the acceleration of follicular growth under the influence of FSH. The follicles begin to secrete estrogen which in turn influences the genital organs. The increasing levels of estrogen suppress the declining levels of progesterone. *Estrus* is marked by the genital organs being under the full influence of estrogen. This is the period of *heat* in which the female will accept the male. *Metestrus* is a transitional stage in which the declining levels of estrogen are counterbalanced by the increasing levels of progesterone. *Diestrus* is that period of the cycle which is under the sole influence of progesterone. Fertilization of the ova and subsequent pregnancy results in a prolonged diestrus. If fertilization is not accomplished, the *anestrus* period follows. This is a period of variable length in which the reproductive organs are relatively quiescent.

The stages of the estrous cycle are of varying lengths in domestic species. Animals are either *monestrous* or *polyestrous*. In monestrous species (dog, cat), one estrous cycle (proestrus, estrus, metestrus, diestrus) is followed by a long period of anestrus. In polyestrous animals (cow, sow, rodents) one estrous cycle terminates in a period of diestrus which merges as the proestrus in the succeeding estrous cycle. In seasonally polyestrous animals (mare, ewe), the terminal diestrus continues as a period of anestrus before the next estrous cycle. The anestrous period in these animals is appreciably shorter than that which occurs in monestrous animals.

Although numerous organs respond to the hormonal activity that characterizes the estrous cycle, the most significant responses are observed in the ovaries, uterus and vagina.

Ovarian Changes. During *proestrus*, the ovaries are influenced by the gonadotrophin, FSH. This results in the rapid growth of the follicles and the initiation of estrogen secretory activity.

During *estrus*, the follicle (or follicles) reaches maturity and estrogen secretory activity is maximum. FSH secretion begins to drop while LH secretion is initiated. This results in ovulation. Ovulation may be considered a transitory period between estrus and metestrus or part of the metestrous stage.

During *metestrus*, the development of the corpus luteum occurs and the secretion of progesterone is initiated.

The *diestrus* is characterized by a maximal development of the corpus luteum and a maximal productivity of progesterone. If pregnancy is not achieved, the latter part of diestrus is characterized by an involution of the corpus luteum spurium and its conversion into a corpus albicans. If pregnancy does occur, the corpus luteum continues its maximal secretory activity.

In *anestrus* the ovary is relatively quiescent. The corpus luteum continues its involution and follicular development is arrested.

Uterine Changes. During *proestrus* the lining epithelium hypertrophies while the uterine glands remain relatively straight (Fig. 22-17). There is an increasing vascularity

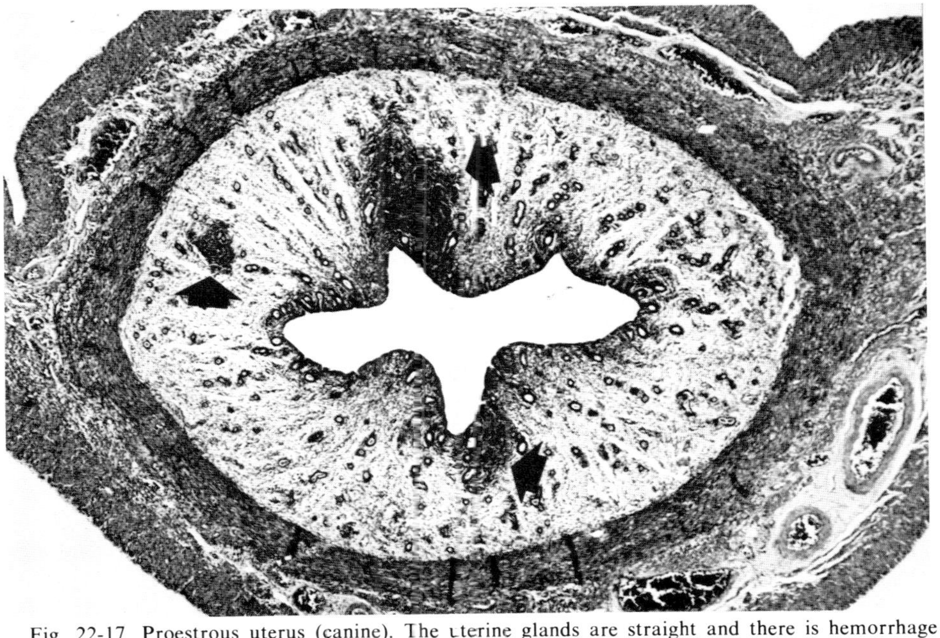

Fig. 22-17. Proestrous uterus (canine). The uterine glands are straight and there is hemorrhage (*arrows*) in the lamina propria. ×10. (Note: the magnifications of Figs. 22-15, 22-16, 22-17 and 22-18 are the same.)

and congestion in the connective tissue space, as well as occasional hemorrhage. Heterophils begin to invade the epithelial lining.

During *estrus* the epithelial and glandular proliferation is continued and is more apparent (Fig. 22-18). Secretory activity of the cells is marked, while agranulocytic infiltration of the epithelium continues. The connective tissue space is marked by maximal congestion, edema and hemorrhage.

Metestrus is characterized by a continuation of glandular hyperplasia through which the coiling of glands is achieved (Fig. 22-19). The high secretory activity continues, while the edema of the connective tissue space declines or disappears.

In *diestrus* maximal glandular hyperplasia is achieved and the glands are extensively coiled. If fertilization occurs, maximal secretory activity is maintained. If fertilization does not occur, the vascularity decreases, the secretory activity is arrested and the lining cells and glands involute.

During *anestrus* the endometrium is thin and lined by a simple cuboidal epithelium (Fig. 22-20). Uterine glands are sparse and assume a simple or branched tubular configuration.

Vaginal Changes. The subsequent description of vaginal changes through the estrous cycle is for the bitch.

The *proestrus* is characterized by a thick epithelium which has many superficial layers of living cells. In a vaginal smear, nucleated epithelial cells are present. Red blood corpuscles are also present as a result of diapedesis from the underlying vascular beds.

During *estrus* the thick epithelium is keratinized and much desquamation of these cells is apparent. In a vaginal smear, keratinized cells predominate or are the only cells present.

In *metestrus*, the epithelium becomes thinner and is invaded by leukocytes. In a vaginal smear during early metestrus the predominant cells are keratinized epithelial cells and leukocytes. In late metestrus, a vaginal smear contains nucleated epithelial cells and leukocytes.

In the *diestrous stage* the epithelium is thin and leukocytes occur in the superficial layers. A vaginal smear during diestrus is similar to one obtained during late metestrus.

In *anestrus* the epithelium is thin and a smear would be characterized by a few nucleated epithelial cells.

Menstrual Cycle. The menstrual cycle of primates includes four phases: *follicular phase*, *luteal phase*, *ischemic phase* and *menstrual phase*.

The *follicular phase* is characterized by those events which occur in proestrus and estrus in other species. The phase is under the influence of FSH and estrogen. It is

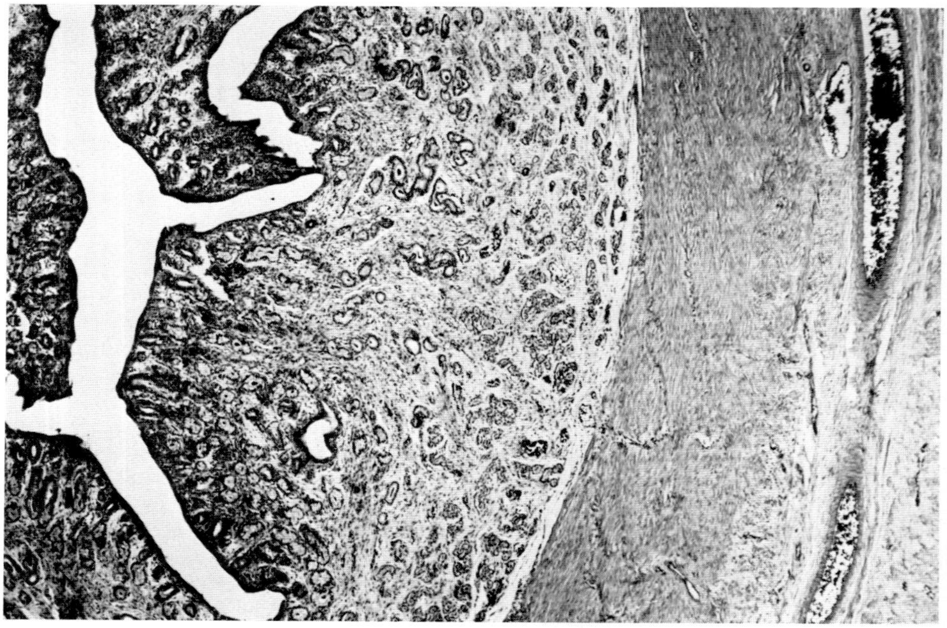

Fig. 22-18. Estrous uterus (canine). Glandular proliferation has occurred. ×10.

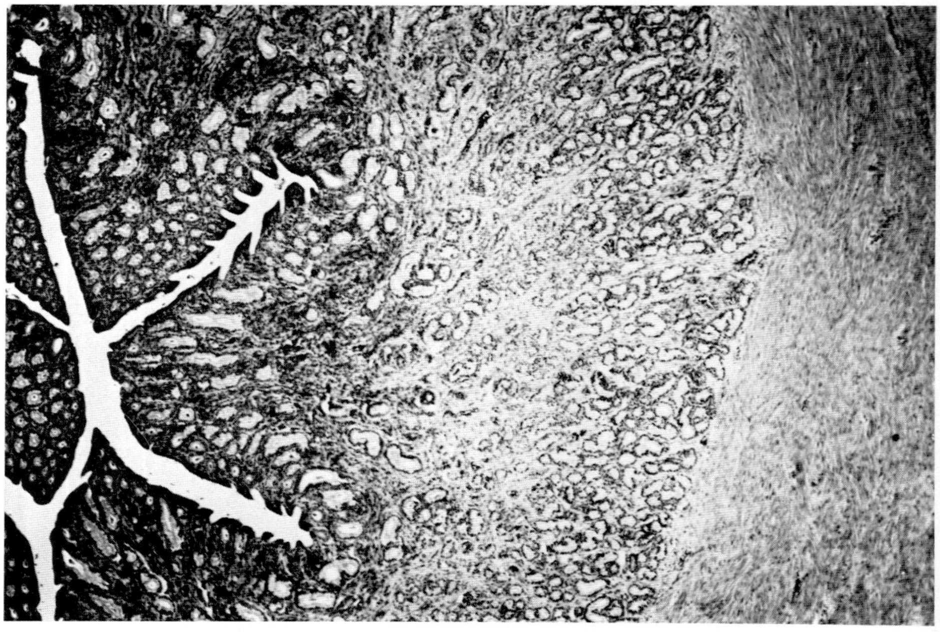

Fig. 22-19. Metestrus uterus (canine). The hyperplasia of the uterine glands is still apparent. ×10.

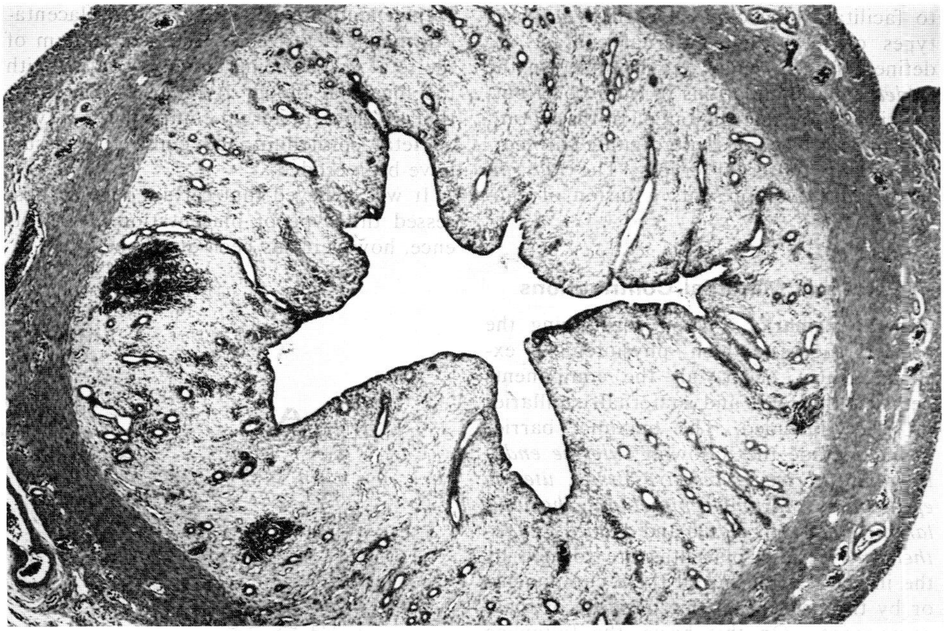

Fig. 22-20. Anestrous uterus (canine). The uterine glands have reduced in number and the endometrium has reduced in size. ×10.

sometimes referred to as the proliferative phase.

The *luteal phase* is also referred to as the *progestational* or *secretory phase*. The events are similar to those of metestrus and diestrus.

The *ischemic* or *premenstrual phase* is characterized by necrotic changes that occur in the endometrium under the declining influence of progesterone.

The *menstrual phase* is characterized by hemorrhage and a loss of a part of the endometrium. Repair is achieved through proliferation of epithelium from the uterine glands and stromal elements from the lamina propria. Then the follicular stage resumes.

Comparative Placentology

Form and Function. The female reproductive tract of mammals is designed to facilitate internal fertilization. Subsequent to that, the system permits the development of the fertilized egg within the uterus. Complex relationships are developed within the uterus between fetal and maternal tissues which ensure nutrition, respiration, removal of waste materials and protection. Besides the important aforementioned functions, the placenta is also an endocrine organ which is responsible for the production of progesterone and relaxin. These functions are ensured by the formation of the *placenta*, a complex structure formed by the union of fetal membranes with the endometrium.

The endometrium was prepared for pregnancy during the metestral and diestral stages of the estrous cycle.

Not all mammals, however, are placental. Nor do all mammals bear live young. The classification of mammals is predicated upon the nature of fetal and maternal relationships. The *prototherian mammals* or *monotremes* include the platypus and echidna. These are egg-laying mammals. The *metatherian mammals* or *marsupials* include such animals as the kangaroo and opossum. These animals form a transitory "yolk sac placenta." However, there is no intimate contact between the fetal membranes and the uterine mucosa. They, in fact, do not form a true placenta.

The remaining extant mammals comprise the *eutherian* subclass. These are the true *placental mammals*. The fetal membranes (chorion, amnion, yolk sac and allantois) and the endometrium contribute to the formation of the placenta. This is accomplished individually or in specified combinations.

Classification. Various means have been devised to classify or characterize certain placental characteristics. These include the distribution of contact, the contributing extraembryonic membranes, the degree of implantation, the configuration of the chorionic attachment and the combination of fetal and maternal tissues which comprise the placenta. These classifications are not mutually exclusive. Rather, they may be used in combination to describe the placenta of a particular species.

Distribution of Chorionic Villi

General Remarks. The chorion is in close contact with the uterine mucosa. Highly vascularized regions, *villi*, project from this extraembryonic membrane and form intimate contact with the endometrium. These projections may occur singly or in groups. The subsequent descriptions refer to the chorioallantoic type of placenta.

Diffuse Placentation. In the *diffuse placenta* the chorionic villi are present over the entire surface of this membrane. The entire chorion, therefore, is attached to the endometrium. This type of placenta is typical of the mare and sow.

Cotyledonary Placentation. The *cotyledonary placenta* or *placenta multiplex* is a multiple structure. The villi are grouped as cotyledons, while the intercotyledonary space is smooth (devoid of villi). The cotyledons attach themselves to the *caruncles* of the endometrium. The *fetal cotyledon* and the *maternal caruncle* comprise the *placentome*. This type of placenta is typical of the cow, ewe and doe.

Zonary Placentation. In the *zonary placenta* the villi are grouped in an area which circumscribes the midportion of the chorion. This type of placenta is characteristic of the dog and cat.

Discoidal Placentation. The *discoidal placenta* is characterized by villi being grouped in one or two disc-shaped regions. This placentation is characteristic of rodents and primates.

Extraembryonic Membrane Contributions

Chorionic Placenta. The *trophoblast* is the outer layer of the blastocyst. During *nidation*, this layer invades the uterine mucosa and serves as a nonvascularized point of attachment. This layer serves to nourish the blastocyst by obtaining nutrients from the uterus until the definitive placenta is formed.

Choriovitelline Placenta. There are two types of yolk sac placenta: *nonvascularized* and *vascularized*. In the *yolk sac, nonvascularized placenta*, the differentiated *yolk sac endoderm* and the *trophoderm* (the trophoblast following the differentiation of the germ layers, chorion) fuse. These layers serve to transport nutrients to the embryo from the uterine mucosa.

In the *yolk sac, vascularized placenta*, the yolk sac endoderm and trophoderm are separated by a layer of mesoderm which contains blood vessels. This is a transitory method of utilizing the embryonic circulation for physiological exchange between fetal and maternal tissues. It is a transitory structure in most eutherian mammals but persists for some time in the horse. This type of exchange organ is the definitive placenta of metatherian mammals.

Chorioallantoic Placenta. The *chorioallantoic placenta* is the definitive or "true" placenta of eutherian mammals. It is formed by the fusion of the *allantoic mesoderm* with the *chorionic mesoderm*. A vascular invasion accompanies the allantoic mesoderm, while the allantoic vesicle may be extensively large or vestigial in size.

Degree of Implantation

General Remarks. The degree of implantation generally defines the extent of the relationship between the fetal and maternal tissues. Through the relationships so established, the shedding or nonshedding of maternal tissues at parturition is established. In those placentas in which a minimal amount of tissue is eroded during the formation of the organ, the placenta is nondeciduate. In those in which an extensive erosion of tissues accompanies the implantation, the placenta is termed deciduate. Maternal tissues are not shed at parturition in a nondeciduate placenta as they are in a deciduate placenta.

Nondeciduate Placenta. The terms *nondeciduate placenta*, *apposed placenta*, *semiplacenta* and *superficial nidation* are used synonymously. The fetal and maternal tissues may be interdigitated and are fused or in apposition to one another. There is, therefore, minimal erosion of the contributing tissues. At parturition, no uterine mucosal elements are lost.

Deciduate Placenta. The *deciduate placenta* is also referred to as a *conjoined placenta* or a *placenta vera. Interstitial nidation* also refers to the formation of this type of placenta. In the formation of this type of placenta, the uterine mucosa and chorion are eroded to varying degrees and subsequently fuse. At parturition, therefore, some maternal tissue is lost.

Decidual Cells. These are multinucleated, round giant cells. They accumulate lipids and glycogen. These cells first appear in the uterine mucosa following the invasion of it by the trophoblast. *The presence or absence of these cells does not imply that a placenta is deciduate or nondeciduate.* The precise function of these cells is not known. They may serve a nutritive function, delineate a cleavage zone at parturition, protect the uterine mucosa against the invading trophoblast or form placental gonadotrophins. These cells are typical of most eutherian mammals but occur minimally or not at all in carnivores and ungulates.

In the mare, masses of cells very similar to decidual cells develop from the mucosa in an interglandular position. These *endometrial cups* may be responsible for the production of gonadotrophins. They regress as gestation progresses.

Configuration of Chorionic Attachments

Folded, Villous and Labyrinthine Attachments. The fetal and maternal tissues are opposed, fused or intimately interdigitated to facilitate physiological exchange. Three types of fetal and maternal contact are defined: folded, villar, labyrinthine. In the *folded type*, undulations of both contributing tissues are interdigitated. In the *villous*, chorionic protrusions interdigitate with corresponding maternal crypts. The *labyrinthine placenta* represents a fusion of chorionic villi.

Fetal and Maternal Contributions

General Remarks. When considering the barriers across which physiological exchange must occur, all the components between the fetal and maternal capillaries must be included. The maximal barrier would include the following: *uterine endothelium, uterine connective tissue, uterine epithelium, chorionic epithelium, chorioallantoic connective tissue* and *allantoic endothelium*. Various placentas are formed by the intact relationship of these components or by the deletion of one or more of these components. On this basis, the following types of placenta are recognized: *epitheliochorial, syndesmochorial, endotheliochorial, hemochorial* and *hemoendothelial* (Fig. 22-21). In the formation of these compound terms, the first term refers to the maternal component, while the second term refers to the fetal component.

Epitheliochorial Placenta. In this type of placenta all six layers are present (Fig. 22-22). The chorionic and uterine epithelia are in contact with one another (Fig. 22-23). This configuration is nondeciduate and is typical of the sow, mare, cow and ewe.

Syndesmochorial Placenta. In this type of placenta the chorionic epithelium is in direct contact with the uterine connective tissue, the uterine epithelium having been eroded. This configuration is also nondeciduate. Although this type of placentation has been described in the ewe, current evidence is contrary to this.

Endotheliochorial Placenta. This type of placentation is characterized by the intimate contact of the chorionic epithelium with the uterine capillaries. Therefore, the uterine epithelium and connective tissue have been eroded. This is a deciduate type of placentation characteristic of carnivores.

Hemochorial Placenta. In hemochorial placentation, the chorionic epithelium is in direct contact with the maternal blood. This is achieved by the erosion of the uterine epithelium, connective tissue and endothelium. Further subdivision of this type of placentation is predicated upon the number of cell layers of the trophoderm in contact with the maternal blood. Thus, *hemomonochorial, hemodichorial* and *hemotrichorial* placentation is recognized.

Hemochorial placentation occurs in primates and rodents.

Hemoendothelial Placenta. This placentation is characterized by the endothelium of the fetal tissues being in direct contact with the maternal blood. It requires, therefore, that all three maternal components, as well as fetal epithelium and connective tissue, have been eroded.

It was believed that certain rodents possessed this type of placentation. Its existence, however, has been questioned.

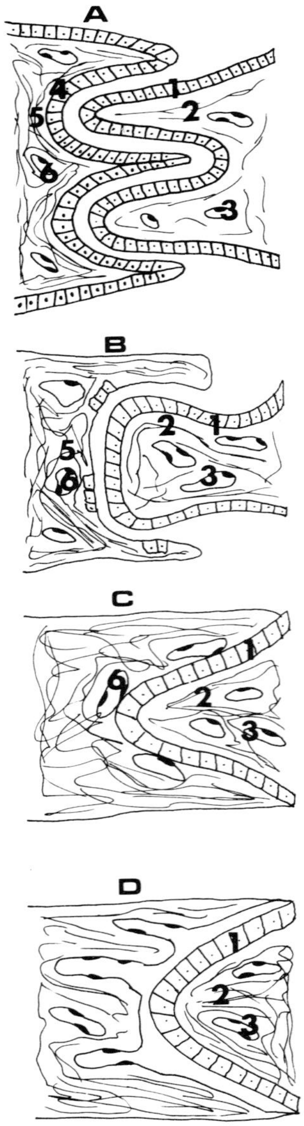

Fig. 22-21. Types of placentation. *A*, epitheliochorial; *B*, syndesmochorial; *C*, endotheliochorial; *D*, hemochorial; *1*, fetal epithelium; *2*, fetal connective tissue; *3*, fetal capillaries; *4*, maternal epithelium; *5*, maternal connective tissue; *6*, maternal capillaries. There is a progressive reduction in the number of maternal components.

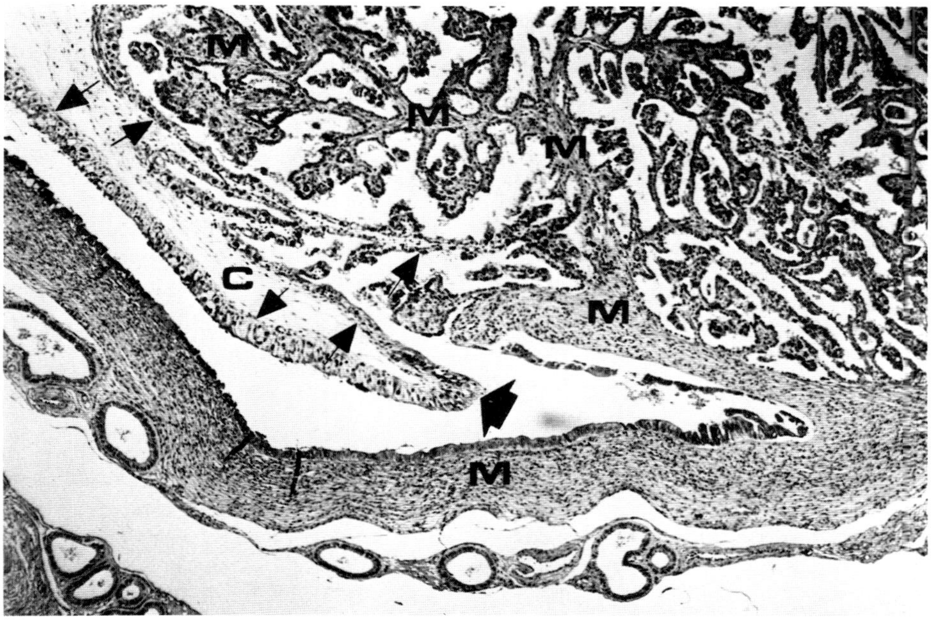

Fig. 22-22. Epitheliochorial placentation (bovine). The chorioallantois (*C*) of the fetus follows (*small arrows*) the villi of the maternal tissue (*M*). The fetal membrane is reflected away from the placentome (*large arrow*). ×13.

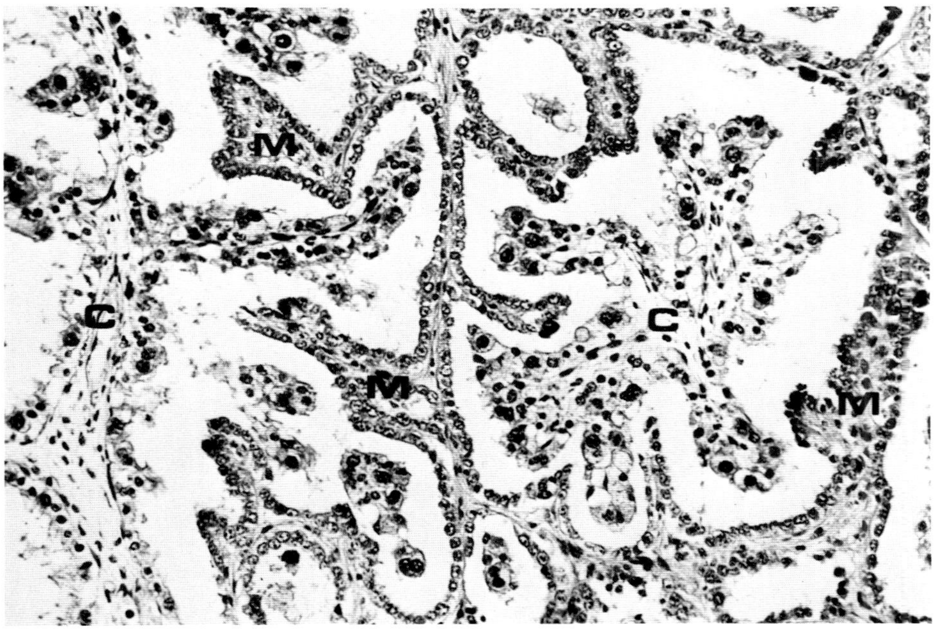

Fig. 22-23. Fetal and maternal tissue relationships in a bovine placentome. The maternal tissue (*M*) is lined by uterine epithelium. The chorioallantois (*C*) of the fetus is lined by trophoblastic cells. The separation between the tissues is artifact. ×50.

Placental Classification in Selected Species. The following unified classification is based upon the previously discussed characteristics:

Swine: diffusely folded, epitheliochorial, nondeciduate.

Horse: diffusely villous, epitheliochorial, nondeciduate.

Ruminants: cotyledonary villous, epitheliochorial, nondeciduate.

Carnivores: zonary labyrinthine, endotheliochorial, deciduate.

Man: discoidal villous, hemochorial, deciduate.

Avian Reproductive System

General Remarks. The avian reproductive system is designed to facilitate internal fertilization as in the mammal. The oviduct and uterus, however, are modified to ensure the survival and development of the offspring outside the body. These structures, therefore, supply the necessary nutrients and enclose the offspring within a protective shell.

Only the left ovary and oviduct are retained in the adult as functional entities.

Ovary. The ovaries of birds are not as compact as those in mammals. Rather, the ovary consists of finger-like projections which are suspended pendulously from the abdominal wall by the mesovarium (Fig. 22-24). A cortex and medulla are distinguishable, but the latter is not well-developed and is diffuse. The cortex consists of "follicles" in various stages of development. Actually, the term follicle is a misnomer because an antrum does not develop. The oocytes and accompanying cells are extremely large structures. The "follicle" contains a primary oocyte, a single layer of membrana granulosa cells, a theca folliculi interna and a theca folliculi externa. The primary oocyte reaches a diameter, in some domesticated species, of approximately 30 mm. Ovulation is not followed by the development of a corpus luteum.

Oviduct. The avian oviduct is divided into five regions: *infundibulum*, *magnum*, *isthmus*, *shell gland* (uterus) and *vagina*.

The *infundibulum* is the funnel-like cranial extension of the oviduct (Fig. 22-25). The tunica mucosa is highly folded and vascularized. The lamina epithelialis mucosae consists of pseudostratified ciliated columnar epithelium with occasional goblet cells (Fig. 22-26). The lamina propria-submucosa is areolar connective tissue. Diffuse lymphatic tissue is commonly encountered. The tunica muscularis and tunica serosa are typical. This portion of the oviduct receives the ova, propels it toward the caudal part of the organ and facilitates fertilization.

The *magnum* is responsible for the deposition of the majority of the egg white (Fig. 22-27). The lamina epithelialis mucosae consists of ciliated columnar cells (Fig. 22-28).

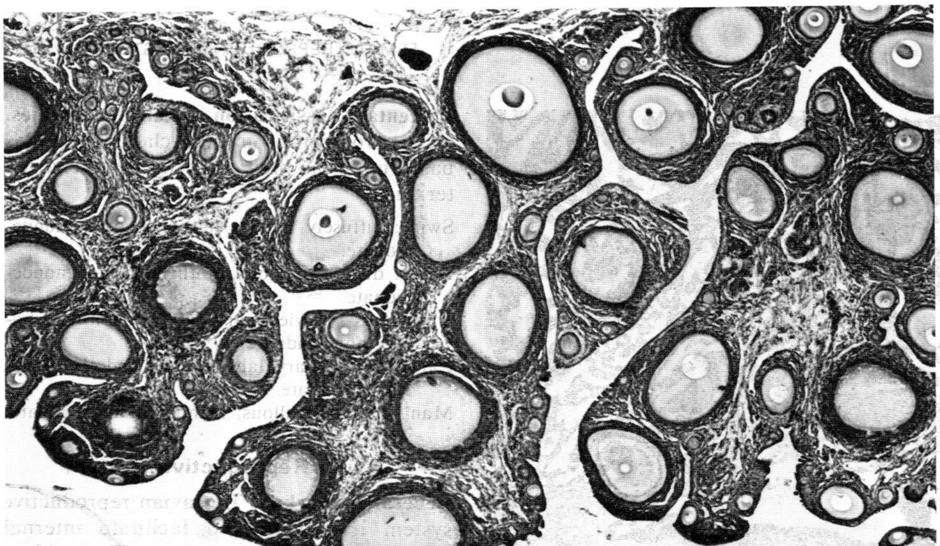

Fig. 22-24. Avian ovary. The ovary is suspended pendulously from the abdominal wall. ×10.

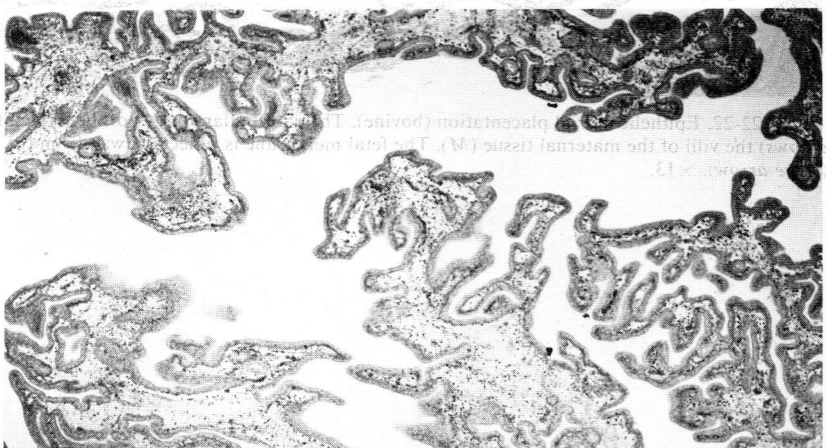

Fig. 22-25. Infundibulum of the avian oviduct. The tunica mucosa is highly folded and devoid of glands. ×10.

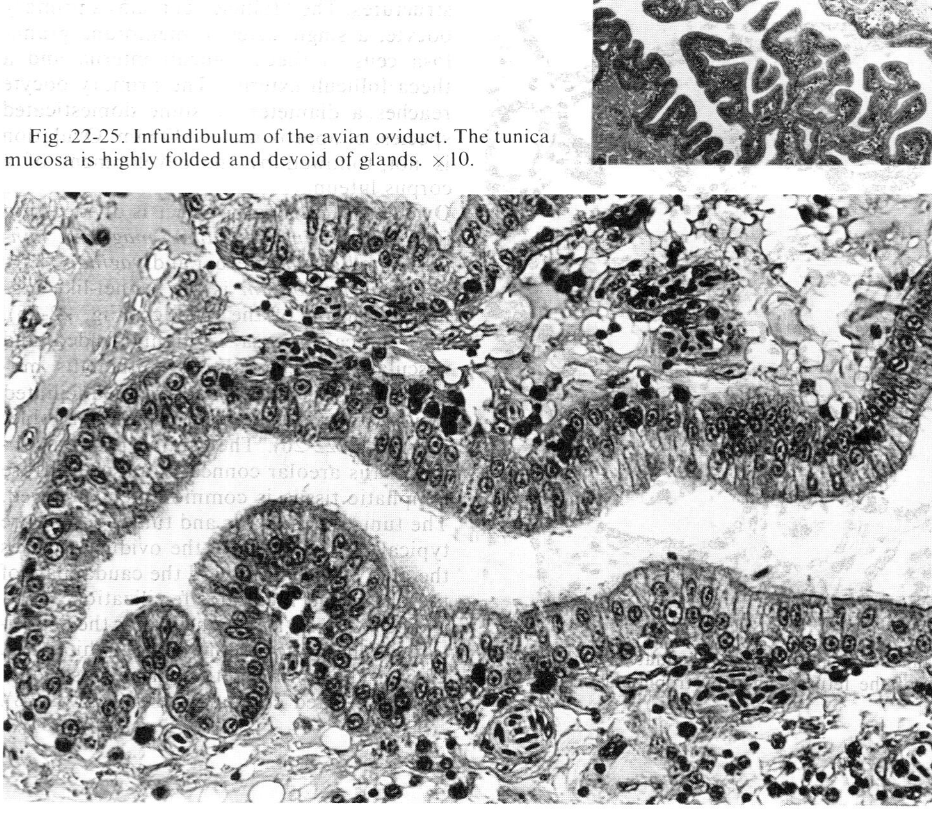

Fig. 22-26. Lining of the avian infundibulum. The lining is pseudostratified ciliated columnar epithelium. Goblet cells may be present, but glands are absent. ×125.

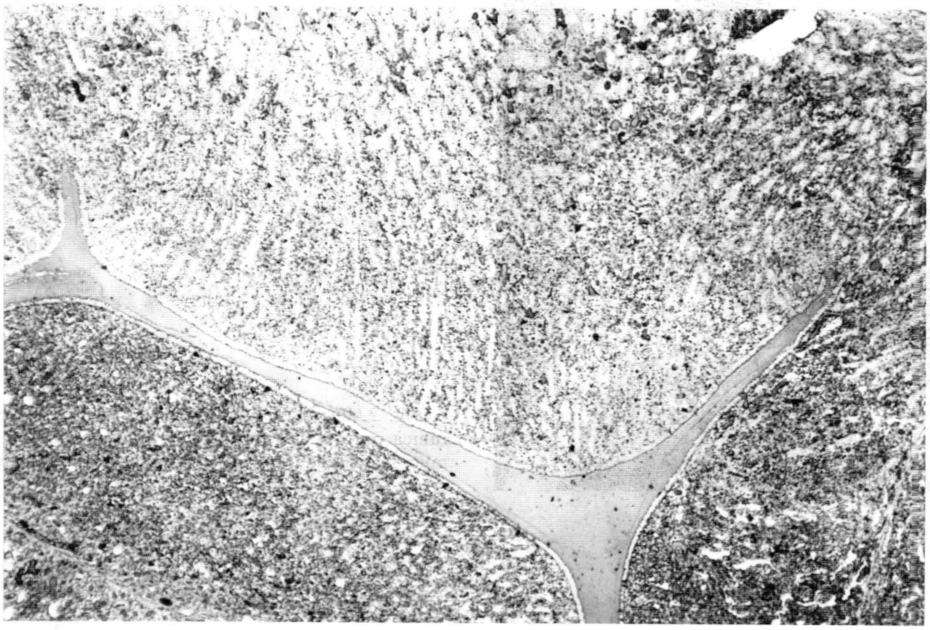

Fig. 22-27. Magnum of the avian oviduct. The tunica mucosa has pronounced folds and numerous branched tubular glands. ×10.

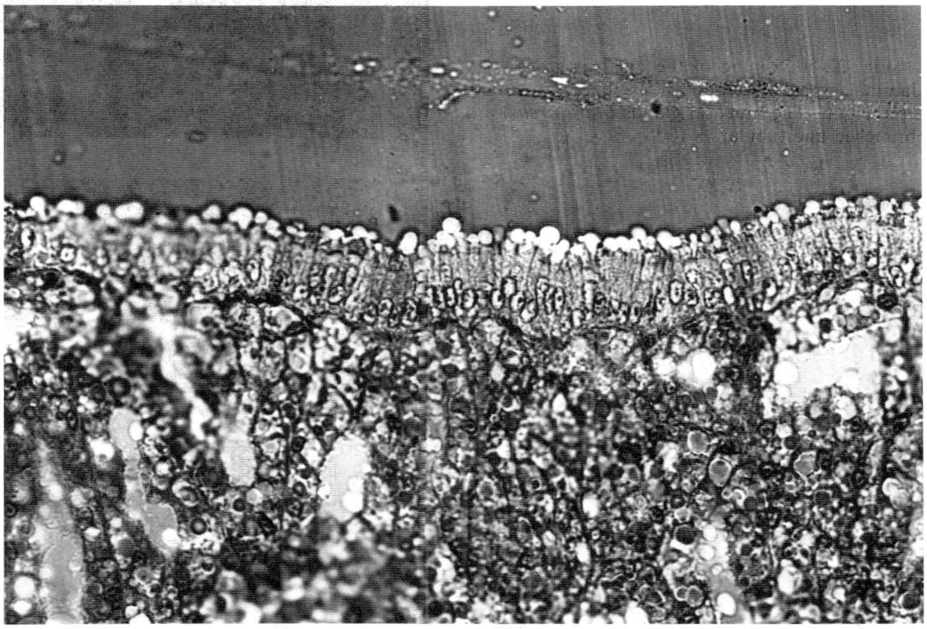

Fig. 22-28. Lining of the avian magnum. The lumen is filled with a protein secretory product. The lamina epithelialis consists of ciliated columnar cells. ×125.

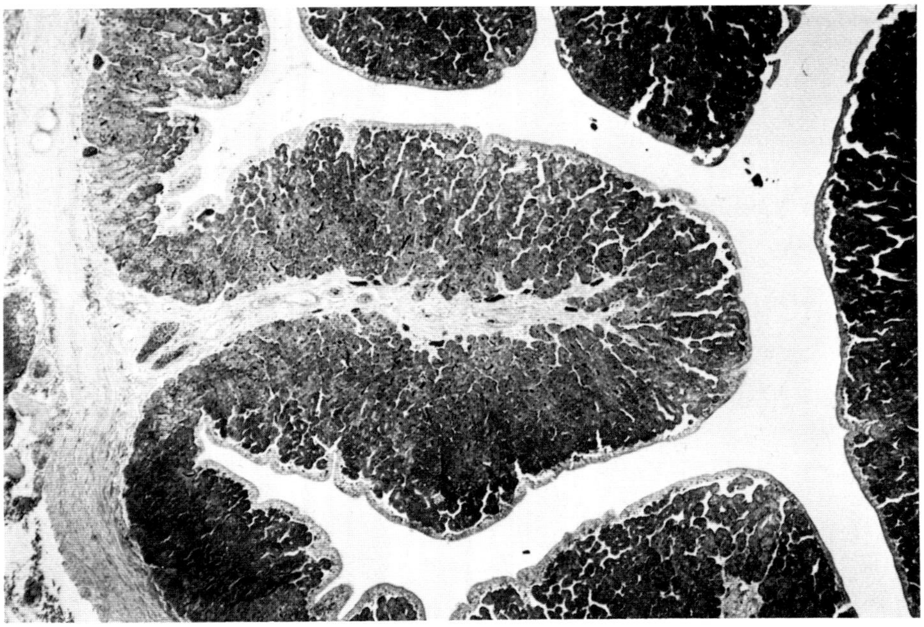

Fig. 22-29. Isthmus of the avian oviduct. The tunica mucosa has pronounced folds. Numerous mucosal glands (*dark areas*) comprise the tunica mucosa. ×10.

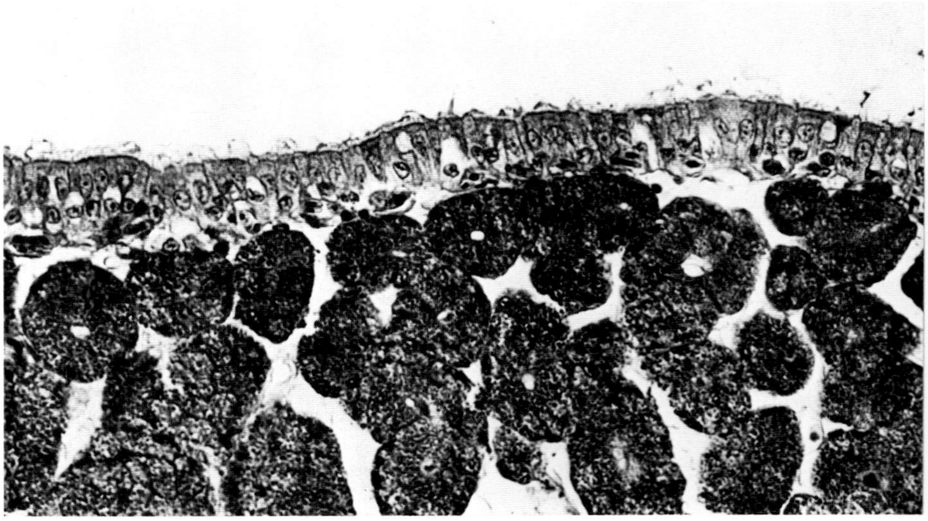

Fig. 22-30. Lining of the avian isthmus. The lamina epithelialis consists of ciliated columnar epithelium. The mucosal glands (*dark areas*) are branched and tubular. ×100.

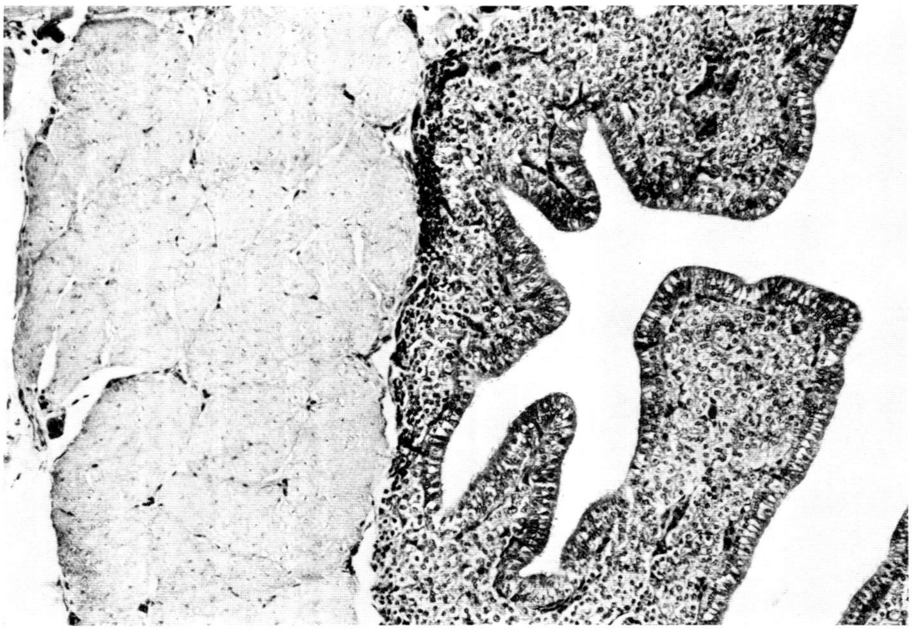

Fig. 22-31. Avian uterus. The tunica mucosa is highly folded. This is the organ that produces the shell of the egg. ×50.

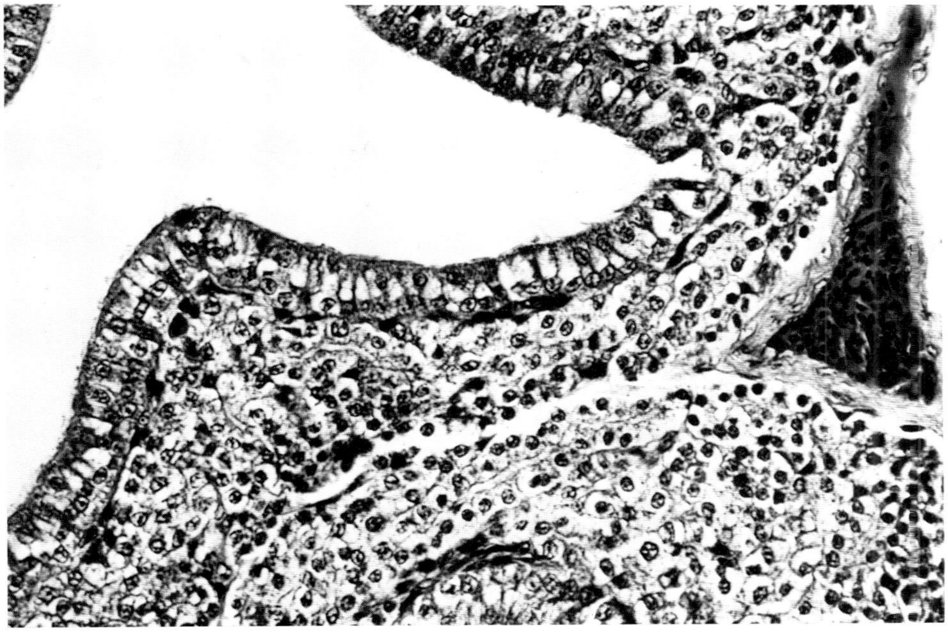

Fig. 22-32. Lining of the avian uterus. The lamina epithelialis is pseudostratified intermittently ciliated columnar epithelium. ×125.

The lamina propria contains numerous branched tubular glands which are lined by a cuboidal or columnar epithelium. Secretory granules are present along the apical border. The connective tissue of the lamina propria-submucosa is areolar with much diffuse lymphatic tissue. The tunica muscularis and tunica serosa are typical.

The *isthmus* is lined by a ciliated columnar epithelium (Fig. 22-29). Numerous branched tubular glands extend into the lamina propria (Fig. 22-30). The glandular lining cells have basally displaced nuclei and apically positioned granules. The remaining layers are similar to those of the magnum. This portion of the oviduct is responsible for the formation of the shell membranes. It may be responsible for the secretion of albuminoids also.

Unlike the mammalian uterus, the avian *uterus* is not designed for the implantation of the fertilized ova. Rather, the avian uterus is the *shell gland* (Fig. 22-31). Its secretory activity is responsible for the formation of the egg shell, as well as for the dilution of the albuminoids.

The lamina epithelialis mucosae consists of pseudostratified intermittently ciliated columnar epithelium (Fig. 22-32). Coiled tubular glands project into the underlying connective tissue. The glandular cells have a centrally placed nucleus, while the cytoplasm may contain apically positioned granules or vacuoles. The remaining portions of the wall are similar to the aforementioned structures.

The *vagina* is the region which follows the shell gland. It is devoid of glands and has a thick muscular tunic. It functions to propel the completed egg to the cloaca for expulsion to the outside environment.

References

Ovary

Baca, M. and Zamboni, L.: The fine structure of human follicular oocytes. J. Ultrastruct. Res. *19*:354, 1967.

Bjersing, L.: On the ultrastructure of the granulosa lutein cells in porcine corpus luteum. Z. Zellforsch. *82*:137, 1967.

Blanchette, E. J.: Ovarian steroid cells. II. The lutein cell. J. Cell Biol. *31*:517, 1966.

Hadek, R.: Morphological and histochemical study on the ovary of the sheep. Amer. J. Vet. Res. *19*:873, 1958.

Hope, J.: The fine structure of the developing follicle of the Rhesus ovary. J. Ultrastruct. Res. *12*:592, 1965.

Weakley, B. C.: Differentiation of the surface epithelium of the hamster ovary. An electron microscopic study. J. Anat. *105*:129, 1969.

Uterus and Associated Structures

Abdalla, O.: Observations on the morphology and histochemistry of the oviducts of the sheep. J. Anat. *102*:333, 1968.

Bal, H. S. and Getty, R.: Changing morphology of the uterine tubes of the domestic pig (*Sus scrofa domesticus*) with age. J. Geront. *25*:347, 1970.

Dessouky, D. A.: Electron microscopic studies of the myometrium of the guinea pig. Amer. J. Obstet. Gynec. *100*:30, 1968.

Ferenczy, A., Richart, R. M., Agate, F. J., Jr., Purkerson, M. L. and Dempsey, E. W.: Scanning electron microscopy of the human fallopian tube. Science *175*:783, 1972.

Ginther, O. J.: Utero-ovarian relationships in cattle: Physiological aspects. J. Amer. Vet. Med. Assoc. *153*:1656, 1968.

Hook, S. J. and Hafez, E. S. E.: A comparative anatomical study of the mammalian uterotubal junction. J. Morph. *125*:159, 1968.

Schultz, R. H., Burcalow, H. B. and Fahning, M. L.: A karyometric study of epithelial cells lining the glands of the bovine endometrium. J. Reprod. Fertil. *19*:169, 1969.

Younes, M. S., Robertson, E. M. and Bencosme, S. A.: Electron microscope observations on Langerhans cells in the cervix. Amer. J. Obstet. Gynec. *102*:397, 1968.

Cyclic Changes in the System

Adams, E. C. and Hertig, A. T.: Studies on the human corpus luteum. I. Observations on the ultrastructure of development and regression of the luteal cells during the menstrual cycle. J. Cell Biol. *41*:696, 1969.

Adams, E. C. and Hertig, A. T.: Studies on the human corpus luteum. II. Observations on the ultrastructure of luteal cells during pregnancy. J. Cell Biol. *41*:716, 1969.

Akins, E. L. and Morrissette, M. C.: Gross ovarian changes during estrous cycle of swine. Amer. J. Vet. Res. *29*:1953, 1968.

Fowler, E. H., Feldman, M. K. and Loeb, W. F.: Comparison of histologic features of ovarian and uterine tissues with vaginal smears of the bitch. Amer. J. Vet. Res. *32*:327, 1971.

Fowler, E. H., Loeb, W. F. and Wilson, G. P.: Vaginal cytologic examination of intact and ovariohysterectomized bitches with mammary neoplasia. Amer. J. Vet. Res. *31*:51, 1970.

Hatch, R. D.: Anatomic changes in the bovine uterus during pregnancy. Amer. J. Vet. Res. *2*:411, 1941.

Peters, H. and Levy, E.: Cell dynamics of the ovarian cycle. J. Reprod. Fertil. *11*:227, 1966.

Sanger, V. L., Engle, P. H. and Bell, D. S.: The vaginal cytology of the ewe during the estrous cycle. Amer. J. Vet. Res. *19*:283, 1958.

Schutte, A. P.: Canine vaginal cytology. II. Cyclic changes. J. Small Anim. Pract. *8*:307, 1967.

Comparative Placentology

Anderson, J. W.: Ultrastructure of the placenta and fetal membranes of the dog. I. The placenta labyrinth. Anat. Rec. *165*:5, 1969.

Ashley, C. A. Study of the human placenta with the electron microscope. Arch. Path. Chicago *80*:377, 1965.

Bjorkman, N. H.: Fine structure of cryptal and trophoblastic giant cells in the bovine placentome. J. Ultrastruc. Res. *24*:249, 1968.

Bjorkman, N. H.: Light and electron microscopic studies on cellular alterations in the normal bovine placentome. Anat. Rec. *163*:17, 1969.

Bjorkman, N. H. *An Atlas of Placental Fine Structure*. Williams & Wilkins Company, Baltimore, 1970.

Davies, J. and Glasser, S. R.: Histological and fine structural observations on the placenta of the rat. Acta Anat. *69*:542, 1968.

Enders, A. C.: A comparative study of the fine structure of the trophoblast in several hemochorial placentas. Amer. J. Anat. *116*:29, 1965.

Avian Reproductive Tract

Brambell, F. W. R.: The oogenesis of the fowl (*Gallus bankiva*). Phil. Trans. Royal Soc. (B). *214*:113, 1926.

Fell, H. F.: Histological studies of the gonads of the Fowl. II. The histogenesis of the so-called "luteal" cells in the ovary. Brit. J. Exp. Biol. *1*:293, 1924.

Fertuck, H. C. and Newstead, J. D.: Fine structural observations on magnum mucosa in quail and hen oviducts. Z. Zellforsch. *103*:447, 1970.

Hewitt, E. A.: The physiology of the reproductive system of the fowl. J. Amer. Vet. Med. Assoc. *95*:201, 1939.

Kohler, P. O., Grimley, P. M. and O'Malley, B. W.: Estrogen-induced cytodifferentiation of the ovalbumin-secreting glands of the chick oviduct. J. Cell Biol. *40*:8, 1969.

Narbaitz, R. and DeRobertis, R. M., Jr.: Postnatal evolution of steroidogenic cells in the chick ovary. Histochemie *15*:187, 1968.

Nevalainen, T. J.: Electron microscope observations on the shell gland mucosa of calcium-deficient hens (*Gallus domesticus*). Anat. Rec. *164*:127, 1969.

23 Eye and Ear

General Characteristics

Form and Function. The eye and ear are part of a special sensory system which is comprised of organs that are involved in the reception of *gustatory*, *olfactory*, *visual*, *auditory* and *positional sensations*. These organs include the taste buds, olfactory epithelium, eye, organ of Corti and the vestibular apparatus (semicircular canals, utriculus and sacculus). The first two organs were included in the chapters on digestive and respiratory organs, respectively.

The special sensory organs are part of a system which includes, besides these organs, those structures involved in general sensibility that are scattered throughout the body (Chapter 12). As an integrated and correlated system, informational input permits the organism to respond to the internal and external environment.

Eye

General Remarks. The eye is a globe-shaped structure which is somewhat flattened (Fig. 23-1). It consists of three layers or tunics: *fibrous layer*, *vascular layer* and *nervous layer*. The outermost *fibrous layer* consists of the *sclera* over most of the eye and the *cornea* rostrally. The middle *vascular layer* or *uveal tract* consists of the *choroid*, *ciliary body* and *iris*. The innermost *nervous tunic* consists of the retina.

The *dioptric media* include the *cornea*, *aqueous humor*, *lens* and *vitreous body*.

The eye is divided into *anterior* and *posterior compartments*. These are separated by the lens and its suspensory fibers. The anterior compartment is subdivided into the *anterior chamber* between the iris and the cornea and the *posterior chamber* between the iris and lens. Both compartments contain aqueous humor. The posterior compartment contains the *vitreous body*.

The primary function of the eye is to transduce visual stimuli into nervous impulses.

Various organs are associated with the eye and are included with the ocular adnexa.

Fibrous Tunic. The fibrous tunic consists of the *sclera* and *cornea*.

The *sclera* is composed of dense white fibrous connective tissue (DWFCT) which is rich in elastic fibers (Fig. 23-2). It is divisible into three zones: *episcleral zone*, *sclera proper* and *lamina fusca*. The outermost *episcleral zone* is fibroelastic tissue which is continuous with the loose connective tissue of *Tenon's space*. This is the space between the globe and the bony structure of the orbit. The loose connective tissue of Tenon's space is continuous with the subdural and subarachnoid cavities and is bounded peripherally by *Tenon's capsule*, a thin layer of DWFCT (fascia bulbi). Blood vessels are present in the episcleral zone.

The *middle portion* or *sclera proper* is a dense fibroelastic connective tissue which is minimally vascularized. It is continued rostrally into the connective tissue of the cornea. This point of transition is termed the *corneoscleral junction* and contains blood vessels and lymphatics. The edge of the cornea at this junction is termed the *limbus*.

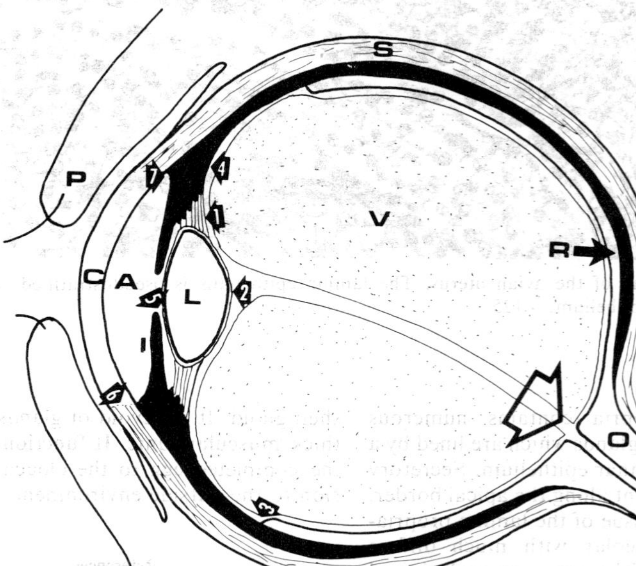

Fig. 23-1. Diagram of the eye. *S*, sclera; *R*, retina; *V*, vitreous body; *A*, anterior chamber; *O*, optic nerve; *L*, lens; *I*, iris; *C*, cornea; *P*, palpebrum; *1*, suspensory ligaments; *2*, lens capsule; *3*, ora ciliaris retinae; *4*, ciliary body and processes; *5*, posterior chamber; *6*, limbus; *7*, filtration angle; *open arrow*, optic papilla. All light micrographs are the original magnifications.

The *inner portion* or *lamina fusca* is a fibroelastic connective tissue which is especially rich in elastic fibers. The presence of chromatophores imparts a brown coloration to this zone.

The *cornea* is the transparent extension of the sclera. It consists of five layers: *epithelium*, *Bowman's membrane*, *substantia propria*, *Descemet's membrane* and *endothelium* (Fig. 23-3).

The *rostral epithelial covering of the cornea* is a nonkeratinized stratified squamous epithelium which is a continuation of the palpebral conjunctival epithelium. It varies in thickness but contains basal cells, intermediate cells and superficial cells. It is richly endowed with naked nerve endings.

Bowman's membrane or the *rostral limiting membrane* is a combination of the basement membrane and a feltwork of fine collagenous fibers. It is most clearly defined in primates but is vaguely defined in other species.

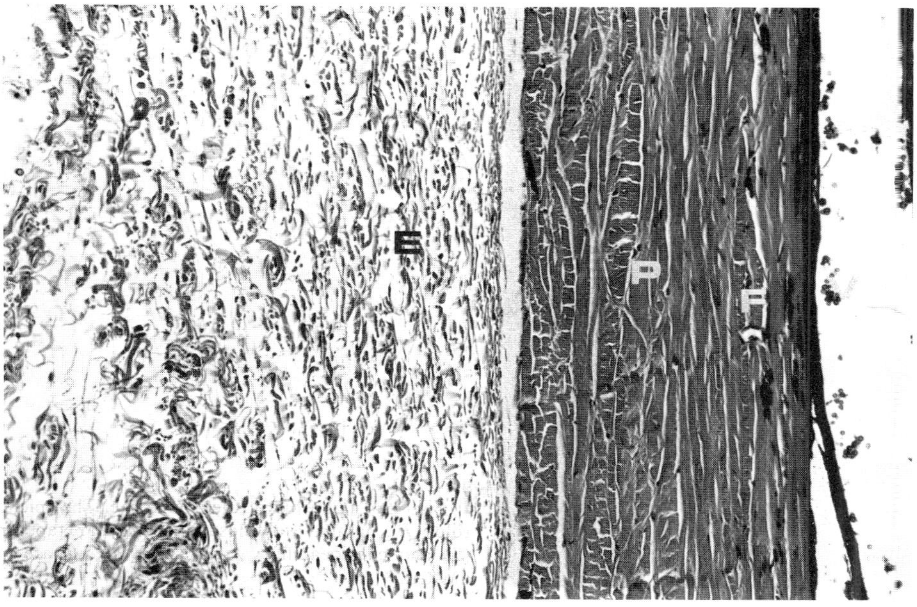

Fig. 23-2. Sclera of the canine eye. The episclera (*E*) is fibroelastic tissue. The sclera proper (*P*) is dense fibroelastic tissue which is minimally vascularized. The lamina fusca (*F*) is fibroelastic tissue which is pigmented. ×40.

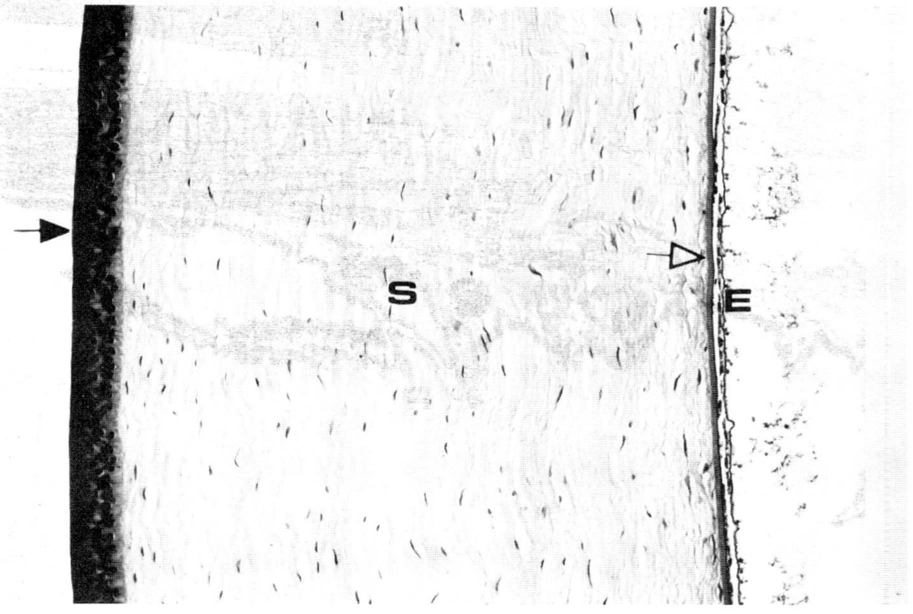

Fig. 23-3. Cornea of the canine eye. The rostral epithelium (*solid arrow*), substantia propria (*S*), Descemet's membrane (*open arrow*) and mesenchymal epithelium (*E*) are indicated. Bowman's membrane is not apparent and the mesenchymal epithelium is artifactually displaced away from the cornea. ×40.

The *substantia propria* forms the bulk of the cornea. It consists of collagenous fibers disposed in platelike configurations. Flattened fibroblasts are contained within the interfibrillar spaces. Numerous unmyelinated nerve fibers are present, but the substantia propria is devoid of blood vessels.

The *caudal limiting membrane* or *Descemet's membrane* separates the substantia propria from the endothelium. Although considered to be a basal lamina, electron microscopic investigations have revealed it to be an ordered, three-dimensional array of atypical collagen.

The *endothelium* or *mesenchymal epithelium* is composed of cuboidal or squamous cells. It separates the cornea proper from the aqueous humor of the anterior chamber.

Vascular Tunic. The *vascular tunic* or *uveal tract* consists of the *choroid coat*, *ciliary body* and *iris*. The uveal tract is not continued rostrally adjacent to the cornea but is reflected as the ciliary body and iris.

The choroid coat is subdivided into five layers: *epichoroid*, *lamina vasculosa*, *tapetum*, *lamina choriocapillaris*, *lamina elastica choroidea* (Fig. 23-4).

The *epichoroid* layer is also referred to as the *suprachoroid* layer. This layer is separated from the lamina fusca by a *perichoroidal* or *suprachoroidal* space. However, collagenous fibers pass through this space and attach the tunics to each other. This avascular layer consists of a loose array of collagenous fibers, chromatophores and fibroblasts.

The *lamina vasculosa* consists of large vessels embedded within a loose connective tissue which contains some chromatophores.

The *tapetum* is either fibrous or cellular. A *fibrous tapetum* consists of collagenous fibers. It is present in the eyes of horses, cattle, sheep and goats. A *cellular tapetum* consists of polygonal cells which contain crystals. This structure is present in the dog and cat and enhances dark-adapted vision. The porcine eye lacks a tapetum.

The *choriocapillary layer* (*lamina capillarium*) is a layer which is rich in capillaries. These are the vascular supply which provide nourishment for the outer part of the tunica nervosa.

The *elastic membrane* is an accumulation of elastic fibers adjacent to the basal lamina of the pigmented epithelium. It is also referred to as ***Bruch's membrane***.

The *ciliary body* is the anterior continuation of the choroid (Fig. 23-5). It consists of contributions from the choroid and retina. The ciliary body begins at the *ora ciliaris retinae*, the point at which the nervous portion of the retina stops (Fig. 23-6). The pigmented epithelium and a non-nervous columnar cell continuation of the retina continue rostrally to cover the ciliary body.

The bulk of the ciliary body consists of

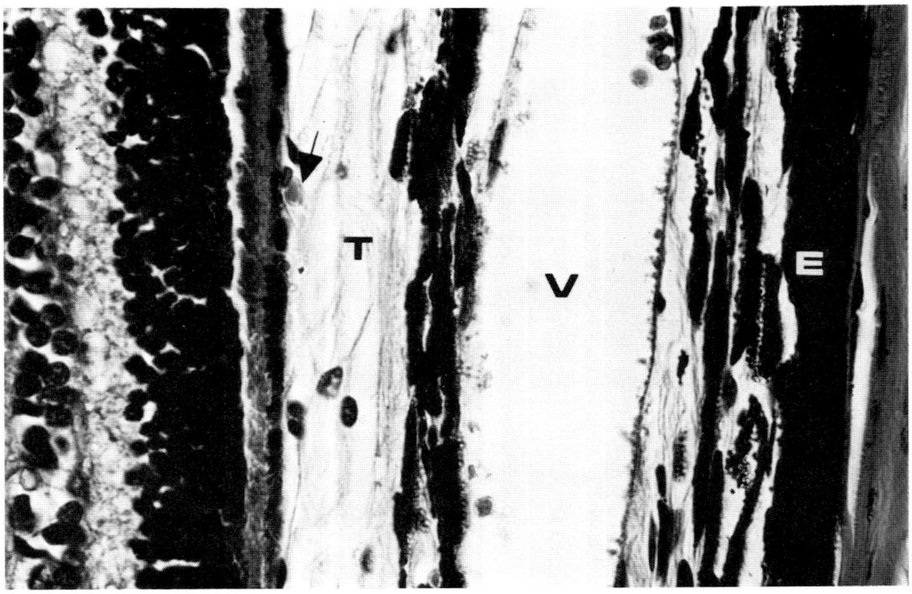

Fig. 23-4. Choroid of the canine eye. The epichoroid (*E*), lamina vasculosa (*V*), cellular tapetum (*T*) and choriocapillary layer (*solid arrow*) are indicated. ×160.

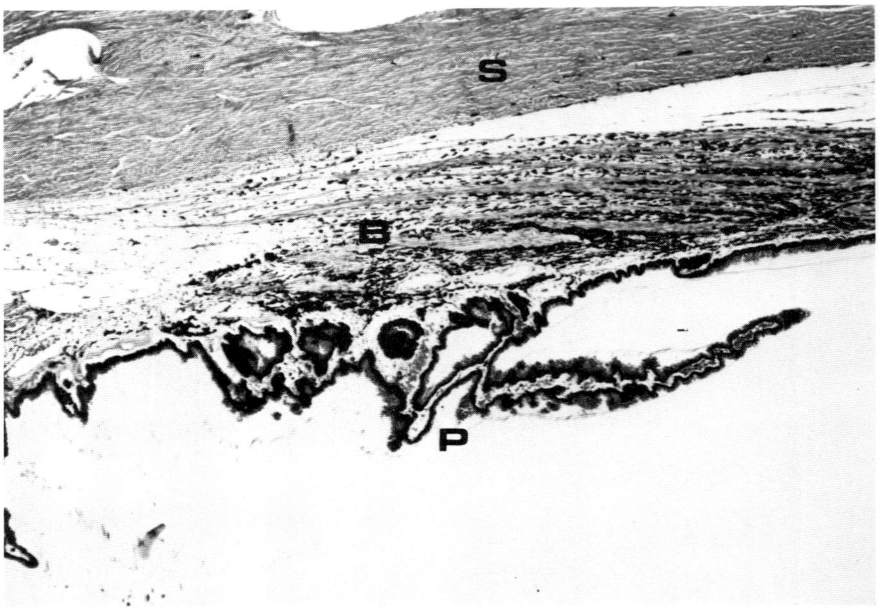

Fig. 23-5. Ciliary body and processes of the canine eye. The ciliary body (*B*) and processes (*P*) are internal to the sclera (*S*). The ciliary body and processes are the anterior continuation of the choroid coat. ×10.

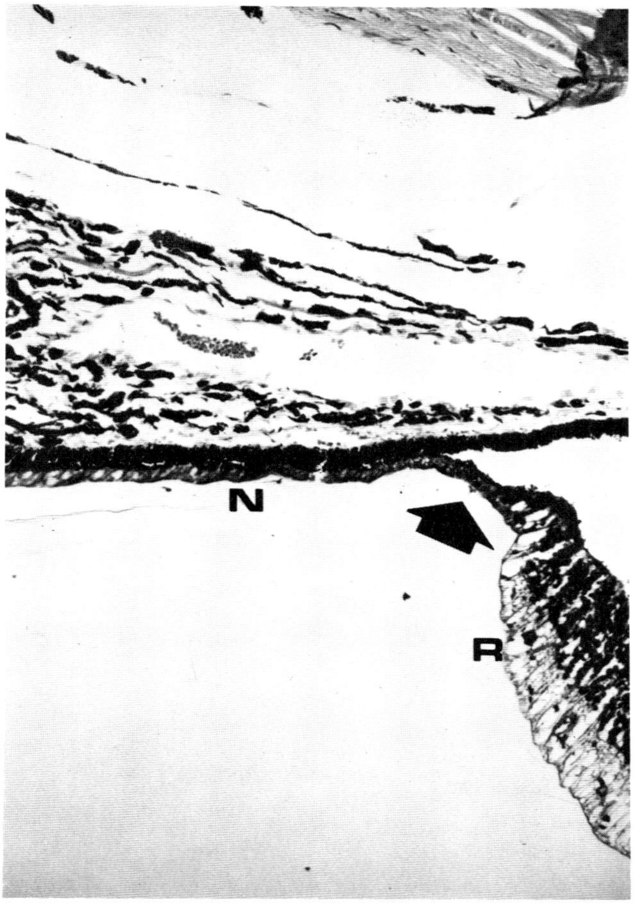

Fig. 23-6. Ora ciliaris retinae of the canine eye. The ora ciliaris retinae (*arrow*) is the continuation of the retina (*R*) as a non-nervous covering (*N*) of ciliary body, ciliary processes and iris. ×40.

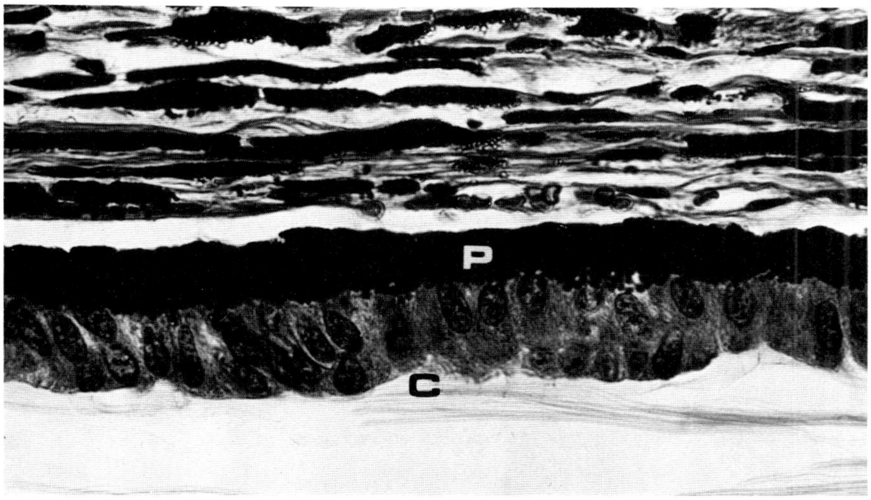

Fig. 23-7. Pars ciliaris retinae of the canine eye. This layer consists of pigmented epithelium (*P*) and ciliary epithelium (*C*). The latter is the non-nervous, anterior continuation of the retina. ×160.

areolar connective tissue rich in elastic fibers, an extensive capillary network and smooth muscle. The smooth muscle, *ciliary muscle*, consists of three layers which arise from the ciliary tendon which is attached to the sclera.

The mass of smooth muscle, areolar connective tissue and vasculature is bounded by an *elastic lamina*. This is the anterior continuation of *Bruch's membrane*. Internal to this membrane is the *basal lamina* of the *pigmented epithelium* of the retina which is continued rostrally. Internal to this cellular layer is the *ciliary epithelium*. This layer of columnar cells is the rostral continuation of non-nervous and nonpigmented cells which began at the *ora ciliaris retinae*. This bilayered sheet of cells is the *pars ciliaris retinae* (Fig. 23-7). The *internal limiting membrane* is a peripheral fibrillar condensation of the vitreous body. It covers the retina and ciliary body, continues rostrally and blends with the fibers which extend from the ciliary process to the lens.

The *ciliary process* is the most rostral extension of the ciliary body at the base of the iris. Zonular fibers extend from it as suspensory fibers of the lens. The extensive capillary network of the ciliary process is probably responsible for the elaboration of aqueous humor into the posterior chamber of the anterior compartment.

Contraction of the ciliary musculature does not stretch the lens and accommodate it for distant vision. Rather, contraction of the muscle fibers causes the sclera to indent slightly. This relieves the tension on the suspensory fibers which causes the lens to thicken for close vision. When these muscle fibers are relaxed the elasticity of the supporting coat flattens the lens for distant vision.

The *iris* is the extension of the choroid coat into the anterior compartment (Fig. 23-8). The iris is oriented radially and its distal margin defines the *pupil*. The rostral border of the iris is covered by *endothelial cells* (*mesenchymal epithelium*) which are reflected from the posterior lining of the cornea. These cells reside on the *rostral limiting layer* which consists of basal lamina, pigmented cells as well as collagenous and reticular fibers. The *iridial stroma* consists of areolar connective tissue, blood vessels, chromatophores and smooth muscle. The *pupillary sphincter* consists of a mass of circumferentially oriented smooth muscle fibers along the pupillary border of the iris. The *pupillary dilator* consists of radially oriented fibers along the caudal border of the iris.

The posterior border of the iris is covered by the same cells as the ciliary body. The cells include the anterior extension of the pigmented epithelium of the retina and the ciliary epithelial cells. These cells form the *pars iridica retinae*.

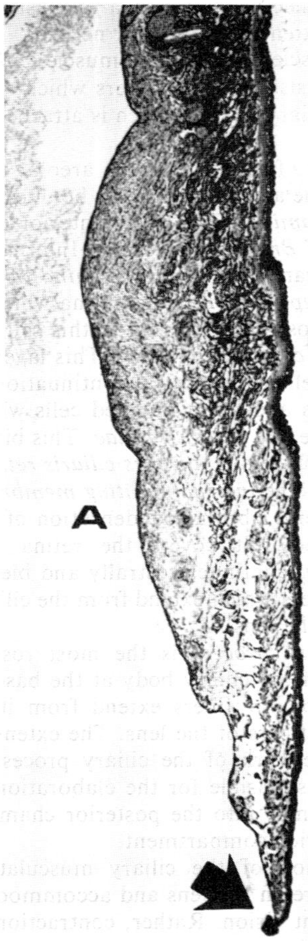

Fig. 23-8. Iris of the canine eye. The pars ciliaris retinae is continued on the posterior (*P*) surface of the iris as the pars iridica retinae. The corpora nigra extend along the pupillary margin (*arrow*) toward the anterior surface. (*A*) × 10.

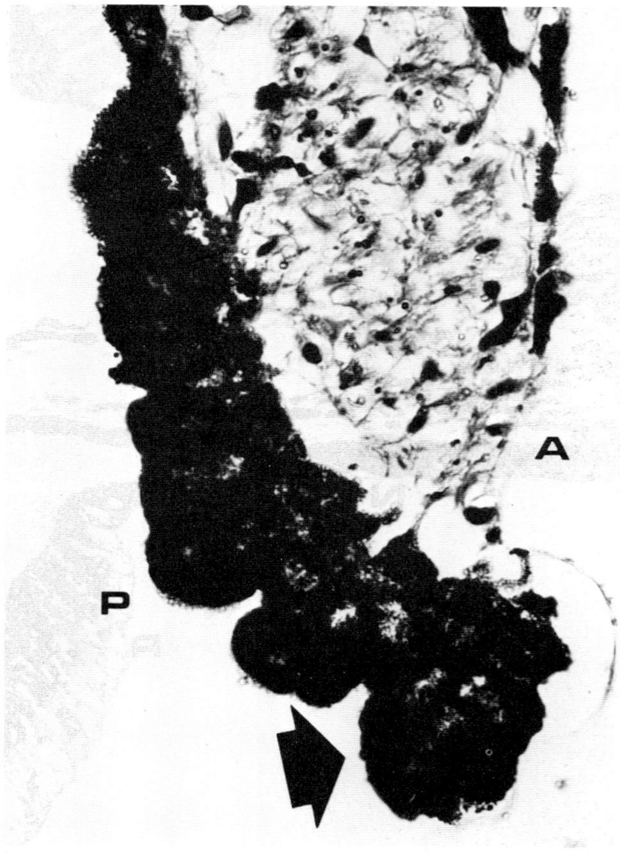

Fig. 23-9. Corpus nigrum of the canine eye. The black body (*arrow*) is an extension of the pigmented epithelium from the posterior surface (*P*) toward the anterior surface (*A*). ×160.

Corpora nigra occur along the pupillary margin of the iris (Fig. 23-9). They are prominences of the posterior pigment epithelium which extend around the pupillary margin.

Compartments of the Eye. The eye is divided, by virtue of the lens and its supportive structures, into anterior and posterior compartments (Fig. 23-1). The anterior compartment is bounded by the cornea, iris and lens. It is subdivided into anterior and posterior chambers. The ciliary process forms aqueous humor as a transudate from the blood. The aqueous humor is added in the posterior chamber. It is removed from the anterior chamber at the *filtration angle* (Fig. 23-10). In domestic species, *spaces of Fontana*, located within the collagenous and reticular fiber network, pick up the aqueous humor wherein it moves to the episcleral vessels. In the ox and man, the *canal of Schlemm*, a modified vein, is present. In other domestic species there is a vascular plexus at the corneoscleral junction which is continuous with the episcleral circulation.

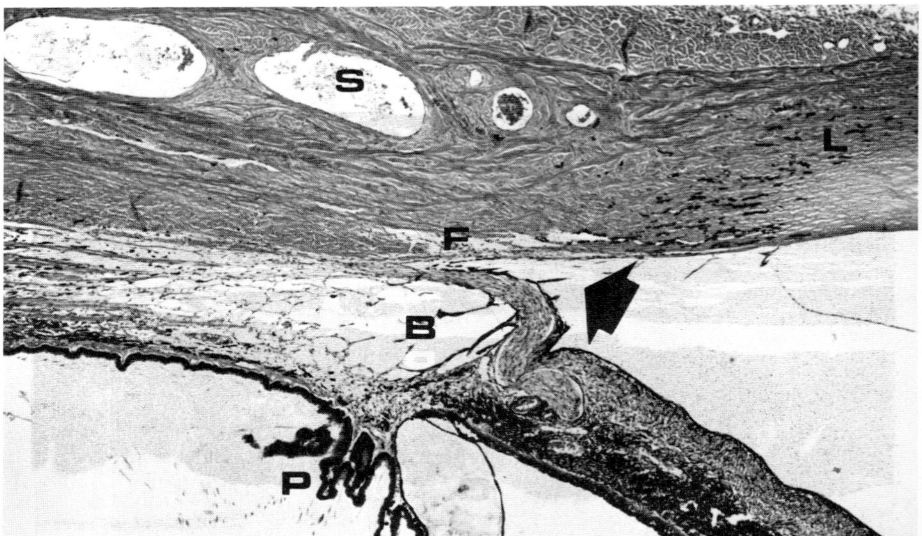

Fig. 23-10. Filtration angle of the canine eye. The filtration angle (*arrow*) is located between th junction of the sclera, iris and ciliary body (*B*). Spaces of Fontana (*F*) are continuous with the sclera plexus (*S*). The limbus (*L*) and ciliary processes (*P*) are apparent also. ×10.

The posterior compartment is filled with a gelatinous fluid, the *vitreous body*, which contains proteins and mucosubstances. It is delineated by the *inner limiting membrane*, which is a condensation of its fibrillar components. The turnover of this material is probably handled by the ciliary body.

Dioptric Media. The *dioptric* or *refractive media* include all those entities through which incoming light rays must pass to reach the photosensitive cells of the retina. These include cornea, aqueous humor, lens, vitreous body and the retina.

The cornea and the lens are responsible for focusing incoming rays on the retina. The lens is a biconcave structure which consists of a *capsule*, *lens epithelium* and *lens fibers* (Fig. 23-11).

The *lens capsule* consists of several layers of collagenous fibers considered to be secreted by the lens epithelium. The suspensory fibers from the ciliary process insert into the lens capsule.

The lens epithelium is composed of cuboidal cells which line the anterior surface of the lens.

The lens fibers, unlike typical connective tissue fibers, are actually converted cells that become stretched at the equator of the lens, lose their nuclei and are converted to an orderly arrangement of parallel hexagonal fibers. These fibers are held together by a cementing material which probably facilitates fiber movement during a change of lens shape. A *lens star*, actually a Y-shaped configuration, is formed near the center of the lens at the point where fibers from the opposite poles of the equator meet one another.

Retina. The *retina* or *nervous tunic* is responsible for the reception and transduction of light stimuli and the transmission of these signals in the form of nerve impulses to the appropriate portions of the brain.

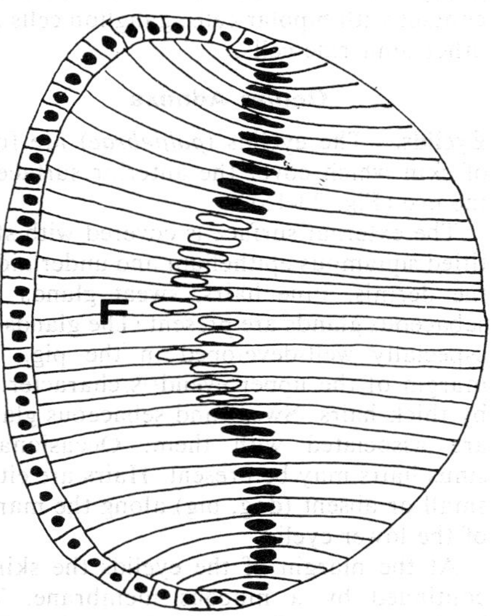

Fig. 23-11. Diagram of the lens. The lens is covered by a capsule of collagenous fibers. The cuboidal epithelium (*E*) lines the anterior surface. The lens fibers (*F*) are converted epithelial cells.

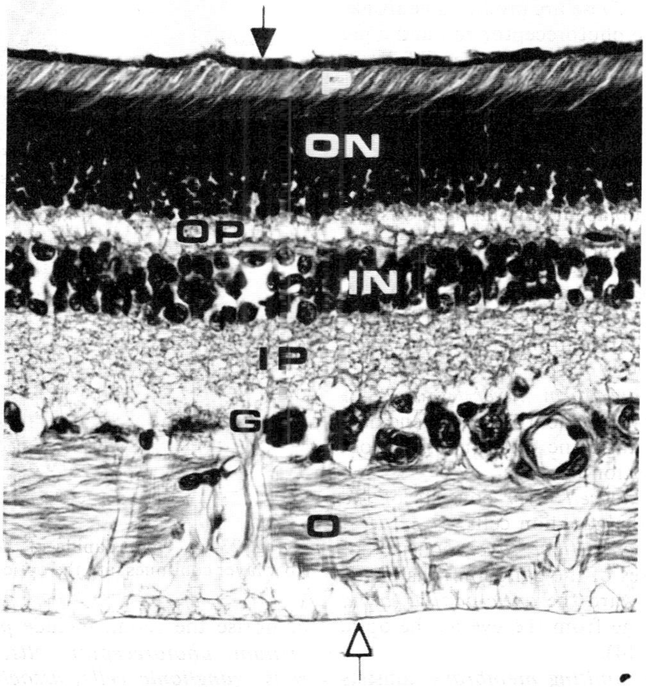

Fig. 23-12. Retina of the canine eye. *P*, photoreceptor cell layer; *ON*, outer nuclear layer; *OP*, outer plexiform layer; *IN*, inner nuclear layer; *IP*, inner plexiform layer; *G*, ganglion cell layer; *O*, optic nerve fiber layer; *solid arrow*, pigment epithelium; *open arrow*, inner limiting membrane. The external limiting membrane is not apparent. ×100. (Note: The photoreceptor cell layer is positioned away from incoming light rays.)

The retina is divisible into ten distinct layers: *pigmented epithelium*, *photoreceptor cell layer*, *external limiting membrane*, *outer nuclear layer*, *outer plexiform layer*, *inner nuclear layer*, *inner plexiform layer*, *ganglionic cell layer*, *optic nerve fiber layer* and *inner limiting membrane* (Figs. 23-12 and 23-13).

The *pigmented epithelium* resides on a basal lamina adjacent to the elastic membrane of the choroid. These cells are cuboidal with a paracentrally positioned nucleus and centrally disposed pigment granules. Long cellular processes extend between the photoreceptors. Under high illumination, pigment moves into the cellular processes and prevents diffusion of the light to adjacent receptors. The intimate contact of the pigmented cells with the photoreceptors is

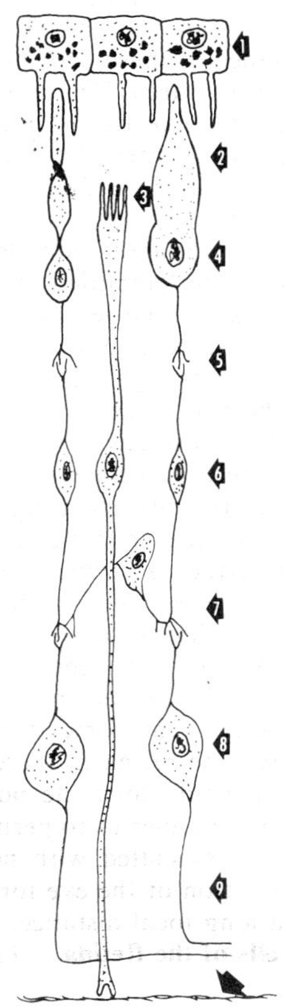

Fig. 23-13. Diagram of the retina. *1*, pigment epithelium; *2*, photoreceptor cell layer; *3*, outer limiting membrane; *4*, outer nuclear layer; *5*, outer plexiform layer; *6*, inner nuclear layer; *7*, inner plexiform layer; *8*, ganglion cell layer; *9*, optic nerve fiber layer; *solid arrow*, inner limiting membrane.

apparently necessary for visual pigment synthesis.

The *photoreceptor layer* consists of the rods and cones. These are modified neuronal processes of the photoreceptor rod and cone cells which will be described in detail following the description of the retinal layers.

The *outer nuclear layer* is comprised of the nuclei of the photoreceptor cells.

The *outer plexiform layer* consists of axons of the photoreceptor cells, the dendrites of the subjacent bipolar neurons, as well as the fibers from association neurons located in this zone or the periphery of the subjacent nuclear zone.

The *inner nuclear layer* contains the cell bodies of bipolar neurons and association neurons.

The *inner plexiform layer* consists of axons of the bipolar neurons, the dendrites of subjacent ganglionic cells and the processes of association neurons.

The *ganglionic cell layer* consists of the cell bodies of the ganglion cells.

The *optic nerve fiber layer* consists of axonal processes of the ganglion cells which are directed toward the *optic papilla* (*blind spot*) and emerge from the eye as the optic nerve (Fig. 23-14).

The *internal limiting membrane* consists of fibrillar material and the conjoined processes of the supporting Müller cells. The *outer limiting membrane*, located just peripheral to the outer nuclear layer, is an incomplete structure formed by the processes of Müller cells forming junctions with the cell bodies of the photoreceptor cells. The cell bodies of these cells are located in the inner nuclear area. The peripheral processes form the external or outer limiting membrane, while their internal processes abut on the outer surface of the inner limiting membrane.

Despite the apparent complexity of the retina, it may be simplified by recognizing that it consists of three neurons in succession with intervening regions of synapses. Also, light must pass through the retina in order to stimulate the photoreceptor cells.

The area of most acute vision in domestic animals is the *area centralis retinae*. Cone cells, bipolar neurons and ganglion cells are increased in number in this area. Although a depression (*fovea centralis*) does not occur in domestic species, this macular region is comparable to that which occurs in man.

The retina of most species is regularly curved along the posterior portion of the globe of the eye. The horse, however, has a *ramp retina*. The retina in these animals is irregularly curved along the posterior surface in such a manner as to permit different axial lengths associated with near and far vision. A rotation of the eye for near vision results in a long focal distance.

Specific Cells of the Retina. The cells that comprise the retina include *pigmented epithelium*, *photoreceptor cells*, *bipolar neurons*, *ganglionic cells*, *association neurons* and *neuroglial elements*.

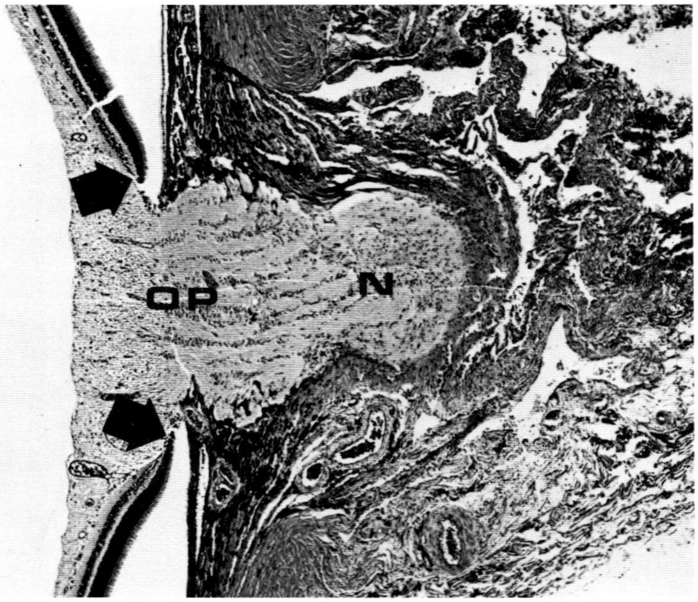

Fig. 23-14. Optic papilla of the canine eye. The nervous retina stops (*arrows*) and the optic nerve fiber layer continues into the optic papilla (*OP*). The fibers continue as the optic nerve (*N*). ×10.

The *photoreceptor cells* are neuroepithelial cells modified for the reception, transduction and transmission of visual stimuli. These cells are the *rod cells* and *cone cells*.

The *rods* consist of an *outer segment*, *connecting cilium*, *inner segment*, *outer rod fiber*, *perikaryon*, *inner rod fiber* and *rod spherule*. The outer segment is an elongated process of the cell which contains numerous double-membraned lamellae and the visual pigment, *rhodopsin*. Nine doublets of microtubules (devoid of a central pair) continue through the *connecting cilium* to terminate in a typical basal body within the expanded inner segment. The inner segment narrows as the outer rod fiber. This is continuous with the perikaryon. The inner rod fiber or axon terminates in a swelling, the *rod spherule*, and synapses with the dendrite of a bipolar neuron.

The *cones* are similar to the rods. The lamellae of the outer segment are often continuous with the plasmalemma. This segment, which is larger than that of the rods, contains *iodopsin*. The connecting cilium is not constricted. The inner and outer segments, therefore, have a conelike appearance. The nucleus of the cones does not contain as much dense chromatin as that of the rods. Also, the cell bodies are located in the outer portion of the outer nuclear layer.

The rods are generally distributed throughout the retina, while the cones are the predominant or only type of photoreceptor in the *area centralis retinae*. This is the region for bright light vision and is the area of most acute vision. The remaining portion of the retina, rich in rods, is for dark-adapted vision. There is wide species variation in the distribution of the type of photoreceptor cells.

Müller cells are neuroglial elements unique to the retina. *Astrocytes*, *oligodendrogliocytes* and *microgliocytes* are present and typical. *Amacrine cells* and *horizontal cells* are association neurons within the retina which serve to modify the visual stimuli from other cells of the retina. The horizontal cells are in contact with groups of rods. The amacrine cells are in contact with bipolar cells, ganglion cells and other amacrine cells.

Ocular Adnexa

Eyelids. The eyelids (*palpebrae*) are folds of skin which cover the anterior surface of the eye (Fig. 23-15).

The external surface is covered with stratified squamous epithelium and underlaid by the dermis. Fine hairs, sweat glands and sebaceous glands are present. The glands are especially well-developed in the pig. The margin of the upper eyelid is characterized by thick hairs. Sweat and sebaceous glands are associated with them. Occasionally, sinus hairs may be present. Hairs are either small or absent (dog, pig) along the margin of the lower eyelid.

At the margin of the eyelids the skin is continued by a mucous membrane. The lamina epithelialis of the internal surface (*conjunctiva*) varies throughout its distribution. It may be stratified columnar or strati-

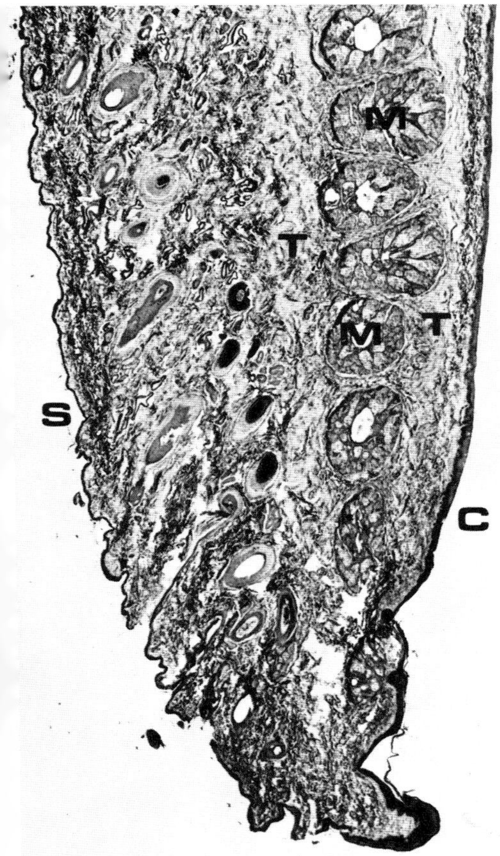

Fig. 23-15. The palpebrum. The skin (*S*) is reflected at the margin of the eye as the palpebral conjunctiva (*C*). The palpebrum contains Meibomian glands (*M*) within a core of DWFCT as the tarsus (*T*). ×4.

fied squamous with goblet cells. At the point of reflection on to the surface of the cornea, it is stratified squamous.

The DWFCT of the dermis and lamina propria fuse centrally as the *tarsus*. The tarsus consists of laminae of collagenous fibers. The extent of the tarsus corresponds to the shape of the eyeball covered by the palpebra. Anterior to the tarsus are bundles of striated muscle fibers and smooth muscle fibers of the *orbicularis oculi* and the *levator palpebrae superioris*.

The *tarsal glands* (*glands of Meibom*) are modified sebaceous glands which open at the margin of the eyelid (Fig. 23-15). Sweat and sebaceous glands of this region are associated with hairs.

Nictitating Membrane. The *nictitating membrane* or *third eyelid* (*palpebra tertia*) is a fold of conjunctiva which contains hyaline cartilage (ruminants, dog) or elastic cartilage (horse, pig, cat). The areolar connective tissue may contain some smooth muscle fibers (cat). Lymphatic nodules are extensive along the bulbar surface (Fig. 23-16).

The *superficial glands* of this organ surround the cartilaginous plate (Fig. 23-17).

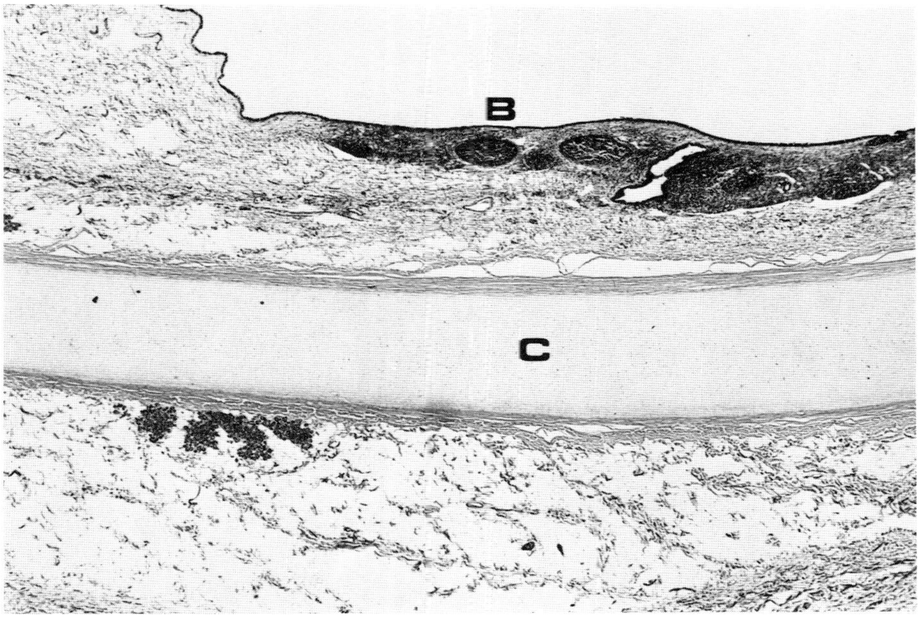

Fig. 23-16. Portion of the bovine nictitating membrane. The bulbar surface (*B*) has lymphatic nodules associated with it. The core of the structure is hyaline cartilage (*C*). ×4.

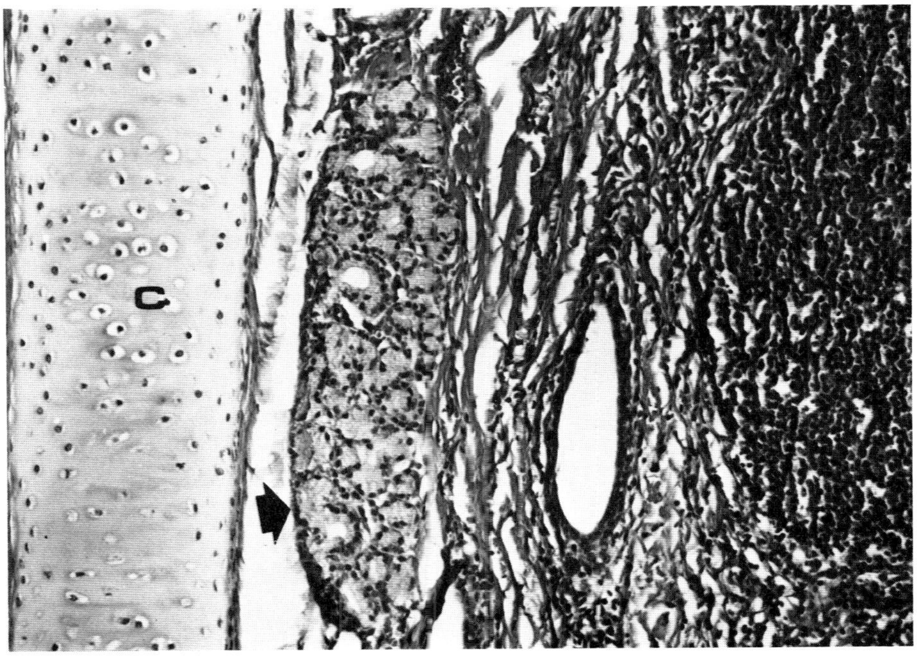

Fig. 23-17. Canine nictitating membrane. The cartilage (*C*) is closely associated with superficial glands of this organ (*arrow*). These are seromucoid glands. ×40.

Their secretion is serous (horse, cat), seromucoid (dog, ruminants) and mucoid (pig). The *deep gland* (*gland of Harder*) is a mixed gland which occurs in the pig and ox (Fig. 23-18).

Lacrimal Apparatus. The lacrimal apparatus consists of the *lacrimal glands*, the *conjunctival sac* and the *lacrimal passages*.

The *lacrimal glands* are located at the dorsolateral margins of the orbit. (Figs. 23-19 and 23-20). In the pig, the glands are mucoid.

The secretion of these glands, *tears*, serves to moisten the conjunctiva, while evaporative water loss is diminished by the mucoid secretion of palpebral goblet cells and the oily secretion of the glands of Meibom.

The fluids of the *conjunctival sac* accumulate in the medial widening of the sac, *lacus lacrimalis*, enter the *lacrimal canaliculi* through the *puncta lacrimalia* and continue to the *lacrimal sac* and thence to the *nasolacrimal duct*. The luminal surfaces of the lacrimal sac and duct are lined by a squamous or columnar epithelium (horse).

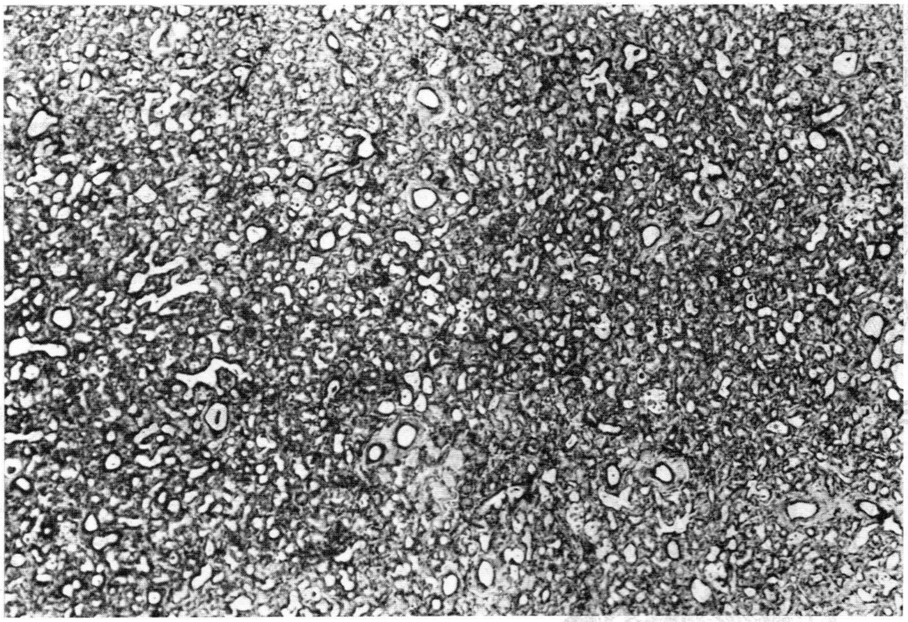

Fig. 23-18. Bovine gland of Harder. It is a seromucoid gland. ×16.

Ear

General Remarks. The ear is responsible for the reception of auditory stimuli, mechanical transduction of the stimuli and the transmission of nerve impulses to appropriate portions of the central nervous system. To accomplish these functions, the ear consists of various components: *auricle*, *auditory meatus*, *tympanic membrane*, *tympanic cavity with ossicles*, *cochlea* and *organ of Corti*.

The ear also functions, however, as an organ of balance. The components of the vestibular portion of the inner ear include *semicircular canals*, *utriculus* and *sacculus*.

External Ear. The external ear includes the *auricle* and *external auditory meatus*.

The *auricle* or *pinna* is a sac of typical skin which contains hairs and associated glands. On the anterior surface (concave side), sebaceous glands are numerous and the frequency of hairs diminishes toward the external auditory meatus. The dermal tissue contained within the sac is typical and contains supportive structures composed of hyaline or elastic cartilage. Striated muscle associated with the movement of the ear is also contained within the fold of integument.

The pinna is the "antenna" of the auditory apparatus. In most species, it also serves the important function of "directional finding."

The *external auditory meatus* or canal is the tubular extension of the auricle. The surface lining of the meatus is typical skin with some hairs and numerous sebaceous and *ceruminous glands*. Ceruminous glands are modified apocrine tubular sweat glands. The combined product of the ceruminous glands and the sebaceous glands, *cerumen*, is

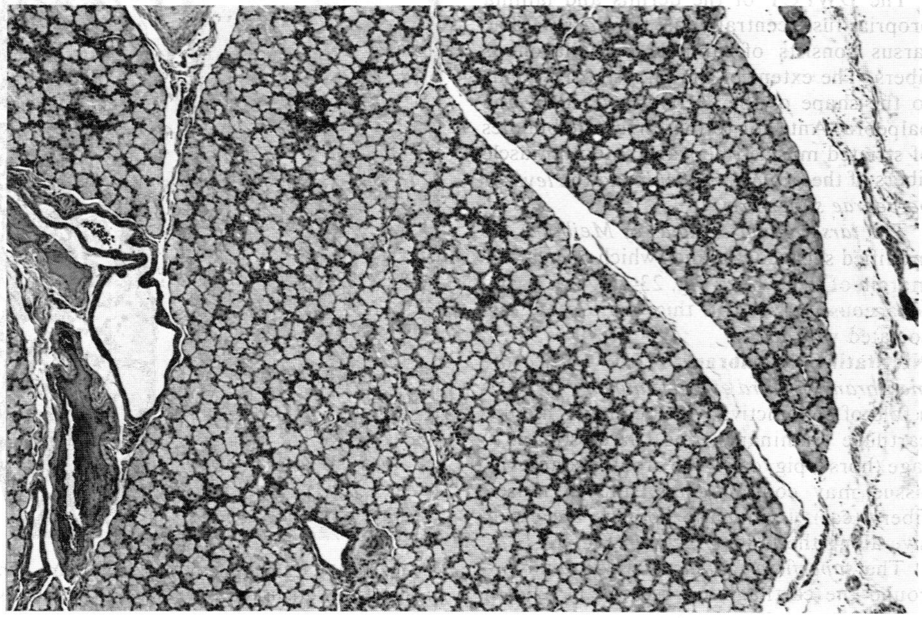

Fig. 23-19. Equine lacrimal gland. These are serous glands. ×16.

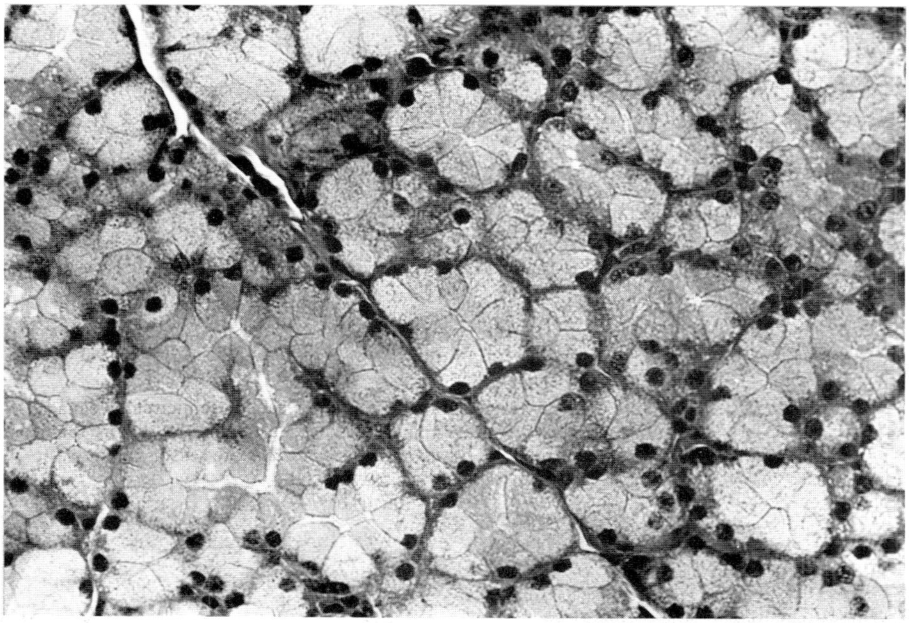

Fig. 23-20. Lining of the equine lacrimal gland. The adenomeres are serous. ×100.

a brown, waxy material which protects the canal and keeps the tympanic membrane moist and pliable.

The underlying dermis is typical and blends with the periosteum or perichondrium of the supportive bone or cartilage.

Middle Ear. The middle ear includes the *tympanic membrane*, *tympanic cavity*, *ear ossicles* and the *internal auditory meatus*. Within the middle ear, the vibrations of the air are transduced to mechanical movement of the ossicles. These, in turn, produce waves in the perilymph of the inner ear via vibrations of the membranous *oval window*.

The *tympanic membrane* consists of an outer and inner epithelium which covers a core of collagenous fibers. The *outer epithelium* is a reflection of the epithelial lining of the external auditory meatus. It is, however, hairless and glandless. The core of connective tissue consists of outer radial and inner circular fibers. The *inner epithelium* is a simple squamous or cuboidal lining which is continuous with that which lines the tympanic cavity.

The *tympanic cavity* is lined by a squamous or cuboidal epithelium. At the opening of the *auditory tube* (*internal auditory meatus*), ciliated columnar cells are present. The cavity contains three *auditory ossicles: malleus* (*hammer*), *incus* (*anvil*) and *stapes* (*stirrup*). These bones are covered by a periosteum and are connected to each other by two diarthroidal joints. The handle of the malleus is embedded in the tympanic membrane, while the stapes is attached to the oval window by a fibrous joint. Two muscles are associated with these ossicles, the *tensor tympani* and *stapedius* muscles. These are striated muscles which serve to dampen the effects of high-frequency vibrations.

The *auditory tube* (*Eustachian tube*, *internal auditory meatus*, *pharyngotympanic tube*) connects the tympanic cavity with the nasopharynx. It is lined by respiratory epithelium—pseudostratified ciliated columnar epithelium. The lamina propria-submucosa consists of areolar connective tissue with diffuse lymphatic tissue and numerous serous and mixed glands. The connective tissue is continuous with the periosteum or perichondrium of the bone and cartilage which lines the canal. During deglutition (swallowing), the tube is opened and the air pressure within the tympanic cavity is equalized with the air pressure in the external auditory meatus.

The *guttural pouches* of the horse are lined by a pseudostratified ciliated columnar epithelium with goblet cells. The supportive lamina propria is rich in smooth muscle fibers, elastic and collagenous fibers, serous and mucous glands, and lymph nodules.

Inner Ear. The inner ear is located within the petrous portion of the temporal bone. The bone forms the *osseous labyrinth*. A *membranous labyrinth* is contained within the osseous chamber. Its shape conforms to that of the osseous labyrinth and consists of squamous epithelium throughout most of its distribution. The membranous labyrinth contains *endolymph* and is surrounded by *perilymph*. It was believed that endolymph is derived from cerebrospinal fluid, since the endolymphatic sac is close to the dura mater near the posterior margin of the petrous temporal bone. However, other areas (*stria vascularis*) have been implicated in the production of endolymph. It is more probable that endolymph is returned to the cerebrospinal fluid via the endolymphatic sac. Perilymph is probably tissue fluid.

The form of the membranous labyrinth is complex, for it is divided into numerous sacs and canals which are interconnected and separated by bone. The subdivisions of the membranous labryinth include *utriculus*, *sacculus*, *endolymphatic duct*, *endolymphatic sac*, *semicircular canals*, *ductus reuniens* and the *ductus cochlearis* (Fig. 23-21). The latter is involved with auditory sensations, while the saccule, utricle and semicircular canals are involved in balance.

Vestibular Apparatus

General Remarks. The vestibular apparatus is that special sensory organ which is concerned with awareness of the position of the body. Two types of sensations are involved in this sense: *static sensation* and *kinetic sensation*. Special sensory regions of the sacculus and utriculus (*macula sacculi* and *macula utriculi*) contain substances which respond constantly to gravity. Other sensory areas (*cristae ampullares*) of the semicircular canals respond to movement of endolymphatic fluid and are probably responsible for the kinetic sensations, e.g., acceleration.

Utriculus and Sacculus. These portions of the membranous labyrinth are lined by a squamous or cuboidal epithelium, except in the sensory areas. The sensory areas are similar to each other, but their orientation is different. They are oriented perpendicular to one another.

The *macula utriculi* and the *macula sacculi* are responsible for the static sensations associated with balance. The epithelium of these sensory areas consists of sensory cells and sustentacular cells (Fig. 23-22). There are two types of sensory cells in the maculae (Fig. 23-23). One type (type I) is a goblet-shaped cell which does not reach the basal surface. Its apical border has numerous stereocilia and one kinocilium. The other type (type II) is a columnar cell with a similar apical morphology. The stereocilia (hairs) and kinocilia of both of these cells are not free in the endolymph. Rather, they are embedded in a gelatinous matrix which contains *otoconia* or *otoliths*. These are concretions of calcium carbonate and protein which move in response to gravity as the position of the head changes. The gelatinous material and otoliths are referred to as the *otolithic membrane*.

The *sustentacular cells* are nonciliated columnar cells. They support and nurture the other cells with which they are associated.

The basal margins of the sensory cells are surrounded by nerve endings which arise from the vestibular branch of the auditory nerve.

Semicircular Canals. The semicircular canals are tubules which arise from the utriculus. The three canals are oriented perpendicular to each other. There are three sensory areas, *cristae ampullares*, located at

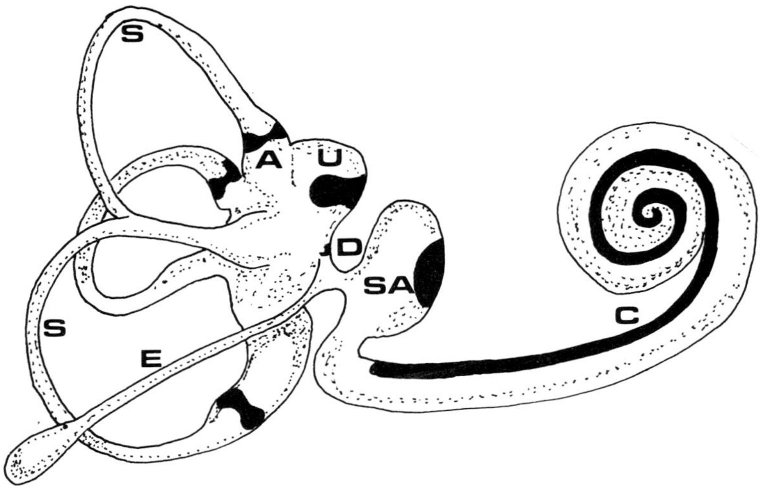

Fig. 23-21. Diagram of the inner ear. *S*, semicircular canals; *A*, ampulla; *E*, endolymphatic duct; *U*, utriculus; *D*, ductus reuniens; *SA*, sacculus; *C*, cochlea. The *black areas* are sensory areas.

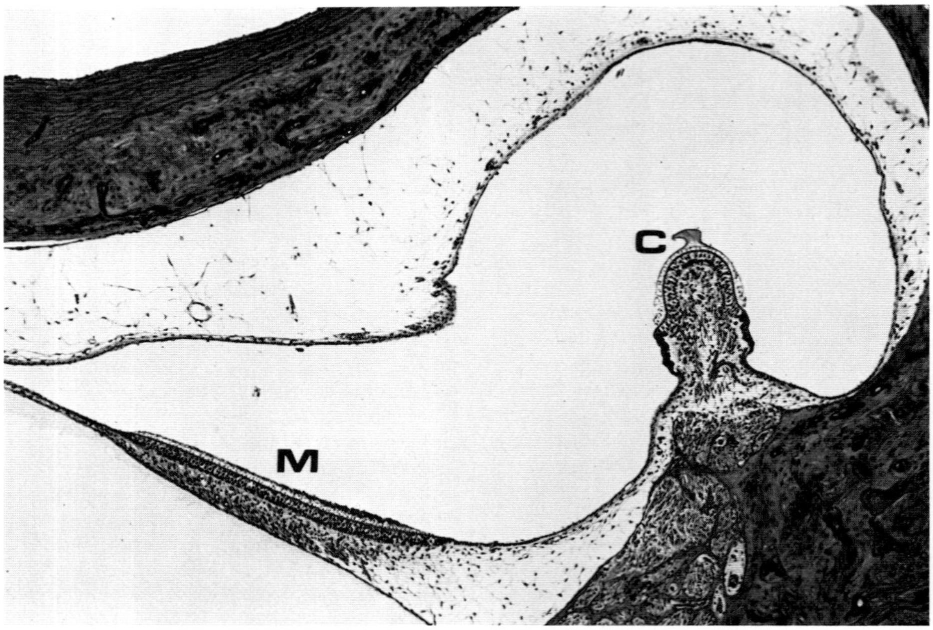

Fig. 23-22. A semicircular canal and utriculus. The macula utriculus (*M*) and one of the cristae ampullares (*C*) are apparent. ×16.

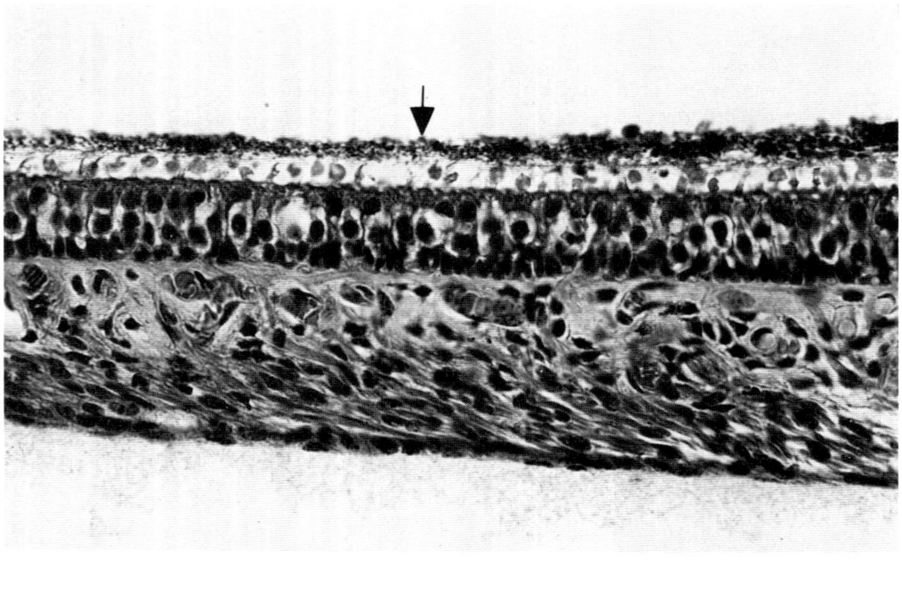

Fig. 23-23. Macula utriculus. Otoconia (*arrow*) occur above the cells. The otoliths are embedded in a gelatinous material. ×100.

the bulbous enlargements (ampullae) of the canals close to the point of contact with the utriculus (Figs. 23-22 and 23-24).

The lining of the semicircular canals is simple squamous or cuboidal. In the sensory areas, the epithelium is thickened and a mound of cells is formed (Fig. 23-25). The constituent cells are similar to those described with the maculae. However, the otoliths are not present and the kinocilia and stereocilia project into a conical mass of gelatinous material, the *cupola*.

The currents of the endolymph during movement probably distort the cupola and embedded hairs, thus accounting for kinesthetic sensation.

Auditory Apparatus

General Remarks. The auditory apparatus is responsible for the reception of auditory stimuli, the transduction of the mechanical signal, the transmission of nerve impulses to the central nervous system and the dissipation of the energy of the auditory signal. This is accomplished through the *ductus cochlearis*, *scala vestibuli* and *scala tympani*.

The cochlear duct is part of the membranous labyrinth and is connected to the vestibular apparatus by the *ductus reuniens*. The scala vestibuli and scala tympani are perilymphatic spaces that surround the cochlear duct. The scala vestibuli is continuous with the scala tympani at the *helicotrema*. This is the apex of the spirally arranged organ.

The movement of the stapes causes a corresponding movement in the oval window. In turn, this causes waves to move through the perilymph of the scala vestibuli. These waves ascend in the scala vestibuli, communicate with the scala tympani at the helicotrema, descend within the perilymph of the scala tympani and dissipate at the round window. The latter is a fibrous covering in the wall of the tympanic cavity.

Cochlea. The cochlear duct, scala vestibuli and scala tympani are disposed in a spiral manner within the osseous labyrinth of the petrous portion of the temporal bone (Fig. 23-26). A central core of bone, the *modiolus*, and its lateral projections, the *bony spiral lamina*, support the membranous subdivisions of the *cochlea*. Fibrous connective tissue extends from the *spiral lamina* to the outer wall of the osseous labyrinth forming the *basilar membrane*. Another fibrous sheath extends from the spiral lamina and passes obliquely to the outer wall of the osseous labyrinth forming the vestibular membrane. The osseous labyrinth, therefore, is subdivided into three membranous compartments (Fig. 23-27). The dorsal compartment, *scala vestibuli*, is lined by a squamous epithelium. The middle compart-

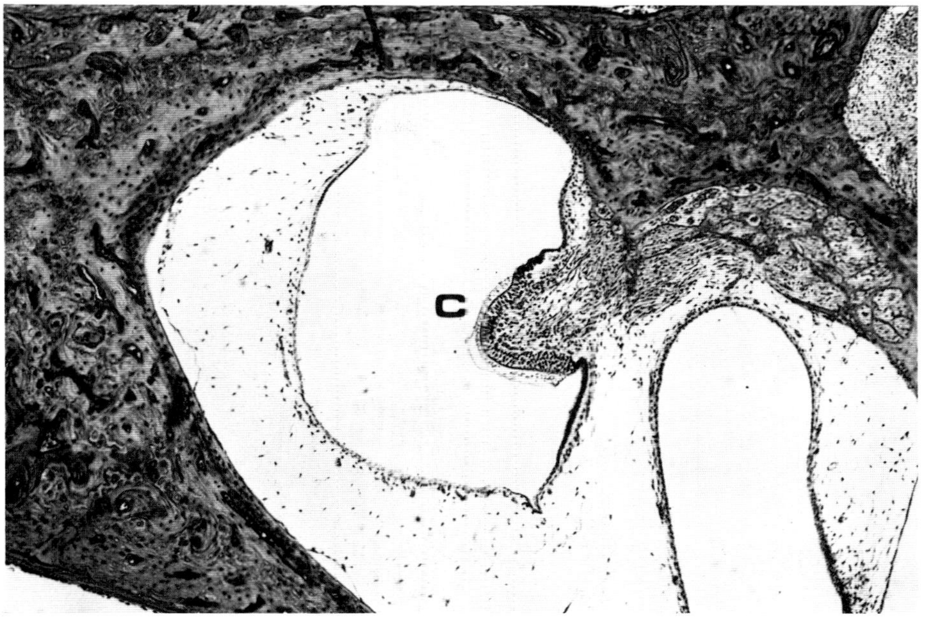

Fig. 23-24. Semicircular canal. One of the cristae ampullares (*C*) protrudes into the endolymphatic space of the canal. ×16.

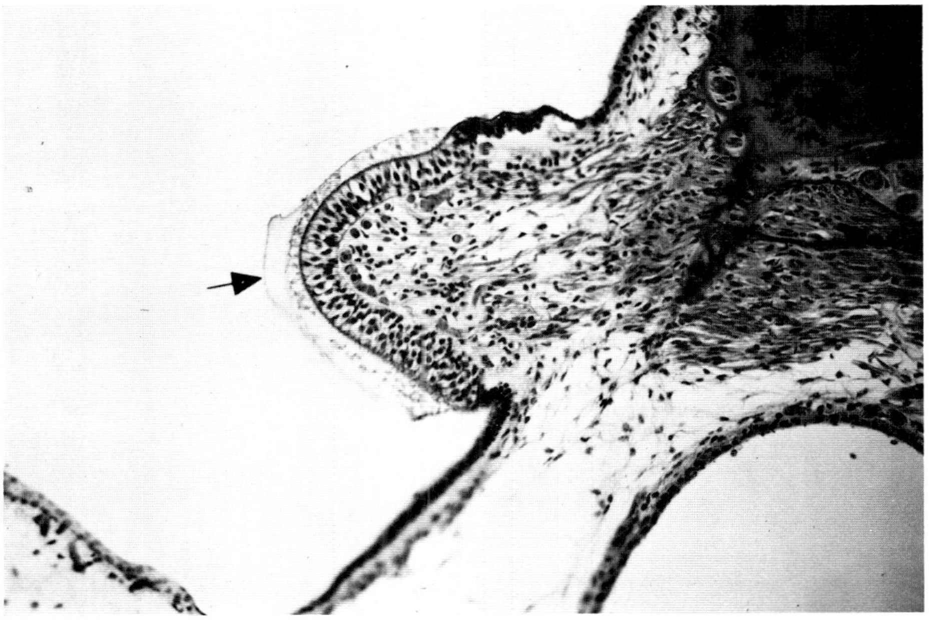

Fig. 23-25. The cupola (*arrow*) is a gelatinous mass devoid of otoliths. ×40.

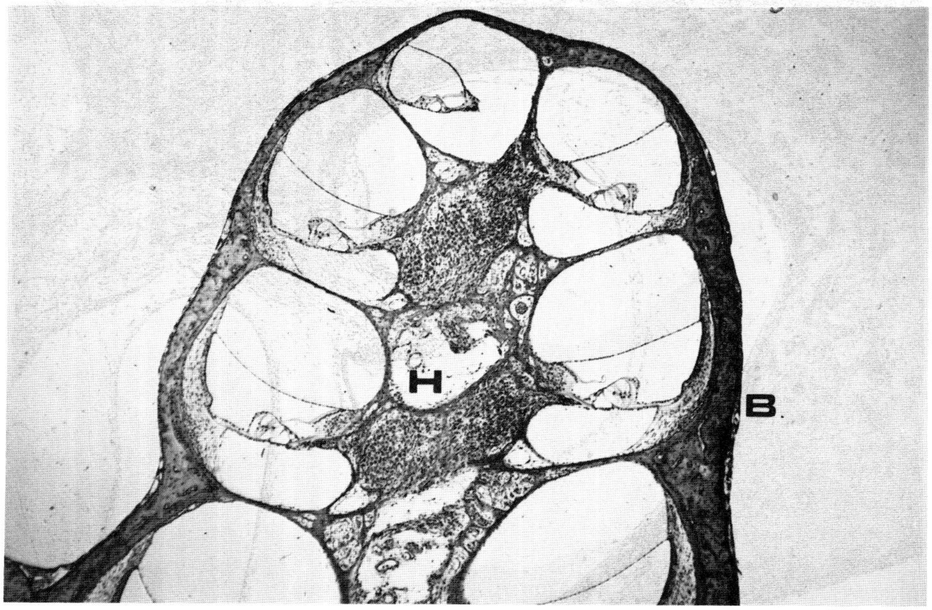

Fig. 23-26. The auditory apparatus. The cochlea is embedded within the bone (*B*) of the temporal bone. The modiolus (*H*) is the central core of supporting bone. ×100.

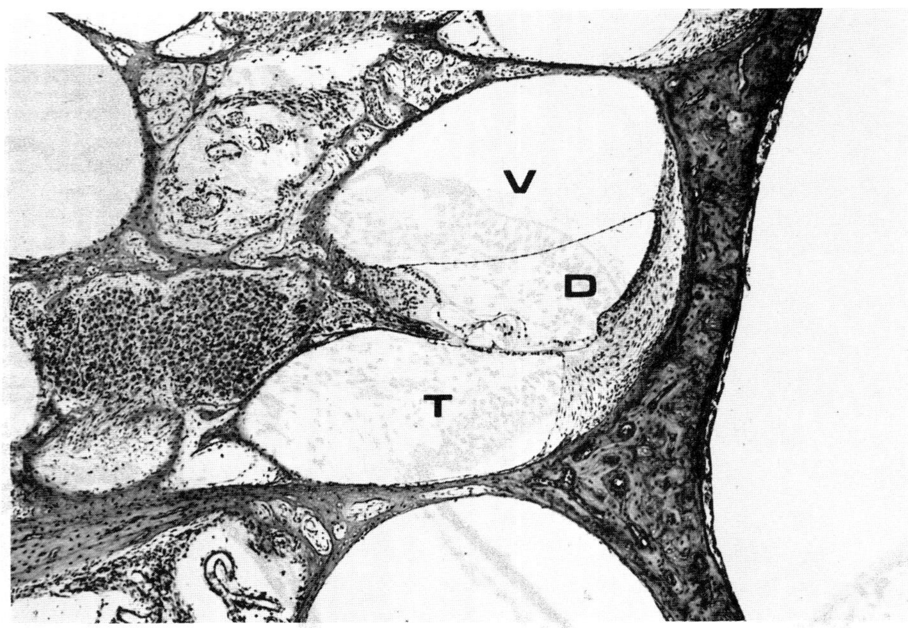

Fig. 23-27. The cochlea. The cochlea consists of a scala vestibuli (*V*), cochlea duct (*D*) and scala tympani (*T*). ×16.

ment, *cochlear duct*, is lined by various epithelial types. Adjacent to the scala vestibuli, the lining is squamous. Thus, the *vestibular membrane* consists of two laminae of squamous cells and a thin central core of collagenous fibers. The lining of the ventral duct, the *scala tympani*, is similar to that of the scala vestibuli.

Nerve fibers of the auditory nerve ascend through the osseous modiolus and pass laterally to the *organ of Corti* which is contained within the cochlear duct.

Cochlear Duct and Organ of Corti. The cochlear duct, as mentioned previously, is an endolymphatic space continuous with the vestibular apparatus through the ductus reuniens (Fig. 23-28). The squamous cells adjacent to the scala vestibuli aid in the formation of the vestibular membrane (*Reissner's membrane*). The lateral or outer wall of the cochlear duct is composed of a bistratified layer of cuboidal or columnar cells. This region is referred to as the *stria vascularis*. It is underlaid by connective tissue, the *spiral ligament*, which is highly vascularized. The stria vascularis is believed to be responsible for the production of endolymph. The basal cells of this region continue as the *spiral prominence* and are continuous with the cuboidal lining cells of the basilar membrane.

The *basilar membrane* is the supportive structure for the *organ of Corti*. The organ of Corti consists of *sensory* (*hair*) *cells*, *sustentacular cells* and a *tectorial membrane*. The hair cells have numerous stereocilia projecting from them arranged in a V pattern. In young organisms a central kinocilium is usually present at the base of the V. It is usually lost in adults. The sustentacular cells are numerous and varied. They, in conjunction with the hair cells, account for the complex morphology of the organ of Corti. The *tectorial membrane* is a fibrous and gelatinous, tonguelike structure which rests upon the hair cells. It is believed to be a secretory product of specific supportive cells, the *interdental cells*.

The following disposition of sensory and sustentacular cells accounts for the complexity of this organ. Besides the neuroepithelial cells, the organ includes: *inner* and *outer pillar cells*, *inner* and *outer phalangeal cells*, *interdental cells*, *border cells*, *cells of Hensen* and *cells of Claudius*. Other structures include the *tectorial membrane*, the *outer tunnel* (*tunnel of Corti*) and the *spiral tunnel* (Figs. 23-28 and 23-29).

The *inner and outer pillar* cells are narrow triangular cells with broad bases and narrow apices. Microtubules are prominent in these cells. These cells are joined at their apices and delimit the *inner tunnel*.

The *inner phalangeal cells* are medial to the inner pillar cells. They are columnar

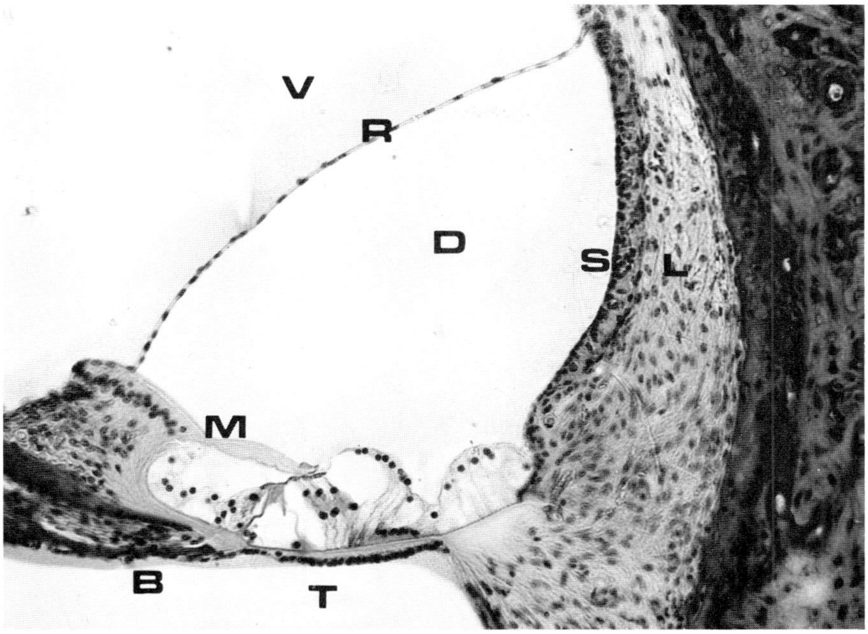

Fig. 23-28. The cochlear duct. The cochlear duct (*D*) is separated from the scala vestibuli (*V*) by Reissner's membrane (*R*). It is separated from the scala tympani (*T*) by the basilar membrane (*B*). The lateral part of the duct consists of the stria vascularis (*S*) and the spiral ligament (*L*). The organ of Corti resides on the basilar membrane covered by the tectorial membrane (*M*). ×40.

cells with a cuplike depression which almost totally surrounds the *inner hair cell.* The inner hair cell is a goblet-like cell. Nerve terminals are associated with it in the space between the hair cell and the inner phalangeal cell. The inner phalangeal cells gradually diminish in size and are transformed into squamous *border cells* which, with the tectorial membrane and inner phalangeal cells, define the spiral tunnel.

The border cells are continuous with columnar cells, *interdental cells,* which probably secrete the tectorial membrane.

The *outer phalangeal cells* are adjacent to the outer pillar cells. They are columnar cells with a cup-shaped depression which supports the outer hair cells. A cytoplasmic process of the outer phalangeal cells reaches the apex of the columnar outer hair cells. Microtubules extend from the base to the apex of the outer phalangeal cells. A smooth border is formed, therefore, above which the stereocilia of the hair cells project to touch the tectorial membrane.

Columnar and polygonal cells, the *cells of Hensen,* are lateral to the outer phalangeal cells. There is a space, the *outer tunnel,* between these cells. Toward the *spiral prominence* the cells are reduced in size to cuboidal cells, the *cells of Claudius.*

Vibrations of the perilymph within the scala vestibuli are transmitted to the vestibular membrane. This causes the endolymph to vibrate. The basilar membrane vibrates accordingly. These vibrations cause a distortion of the hairs which are resting against the tectorial membrane. This distortion results in the transduction of the stimulus and the generation of a nerve impulse. This is carried via the auditory branch of the eighth cranial nerve to the spiral ganglia, which are contained within the osseous labyrinth, and thence to appropriate centers in the brain.

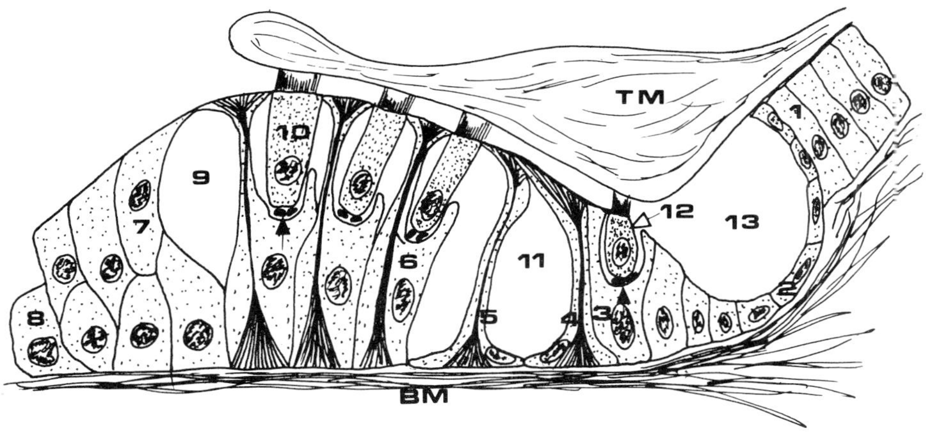

Fig. 23-29. Organ of corti. *1*, interdental cells; *2*, border cells; *3*, inner phalangeal cell; *4*, inner pillar cell *5*; outer pillar cell; *6*, outer phalangeal cell; *7*, cells of Hensen; *8*, cells of Claudius; *9*, outer tunnel; *10*, outer hair cells; *11*, inner tunnel; *12*, inner hair cell; *13*, spiral tunnel; *BM*, basilar membrane; *TM*, tectorial membrane; *arrows*, nerve terminals.

References

Eye

Jakus, M. A.: *Ocular Fine Structure.* Churchill, Ltd., London, 1964.

Pedler, C. M. H. and Tilly, R.: The fine structure of photoreceptor discs. Vision Res. *7*:829, 1967.

Prince, J. H., Diesem, C. D., Eglitis, I. and Ruskell, G. L: *Anatomy and Histology of the Eye and Orbit in Domestic Animals,* C. C Thomas, Springfield, Ill., 1960.

Tripathi, R. C.: Ultrastructure of Schlemm's canal in relation to aqueous outflow. Exp. Eye Res. *7*:335, 1968.

Villegas, G. M.: The ultrastructure of the human retina. J. Anat. *98*:501, 1964.

Young, R. W.: The renewal of photoreceptor cell outer segments. J. Cell Biol. *33*:61, 1967.

Ear

Bredberg, G., Lindemann, H. H., Ades, H. W. and West, R.: Scanning electron microscopy of the organ of Corti. Science *170*:861, 1970.

Hinojosa, R. and Rodriguez-Echandia, E. L.: The fine structure of the stria vascularis of the cat inner ear. Amer. J. Anat. *188*:631, 1966.

Iurata, S.: *Submicroscopic Structure of the Inner Ear.* Pergamon Press, Oxford, 1967.

Index

Page numbers in **boldface** refer to illustrations.